NURSING LEADERSHIP
& MANAGEMENT

Dedication

This book is dedicated to my wonderful husband, Paul; my loving dad and mom, Ed and Jean Kelly; to my super sisters, Tessie Dybel and Kathy Milch; to my dear aunts and uncles, Aunt Verna and Uncle Archie Payne and Aunt Pat and Uncle Bill Kelly; to my nieces, Natalie Dybel Bevil, Melissa Milch, and Stacey Milch; my nephew, John Edward Milch; and grandnephew, Brock Aaron Bevil; to my dear friends Patricia Wojcik, Florence Lebryk, and Lee McGuan; to my nursing mentors, Dr. Imogene King, Dr. Joyce Ellis, and Nancy Weber; and to my wonderful nursing friends, Zenaida Corpuz, Dr. Mary Elaine Koren, Dr. Barbara Mudloff, Dr. Patricia Padjen, Jane McKeon, and especially to Gerri Kane, Julie Martini, Sylvia Komyatte, and Janice Klepitch, who have supported me throughout this book and during our 40 years together as nurses.

Nursing Leadership & Management

Patricia Kelly-Heidenthal,
RN, MSN

Professor Emerita
Purdue University Calumet
Hammond, Indiana

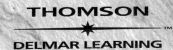

THOMSON

DELMAR LEARNING

™ Australia Canada Mexico Singapore Spain United Kingdom United States

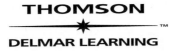

THOMSON

DELMAR LEARNING

Nursing Leadership & Management
by
Patricia Kelly-Heidenthal

Executive Director:
William Brottmiller

Executive Editor:
Cathy L. Esperti

Acquisitions Editor:
Matthew Filimonov

Senior Developmental Editor:
Elisabeth F. Williams

Executive Marketing Manager:
Dawn F. Gerrain

Channel Manager:
Jennifer McAvey

Editorial Assistant:
Patricia Osborn

Production Manager:
Barbara A. Bullock

Art/Design Coordinator:
Jay Purcell

Project Editors:
Maureen M. E. Grealish
Shelley Esposito

Production Coordinator:
Catherine Ciardullo

Library of Congress Cataloging-in-Publication Data

Nursing leadership & management / by Patricia Kelly-Heidenthal.

   p. ; cm.
Includes bibliographical references and index.
  ISBN 0-7668-2508-6 (soft cover)
  1. Nursing services—Administration.
  [DNLM: 1. Nursing Services—organization & administration—United States. 2. Delivery of Health Care—United States. 3. Leadership—United States. 4. Nurse Administrators—United States. 5. Nursing Care—organization & administration—United States. WY 105 N974745 2003] I. Title: Nursing leadership and management. II. Kelly-Heidenthal, Patricia.
  RT89 .N794 2003
  362.1'73'068—dc21

                                        2002004364

CONTENTS

UNIT III
PLANNING CARE

UNIT IV
MANAGING CARE

UNIT V
EVALUATION

CHAPTER 19

**Managing Outcomes Using an
Organizational Quality
Improvement Model / 376**

CHAPTER 20

**Strategies to Improve Patient Care
Outcomes / 398**

CHAPTER 21

Decision Making / 428

CONTRIBUTORS

Rinda Alexander, PhD, RN, CS
Professor of Nursing
Purdue University Calumet
Hammond, Indiana
and
Professor of Nursing
University of Florida
College of Nursing
Gainesville, Florida
Chapter 3: Evidence-Based Health Care

Margaret M. Anderson, EdD, RN-C, CNAA
Associate Professor and Chair
Department of Nursing
Northern Kentucky University
Department of Nursing
Highland Heights, Kentucky
Chapter 16: Change and Conflict Resolution

Ida M. Androwich, PhD, RN-C, FAAN
Professor
Community, Mental Health,
and Administrative Nursing
Niehoff School of Nursing
Loyola University Chicago
Chicago, Illinois
Chapter 2: Basic Clinical Health Care Economics
Chapter 9: Strategic Planning and
Organizing Patient Care

Anne L. Bernat, RN, BSN, MSN, CNAA
Consultant
Arlington, Virginia
Chapter 12: Allocation of Human Resources
for Effective Staffing

Sister Kathleen Cain, OSF, JD
Attorney
Franciscan Legal Services
Baton Rouge, Louisiana
Chapter 22: Legal Aspects of Patient Care

Corinne Haviley, RN, MS
Director, Ambulatory Care Services
Northwestern Memorial Hospital
Chicago, Illinois
Chapter 11: Budget Concepts for Patient Care

Paul Heidenthal, MS
Consultant
Austin, Texas
Chapter 15: Patient Teaching

Karen Houston, RN, MS
Director of Quality and Continuum of Care
Albany Medical Center
Albany, New York
Chapter 19: Utilizing an Organizational
Performance Improvement Model

Mary Anne Jadlos, MS, ACNP-CS, CWOCN
Acute Care Nurse Practitioner
Wound, Skin, Ostomy Service
Northeast Health Acute Care Division
Troy, New York
Chapter 20: Strategies to
Improve Patient Care Outcomes

Stephen Jones, MS, RN-C, PNP, ET
Pediatric Clinical Nurse Specialist/Nurse Practitioner
The Children's Hospital at Albany Medical Center
Albany, New York
and
Founder and Principal
Pediatric Concepts
Averill Park, New York
Chapter 27: Emerging Opportunities

Glenda Kelman, PhD, ACNP-CS
Chair, Division of Nursing
The Sage Colleges
Troy, New York
and
Acute Care Nurse Practitioner
Wound, Skin, Ostomy Service
Northeast Health Acute Care Division
Troy, New York
Chapter 20: Strategies to Improve Patient
Care Outcomes

Mary Elaine Koren, RN, DNSc
Assistant Professor
School of Nursing
Northern Illinois University
DeKalb, Illinois
Chapter 29: Healthy Living: Integrating Personal
and Professional Needs

Lyn LaBarre, MS, RN, CEN
Nurse Manager, Emergency Department
Albany Medical Center
Albany, New York
Chapter 28: Your First Job

Linda Searle Leach, PhD, RN, CNAA
Assistant Professor of Nursing
California State University
Fullerton, California
Chapter 8: Leadership and Management

Camille B. Little, RN, MS
Instructional Assistant Professor
Mennonite College of Nursing
Illinois State University
Normal, Illinois
Chapter 23: Ethical Dimensions of Patient Care

Sharon Little-Stoetzel, RN, MS
Assistant Professor of Nursing
Graceland University
Independence, Missouri
Chapter 21: Decision Making

Patsy L. Maloney, RN-C, MSN, EdD, CNAA
Associate Professor and Director of Continuing
Nursing Education
School of Nursing
Pacific Lutheran University
Tacoma, Washington
Chapter 18: Time Management

Maureen T. Marthaler, RN, MS
Assistant Professor
Purdue University Calumet
Hammond, Indiana
Chapter 13: Delegation of Nursing Care

Judith W. Martin, RN, JD
Attorney
Franciscan Legal Services
Baton Rouge, Louisiana
Chapter 22: Legal Aspects of Patient Care

Mary McLaughlin, RN, MBA
Project Specialist
Albany Medical Center
Albany, New York
*Chapter 19: Utilizing an Organizational Performance
Improvement Model*

Terry W. Miller, PhD, RN
Dean and Professor
School of Nursing
Pacific Lutheran University
Tacoma, Washington
and
Professor Emeritus
San Jose State University
San Jose, California
Chapter 7: Politics and Consumer Partnerships
Chapter 17: Power

Leslie H. Nicoll, PhD, MBA, RN
Consultant
and
Editor in Chief, *Computers in Nursing*
and
Editor, *Journal of Hospice and Palliative Nursing*
Portland, Maine
Chapter 4: Nursing and Health Care Informatics

Laura J. Nosek, PhD, RN
Adjunct Associate Professor of Nursing
Frances Payne Bolton School of Nursing
Case Western Reserve University
Cleveland, Ohio
and
Course Facilitator, Graduate Teaching Faculty
Excelsior College
Albany, New York
Chapter 2: Basic Clinical Health Care Economics

Amy Androwich O'Malley, RN, MSN
Director of Nursing Resources
Children's Memorial Hospital
Chicago, Illinois
*Chapter 9: Strategic Planning and
Organizing Patient Care*

Karin Polifko-Harris, PhD, RN, CNAA
Vice President
Organization Development and Research
Naples Community Healthcare System
Naples, Florida
Chapter 10: Effective Team Building
Chapter 24: Cultural Diversity and Spirituality
Chapter 26: Career Planning

Jacklyn L. Ruthman, PhD, RN
Assistant Professor
Bradley University
Peoria, Illinois
Chapter 6: Personal and Interdisciplinary Communication

Patricia M. Lentsch Schoon, MPH, RN
Assistant Professor
College of St. Catherine
St. Paul, Minnesota
Chapter 5: Population-Based Health Care Practice

Kathleen Fischer Sellers, PhD, RN
Assistant Professor
SUNY at Utica/Rome
Utica, New York
Chapter 14: First-Line Patient Care Management

Janice Tazbir, RN, MS, CCRN
Assistant Professor
Purdue University Calumet
Hammond, Indiana
Chapter 25: Collective Bargaining

REVIEWERS

Sandra C. Baird, RN, MSN, PhD
Director and Professor
School of Nursing
University of Northern Colorado
Greeley, Colorado

Janet Barrett, RN, BSN, MSN, PhD
Professor and Academic Dean
Deaconess College of Nursing
St. Louis, Missouri

Vera Cull, RN, DSN
Assistant Professor
School of Nursing
University of Alabama
Birmingham, Alabama

David Derrico, RN, MSN
Assistant Clinical Professor
College of Nursing
University of Florida
Gainesville, Florida

Mary Fisher, RN, PhD, CNAA
Associate Professor
School of Nursing
Indiana University
Indianapolis, Indiana

Melanie King-Gulliver, RN, MS
Broward Community College
Coconut Creek, Florida

Hope Laughlin, RN, BSN, MS, MSN, EdD
Professor of Nursing
Pensacola Junior College
Pensacola, Florida

Patty Leary, MEd
Mecosta Osceola Career Center
Big Rapids, Michigan

Carrie McCoy, RN, PhD, MSPH, CEN
Associate Professor of Nursing
Northern Kentucky University
Highland Heights, Kentucky

Alice Neid, RN, MSN
Director of Nursing
Highland Community College
Freeport, Illinois

Margaret B. Payne, RN, MNSc
Assistant Professor
School of Nursing
William Cary College
Hattiesburg, Mississippi

**Patricia Dianne Padjen,
RN, BSN, MBA, MS, EdD**
Emergency Medical Services Program Manager
University of Wisconsin Hospital and Clinics
Madison, Wisconsin

Dolores M. Zygmont, RN, PhD
Assistant Professor of Nursing
College of Allied Health
Temple University
Philadelphia, Pennsylvania

Nursing Leadership & Management is designed to help students and beginning nurses develop the knowledge and skills to lead and manage nursing care delivery in the 21st century. Every nurse today must lead and manage nursing care delivery, and the need for nurse leaders and nurse managers has never been greater. The nursing shortage is pressuring health care organizations to require nurses to do more with less, and to adapt quickly to change.

Indeed, the Pew Health Professions Commission, in its *Fourth Report on Competencies for the 21st Century* (Bellack & O'Neil, 2000), calls for nursing, medical, and other health care curricula to change and move into the 21st century. Some of the recommendations for the health care profession highlight the need for nurses to be educated in a broader way, including education in the areas of interdisciplinary teamwork, population-based health care, evidence-based practice, informatics, ethics, quality improvement, culture, and change, to name just a few.

This text addresses many of the topics mentioned in the report, along with others, to prepare the beginning nurse leader and manager to successfully function in the modern health care system. Many of the chapters are written by nursing faculty. Others are written by clinical nurses who are specialists in their fields, such as nurse lawyers, nurse practitioners, wound and ostomy care nurses, nurse entrepreneurs, and so on. One chapter is written by an educator with many years of experience teaching and developing computer software training for state agencies throughout the United States. Another chapter is written by the editor in chief of *Computers in Nursing* and editor of the *Journal of Hospice and Palliative Nursing*. These contributors are from various areas of the United States, thus allowing them to offer a broad view of nursing leadership and management.

ORGANIZATION

Nursing Leadership & Management consists of 29 chapters grouped into seven units. These seven units will provide beginning nurse leaders and managers with the expertise needed to succeed in today's health care environment. They are arranged as follows:

- **Unit I** presents the changing health care environment and basic clinical economics.
- **Unit II** outlines a new health care model, emphasizing the role of evidence-based health care, nursing and health care informatics, population-based health care practice, interdisciplinary and personal communication, and politics and consumer partnerships in health care today.
- **Unit III** discusses planning care through leadership and management, strategic planning and organizing patient care, effective team building, budget concepts for patient care, the allocation of human resources for effective staffing, and delegation of patient care.
- **Unit IV** discusses organizing and coordinating care. It presents first-line patient care management, patient teaching, change and conflict resolution, power, and time management.
- **Unit V** covers evaluation of care, including managing outcomes using an organizational performance improvement model; strategies to improve patient care outcomes; and decision making.
- **Unit VI** presents other professional considerations such as legal aspects of patient care, ethical dimensions of patient care, cultural diversity and spirituality, and collective bargaining.
- **Unit VII** presents preparation for entry-level nursing practice. It discusses career planning, emerging nursing opportunities, your first job, and integrating personal and professional needs.

An appendix outlines how to prepare for the NCLEX examination. Additional appendices, including the Baldrige Health Care Quality Award, and two appendices by nurse entrepreneurs are offered in the text's online companion, available at www.delmarhealthcare.com.

The textbook uses graphics and color photographs to engage readers and enhance their learning. Full-color photographs provide visual reinforcement of concepts such as teamwork and the changes occurring in health care settings today while adding visual interest. Figures and tables depict concepts and activities described in the text. Colors are used consistently throughout the text to help the reader identify the various chapter elements.

FEATURES

Each chapter includes several pedagogical features that provide the reader with a consistent format for learning and an assortment of resources for understanding and applying the knowledge presented. These features include the following:

- Objectives state each chapter's learning goals.
- An introduction to each chapter briefly describes the purpose and scope of the chapter.
- A bulleted list of key concepts at the end of each chapter assists the reader in remembering and using the material presented.
- Review questions and review activities encourage students to think critically about how to apply chapter content to the workplace and other real-world situations. They provide reinforcement of key leadership and management skills. Exercises are numbered in each chapter to facilitate using them as assignments or activities.
- Key terms appear in bold type in each chapter and are designed to encourage understanding of new terms presented in the chapter.
- References are the key to finding the sources of the material presented in each chapter.
- Suggested readings help the reader to find additional information concerning the topics covered in each chapter.

Special features are used throughout the text to emphasize key points and to provide specific types of information. Features include the following:

- An opening quote by a nursing or health care theorist gives a professional perspective on the chapter's topic.
- An opening scenario with thought-provoking questions opens each chapter and establishes the background for the reader's approach to the chapter.
- Critical Thinking sections encourage critical thinking and personal reflection about important topics.
- Interviews with staff nurses, nurse practitioners, nursing managers and leaders, nursing adminis-

trators, nursing risk managers, nursing faculty, doctors, patients, and a hospital administrator are sprinkled throughout the chapters to illustrate various points of view. Interviews with Loretta Ford, Tim Porter-O'Grady, and other nursing leaders are included in some chapters.

- Literature applications illustrate the applicability of current literature for practice.
- Case studies provide real-world illustrations of the chapter's topic.
- Web exercises guide the reader to the Internet and give Internet addresses for the latest information related to the chapter content.

ELECTRONIC CLASSROOM MANAGER (ECM)
Order # 0-7668-2509-4

An *Electronic Classroom Manager* is available to adopters of the text. It is designed to assist faculty in presenting to nursing students the essential skills and information that are needed to help them secure a position as a beginning nursing manager and leader. The ECM will assist faculty in planning and developing their programs and classes for the most efficient use of time and resources. The ECM includes three elements:

1. An instructor manual offers practical resources for presenting material in the text and includes suggested answers to the text review questions, review activities, and case studies.
2. PowerPoint® templates serve as guides for presentation in the classroom.
3. A test bank offers approximately 900 questions in multiple-choice format.

REFERENCES

Bellack, J. P., & O'Neil, E. H. (2000). Recreating nursing practice for a new century: Recommendations and implications of the Pew Health Professions Commission's final report. *Nursing and Health Care Perspectives, 21*(1), 14–21.

ACKNOWLEDGMENTS

Many people must work together to produce any book. A comprehensive book such as this requires even greater effort and the coordination of many people with various areas of expertise. I would like to thank all the contributors for their time and effort and for sharing their knowledge gained through years of experience in both the clinical and academic setting. I thank them all for being responsive, making the necessary revisions, and sounding happy to hear from me whenever I e-mailed or called them. I also thank the reviewers for their time spent critically reviewing the manuscript and providing the valuable comments that have added to this text.

I would like to acknowledge and sincerely thank the team at Delmar Learning who have worked to make this textbook a reality. Matthew Filimonov, acquisitions editor, and Elisabeth F. Williams, senior developmental editor, are great people who have worked tirelessly and brought knowledge, guidance, humor, and attention to help keep me motivated and on track throughout the project. Thanks to Eve Minkoff, project manager at Argosy. Thanks to Barbara A. Bullock, production manager, and Shelley Esposito and Maureen Grealish, project editors, as well. Finally, thanks to Melissa Longo and Patricia Osborn, editorial assistants, who also supported me every step of the way.

I would like to thank Edward P. Robinson, hospital administrator, The Community Hospital, Munster, Indiana, for sharing his insights on health care and allowing me to use the hospital's facilities in shooting several of the photographs that appear in this book. Special thanks to Janice L. Ryba, director of quality management at Munster Community Hospital, for sharing her perceptions about health care, reviewing Chapter 1, and offering helpful suggestions. Thanks also to Sharon Desancic, division director of patient care services; Sharon Rundle, associate director of patient services; Mylinda Cane, director of public relations; Sherri Holtz, marketing/public relations assistant; and Pam Kaczmarski, executive assistant to the administrator, at Munster Community Hospital for helping set up the photos. Thanks to Matt Zaucha for his critique of Chapter 1's content. And thanks to Sparky for his support. Thanks to Janice Tazbir and Maureen Marthaler, textbook contributors and nursing faculty at Purdue University Calumet, Hammond, Indiana, as well as their students, for their help in setting up many of the photographs. Thanks to Dr. Patricia Dianne Padjen for her reviews and for developing the test bank.

A special huge thank you goes to my husband and best friend, Paul, for helping me with every stage of the book, including writing the Patient Teaching chapter, developing Power Point templates for the instructor manual, organizing my computer efforts, and just supporting me through each stage of the project. I could not have done this project without his help—he is my rock!

ABOUT THE AUTHOR

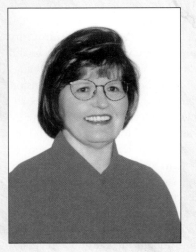

Patricia Kelly-Heidenthal earned a diploma in nursing from St. Margaret Hospital School of Nursing, Hammond, Indiana; a baccalaureate in nursing from DePaul University in Chicago; and a master's degree in nursing from Loyola University in Chicago. She has worked as a staff nurse and school nurse. Pat has traveled extensively, teaching conferences for the Joint Commission on Accreditation of Healthcare Organizations (JCAHO). She was director of quality improvement at the University of Chicago Hospitals and Clinics.

Pat has taught at Wesley-Passavant School of Nursing, Chicago; Chicago State University; and Purdue University Calumet in Hammond, Indiana. She is professor emerita, Purdue University Calumet. Pat has taught fundamentals of nursing, adult nursing, nursing leadership and management, nursing issues, nursing trends, and legal aspects of nursing. She has taught nursing conferences on quality improvement in almost every U.S. state, as well as in Canada and Puerto Rico. Pat also teaches NCLEX reviews nationally and is a member of Sigma Theta Tau and the American Nurses Association. She is listed in *Who's Who in American Nursing, 2000 Notable American Women*, and the *International Who's Who of Professional and Business Women*.

Pat has served on the board of directors of both Tri City Community Mental Health Center, East Chicago, Indiana, and St. Anthony's Home, Crown Point, Indiana. She was on the board of directors for the nursing newsletter, *Quality Connection*. She contributed a chapter on "Preparing the Undergraduate Student and Faculty to Use Quality Improvement in Practice" to the book *Improving Quality: A Guide to Effective Programs*. Pat has written several articles, including one on chest x-ray interpretation and many on various elements of quality improvement. She is an active disaster volunteer for the American Red Cross. Throughout most of her career, she has taught nursing at the university level and has continued to work part time as a staff nurse in the Emergency Department. This has allowed her to wear several hats and see nursing from many points of view.

Pat has been licensed as an RN in many states over her career, including Indiana, Illinois, Wisconsin, Oklahoma, New York, and Pennsylvania. She worked as a nurse in these states as she accompanied her husband, Paul, in his consulting assignments. Pat and her husband recently moved to Austin, Texas, where Pat can be reached at PATKH1@aol.com.

HOW TO USE THIS BOOK

When delegating a task, be sure you're clear on the nursing knowledge components of the task. (Mary Ann Boucher, instructor at Frances Payne Bolton School of Nursing)

Quote A nursing or health care theorist quote gives a professional's perspective regarding the topic at hand; read this as you begin each new chapter and see whether your opinion matches or differs, or whether you are in need of further information.

Chapter Objectives These goals indicate to you the performance-based, measurable objectives that are targeted for mastery upon completion of the chapter.

OBJECTIVES

Upon completion of this chapter, the reader should be able to:

1. Review the history of delegation.
2. Define delegation, accountability, responsibility, authority, and assignment making.
3. Identify responsibilities the health team members can perform.
4. List the five delegation rights.
5. Identify three potential delegation barriers.
6. List six cultural phenomena that affect transcultural delegation.

In a large teaching hospital, a patient you are caring for says he does not want to go on living. He has had cancer for several years and states he is tired of being sick. When you ask him whether he has shared these feelings with his family, he says that he does not want them to think he is giving up. You report the patient's statements to the next shift and explain how you encouraged him to talk with his family and his doctor. That evening, the patient suddenly arrests and a code is called. The patient ends up on a ven-

Opening Scenario This mini case study with related critical thinking questions should be read prior to delving into the chapter; it sets the tone for the material to come and helps you identify your knowledge base and perspective.

Case Study These short cases with related questions present a beginning clinical nursing management situation calling for judgment, decision making, or analysis in solving an open-ended problem. Familiarize yourself with the types of situations and settings you will later encounter in practice, and challenge yourself to devise solutions that will result in the best outcomes for all parties, within the boundaries of legal and ethical nursing practice.

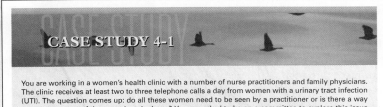

CASE STUDY 4-1

You are working in a women's health clinic with a number of nurse practitioners and family physicians. The clinic receives at least two to three telephone calls a day from women with a urinary tract infection (UTI). The question comes up: do all these women need to be seen by a practitioner or is there a way to manage some of the cases by telephone? You are asked to be on a committee to explore this issue and possibly come up with a protocol. Where do you begin? Is a protocol for telephone management of UTI realistic?

Literature Application Study these key findings from nursing and health care research, theory, and literature, and ask yourself how they will influence your practice. Do you see ways in which your nursing could be affected by these literature findings and research results? Do you agree with the conclusions drawn by the author?

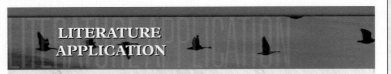

LITERATURE APPLICATION

Citation: Bauer, H. M., Rodriguez, M. A., Quiroga, S. S., & Flores-Ortiz, Y. G. (2000). Barriers to health care for abused Latina and Asian immigrant women. *Journal of Health Care for the Poor and Underserved, 11*(1), 33–44.

Discussion: This qualitative study included 28 abused Latina and Asian immigrant women. Data were collected using four semistructured, ethnic-specific focus group interviews. Many sociopolitical and sociocultural factors were identified as barriers to seeking help and patient-provider communication. Sociopolitical barriers included social isolation, language barriers, discrimination, and fear of deportation. Sociocultural barriers included dedication to children and family unity, shame related to the abuse, and the cultural stigma of abuse.

Implications for Practice: Nurses must be aware not only of those who seek care but also those who do not. Culturally competent outreach and case finding programs are needed to identify and serve hidden underserved populations. Nurses can play a strong advocacy role in the process.

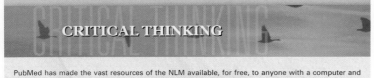

CRITICAL THINKING

PubMed has made the vast resources of the NLM available, for free, to anyone with a computer and Internet hookup. Some argue that scientific publications, such as the *New England Journal of Medicine,* are too technical and sophisticated for laypeople. Others contend that the resources of the NLM are maintained with taxpayer dollars and, therefore, should be available to all taxpayers.

Which point of view do you support? Why? As a health care professional, what resources for understanding and clarification would you suggest to your patients who are accessing abstracts and article citations from the professional health care literature?

Critical Thinking Ethical, cultural, spiritual, legal, delegation, and performance improvement considerations are highlighted in these boxes. Before beginning a new chapter, page through and read the Critical Thinking sections and jot down your comments or reactions, then see whether your perspective changes after you complete the chapter.

Real World Interviews RWI Interviews with well-known nursing leaders, such as Dr. Loretta Ford, Dr. Tim Porter O'Grady, and others are included as well as interviews with nurses, doctors, hospital administrators, staff, patients, and family members. As you read these, ask yourself whether you had ever considered that individual's point of view on the given topic. How would knowing another person's perspective affect the care you deliver?

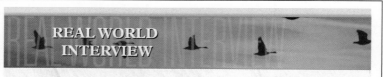

REAL WORLD INTERVIEW

It is amazing what some people have gone through. I work at a free clinic and I couldn't believe some of the things I ran into such as the torture experienced by Mexicans trying to cross the border. We work with illegal immigrants who need us to provide everything they need, including free health visits and free medications. If we set up a free referral to a specialty, they need us to provide transportation and an interpreter. For the most part, the immigrants I have met are grateful for what we do for them.

Anita M. Matos, RN
Degree Completion Nursing Student

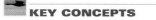
Key Concepts This bulleted list serves as a review and study tool for you as you complete each chapter.

Key Terms Study this list prior to reading the chapter, then again as you complete a chapter, to test your true understanding of the terms and concepts covered. Make a study list of terms you need to focus on to thoroughly appreciate the material of the chapter.

Review Questions These questions will challenge your comprehension of objectives and concepts presented in the chapter and will allow you to demonstrate content mastery, build critical thinking skills, and achieve integration of the concepts.

Review Activities These thought-provoking activities at the close of a chapter invite you to approach a problem or scenario critically and apply the knowledge you have gained.

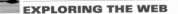
Exploring the Web Internet activities encourage you to use your computer and reasoning skills to search the Web for additional information on quality and nursing leadership and management.

References Evidence-based research, theory, and general literature, as well as nursing, medical, and health care sources, are included in these lists; refer to them as you read the chapter and verify your research.

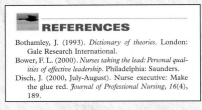

REFERENCES

Bothamley, J. (1993). *Dictionary of theories*. London: Gale Research International.

Bower, F. L. (2000). *Nurses taking the lead: Personal qualities of effective leadership*. Philadelphia: Saunders.

Disch, J. (2000, July-August). Nurse executive: Make the glue red. *Journal of Professional Nursing, 16*(4), 189.

Suggested Readings These entries invite you to pursue additional topics, articles, and information in related resources.

SUGGESTED READINGS

American Nurses Association. (1985). *Nursing's social policy statement*. Washington, DC: American Nurses Publishing.

Benner, P. E. (2000). *From novice to expert: Excellence and power in clinical nursing practice* (Commemorative edition). Upper Saddle River, NJ: Prentice Hall.

Photos Tables, and Figures
These items illustrate key concepts.

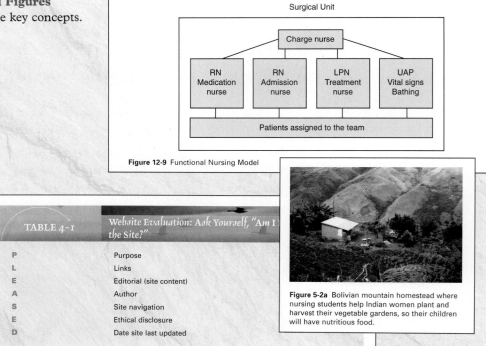

Surgical Unit

Charge nurse

| RN Medication nurse | RN Admission nurse | LPN Treatment nurse | UAP Vital signs Bathing |

Patients assigned to the team

Figure 12-9 Functional Nursing Model

TABLE 4-1	Website Evaluation: Ask Yourself, "Am I ___ the Site?"
P	Purpose
L	Links
E	Editorial (site content)
A	Author
S	Site navigation
E	Ethical disclosure
D	Date site last updated

Figure 5-2a Bolivian mountain homestead where nursing students help Indian women plant and harvest their vegetable gardens, so their children will have nutritious food.

CHAPTER 1

For us who Nurse, our Nursing is a thing, which, unless in it we are making progress every year, every month, every week, take my word for it, we are going back. (Florence Nightingale, 1872)

America's Health Care Environment

Patricia Kelly-Heidenthal, RN, MSN

OBJECTIVES

Upon completion of this chapter, the reader should be able to:

1. Identify how health care is organized and funded in America.
2. Review the movement toward population-based health care and disease management.
3. Discuss health care variation, evidence-based practice, and malpractice.
4. Review the Institute of Medicine's Committee on Health Care Reports.
5. Identify recent changes and current forces and trends influencing the development of caring, transdisciplinary nursing and health care delivery in America.

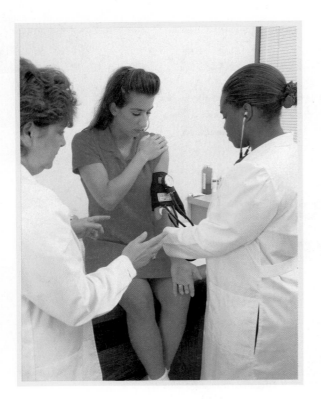

You stop to eat at a local restaurant and see an old friend and her husband. They tell you they had to take their 2-year-old boy to the Emergency Department that past week for a temperature of 104°. Though the boy is better now, they are worried about the hospital bill. They are both working, but have not been able to afford health insurance. This scene occurs over and over again in today's health care environment as Americans struggle to find a way to ensure access to cost-effective, quality care for all.

What are your thoughts about this situation?

What advice do you have for your friend?

How can you contribute to improving access to affordable health care for your friend and for the community?

Health care delivery in the United States is a combination of public and private initiatives organized to provide citizens with access to cost-effective, quality health care. Most Americans are in good health, but many citizens are children, elderly, sick, disabled, or otherwise in need of access to quality health care services at a reasonable cost. The need for access, quality, and cost-effectiveness has driven various initiatives to improve health care in the past and present.

Present-day nursing's role in quality health care began to develop in the United States in the after-

math of Florence Nightingale's efforts in London. Nightingale's emphasis on cleanliness, fresh air, regular patient observation, and monitoring of mortality rates, though familiar today, was radical in the management of patient care at that time. Nightingale illustrated mortality rates with a coxcomb diagram (Figure 1-1).

Nightingale used these coxcomb diagrams to dramatize the number of preventable deaths in the Crimean war campaign. The dark gray wedges on the coxcomb measured from the center of the circle represent the deaths from preventable diseases. It is important to note that while Nightingale managed patients and their environment closely, she also emphasized health promotion and disease prevention. She paid close attention to physicians and government policy makers, recognizing their influence on her freedom to practice (Simms, Price, & Ervin, 2000). Nightingale's ideas spread from England to the United States in the 1870s. Today's nurse can improve the quality of patient care by understanding and dealing with many of these same issues affecting today's health care system and the nursing profession.

This chapter discusses how American health care is organized, funded, and accredited. It discusses population-based health care and disease management. It then explores clinical variation and malpractice. It reviews two Institute of Medicine Committee on Health Care Reports. Finally, it discusses recent changes and current trends and forces affecting health care and the development of caring, transdisciplinary nursing.

ORGANIZATION OF HEALTH CARE

The health care system in the United States today has developed within a political context. Elazar (1966) describes the political culture of this country as being one of (1) individualism; (2) civil liberties; (3) equality of process, not outcomes; (4) popular sovereignty and representative democracy; (5) belief in private property, capitalism, and the free market; (6) rationality, which is reflected in self-interest and competition; (7) a Protestant work ethic; and (8) separation of church and state. Further, Americans believe in the decentralization of power throughout the various levels of federal, state, county, and local government (Lockart, 1999).

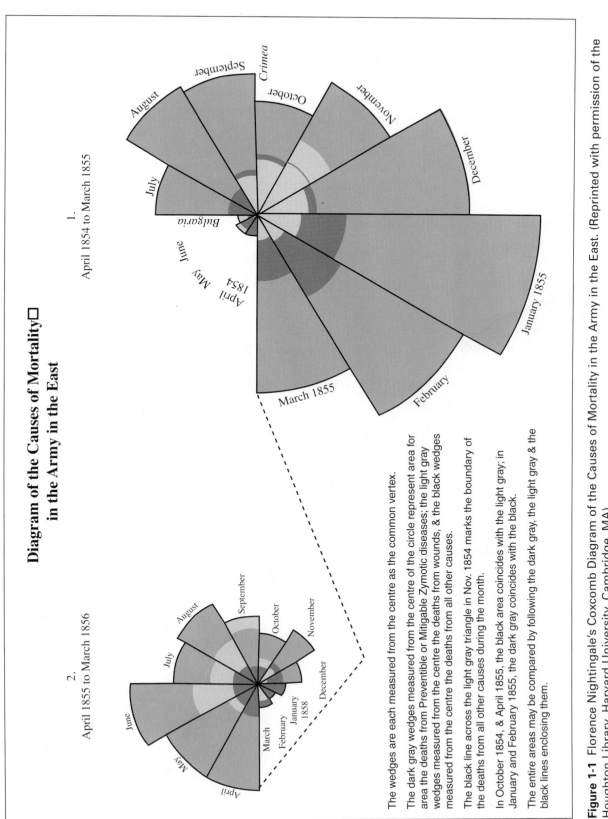

Diagram of the Causes of Mortality in the Army in the East

1. April 1854 to March 1855

2. April 1855 to March 1856

The wedges are each measured from the centre as the common vertex.

The dark gray wedges measured from the centre of the circle represent area for area the deaths from Preventible or Mitigable Zymotic diseases; the light gray wedges measured from the centre the deaths from wounds, & the black wedges measured from the centre the deaths from all other causes.

The black line across the light gray triangle in Nov. 1854 marks the boundary of the deaths from all other causes during the month.

In October 1854, & April 1855, the black area coincides with the light gray; in January and February 1855, the dark gray coincides with the black.

The entire areas may be compared by following the dark gray, the light gray & the black lines enclosing them.

Figure 1-1 Florence Nightingale's Coxcomb Diagram of the Causes of Mortality in the Army in the East. (Reprinted with permission of the Houghton Library, Harvard University, Cambridge, MA)

These beliefs have fostered the development of a health care system in the United States that has varied and differing resources. Some parts of this system include highly sophisticated research and technology programs, while other parts offer little to patients. Coordinated health care quality, access, and reasonable cost are not available to all. Americans have resisted the development of a coordinated, centralized, national health care system or any other health care system that could provide access to cost-effective quality health care for all.

Types of Health Care Services

Health care can be categorized into three levels (Table 1-1): primary, secondary, and tertiary (Joel & DeLaune, 2002). **Primary health care** services emphasize health promotion and the prevention of illness or disability. **Secondary health care** services emphasize detection and early intervention to prevent further illness and disability. Finally, **tertiary health care** services provide restorative or rehabilitation services for patients with chronic or irreversible conditions.

Stakeholders

Public and private stakeholders, both voluntary and involuntary, affect the delivery of health care services in a variety of settings in the United States. Figure 1-2 shows some of the stakeholders in a large U.S. hospital.

Subcultures of Health Professionals

Several subcultures of individual disciplines work in the various health care settings of health care—nursing, medicine, physical therapy, social work, hospital administration, dietary, pharmacy, to name a few. These subcultures affect patient care delivered in

TABLE 1-1	Types of Health Care Services	
Type of Care	**Description**	**Examples**
Primary	*Goal:* To decrease the risk to a client (individual or community) for disease or dysfunction	Lifestyle modification for health (e.g., smoking cessation, nutritional counseling)
		Referrals
		Immunization
	Explanation: General health promotion Protection against specific illnesses or disability	Promotion of a safe environment (e.g., sanitation, protection from toxic agents)
Secondary	*Goal:* To alleviate disease and prevent further disability through early intervention	Screenings Acute care Surgery
	Explanation: Early detection and intervention	
Tertiary	*Goal:* To minimize effects and permanent disability of chronic or irreversible condition	Education and retraining Provision of direct care Environmental modifications (e.g., advising on necessity of wheelchair accessibility for a person who has experienced a cardiovascular accident [stroke])
	Explanation: Restorative and rehabilitative activities to obtain optimal level of functioning	

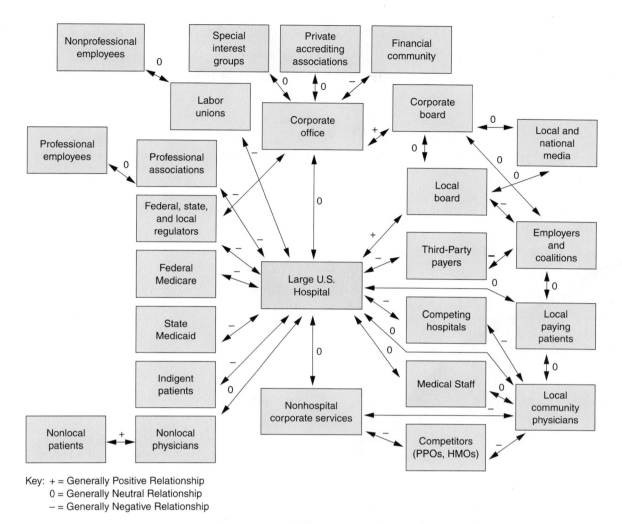

Figure 1-2 Stakeholders in a Large U.S. Hospital (From Fottler M. D., Blair, J. D., Whitehead, C. J., Laus, M. D., & Savage, G. T. Assessing key stakeholders: Who matters to hospitals and why? *Hospital and Health Services Administration.* Winter 1989; 34: 530. Copyright 1989. Foundation of the American College of Healthcare Executives.)

the various settings. Table 1-2 lists generalized characteristics of three of these subcultures of health professionals identified by Byers (1997). These characteristics are dynamic and constantly changing the culture of the health care organization and the way these groups work with each other to provide quality health care.

HEALTH CARE SPENDING

The United States spends heavily on health care services, yet ranks 18th in overall health compared with all other countries in the world (Strasen, 1999). Americans' health care needs are covered by Medicare, Medicaid, insurance companies, and managed care companies, but 44.3 million people— 16.3% of the U. S. population—are not insured. These Americans pay for health care themselves as the need arises, and they are often forced to go to the Emergency Department (ED) of their local hospital when ill. Any person in the United States can go to the ED of a hospital when ill, and, under the 1986 Emergency Medical Treatment and Active Labor Act (EMTALA), no one can be refused treatment. EMTALA requires that hospitals provide patients with a medical screening exam and stabilize patients

TABLE 1-2	Generalized Characteristics of Three Subcultures of Health Professionals		
Characteristics	**Nursing**	**Medicine**	**Health Care Administration**
Major task	Patient care	Diagnosis and treatment of disease	Organizational continuity, managing change and stability
Membership	Historically female, white, middle class; humanistic	Historically male, white, middle and upper class; scientific	Historically male-dominant,* rational
Leading role strength	Comforter, nurturer, health educator	Life-saver and problem-solver; miracle-worker	Keeper of the house, protector
Role centrality	Coordinator of health services	Gatekeeper of health services	Proprietor of health services; holder of the purse strings
Relationships with other professional groups	Collaborative ethic	Autonomy; directing the team	Negotiating, seeks cooperation
Model of authority within profession	Hierarchy	Collegiality, equality	Hierarchy
Perspective	Patient-centered, clinical unit/area	Patient- and practice-centered	Hospital's business and market relations
Conflict management	Interpersonal approach	Use leverage available, e.g., resources and authority, to maintain control	Structural and rational approach
Core dilemmas in era of health care reform	Degree of proactivity within context of high uncertainty; traditional vs. new role initiatives	Choice of organizational and network affiliations, and the conditions and extent of affiliation; the future destiny of medical specialists	Where to invest strategic resources in an era of high future uncertainty
Major threats (current)	Decrease in job security; constraints on staffing levels and other resources; (undesirable) changes in role	Health economics; changes in role; losses in authority, income; malpractice	Organizational survival, job security

*The management of Catholic hospitals, typically run by orders of Catholic sisters, is a notable exception to the generalizations about health care administrators.

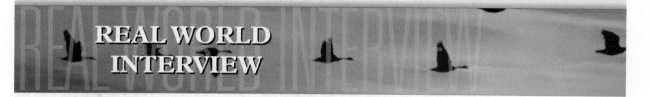

REAL WORLD INTERVIEW

I became involved with the local American Red Cross (ARC) of Northwest Indiana chapter as a volunteer and certified instructor during high school. I taught health and safety, CPR, and first aid. This was the beginning of a lifetime connection between Red Cross and my nursing career. Much later, when I began working as an employed ARC corporate health and safety instructor, I began to see the importance of my nursing education in improving the delivery of emergency services to local community disaster victims. I noticed more and more the community lifeline linkage between nursing and the Red Cross service areas of Blood, Emergency Services for Disaster and Military, and Health and Safety. Red Cross works hard to meet the needs of our patients. There are patient satisfaction surveys for our programs and services. These are assessed and reviewed by the National Red Cross Headquarters. There are also standardized National Red Cross clinical practice guidelines, both physical and mental, to be used as protocols for disaster health service professionals to follow in order to provide quality care to local and national disaster victims. It has been exciting to see that nursing interlinks with Red Cross community services to advance improvements in health service delivery for our communities.

Carol Marie Dahms, RN, MS
American Red Cross of Northwest Indiana

prior to transferring them to any other health care facility. Going to the ED, however, is not a very effective or efficient way to provide health care. It uses expensive emergency care to provide service to those with less serious needs simply because they often have no other place to go.

Medicare and Medicaid

In 1965, Title XVIII of the Social Security Act Amendments created Medicare, and Title XIX created Medicaid. Medicare provided financing of health care services for citizens over the age of 65 and for the disabled. Medicaid provided financing of health care services for the medically indigent. Under Medicare/Medicaid, physicians and hospitals were reimbursed for their services based on the amount of service they delivered to patients. This process was called fee for service. In a **fee-for-service reimbursement** system, the total number of fees increases when the number of patient services increases. Unfortunately, this fee-for-service system may have provided an incentive to increase the number of services provided by physicians and hospitals, especially in an age of increased consumer demand

for health care services and advances in the availability of costly technologies.

Managed Care

In 1973, the U.S. Congress passed the Health Maintenance Organization Act, which encourages the formation and proliferation of health maintenance organizations (HMOs). The intent of this legislation was cost containment. These managed care organizations were responsible for delivering health care to a specific group of patients for a preset (capitated) fee. **Capitation** is the payment of a fixed dollar amount, per person, for the provision of health services to a patient population for a specified period of time (e.g., 1 year). Under capitation, health care organizations benefit from using their financial resources to keep people well. HMOs lose money when their members are hospitalized.

Competition and cost-containment efforts in HMOs have led to more rigorous peer review of quality and the development of standard diagnostic and clinical treatment guidelines for common conditions. Comparing clinical outcomes among HMOs is also becoming an important measure of the quality of care. Cost-containment restrictions in managed care

CRITICAL THINKING

You work in an ED that sees 2,000 patients a month. Patients are charged $200 per visit plus charges for tests and medications. Thus, these 2,000 patients can generate $400,000 per month in gross revenue for the hospital. Consider that there are five registered nurses (RNs) making $20 per hour and 2 medical doctors (MDs) making $100 per hour working each shift. Salaries for the RNs total $2,400 per day. Salaries for the MDs total $4,800 per day. The total salary for these two groups is $7,200 per day or $216,000 per month ($7,200 × 30 days).

Fifty percent of these patients have Medicare/Medicaid, and 45% of the patients are covered by managed care or insurance. Five percent of these patients have no insurance. Thus, just 95% of patients can pay their bills. The other 5% of patients' bills are written off by the hospital as bad debt. Medicare/Medicaid/managed care/insurance companies often pay only 55% of the bills for these patients. They often deny payment for 45% of the bills. Thus, for the $380,000 (95% of $400,000) billed, the hospital will receive approximately $209,000 (55% of the $380,000 billed). Approximately $171,000 of the bill will not be paid by Medicare/Medicaid/managed care/insurance. Consider the following:

What other expenses besides salary must the hospital pay out of the $209,000 that it receives? Consider hospital space, liability insurance, technology costs, and so on.

Notice the effect that increasing the volume of patients has on budget figures. What happens to the budget if the patient volume goes to 2,500 patient ED visits per month and staffing stays the same? What happens if the fee rises to $300 per visit?

Are patients receiving useful information about future illness prevention and healthy living practices in the ED?

Is this a cost-effective way to deliver health care? How could we better serve the health care needs of 44 million Americans?

may include limiting patient referrals to specialists and limiting expensive diagnostic tests. Some HMOs have given their providers financial incentives to reduce the amount of unneeded services (Raffel, 1997). These patient service limits have also led to calls by some groups for the right to sue HMOs. Texas, California, and Georgia have authorized HMO enrollees to sue their company-sponsored health care plans in state court (Coile, 1999). Congress is debating competing versions of a national Bill of Rights to safeguard patient rights, and a majority of states have enacted managed care reform legislation. Lately, there is some evidence that HMOs are responding to consumer concerns. Blue Cross of California recently announced it would begin paying bonuses to doctors based on how good

they are at maintaining patient satisfaction—not how well they hold down cost.

Prospective Payment

In other attempts to curtail health care costs, Congress passed the Tax Equity and Fiscal Responsibility Act of 1982 (TEFRA). This act put a ceiling on Medicare reimbursement for hospital services and set the stage for the 1983 Social Security Amendments, which mandated a prospective payment system (PPS). PPS focused on in-hospital Medicare charges (often known as Part A). A result of PPS was the establishment of diagnosis-related groups (DRGs) to permit the comparison of like admissions and the regulation of their cost. In 1990,

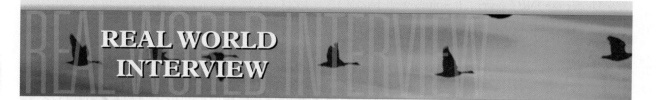

REAL WORLD INTERVIEW

I was admitted to the hospital in December for what was later diagnosed as angina. After being stabilized in the emergency room, I was admitted to the cardiac care unit. A series of tests was ordered by my cardiologist to determine enzyme levels in my blood. This would show if I had suffered a heart attack. Blood was drawn every 8 hours for 24 hours. The news was good—no heart attack—until I received the bill. I thought I had good insurance, but my insurance company said the enzyme tests were not necessary and they would not pay. I had my cardiologist write a letter of explanation, saying the tests he ordered were routine for determining a diagnosis. After this second appeal, the insurance company rejected my payment claim again. After several more appeals, my insurance company ultimately paid the laboratory bill for these tests but would not pay the pathologist for his interpretation of the blood tests. It has now been 6 months since I received my initial bill, and the hospital and pathologist's office have turned my case over to a collection agency. They did not take into consideration the fact that I was appealing the bill. They wanted me to pay up front and then appeal. That was not going to happen.

Kathleen A. Milch
Patient

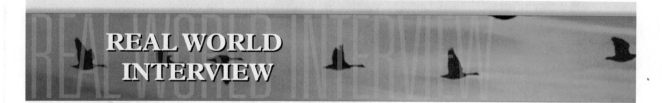

REAL WORLD INTERVIEW

Three years ago, I went to the hospital with excruciating pain. They admitted me to the hospital and I had tests and x-rays for 9 days before they found the cause. I had cancer in my left kidney, and I needed immediate surgery. I had the surgery and was discharged on my 18th hospital day. Thank heaven, I was now cancer free.

The hospital bill for this stay was $18,689.20. The radiologist and surgeon submitted additional bills. I was glad that I had Medicare and Blue Cross insurance, which paid it all. The only charge I had to pay was $25 per day for a private room. When I looked at the hospital bill, there were many charges for medications and treatments I never received. There were even charges for the day after I was discharged. I wonder how the hospital makes out the bill. I also wonder how people with no insurance pay these kinds of hospital bills.

Leona McGuan
Patient

Medicare was further reformed with the establishment of the Resource-Based Relative Value Scale (RBRVS) for reimbursement of physician services (often known as Medicare Part B). RBRVS is an extension of PPS, and its intent is also cost containment (Fos & Fine, 2000).

Under the DRG system, hospitals were paid a predetermined standard fee for each case within a given DRG, regardless of the length of stay (Bull, 1997). For example, a hospital would be paid a set fee for each patient with diabetes, regardless of whether it were a simple case of diabetes or a complicated case of diabetes. If the hospital could provide care at a cost lower than the DRG payment, the hospital kept the difference. If the cost of care exceeded the DRG payment, the hospital had to bear the additional cost in all but exceptional cases. The DRG system has limited services to patients by reducing hospital admissions and reducing hospital length of stays. DRGs have also reduced the amount of diagnostic testing. A positive effect of DRGs is that by collecting data on patients by diagnostic groups, DRGs laid the groundwork for the later comparison of data about the clinical outcomes of various patient groups receiving health care across the country.

Balanced Budget Act

Comprehensive reform of the Medicare program was enacted via the Balanced Budget Act (BBA) of 1997. The changes to Medicare under the BBA include expansion of Medicare's offerings of health care plans and changes in the way plans are paid, extension of the prospective payment system to ambulatory and post acute care organizations and providers, correction of numerous payment policies governing physicians and graduate medical education, availability of new preventive services for beneficiaries, and strengthening of fraud and abuse regulations and provisions (Simms, Price, & Ervin, 2000). In addition, the BBA designated nurse practitioners as fully qualified providers of all Medicare Part B services, with reimbursement being 85% of physician fee schedules.

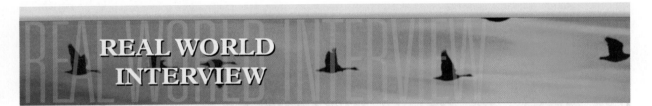

REAL WORLD INTERVIEW

I feel that all people should have ready access to primary health care services close to their homes. Information technologies—telephone systems, e-mail, Web, faxes, wireless, computers, audiovisual equipment—all promise to assist primary care physicians in being available and in providing improved quality of care. However, the goal of achieving high percentage levels of access to care is actually being hindered by inadequate and even improper implementation of technology at local levels. For example, automated telephone systems often place people into dead ends without a rescuer and with no accurate feedback about messages left on them. Answering systems that give a second and then a third number for calling dismay all, but especially pay-phone and elderly callers. E-mail messaging is not utilized for several reasons. Some of these include the cost of installing e-mail services in patient homes and physicians' offices, as well as the steep learning curve required to get all e-mail users able to use the equipment. In addition, serious concerns exist related to privacy protection of patient information.

Finally, systems like nurse triage centers sponsored by many hospitals to provide information about primary care access are not present in all communities and have different names in various communities, leaving the members of our mobile society to fend as best they can when they have no local primary provider.

What can be said about the United States health care system is that it is not really a system, but rather a hodgepodge of systems, some great, some not so great, with a "sometimes" desire for universal service but with also the fierce energy of independent individuals seeking autonomy.

Ellyn Stecker, MD

Health Care Rationing

Data about patient outcomes is being used in decisions about rationing of care, based on results of cost-effectiveness studies. In addition, patients may use effectiveness results to rank different types of care, and may pay only for those services above a particular cutoff. The State of Oregon has used cost-effectiveness analysis to develop a priority list of reimbursable health care services delivered to Medicaid patients. This list is based on a ranking method that considers both community input and the relative cost-effectiveness of all services. A cutoff of ranked services is used to select services on the priority listing that will be paid by Medicaid (Fos & Fine, 2000).

MOVEMENT TOWARD POPULATION-BASED HEALTH CARE, INTEGRATED DELIVERY SYSTEMS, AND DISEASE MANAGEMENT

Population-based health care, integrated health care delivery, and disease management have begun to develop as an approach to health care in the United States.

Population-Based Health Care

Population-based health care addresses the health care needs of a population of people and patients rather than focusing only on care delivery to individual patients. It directs attention to the causes of death in the general population. The top 10 underlying common causes of death in the United States are identified in Table 1-3 (McGinnis & Foege, 1993).

These underlying causes or determinants of death and disease contribute significantly to the mortality rate in the United States. Research into health and illness has now recognized the contribution of social, economic, and environmental factors to health, and a critical body of evidence is beginning to document the influence of these factors on morbidity and mortality (Gruman & Chesney, 1995). Table 1-4 summarizes what selected evidence-based studies have found.

Populations do not get healthier with just large investments in clinical care after illness has begun. Populations get healthier when we invest in preventing illness and keeping people healthy. A United Nations study of 15 developing countries showed that 1 additional year of mothers' schooling resulted in a 3.4% decrease in infant mortality. Thus, the educational resources available in a community can profoundly affect the health of the community. Note that expenditures for health care and education each consumed 6% of the U.S. gross national product in 1965. By 1995, expenditures for health care increased to 14% while expenditures for education remained at 6%.

If our society really wants to increase health, perhaps resources would be better directed toward strengthening the determinants of health: health care system influences (e.g., access to medical care, cost, etc.); individual influences (lifestyle, genetics, etc.); interpersonal, social, and work influences (job satisfaction, social support, etc.); community influences (services, programs, etc.); and environmental influences (air, water, etc.) (Donatelle & Davis,

TABLE 1-3	Top 10 Underlying Causes of Death in the United States in 1990

1. Tobacco
2. Poor diet
3. Lack of exercise
4. Alcohol
5. Infectious agents
6. Firearms
7. Sexual behavior
8. Motor vehicles
9. Illicit drug use
10. Pollutants/toxins

©McGinnis, J. M., & Foege, W. H. Actual causes of death in the United States. Journal of the American Medical Association, 270(18), p. 2207–2212.

TABLE 1-4	*Evidence-Based Studies: What They Show*

- In a study examining 232 elderly patients who had elective open-heart surgery, those who did not participate in any group and did not receive strength and comfort from religion had three times the risk of dying as those who did (Oxman,1995).

- A 7-year follow-up of women diagnosed with breast cancer showed that those who confided in at least one person in the 3 months after surgery had a 7-year survival rate of 72.4%, as compared to 56.3% for those who did not have a confidant (Maunsell, Brisson, & Deschenes, 1995).

- In a large study covering 13 years, depressed and socially isolated persons were four times more likely to have a heart attack than those who were not depressed or isolated (Pratt, Ford, Crum, Annenian, Gallo, & Eaton, 1996).

- In a study examining the correlation of social ties to susceptibility to common cold viruses, increased diversity in types of ties to friends, family, work, and community was significantly associated with increased host resistance to infection (Cohen, Doyle, Skoner, Rabin, & Gwaltney, 1997).

1998). A society that spends so much on medical care that it cannot or will not spend adequately on other health-enhancing activities may actually be reducing the health of its population (Evans & Stoddard, 1990).

Public health has begun to direct some of its efforts to population-based interventions designed to improve the health of populations by reducing smoking, substance abuse, violence, risky sexual behaviors, and obesity. Healthy People 2010 indicators, issued by the United States Department of Health and Human Services (USDHHS, 2000), are a major public health initiative to provide a snapshot of the health of the nation. Communities are showing increased interest in disease screening, prenatal and child care, health education, and immunization. Planning and implementation of such services is centered at the community or larger population levels, rather than individuals. Shortell and Kaluzny (2000) have identified features of the new role of health care management in such a population-based health system (Table 1-5).

TABLE 1-5	*Features of the New Role of Health Care Management in a Population-Based Health System*

- Emphasis on the continuum of care
- Emphasis on maintaining and promoting wellness
- Accountability for the health of defined populations
- Differentiation based on ability to add value
- Success achieved by increasing the number of covered lives and keeping people healthy
- Goal is to provide care at the most appropriate level
- Integrated health delivery system
- Managers oversee a market
- Managers operate service areas across organizational borders
- Managers actively pursue quality and continuous improvement

Integrated Health Care Delivery Systems

An **integrated delivery system** is a network of health care organizations that provides or arranges to provide a coordinated continuum of services to a defined population and is willing to be held clinically and fiscally accountable for the outcomes and the health status of the population served (Shortell, 1996).

A coordinated continuum of health care services includes prevention, wellness, and health promotion services, as well as acute, restorative, and maintenance care to serve the needs of a population of patients in a specific geographic area. These services are delivered by a network of organized, community-oriented health and social service systems focused on broad aspects of health care and chronic disease management. This network can include hospitals and nursing homes, as well as schools, public health departments, and social and community health organizations that provide service and education programs to address smoking cessation, exercise, and other illness prevention and health promotion initiatives.

Horizontal and Vertical Integration

Health care networks can be horizontally or vertically integrated. **Horizontal integration** occurs when a health care system contains several organizations of one type, such as hospitals. Health care networks can also be vertically integrated. **Vertical integration** occurs when different stages of health care are linked and delivered by one agency. For example, a single organization grows and offers services along the continuum of care for wellness, prevention, acute and chronic care, disease management and rehabilitation, ambulatory care, long-term and home care, and hospice care (Byers, 1997).

In the year 2000, many integrated health care delivery systems are contracting with HMOs for the provision of capitated health care services. Lando (2000), though, cites the Balanced Budget Act of 1997 as a key element pressuring organizations to halt the often costly mergers associated with developing integrated delivery systems, so it is unclear at this time whether the growth of integrated health care systems will continue.

Disease Management

Increasingly, health care centers are developing disease management (DM) programs. **Disease management** is a "systematic, population-based approach to identify persons at risk, intervene with specific programs of care, and measure clinical and other outcomes" (Epstein & Sherwood, 1996). An objective of disease management is cost containment, and research indicates that this is occurring. A study of nurses who managed patients with congestive heart failure in an aged population showed significantly lower numbers of patient readmissions and costs (Rich et al., 1995). Disease management can be classified as either a contracted carve-out or a primary care model. The carve-out model is characterized by the provision of care to patients by contracting with disease management companies. The term *carve-out* refers to the separation of specialized care from a primary care model (Fos & Fine, 2000).

DM can be as simple as a pharmaceutical pamphlet describing how best to use a medication or as complex as nurse managers developing individualized care plans and regularly contacting patients to ensure compliance with the plans.

Disease management strategies use a variety of methods, including telephone, the Internet, and in-person visits, to keep high-risk, high-cost patients out of the hospital. These DM strategies collect data from and send reminders to patients who need constant monitoring. They also provide information systems that help caregivers develop care plans and gather data for clinical improvement initiatives.

ACCREDITATION

The Joint Commission on Accreditation of Healthcare Organizations (JCAHO) is the current national organization that develops standards and accredits health care organizations. This accreditation is important to hospitals because it is one of the ways hospitals can be certified to receive federal government Medicare and Medicaid reimbursement for delivery of patient care services.

As many as 50% of the JCAHO's hospital accreditation standards were written to correspond with Medicare's conditions of participation, a comprehensive set of criteria that hospitals and other care

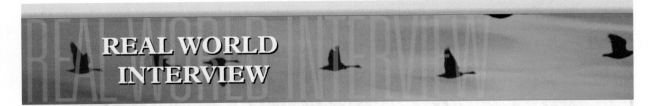

REAL WORLD INTERVIEW

Community Hospital in Munster, Indiana, has grown from 99 inpatient beds in 1973 to 373 beds with 22,000 admissions, 105,000 patient days, and over 200,000 outpatient visits annually and has become the "Hospital of Choice in Northwest Indiana." This has been accomplished by concentrating on our mission, which is to operate an accredited, financially sound health care organization to serve the needs of the community, physicians, and hospital staff with the highest possible quality care.

"A hospital is not a business but it must be run in a businesslike manner," is an important criterion for Munster Community Hospital. It is essential that a hospital must be financially viable in order to provide the services necessary for the well-being of the community.

The Community Hospital payor mix, which includes Medicare and Medicaid, managed care, commercial insurance companies, and private-pay patients, reimburses the hospital only $0.53 for every $1.00 of billed services due to contractual agreements. The hospital must continually evaluate expenses, including salaries and supplies, and eliminate duplication as much as possible. The hospital must meet its responsibilities in order to stay in business. These responsibilities must be met at 100 cents on the dollar to vendors and to pay employee salaries even though reimbursement is 53 cents on the dollar. Efficient management makes the difference.

The hospital's current payor mix includes approximately 45% Medicare/Medicaid, 53% managed care and commercial insurance, with about 2% uncollectibles. The financial bottom line is dependent, to a great deal, on the ability to negotiate with managed care companies to maximize their reimbursement to the hospital, since they do not pay 100% of claims.

Community Hospital has maintained its success by being cognizant of the needs of the patients, the community, the medical and hospital staff and by establishing necessary services, such as a linear accelerator, open heart surgery, neurosurgery, neonatology, etc., in the community so that patients do not have to travel to Chicago and can be treated near their homes. The hospital has always met the needs for new services rather than trying to create a need that doesn't exist. The criterion of a good hospital means that it is a place where you would unhesitatingly bring your family for care.

Edward P. Robinson
Community Hospital Administrator

providers must meet to qualify for reimbursement. The JCAHO's adherence to the conditions stems from its "deemed" status with Medicare, which means that JCAHO-accredited hospitals are assumed to have met the Medicare participation standards. Hospitals pay an average of $20,000 for a JCAHO survey (Lovern, 2001c). See Table 1-6 for the list of chapters in the accreditation manual. Each chapter highlights a hospital function and how quality is reviewed for that function. All hospitals and long-term care organizations seeking JCAHO accreditation monitor patient outcomes and use a performance measurement system to provide data about these patient outcomes and other indicators of care.

Submission of data about quality outcomes and performance measures has been controversial in the health care community. Some problems that have been identified in the mass submissions of outcome data include the need to make adjustments for the patient's initial severity of illness and the need to standardize definitions used by different facilities for the collection of data about the indicators.

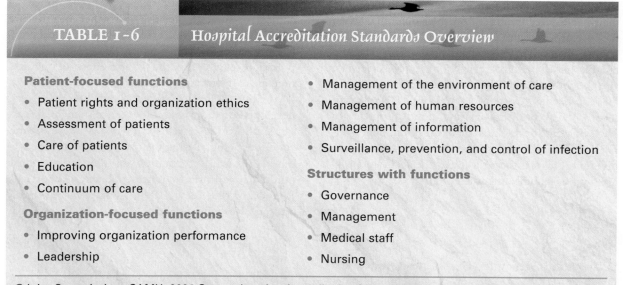

TABLE 1-6	Hospital Accreditation Standards Overview

Patient-focused functions

- Patient rights and organization ethics
- Assessment of patients
- Care of patients
- Education
- Continuum of care

Organization-focused functions

- Improving organization performance
- Leadership

- Management of the environment of care
- Management of human resources
- Management of information
- Surveillance, prevention, and control of infection

Structures with functions

- Governance
- Management
- Medical staff
- Nursing

©Joint Commission: *CAMH: 2001 Comprehensive Accreditation Manual for Hospitals*. Oakbrook Terrace, IL: Joint Commission on Accreditation of Healthcare Organizations, 2001. Reprinted with permission.

For example, a mortality indicator may be defined as death within 48 hours, death within 72 hours, death within 7 days, or death within 30 days, depending on who is collecting the data. These differences in data collection and reporting could make the performance of one hospital appear artificially more favorable than the performance of another hospital. For example, if one hospital reported mortality rates after heart surgery based on the death rate in the first 24 hours postoperative, this would make the data from another hospital that reports death rates within 30 days postoperatively look very different. To compare the death rates fairly, the data definitions must be similar. Despite these difficulties, many clinicians agree with the need to use and improve on outcome measures for quality assessments (Wolper, 1999).

HEALTH CARE VARIATION, EVIDENCE-BASED PRACTICE, AND MALPRACTICE

Research on variation in medical care practice first began to be reported in the 1970s (Wennberg & Gittelsohn, 1973). Depending on what part of the country you lived in, patient outcomes and costs var-

ied significantly for the same health care condition. Studies on unnecessary surgery (Leape, 1987) and the occurrence of preventable complications in patients (Adams, Fraser, & Abrams, 1973) led to more research into variations in physician practice patterns. Nursing and physician clinicians, as well as patients, began to consider what health care practices led to good health care outcomes. Prior to this time, there was little study of the effect of various interventions on patient outcomes.

Variation in Patient Outcomes

Many variables affect patient outcomes including the severity of the patient's illness. As mentioned earlier, data on health care outcome findings must be adjusted to allow for these variables. The process of statistically adjusting patient data to reflect significant patient variables is called **risk adjustment**. One of the difficulties with data about groups of patient outcomes is that the condition of different patients in that group is variable, even in patients admitted for the same diagnosis. For example, the condition of each of two diabetic patients can be very different. One patient can be a new diabetic patient with few complications. The other patient can be a more seriously ill diabetic patient with many complications.

This makes it very difficult to identify the impact of their health care treatment on their outcomes when they are grouped and compared. Add to this the difficulties involved in gathering data based on valid and reliable patient record review by trained reviewers, and the difficulties involved in using risk adjustment on data become clear (Wolper, 1999). If all patient record reviewers do not extract identical data from reviewing patient records, the figures from data compilation from different record reviewers will be quite different. This significantly affects the accurate measurement of patient outcomes.

Agency for Healthcare Research and Quality

In 1989, the Agency for Healthcare Research and Quality (AHRQ), an agency of the United States Public Health Service, was formed. The AHRQ began to develop clinical practice guidelines using the best available evidence as a basis. National committees of clinical nurses, physicians, and other health care experts worked on these evidence-based clinical practice guidelines for various topics. The AHRQ also supported research into the effectiveness of medical practice (McCormick, Cummings, & Kovner, 1997).

Today, clinical practice guidelines are being developed by more than 60 organizations in at least 10 countries (Rogers, 1995). Most of these organizations are emphasizing the use of the best evidence-based clinical information in developing these guidelines (Titler, Mentes, Rakel, Abbott, & Baumler, 1999; Lang, 1999; Lohr & Carey, 1999; Sackett, Rosenberg, Gray, Haynes, & Richardson, 1996).

Malpractice Concerns

A significant factor driving the quest for quality, access, and reasonable cost is the United States legal

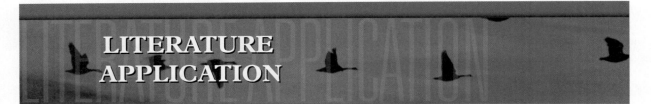

LITERATURE APPLICATION

Citation: McCormick, K. A., Cummings, M. A., & Kovner, C. (1997). The role of the Agency for Health Care Policy and Research in improving outcomes of care. *Nursing Clinics of North America, 32*(3), 521–526.

Discussion: The Agency for Healthcare Policy and Research (AHCPR), recently renamed the Agency for Healthcare Research and Quality (AHRQ), was established in 1989 and does research on quality, cost, and access to health care. It supports research on outcomes, effectiveness, and efficiencies in health care, and the development of clinical practice guidelines. Some of the AHRQ's activities include funding large projects known as Patient Outcome Research Teams (PORTs) to study topics such as prostate disease. Other studies include research on pharmaceutical outcomes and minority populations. The AHRQ has developed many clinical practice guidelines and now has a Clinical Improvement Program to assist with clinical practice guideline development by various health care groups. The Clinical Improvement Program has three new initiatives, including an Evidence-Based Practice Center, a National Guideline Clearinghouse, and Product Research and Evaluation. The AHRQ has also supported the development of computerized patient records and computer decision support services for clinical practice. Other outcome initiatives, such as the National Committee on Quality Assurance's Health Plan Employer Data and Information Set (HEDIS), the Foundation for Accountability, Health Outcomes, and the National Cancer Institute, are discussed in the article.

Implications for Practice: Nurses can help their work with patients by participating in and being knowledgeable about national initiatives to improve patient outcomes and identify the most effective clinical practices.

system. In particular, the case of Darling v. Charleston Community Memorial Hospital (1963) established that hospitals have a legal responsibility to know about problems in patient care. Further, the court stated that hospitals can be held independently liable for negligence in failing to establish a system of safe practices in the hospital (McLaughlin & Kaluzny, 1999). Because of such influences as the Darling case and other legal cases like it, hospitals today develop protocols for staff use in reporting problems in health care quality in an organization. In addition, many hospitals guide staff in quality health care delivery through the use of patient care standards, clinical practice guidelines and protocols, policy and procedures, and an active orientation and training program.

INSTITUTE OF MEDICINE COMMITTEE ON HEALTH CARE QUALITY REPORTS

In 1999, the Institute of Medicine (IOM) released a report titled *To Err Is Human: Building a Safer Health System.* The report concluded that more people die annually from medication mistakes than from highway accidents, breast cancer, or AIDS (Kohn, Corrigan, & Donaldson, 1999).

A second IOM committee report released in 2001, *Crossing the Quality Chasm: A New Health System for the 21st Century* (Kohn, Corrigan, & Donaldson, 2001) recommends that "all health care organizations, professional groups, and private and public purchasers should adopt as their own the explicit purpose of reducing the burden of illness, injury, and disability, and improving the health and functioning of the people of the United States." Health providers should pursue six major areas for improvement of health care (Maddox, 2001); see Table 1-7.

The Second IOM Report identified four major areas to target for change in the health care environment. These areas include information technology, payment, clinical knowledge, and the professional workforce (Kohn, Corrigan, & Donaldson, 2001).

New JCAHO Patient Safety Standard

Under the JCAHO's new patient safety and medication error reduction standard, accredited hospitals are required to implement an organization-wide patient safety program complete with procedures for immediate response to medical errors. Hospitals must also inform patients and, when appropriate, their families whenever results of care differ significantly from anticipated outcomes (Lovern, 2001a).

TABLE 1-7	*Major Areas to Be Pursued in Health Care — Second IOM Report*

Health care should be:

- Effective—providing services based on scientific knowledge to all who could benefit and refraining from providing services to those not likely to benefit (avoiding overuse and underuse).

- Patient-centered—providing care that is respectful of and responsive to individual patient preferences, needs, and values and ensuring that patient values guide all clinical decisions.

- Timely—reducing waits and sometimes harmful delays for both those who receive and those who give care.

- Efficient—avoiding waste, in particular waste of equipment, supplies, ideas, and energy.

- Safe—avoiding injuries to patients from care intended to help them.

- Equitable—providing care that does not vary in quality because of personal characteristics, such as gender, ethnicity, geographic location, and socioeconomic data.

CRITICAL THINKING

Nurses who work in large health care settings can sometimes feel lost and wonder how they and their system can deliver quality in the midst of rapid change. What can nurses do to ensure safe, high-quality care? Political events of the recent past can remind us each to "light a small candle." Thinking about the following may be useful:

What can I do at my level to manage care and support and contribute to the quality of health care in my organization and community? How can I work well with other people in my nursing unit, the organization, and the community? Where can I find "best evidence" clinical practice guidelines to apply to patient care in my organization and community? How much do I control care or anything else at a beginning level? I want to be optimistic, yet realistic!

QUALITY HEALTH CARE

It is useful to consider a basic framework for quality health care. Donabedian (1966) conceptualized such a framework (Bull, 1997). This framework is composed of the elements of structure, process, and outcome.

Structure, Process, Outcome

Using Donabedian's framework, a health care organization that wishes to develop quality will organize or structure itself for quality. Quality patient care does not just happen. It must be planned. Quality is the result of assessing patient needs and delivering care to meet those needs. Donabedian's framework has three elements: structure, process, and outcome.

Structure elements of quality lay a foundation for quality health care by identifying what structures must be in place in a health care system to deliver quality. Structure elements consist of such things as a well-constructed hospital, quality patient care standards, quality staffing policies, environmental standards, and the like.

Process is the next element of the quality framework. Process elements of quality build on the structure elements and take quality a step further. Process elements identify what nursing and health care interventions must be in place to deliver quality. Process elements are such things as manag-

ing the health care process and utilizing clinical practice guidelines and standards for nursing and medical interventions—passing medications and the like.

Finally, an outcome element completes the quality framework. Outcome elements of quality are the end results of quality care. Outcome elements review the status of patients after health care has been delivered. Outcomes reflect the presence of structure and process elements of quality. Outcomes ask whether the patient is better as a result of health care. If a quality hospital (structure) and quality standards (process) are in place, patients should experience good health (outcome). See Table 1-8 for examples of structure, process, and outcome quality performance measures in three domains of activity: clinical care, financial management, and human resources management.

For quality to occur, monitors of all three elements of Donabedian's framework—structure, process, and outcome—should be in place. Many people today who review quality focus initially on outcome evaluation. Quality outcomes are considered to be at least partially reflective of having quality structures and quality processes in place. For example, if a patient is breathing better after health care interventions for an asthma attack, this is a quality outcome and may be a reflection of quality structures (good equipment and medications) and quality processes (nursing and medical interventions). Of course, the patient's overall initial health status, as

TABLE 1-8 *Examples of Performance Measures by Category*

Domain of Activity

	Clinical Care	Financial Management	Human Resources Management
Structure	*Effectiveness* • Percent of active physicians who are board certified • JCAHO accreditation • Number of residencies and filled positions • Presence of council for quality improvement planning	*Effectiveness* • Qualifications of administrators in finance department • Use of preadmission criteria • Presence of an integrated financial and clinical information system	*Effectiveness* • Ability to attract desired registered nurses and other health professionals • Size (or growth) of active physician staff • Salary and benefits compared to competitors • Quality of inhouse staff education
Process	*Effectiveness* • Rate of medication error • Rate of nosocomial infection • Rate of postsurgical wound infection • Rate of normal tissue removed *Productivity* • Ratio of total patient days to total full-time equivalent (FTE) nurses • Ratio of total admissions to total FTE staff • Ratio of physician visits to total FTE physicians *Efficiency* • Average cost per patient • Average cost per admission	*Effectiveness* • Days in accounts receivable • Use of generic drugs and drug formulary • Market share • Size (or growth) of shared service arrangements *Productivity* • Ratio of collection to FTE financial staff • Ratio of total admissions to FTE in finance department • Ratio of new capital to fund-raising staff *Efficiency* • Cost per collection • Debt/equity ratio	*Effectiveness* • Grievances • Promotions • Organizational climate *Productivity* • Ratio of line staff to managers *Efficiency* • Cost of recruiting
Outcome	*Effectiveness* • Case-severity-adjusted mortality • Patient satisfaction • Patient functional health status	*Effectiveness* • Return on assets • Operating margins • Size (or growth) of federal, state, or local grants for teaching and research • Bond rating	*Effectiveness* • Turnover rate • Absenteeism • Staff satisfaction

well as other factors, affects the outcome also. When outcomes are not good, nurses and other health care leaders must examine the structure and process elements critically. Change in these elements may be needed to improve health care quality. See Chapter 20 for examples of other indicators of the quality of nursing care.

Malcolm Baldridge National Quality Award

In 1999, health care organizations were eligible to consider another framework for health care quality and to apply for the Malcolm Baldridge National Quality Award. In 1995, 46 health care organizations and 19 educational institutions participated in a pilot program for health care and education. The Baldridge Award highlights the importance of leadership; strategic planning; and a focus on patients, other customers, and markets in building a quality health care system. Baldridge also stresses the importance of focusing on staff and monitoring organizational performance results (Baldridge National Quality Program, 2000). The importance of collecting good data and analyzing information using tools is also emphasized. See Appendix for more information on the Baldridge Award.

Outcome Measurement

Outcome measurements can be done indicating an individual's clinical state, such as their severity of illness, course of illness, and the effect of interventions on their clinical state. Outcome measures involving a patient's functional status evaluate a patient's ability to perform activities of daily living (ADLs). These can include measures of physical health in terms of function, mental and social health, cost of care, health care access, and general health perceptions. The measures can distinguish the concepts of physical and mental health and identify the five indicator categories of clinical status, functioning, physical symptoms, emotional status, and patient/family evaluation and perceptions about quality of life. Selected quality-of-life measures include quality-adjusted life years (QALY), quality-adjusted life expectancy (QALE), and quality-adjusted healthy life years (QUALY) (Drummond, Stoddart, & Torrance, 1994).

The Medical Outcomes Study (MOS) "Short Form 36" Health Survey is one of the many health indices that have been developed since 1950. The SF-36, as it is commonly known (Ware & Sherbourne, 1992), measures physical functioning, role limitations due to physical health, bodily pain, social functioning, general mental health, role limitations due to emotional problems, vitality, and general health perceptions.

Other Health Assessment Tools

Other health status assessment surveys in use today include the Quality of Life Index (Spitzer, 1998), developed to measure the general health and well-being of terminally ill individuals; the COOP Charts for primary care practice patients; the functional status questionnaire (Jette & Cleary, 1987), a self-administered general health and social well-being survey for ambulatory patients; the Duke Health Profile (Parkerson, Broadhead, & Tse, 1990), which evaluates health status in primary care patients; the Sickness Impact Profile (Bergner, Bobbit, Carter, & Gilson, 1981), which was developed to measure changes in an individual's behavior as a result of illness; and the Nottingham Health Profile (Hunt, McKenna, McEwen, Williams, & Papp, 1981), developed as a measure of perceived general health status for primary care patients and general population health surveys.

RECENT CHANGES IN HEALTH CARE

Several changes have taken place recently in health care; these are discussed below.

Health Insurance Portability and Accountability Act

The Health Insurance Portability and Accountability Act of 1996 (HIPAA) includes measures to standardize and computerize the business transactions of health care billing, claims processing, and reimbursement. The law dictates that patients' data be transmitted securely and handled confidentially, all of which will require fundamental changes in administrative operations and information services for most providers (Morrissey, 2001). Table 1-9 includes HIPAA privacy regulations.

TABLE 1-9	HIPAA *Privacy Regulations*

- Allows patient to review and request amendments to their medical records
- Gives consumers control over how their personal health information is used and limits the release of information without a patient's consent
- Restricts the amount of patient information shared between physicians and other caregivers to the "minimum necessary"
- Requires privacy-conscious business practices, such as hiring a privacy officer and training employees about patient confidentiality
- Requires that paper records and oral communications be protected from privacy breaches

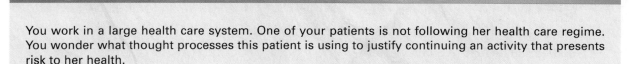

CRITICAL THINKING

You work in a large health care system. One of your patients is not following her health care regime. You wonder what thought processes this patient is using to justify continuing an activity that presents risk to her health.

How can you best assist the patient in your health care system and community? What kinds of structures, processes, and outcomes will your system want to develop to improve care to this patient and the population of patients that your system serves? How could you work in the community to enhance the population's choices for diet, exercise, or lifestyle?

Public Information about the Quality of Health Plans

Public dissemination of data on the quality of care that patients receive from health plans has become increasingly common. Several states, the Department of Health and Human Services, the Centers for Disease Control, and the Agency for Healthcare Research and Quality, as well as several for-profit health care firms, have become involved in these data efforts (Guadagnoli et al., 2000). These projects have the potential to improve care through comparison of data about health care across health care delivery sites. It is important when reviewing this data to ensure that it is accurate, valid, and reliable.

Centers for Medicare and Medicaid Services Quality of Care Ranking

The first national Medicare quality of care study from the Centers for Medicare and Medicaid Services (CMS), formerly the Health Care Financing Administration (HCFA), released in October 2000, ranked states from best to worst and brought attention to the tremendous variation among providers in adhering to clinical best practices (Lovern, 2001b). These rankings are published and widely distributed throughout the United States, and rankings are used for many purposes, including serving as hospital report cards.

Health Care Ratings

Solucient, a health care information company based in Evanston, Illinois, has reviewed the clinical and financial performance of some 6,000 acute care hospitals of all types and sizes. It annually publishes a listing of the 100 top hospitals nationally, both generally and in selected specialties ("100 Top Hospitals," 2001). *U.S. News and World Report* annually publishes a list of the top hospitals nationally ("America's Best Hospitals," 2001).

The Pew Health Professions Commission Report

In 1998, the Pew Health Professions Commission published its *Fourth Report on Competencies for the 21st Century* (Bellack & O'Neil, 2000). The report calls for nursing, medical, and other health care curriculums to change and move into the 21st century. Table 1-10 includes the competency recommendations for the health professions.

TABLE 1-10	*Pew Health Professions Competencies*

1. Embrace a personal ethic of social responsibility and service.
2. Exhibit ethical behavior in all professional activities.
3. Provide evidence-based clinically competent care.
4. Incorporate the multiple determinants of health in clinical care.
5. Apply knowledge of the new sciences.
6. Demonstrate critical thinking, reflection, and problem-solving skills.
7. Understand the role of primary care.
8. Rigorously practice preventive health care.
9. Integrate population-based care and services into practices.
10. Improve access to health care for those with unmet health needs.
11. Practice relationship-centered care with individuals and families.
12. Provide culturally sensitive care to a diverse society.
13. Partner with communities in health care decisions.
14. Use communication and information technology effectively and appropriately.
15. Work in interdisciplinary teams.
16. Ensure care that balances individual, professional, system, and societal needs.
17. Practice leadership.
18. Take responsibility for quality of care and health outcomes at all levels.
19. Contribute to continuous improvement of the health care system.
20. Advocate for public policy that promotes and protects the health of the public.
21. Continue to learn and help others learn.

©O'Neil, E. H., and the Pew Professions Commission. *Recreating Health Professional Practice for a New Century.* San Francisco, CA: Pew Health Professions Commission. December, 1998, p. 29–43.

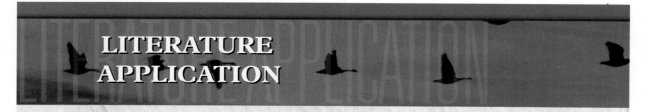

LITERATURE APPLICATION

Citation: Soukup, S. M. (2000). Preface to section on evidence-based nursing practice. *Nursing Clinics of North America, 35*(2), xvii–xviii.

Discussion: Author discusses a nurse's response to queries as to whether she has integrated evidence-based practice. The nurse responds, "Yes, I practice state-of-the-art nursing. My education and professional practice experiences have prepared me to care for more than 700 chronically ill patients annually, in the past 5 years. These patients have an average reported expected pain rating of 6.9 (using a scale of 1 to 10, with 10 being severe pain), and my pain management interventions have kept these patients, during my hours of care, at a reported actual pain rating of 4. Also, as a team member, these patients have not had any known pressure ulcers, skin tears, or catheter-related infections. On two occasions, for patients who were dying, I created a humanizing environment for these patients and their families when they were rapidly transferred from the critical care unit. My documentation has met organizational standards during monthly peer reviews; I have provided leadership for emergencies with positive outcomes; and physician and patient satisfaction rating for clinical practice on our unit is 9.5 on a scale of 10, with 10 being the highest. Our unit-based team has not had a needle-stick-related or back-related injury during the past 2 years. This has contributed to a significant cost avoidance and benefit to the organization."

Implications for Practice: Nurses practicing in the 21st century must embrace the principles of evidence-based practice as an approach to clinical care and professional accountability.

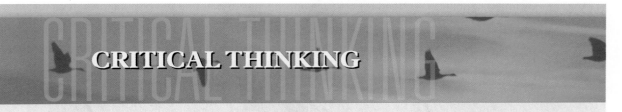

CRITICAL THINKING

Review the ratings of hospitals in your area of the country on the following web sites: *www.healthgrades.com* or *www.100tophospitals.com*.

What kinds of ratings are given to hospitals in your area? Review the criteria and evaluation system used to rate the hospitals. Is it valid and reliable? Are the criteria important to quality and patient satisfaction? Will you choose a hospital for your own family's care using a rating system like this?

OTHER FORCES INFLUENCING HEALTH CARE

Shortell & Kaluzny (2000) identify nine major forces influencing health care (Table 1-11). Such forces as capitation; payment of clinicians based on performance using clinical practice guidelines; new technology; the aging population; genetic engineering; increasing cultural diversity; new diseases; information management; and the globalization of the world economy continue to shape health care in the

TABLE 1-11	Nine Forces Influencing Health Care Delivery and Their Implications for Management
External Force	**Management Implication**
1. Capitated payment, expenditure targets, or global budgets for providing care to defined populations	• Need for increased efficiency and productivity • Redesign of patient care delivery • Development of strategic alliances that add value • Increased growth of networks, systems, and physician groups
2. Increased accountability for performance	• Information systems that link financial and clinical data across episodes of illness and "pathways of wellness" • Effective implementation of clinical practice guidelines • Ability to demonstrate continuous improvements of all functions and processes
3. Technological advances in the biological and clinical sciences	• Expansion of the continuum of care, need for new treatment sites to accommodate new treatment modalities • Increased capacity to manage care across organizational boundaries • Need to confront new ethical dilemmas
4. Aging of the population	• Increased demand for primary care, wellness, and health promotion services among the 65 to 75 age group • Increased demand for chronic care management among the 75 plus group • Challenge of managing ethical issues associated with prolongation of life
5. Increased ethnic or cultural diversity of the population	• Greater difficulty in understanding and meeting patient expectations • Challenge of managing an increasingly diverse health services workforce
6. Changes in the supply and education of health professionals	• Need for creative approaches in meeting the population's need for disease prevention, health promotion, and chronic care management services • Need to compensate for shortages in some categories of health professionals (i.e., physical therapy, pharmacy, and some areas of nursing) • Need to develop effective teams of caregivers across multiple treatment sites
7. Social morbidity (AIDS, drugs, violence, "new surprises")	• Ability to deal with unpredictable increases in demand • Need for increased social support systems and chronic care management • Need to work effectively with community agencies
8. Information technology	• Training the health care workforce in new information technologies • Increased ability to coordinate care across sites • Challenge of managing an increased pace of change due to more rapid information transfer • Challenge of dealing with confidentiality issues associated with new information technologies
9. Globalization and expansion of the world economy	• Need to manage cross-national and cross-cultural tertiary and quaternary patient care referrals • Increasing the competitiveness and productivity of the American labor force • Managing global strategic alliances, particularly in the areas of biotechnology and new technology development

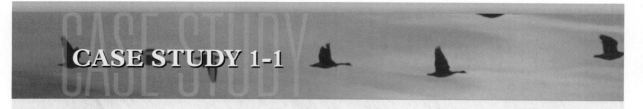

CASE STUDY 1-1

Mrs. Williams comes to your unit from the Emergency Department (ED). Her admitting diagnosis is asthma. Her husband tells you she was really frightened and could not breathe when she came to the ED. They belong to a health maintenance organization. Mrs. Williams and her husband feel better now. They ask you how long she will be in the hospital and what will happen next. You give them a copy of your unit's asthma clinical practice guideline and go over it with them.

How can you try to ensure a smooth transition home?

How will you work with your health care system and the community you serve to ensure that Mrs. Williams and other asthma patients in the community are not admitted with asthma again soon? What kind of teaching will Mrs. Williams need to prevent future attacks?

new millennium. These changes, as well as the emergence of terrorism and bioterrorism, continue to call for ongoing changes in the education of health care professionals.

TRENDS IN AMERICAN HEALTH CARE AND THE NEED FOR CARING, TRANSDISCIPLINARY NURSING

American health care quality, cost, and access needs continue to develop. Nurses who work in health care today continue the tradition of nursing caring and excellence that began with Nightingale. Nightingale served patients in her time by meeting their needs. Today's nurse will prosper by continuing this commitment to a personal ethic of social responsibility, service, and caring. Caring is the core of nursing practice because it renders technical, curative procedures tolerable and safe, helping patients and families weather their illness and sustain or regain familiar life worlds (Benner, 2000).

Nursing Role

Nursing has come a long way in this century. Six characteristics are commonly used to assess whether a job is a profession. These characteristics include maintaining quality education of the practitioner, having a code of ethics, receiving compensation commensurate with the work, being organized to promote a needed service, having autonomy in practice, and being recognized by the government with licensure (Pinkerton, 2001). Nursing is recognized as a profession in most circles today, though nurse-physician work relationships continue to evolve. In the late 1990s, some nurses still reported "knowing the right thing to do and having no support or authority to carry it out" (Aroskar, 1998). Development of the nurse-physician relationship must be part of improving the health care delivery system, particularly because it has been documented that when nurses and physicians work together, patient care improves (Baggs & Ryan, 1990).

Transdisciplinary Nursing

Health needs of the future will require a professional nurse who can demonstrate caring, competency, and practice in a transdisciplinary fashion, planning for the changing health care delivery system. Transdisciplinary practice brings nurses to the table with more-equal footing and diminishes the notion that the team needs a captain to function. With each discipline bringing its unique talents to the job of providing care for a patient and that patient's family, transdisciplinary practice removes the gatekeeper and

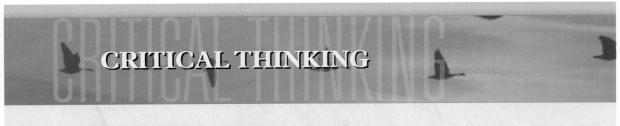

CRITICAL THINKING

Go to the Web site for Healthy People 2010 (*http://www.health.gov/healthypeople/*).

Click on "Leading Health Indicators" and on "Healthfinder." What did you find?

How is your state doing on the Healthy People 2010 indicators?

How could you work with leaders in your community and state to improve your state's performance?

allows patients access to all caregivers based on what expertise is needed. Success in transdisciplinary practice will depend on each profession maintaining the highest standards, including expectations of advanced education, some sort of certification, and requirements for continuing education to maintain competency (Carroll-Johnson, 2001). The health care of the future will increasingly be outcome focused, evidence based, wellness oriented, population based, technology intensive, and highly cost aware. Nursing must be ready to meet this challenge.

KEY CONCEPTS

- American health care has developed within a political context. It can be highly sophisticated, but it does not deliver the same level of health care, access, and cost-effective quality to all its citizens.
- Various groups deliver American health care in a variety of settings.
- American health care is paid for by a variety of public and private groups. Medicare is the largest purchaser of health care.
- Health care can be categorized into three levels: primary, secondary, and tertiary.
- The JCAHO is the national organization that accredits health care organizations. This accreditation is one of the ways hospitals can be certified to receive federal government reimbursement for health care delivery to Medicare patients.

- In 1965, Title XVIII of the Social Security Act Amendments created Medicare, and Title XIX created Medicaid. Health care costs began to rise faster than the rate of inflation after the passage of these amendments.
- Research in the 1970s revealed much variation in health care, and clinical practice guidelines based on the best available evidence were developed by the AHRQ to guide and improve care.
- Malpractice concerns have influenced hospitals and nurses to improve quality of and access to care for patients.
- Donabedian developed a framework for quality. He identified structure, process, and outcome elements of quality. When outcomes are not good, nurses must review the structure and process of health care.
- The Malcolm Baldridge National Quality Award provides a framework for the delivery of quality health care.
- Efforts to improve health care must address the underlying causes of death and the multiple determinants of health in the United States.
- The Pew Health Professions Commission identified 21 competencies for the 21st century for health care providers. Nursing and other health care professions will have to adapt to a fast-changing environment in the future.
- Various forces are affecting health care in the new millennium.
- Caring, transdisciplinary nursing practice promises to be an important part of nursing's future role in health care.

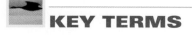

KEY TERMS

capitation
disease management
fee-for-service
  reimbursement
horizontal integration
integrated delivery
  system
outcome elements
  of quality

primary health care
process elements of
  quality
risk adjustment
secondary health care
structure elements of
  quality
tertiary health care
vertical integration

REVIEW QUESTIONS

1. Diagnosis-related groups (DRGs) often cause which of the following?
   A. Increased laboratory and x-ray testing
   B. Decreased length of stay in hospital
   C. Increased use of new technology
   D. Decreased patient turnover in hospitals

2. The national organization that accredits health care organizations is known as which of the following?
   A. American Nurses Association
   B. Pew Health Professions Commission
   C. Agency for Healthcare Research and Quality
   D. Joint Commission on Accreditation of Healthcare Organizations

3. The largest purchaser of health care in America is which of the following?
   A. Private individuals
   B. Private insurance companies
   C. Health maintenance organizations
   D. Medicare, Medicaid, and other governmental programs

4. Who identified a structure, process, and outcome framework for quality?
   A. Titler
   B. Elazar
   C. Wennberg
   D. Donabedian

5. Which of the following is the name of a National Award for Quality?
   A. Hill Burton
   B. Malcolm Baldridge
   C. Foundation for Accountability
   D. National Committee on Quality Assurance

REVIEW ACTIVITIES

1. You have just graduated from your nursing education program and have begun working on a new patient care unit. Your nurse manager asks you to serve on the team to develop and improve the unit. Give examples of the three elements of quality that you will consider. Consider structure, process, and outcome examples in your answer. How will you monitor the effects of your improvements?

2. Your uncle is a quality improvement director at a local manufacturing company. He comments on some of the activities the manufacturing company does to improve quality. What could you tell him about the quality improvement activities done by a patient care unit on which you have recently given clinical care?

3. Review the Pew Health Professions Commission competencies. Consider how you can improve your own knowledge level in any of the competency areas in which you do not feel comfortable.

EXPLORING THE WEB

- What sites could you recommend to patients and families seeking information about self-help, hospital accreditation, research, and clinical practice guidelines, for example, the JCAHO and the Agency for Healthcare Research and Quality?
  http://www.selfhelpweb.org
  http://www.jcaho.org
  http://www.ahrq.gov
  http://www.centerwatch.com
  http://www.guideline.gov
  http://www.cdc.gov
  http://www.netdoctor.co.uk

- Go to the sites for the Malcolm Baldridge National Quality Award and the IOM Report. What information did you find there?
  http://www.www.quality.nist.gov/
  http://www.www.nas.edu

- Where can you find statistics on health care spending?
  http://www.www.hcfa.gov/stats/nhe-oact/tables/chart.htm

- Search the Web, checking these sites: Medicare, National Institute of Health, American Nurses Association, National League for Nursing, American Cancer Society, American Heart Association, diabetes, Ellis Island records, Delmar Learning. What did you find?
  http://www.www.medicare.gov
  http://www.www.nih.gov
  http://www.www.ana.org
  http://www.www.nln.org
  http://www.www.cancer.org
  http://www.www.americanheart.org
  http://www.www.diabetes.org
  http://www.www.delmarnursing.com
  http://www.www.ellisislandrecords.org

- Go to Pubmed. What did you find there? Can you access nursing and medical journals? Would you recommend this site to patients?
  http://www.ncbi.nlm.nih.gov/PubMed/

- What are some helpful sites for nurses?
  http://www.allnurses.com
  http://www.nursingworld.org
  http://www.continuingeducation.com
  http://www.hotnursejobs.com
  http://www.www.freelawyer.co.uk
  http://www.nln.org
  http://www.hospitalsoup.com

- Where could you go for information on the eHealth Internet Code of Ethics?
  http://www.ihealthcoalition.org

- What are some sites to check on HIPAA information?
  U.S. Department of Health and Human Services: *aspe.hhs.gov/admnsimp/*
  Workgroup for electronic data interchange: *http://www.wedi.org*
  X12N insurance industry implementation guides: *http://www.wpc-edi.com.hipaa*
  X12N home page: *http://www.disa.org*

REFERENCES

Adams, D. F., Fraser, D. B., & Abrams, H. L. (1973). The complications of coronary arteriography. *Circulation, 48*(3), 609–618.

America's best hospitals. (2001, July 23). *U.S. News and World Report,* 44–105.

Aroskar, M. (1998). Ethical working relationships in patient care. *Nursing Clinics of North America, 33*(2), 313–323.

Baggs, J. G., & Ryan, S. A. (1990). ICU Nurse-physician collaboration and nursing satisfaction. *Nursing Economic$, 8*(6), 386–392.

Baldridge National Quality Program. (2000). *Health care criteria for performance excellence.* Gaithersburg, MD: Baldridge National Quality Program.

Bellack, J. P., & O'Neil, E. H. (2000). Recreating nursing practice for a new century: Recommendations and implications of the Pew Health Professions Commission's final report. *Nursing and Health Care Perspectives, 21*(1), 14–21.

Benner, P. (2000). The wisdom of our practice. *American Journal of Nursing, 100*(10), 99–103.

Bergner, M., Bobbit, R. A., Carter, W. B., & Gilson, B. S. (1981). The Sickness Impact Profile: Development and final revision of a health status measure. *Medical Care, 19*(8), 787–805.

Bull, M. J. (1997). Lessons from the past: Visions for the future of quality care. In C. G. Meisenheimer, *Improving quality* (2nd ed., pp. 3–16). Gaithersburg, MD: Aspen.

Byers, S. A. (1997). *The executive nurse—leadership for new health care transitions.* Clifton Park, NY: Delmar Learning.

Carroll-Johnson, R. (2001). Redefining interdisciplinary practice. *Oncology Nursing Forum, 28*(4), 619.

Cohen, S., Doyle, W. J., Skoner, D. P., Rabin, B. S., & Gwaltney, J. M., Jr. (1997). Social ties and susceptibility to the common cold. *Journal of the American Medical Association, 277*, 1940–1944.

Coile, R. C., Jr. (1999, October). Managed care in the millennium. New forecast for the "five stages of managed care." *Russ Coile's Health Trends, 11*(12), 1, 3–7.

DeLaune, S. C., & Ladner, P. K. (2002). *Fundamentals of nursing* (2nd ed.). Clifton Park, NY: Delmar Learning.

Donabedian, A. (1966). Evaluating the quality of medical care. *Milbank Memorial Fund Quarterly, 44*, 194–196.

Donatelle, R., & Davis, L. G. (1998). *Access to health* (8th ed.). Needham Heights, MA: Allyn & Bacon.

Drummond, M. F., Stoddart, F. L., & Torrance, G. W. (1994). *Methods for the economic evaluation of health care programmes.* Oxford, England: Oxford University Press.

Elazar, D. (1966). *American federalism: A view from the states.* New York: Crowell.

Epstein, R. S., & Sherwood, L. M. (1996). From outcomes research to disease management: A guide for the perplexed. *Annals of Internal Medicine, 124,* 832–837.

Evans, R., & Stoddard, G. (1990). Consuming health care, producing health. *Social Science and Medicine, 31*(12), 1347–1363.

Fos, P. J., & Fine, D. J. (2000). *Designing health care for populations.* San Francisco: Jossey-Bass.

Fottler, M. D., Blair, J. D., Whitehead, C. J., Laus, M. D., & Savage, G. T. (1989). Assessing key stakeholders: Who matters to hospitals and why? *Hospital and Health Services Administration, 34*(530).

Gruman, J., & Chesney, M. (1995). Introduction for superhighways for disease. *Psychosomatic Medicine, 57,* 207.

Guadagnoli, E., Epstein, A. M., Zaslavsky, A., Shaul, J. A., Veroff, D., Fowler, F. J., Jr., & Cleary, P. D. (2000). Providing consumers with information about the quality of health plans: The consumer assessment of health plans demonstration in Washington State. *Joint Commission Journal on Quality Improvement, 26*(7), 410–420.

Hitchcock, J. E., Schubert, P. E., & Thomas, S. A. (1999). *Community health nursing.* Clifton Park, NY: Delmar Learning.

Hunt, S. M., McKenna, P., McEwen, J., Williams, J., & Papp, E., (1986). The Nottingham Health Profile: Subjective health status and medical consultations. *Social Science and Medicine, 15*(3, Pt. 1), 221–229.

Jette, A. M., & Cleary, P. D. (1987). Functional disability assessment. *Physical Therapy, 67,* 1854–1859.

Joel, L., & DeLaune, S. C. (2002). The health care delivery system. In S. C. DeLaune & P. K. Ladner, *Fundamentals of nursing* (2nd ed.). Clifton Park, NY: Delmar Learning.

Joint Commission on Accreditation of Healthcare Organizations. (2001). *Manual for hospitals.* Chicago: Author.

Kohn, L., Corrigan, J., & Donaldson, M. (Eds.). (1999). *To err is human: Building a safer health system.* Washington, DC: Committee on Quality of Care in America, Institute of Medicine, National Academy Press.

Kohn, L., Corrigan, J., & Donaldson, M. (Eds.). (2001). *Crossing the quality chasm: A new health system for the 21st century.* Washington, DC: Committee on Quality of Care in America, Institute of Medicine, National Academy Press.

Lando, M. (2000, May/June). The framework for a successful merger. *Healthcare Executive,* 6–11.

Lang, N. M. (1999). Discipline approaches to evidence-based practice: A view from nursing. *Joint Commission Journal on Quality Improvement, 25*(10), 539–544.

Leape, L. (1987). Unnecessary surgery. *Health Services Research, 24*(3), 351–407.

Lockart, C. A. (1999). Health care delivery in the United States. In J. E. Hitchcock, P. E. Schubert, & S. A. Thomas, *Community health nursing.* Clifton Park, NY: Delmar Learning.

Lohr, K. N., & Carey, T. S. (1999). Assessing "best evidence": Issues in grading the quality of studies for systematic reviews. *Joint Commission Journal on Quality Improvement, 25*(9), 470–479.

Lovern, E. (2001a, January 1). JCAHO's new tell-all. Standards require that patients know about below-par care. *Modern Healthcare, 31*(1), 2, 15.

Lovern, E. (2001b, May 7). Another makeover. JCAHO moves to rewrite many rules to lessen hospitals' regulatory burden. *Modern Healthcare, 31*(19), 5, 16.

Lovern, E. (2001c, May 28). Oh no, not that type of review. JCAHO singling out more hospitals for non-compliance with standards. *Modern Healthcare, 31*(22), 4–5.

Maddox, P. (2001). Update on national quality of care initiatives. *Nursing Economic$, 19*(3), 121–124.

Maunsell, E., Brisson, J., & Deschenes, L. (1995). Social support and survival among women with breast cancer. *Cancer, 76,* 631–637.

McCormick, K. A., Cummings, M. A., & Kovner, C. (1997). The role of the Agency for Health Care Policy and Research in improving outcomes of care. *Nursing Clinics of North America, 32*(3), 5.

McGinnis, J. M., & Foege, W. H. (1993). Actual causes of death in the United States. *Journal of the American Medical Association, 270*(18), 2207–2212.

McLaughlin, C. P., & Kaluzny, A. D. (1999). *Continuous quality improvement in health care* (2nd ed.). Gaithersburg, MD: Aspen.

Morrissey, J. (2001, January 1). Slow down: HIPAA ahead. *Modern Healthcare,* 30.

Nightingale, F. (1914). Florence Nightingale to her nurses: A selection from Miss Nightingale's addresses to probationers and nurses of the Nightingale School at St. Thomas's Hospital [p. 1; Address in May 1872]. London: Macmillan.

100 top hospitals. (2001, February). *Modern Healthcare,* 6–29.

Oxman, T. E. (1995). Lack of social participation or religious strength and comfort as risk factors for death after cardiac surgery in the elderly. *Psychosomatic Medicine, 57,* 5–15.

Parkerson, G. R., Jr., Broadhead, W. E., & Tse, C.-K. J. (1990). The Duke health profile: A 17 item measure of health and dysfunction. *Medical Care, 28,* 1056–1072.

Pinkerton, S. (2001). The future of professionalism in nursing. *Nursing Economic$, 18*(3), 130–131.

Pratt, L. A., Ford, D. E., Crum, R. M., Annenian, H. K., Gallo, J. J., & Eaton, W. W. (1996). Depression, psychotropic medication, and risk of myocardial infarction. Prospective data from the Baltimore ECA follow-up. *Circulation, 94,* 3123–3129.

Raffel, M. (Ed.). (1997). *Health care and reform in industrialized countries.* University Park: The Pennsylvania State University Press.

Rich, M. W., Beckham, V., Wittenberg, C., Leven, C. L., Freedland, K. E., & Carney, R. M. (1995). A multidisciplinary intervention to prevent readmission of elderly patients with congestive heart failure. *New England Journal of Medicine, 333,* 1190–1195.

Rogers, E. M. (1995). Lessons for guidelines from the diffusion of innovations. *Joint Commission Journal on Quality Improvement, 21*(7), 324–328.

Sackett, D. L., Rosenberg, W. M. C., Gray, J. A. M., Haynes, R. B., & Richardson, W. S. (1996). Evidence-based medicine: What it is and what it isn't. *British Medical Journal, 312*(7023), 71–72.

Shortell, S. M. (1996). *Remaking health care in America: Building organized delivery systems.* San Francisco: Jossey-Bass.

Shortell, S. M., & Kaluzny, A. D. (2000). *Health care management* (4th ed.). Clifton Park, NY: Delmar Learning.

Simms, L. M., Price, S. A., & Ervin, N. E. (2000). *Professional practice of nursing administration* (3rd ed.). Clifton Park, NY: Delmar Learning.

Soukup, S. M. (2000). The Center for Advanced Nursing Practice evidence-based practice model: Promoting the scholarship of practice. *Nursing Clinics of North America, 35*(2), 301–309.

Spitzer, W. O. (1998). Quality of life. In D. Burley & W. H. W. Inman (Eds.), *Therapeutic risk: Perception, measurement, and management.* New York: Wiley.

Strasen, L. (1999). The silent health care revolution: The rising demand for complementary medicine. *Nursing Economic$, 17*(5), 246–256.

Titler, M. G., Mentes, J. C., Rakel, B. A., Abbott, L., & Baumler, S. (1999). From book to bedside: Putting evidence to use in the care of the elderly. *Joint Commission Journal on Quality Improvement, 25*(10), 545–546.

U.S. Department of Health and Human Services. (2000). *Healthy people 2010* [Conference edition, in two volumes]. Washington, DC: U.S. Government Printing Office.

Ware, J. E., & Sherbourne, C. D. (1992). The MOS 36-item short form health survey I: Conceptual framework and item selection. *Medical Care, 30,* 473–478.

Wennberg, J. E., & Gittelsohn, A. M. (1973). Small area variations in health care delivery. *Science, 182*(117), 1102–1108.

Wolper, L. F. (1999). *Health care administration: Planning, implementing, and managing organized delivery systems* (3rd ed.). Gaithersburg, MD: Aspen.

SUGGESTED READINGS

American Nurses Association. (1995). *Nursing's social policy statement.* Washington, DC: American Nurses Publishing.

Berman, S. (2000). The AMA clinical quality improvement focus on addressing patient safety. *Joint Commission Journal on Quality Improvement, 26*(7), 428–433.

Berwick, D. M. (1994). Eleven worthy aims for clinical leadership of health system reform. *Journal of the American Medical Association, 272,* 797–802.

Boggs, P. B., Hayati, F., Washburne, W. F., & Wheeler, D. A. (1999). Using statistical process control charts for the continual improvement of asthma care. *Joint Commission Journal on Quality Improvement, 25*(4), 163–170.

Codman, E. (1914). The product of a hospital. *Surgical Gynecology and Obstetrics, 18,* 491–494.

Couch, J. B. (1999). *The health care professional's guide to disease management.* Gaithersburg, MD: Aspen.

Dienemann, J. A. (Ed.). (1998). *Nursing administration: Managing patient care* (2nd ed.). Upper Saddle River, NJ: Prentice Hall Health.

Drummond, H., & Stoddart, G. (1995). Assessment of health producing measures across different sectors. *Health Policy, 33,* 219–231.

Ellwood, P. M. (1998). Outcomes management: A technology of patient experience. *New England Journal of Medicine, 318,* 1549–1556.

Enthoven, A. C., & Kronick, R. (1994). Universal health insurance through incentive programs. In P. Lee & C. Ester (Eds.), *The nation's health* (4th ed.). Boston: Jones and Bartlett.

Erickson, P., Wilson, R., & Shannon, I. (1995). *Years of healthy life* [NCHS Healthy People Statistical Notes #7]. Rockville, MD: U.S. Public Health Service.

Ferguson, S. L. (1999). Institute for Nursing Leadership: A new program to enhance the leadership capacity of all nurses. *Nursing Outlook,* 91–92.

Ginsberg, E. (1996). *Tomorrow's hospital: A look to the twenty-first century.* New Haven, CT: Yale University Press.

Grol, R., & Grimshaw, J. (1999). Evidence-based implementation of evidence-based medicine. *Joint Commission Journal on Quality Improvement, 25*(10).

Hamer, R. (1999). Goals 2000: For MDs: Managerial competency. For HMOs: Administrative retooling. *Managed Care, 8*(11), 38.

Heller, B. R., Oros, M. T., & Durney-Crowley, J. (2000). The future of nursing education: Ten trends to watch. *Nursing and Health Care Perspectives, 21*(1), 9–13.

Kelly, L. Y., & Joel, L. A. (1999). *Dimensions of professional nursing* (8th ed.). McGraw-Hill.

Kindig, D. A. (1999). Purchasing population health: Aligning financial incentives to improve health outcomes. *Nursing Outlook,* 15–22.

Lancaster, J. (1999). *Nursing issues in leading and managing change.* St. Louis, MO: Mosby.

Lea, D. H., & Lawson, M. T. (2000). A practice-based genetics curriculum for nurse educators: An innovative approach to integrating human genetics into nursing curricula. *Journal of Nursing, 39*(9), 418–421.

Lindeman, C. A. (2000). The future of nursing education. *Journal of Nursing Education, 39*(1), 5–12.

Mariner-Tomey, A., & Alligood, M. R. (1998). *Nursing theorists and their work* (4th ed.). St. Louis, MO: Mosby.

McCloskey, J. C., Maas, M. L., Huber, D. G., Kasparek, A., Specht, J. P., Ramler, C. L., Watson, C., Blegen, M. A., Delaney, C., Ellerbe, S., Etsheidt, C., Gongawera, C., Johnson, M. R., Kelly, K. C., Mehmert, P., & Clougherty, J. (1996). Nursing management innovations: A need for systematic evaluation. In K. C. Kelly & M. L. Maas (Eds.), *Outcomes of effective management practice* (pp. 3–19). Thousand Oaks, CA: Sage.

Milstead, J. A. (Ed.). (1999). *Health policy and politics: A nurse's guide* (3rd ed.). Gaithersburg, MD: Aspen.

Murray, C. J. L. (1994). Quantifying the burden of disease: The technical basis for disability-adjusted life years. *Bulletin of the World Health Organization, 72,* 429–445.

Nelson, E. C., Splaine, M. E., Godfrey, M. M., Kahn, V. V., Hess, A., Batalden, P., & Plume, S. K. (2000). Using data to improve medical practice by measuring processes and outcomes of care. *Joint Commission Journal on Quality Improvement, 26*(12), 667–685.

Norton, D., & Kaplan, R. (2001). *The strategy-focused organization: How balanced scorecard companies thrive in the new business environment.* Boston: Harvard Business School Press.

O'Grady, E. (2000). Access to health care: An issue central to nursing. *Nursing Economic$, 18*(2), 88–90.

Oregon Process Board. (1994). *Oregon benchmarks: Standards for measuring statewide progress and institutional performance.* Portland: State of Oregon.

Ozbolt, J. G., Fruchtnight, J. N., & Hayden, J. R. (1994). Toward data standards for clinical nursing information. *Journal of the American Medical Informatics Association, 1*(2), 175–185.

Pesut, D. J., & Rezmerski, C. J. (2000). Future think. *Nursing Outlook, 48*(1), 9.

Schor, E. L., & Menaghan, E. (1995). Family pathways to child health. In B. C. Amick, *Society and health.* New York: Oxford University Press.

Schroeder, P. (1994). *Improving quality and performance: Concepts, programs, and techniques.* St. Louis, MO: Mosby.

Springhouse Corporation. (1999). *Nurse's handbook of alternative and complementary therapies.* Springhouse, PA: Author.

Springhouse Corporation. (2000). *Nurse's legal handbook* (4th ed.). Springhouse, PA: Author.

Stevens, K. R., & Cassidy, V. R. (1999). *Evidence-based teaching.* NLN Press. Boston: Jones and Bartlett.

Sullivan, E. J. (1999). *Creating nursing's future: Issues, opportunities, and challenges.* St. Louis, MO: Mosby.

Tengs, T., Adams, M., Pliskin, J., Safron, D., Siegel, J., Weinstein, M., & Graham, J. (1995). Five hundred life-saving interventions and their cost effectiveness. *Risk Analysis, 15,* 369–390.

Tieman, J. (2001, July 9). Coming of age. Disease management making a case for itself clinically and financially. *Modern Healthcare, 31*(28), 26, 27, 38.

Tieman, J., & Bellandi, D. (2001, January 1). HIPAA will be no holiday. Experts say exhaustive rules may require significant cultural and administrative changes. *Modern Healthcare, 31*(1), 3, 15.

Trofino, J. (1997). The courage to change—reshaping health care delivery. *Nursing Management, 28*(11), 50–53.

Weeks, W. B., Hamby, L., Stein, A., & Batalden, P. B. (2000). Using the Baldridge Management System framework in health care: The Veterans Health Administration experience. *Joint Commission Journal on Quality Improvement, 26*(7), 379–387.

Wilson, L. M. (1999). Healthy people—a new millennium. *Journal of Nursing Administration's Healthcare Law, Ethics, and Regulation, 1*(2), 29–32.

CHAPTER 2

The purpose of creating and analyzing records of what transpires in hospitals is to know how the money is being spent; whether it is, in fact, doing good, or whether it is doing mischief. (Florence Nightingale, 1859)

Basic Clinical Health Care Economics

Laura J. Nosek, PhD, RN
Ida M. Androwich, PhD, RNC, FAAN

OBJECTIVES

Upon completion of this chapter, the reader should be able to:

1. Discuss why health care is managed as a business.
2. Identify at least three reasons why cost is an important consideration in choosing among health care options.
3. Critically discuss three to five issues that influence basic health care economics.

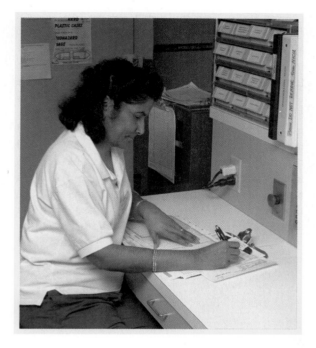

You and your spouse take an island vacation for 15 days with a 4-night extension in a European capital. Your spouse, an insulin-dependent diabetic for 12 years, runs out of insulin the day before you are scheduled to leave the island for the mainland but refuses to consult the local physician. On day 5 without insulin, your spouse is weak and "spacey." You go to a pharmacy with the empty insulin container and purchase the local equivalent of insulin after consulting with the English-speaking pharmacist. Your spouse no sooner takes the insulin than the pharmacist appears at the door of your hotel room frantic that the strength of the insulin you bought is incorrect; it is 10 times too strong. You convince your spouse to go to a nearby hospital Emergency Department where, with your sparse local language and the help of one person who speaks English, you discover that all health care is socialized and provided free to all citizens. You are told there is no provision for using your health insurance and no provision for paying cash.

What does the hospital perceive the problem to be?

Do you perceive the problem to be the same as the hospital does?

When cost is removed from the equation, what drives the decision to provide or not provide health care?

Is that driver a universal value, or is it culturally dependent?

If cost were not a driving consideration in providing health care in the United States, what would the health care system be like?

Regardless of how expert, creative, collaborative, and altruistic a health care system may be, it cannot function without money. Over the ages, that money has flowed from varying sources, including philanthropy, volunteerism, fees for services, insurance, and government subsidies. Securing the bottom line is basic to achieving the mission of providing health care and is now viewed as the shared responsibility of humans around the world.

It was once thought that nurses need only be educated in the art and the science of providing clinical care to patients. Today, it is recognized that nurses must be much more broadly educated. In addition to clinical care expertise, they must demonstrate minimal competence in the humanities, management science, and computer science, as well as be skilled in evaluating and applying new knowledge suggested by scientific research.

The United States spends more per capita on health care than any other country in the world (Wolper, 1999), yet morbidity and mortality statistics, in terms of improved health outcomes, lead us to question the value that we receive for our dollars. Nightingale's early search for the "good" versus "mischievous" outcomes of the money spent on health care may have initiated an unspoken commitment to financial stewardship among nurses. It seems fitting, then, that all nurses be required to participate knowledgeably in designing care systems that provide the best possible care at the lowest cost (Chang, Price, & Pfoutz, 2001). Consequently, every nurse today needs to have a basic understanding of clinical health care **economics**—the study of how scarce resources are allocated among possible uses—in order to make appropriate choices among the increasingly scarce resources of the future.

The study of economics is based on three general premises: (1) scarcity—resources exist in finite quantities and consumption demand is typically greater than resource supply; (2) choice—decisions are made about which resources to produce and consume among many options; and (3) preference—individual and societal values and preferences influence the decisions that are made. In a traditional market economy, the sellers sell to the buyers who buy, with each trying to maximize their gains from the transactions. Health care does not fit well in this model. For example, consider the concept of price elasticity, which is related to the price that an individual is willing to pay for a given item. Normally, as the price goes up, the demand goes down. When the purchase is health care, however, the price may be viewed as irrelevant to the decision to purchase. Think of a wristwatch that you might always purchase for $5, would likely not buy at $50, and would never consider at $500. Now, imagine that instead of a wristwatch, the item in question is a medication or therapy needed to save your sick child. Now the consideration of price in the decision-making process is likely quite different. Thus, health care is much less "elastic" with reference to price than many other consumer goods.

Another aspect of health care's difference from the traditional economic model relates to the knowledge of options and payment mechanisms available to the consumer. In a typical market, the buyer is also the payer. In health care, the health care provider (buyer) ordering a hospitalization or treatment is a doctor or nurse. The provider is not the payer, nor is the patient (buyer) using the hospital or treatment the payer. The actual **payer** is the third-party reimburser (insurance company or government). Consequently, the financial impact of the decision on the provider (buyer) and the patient user (buyer) is skewed. Neither of these buyers is the payer.

This chapter presents basic clinical health care economics concepts that are important to the novice nurse entering clinical practice. Included are perspectives on the role cost has played and will play in directing health care delivery, the methods for determining the cost of delivering nursing care, and the effect of health care policy on the delivery of nursing care. Recognized nurse experts provide projections for the future impact of economics on clinical nursing.

TRADITIONAL PERSPECTIVE ON THE COST OF HEALTH CARE: HEALTH CARE AS ALTRUISM

The long-standing tradition of health care is to help people achieve their optimal level of health so that they can enjoy their maximum quality of life. **Altruism**, the unselfish concern for the welfare of others, and **ethics**, the doctrine that the general welfare of society is the proper goal of an individual's actions as opposed to **egoism**, the tendency to be self-centered or to consider only oneself and one's own interests

(Agnes, 2000), drove the way health care was viewed and provided. Several early nursing leaders, including Florence Nightingale and Isabel Adams Hampton Robb, were members of socially prominent families instilled with the value that altruistic service was the expected role of the privileged. Such feelings of dedication to the less fortunate stemmed from medieval infirmaries established by convents and monasteries to care for the aged, orphaned, poor, and disabled. The first hospitals to care for the sick and injured were also charitable institutions established around the 14th century to provide illness care to those who did not have a home or who could not afford home care (Nosek, 1986). The people cared for in hospitals were called patients from the Latin *patiens*, meaning "to suffer" (vos Savant, 2001).

Need for Health Care Determined by Provider

Health care traditionally was delivered from a paternalistic model of governance and control. Health professionals, led by physicians, controlled a vast body of scientific knowledge and skill rendered awesome and mystical by complex scientific language. Command of that scientific knowledge and skill required extensive and expensive education and was not shared with "outsiders." The physician determined what health care was needed independent of the patient and even independent of professional colleagues. The physician also decided how much to charge for that care. Decision making about all aspects of health care was the exclusive domain of the professionals.

Right to Health Care at Any Cost

The cost of health care was not considered, let alone questioned, until the early 1960s. The American belief system firmly held that every individual was entitled to all the knowledge, skill, and technology related to health care at any cost. It was claimed to be a "right"; it was the "American way." The spiraling cost of providing health care was noted, but it was antithetical to the American value system to consider rationing health care. In an attempt to control costs, the U.S. government stepped up in 1965 and enacted

Titles XVIII and XIX, amendments to the Social Security Act, commonly referred to as the Medicare and Medicaid programs, which provide health care coverage for the elderly and the indigent, respectively. It was anticipated that by requiring health care providers to account for the cost of Medicare and Medicaid patients' care, spending would be curbed. Other insurers soon followed with their own requirements, launching the overall budgeting of health care.

Cost Plus

Despite the initiation of budgets in the late 1960s, the cost of health care continued to spiral upward as hospitals became the preferred site for provision of intermediate care and the high technology necessary for state-of-the-art illness care (Nosek, 1986). That cost was determined by the actual cost the provider incurred for the care plus a profit incentive for being in the business. The method was known as "cost plus," and clearly the incentive was "the more you spend, the more you get," not "how can this be accomplished more economically?"

CONTEMPORARY PERSPECTIVE ON COST OF HEALTH CARE: HEALTH CARE AS A BUSINESS

Possibly the most common reason given for entering a health care profession still was "to help people." Virginia Henderson, viewed by some as the contemporary Florence Nightingale, defined nursing as

> primarily helping people (sick or well) in the performance of those activities contributing to health, or its recovery (or to peaceful death) that they would perform unaided if they had the necessary strength, will, or knowledge. It is likewise the unique contribution of nursing to help people to be independent of such assistance as soon as possible. (Henderson & Nite, 1978)

Nurses fervently believed and stated that this definition applied irrespective of the site where nursing care was given. Yet, nurses also began to recognize that the cost of providing care in the traditional altruistic way was prohibitive and that achieving independence from nursing care as quickly as possible conserves scarce nursing resources.

Taxes to cover the ever-increasing costs of the government health care programs were climbing. Medicare insolvency was a threat. Again, the government, the major payer, stepped in. The Health Care Financing Administration (HCFA), the department responsible for the Medicare and Medicaid programs, was authorized to change the way it paid for health care. The Tax Equity and Fiscal Responsibility Act (TEFRA) of 1982 established new payment regulations. Instead of reimbursing the provider's cost, the government would henceforth pay a flat rate stated up front. The new system would therefore be called the prospective payment system.

The new payment system considerably changed institutions' incentives for spending. If the provider was able to provide the care for less than the prospective payment, the provider could make a profit. If the provider spent more than that payment, the provider lost money. Because length of hospital stay is a surrogate measure of hospital cost, reducing length of stay was seen as the easiest and most logical way to reduce the cost of care enough to ensure adequacy of the payment.

One of the first hospital lengths of stay to be shortened was that for obstetrical patients. It was an unforgettable October morning in 1983 when the headlines of the *Cleveland Plain Dealer* shocked the city with the news. Effective immediately, hospital care for those experiencing normal vaginal delivery would be 3 calendar days starting with the day of admission, the story read. At that time in that city, the usual stay for a normal vaginal delivery was 5 days; for a Cesarean delivery, it was 7 days. If a woman were admitted shortly before midnight, that constituted day 1. If she experienced a long labor, she could end up being discharged on her first postpartum day. Patients were crying in the halls. Nurses were outraged, trying to figure out how they could possibly teach breastfeeding when breast milk does not come in until postpartum day 3. Physicians were threatening a variety of actions, citing unsafe care.

Out with altruism. In with health care that clinicians had to recognize was truly a business. In with a whole new language, that of business and consumers and profit and margin and competition and cost, *cost*, COST. The bottom line (cost) became the focus, not only of managers and administrators but of all employees at all levels of all health care enti-

Everyone needed to question what they did, how they did it, and how many it took to do it in order to determine whether it was required for safe care and quality outcomes and whether there was a less costly way of attaining a safe, quality outcome. In 1960, Abdellah had challenged health care providers to determine the care that was needed and to provide no more, no less (Abdellah, Beland, Martin, & Matheney, 1960). Nearly 25 years later, health care providers were trying to come to grips with just that. Yet, there was alarm that safety and quality, the cornerstones of professional practice, were being sacrificed.

Need for Health Care Determined by the Consumer

Attention shifted toward safety and quality and the need for measurable outcomes. Total quality improvement (TQI) and continuous quality improvement (CQI) programs were initiated to assure society that cost management was not compromising safety or quality. These programs required all stakeholders, including patients, to work together to evaluate and improve outcomes. The expertise of allied health care providers was recognized, and through the growing access to information technology, consumers were empowered to better understand their own health, the complex technologies available, their options for choosing to manage the decisions about their care, and the cost implications of those decisions (Hein, 2001). No longer was health care the exclusive realm of the physician and other professionals.

Right to Health Care at a Reasonable Cost

The contemporary value system holds that individuals have the right to health care at a reasonable cost. Reasonable cost is determined by insurers. When it refers to fees charged for services, a *reasonable cost* is the usual and customary fee charged in the region. When referring to technology; complex and expensive procedures; or expensive, extensive pharmacologic therapies, there is no established standard for how much it should cost to provide someone enhanced quality of life over time. Clearly, the lack of consensus on what constitutes reasonable cost is at the heart of the controversies between insurers and patients and their professional providers.

Managed Care

The effort to control cost through the Medicare and Medicaid programs marked the beginning of health care reform. There was keen anticipation that if the care of the neediest—the elderly and the poor—was managed centrally, access, cost, and quality would be optimally controlled. When it became evident that the program costs had been woefully underestimated, health maintenance organizations (HMOs), or managed care, emerged as the answer to cost-efficient and quality care (Hein, 2001).

Managed care is not easily defined and categorized. It is the product of a series of efforts to establish an effective program for all **stakeholders** (providers, employers, customers, patients, and payers who may have an interest in, and seek to influence, the decisions and actions of an organization) that has resulted in a complex, still-evolving array of structures and processes to deliver health care. Managed care has two distinct characteristics as viewed by Chang, Price, and Pfoutz (2001). First, managed care integrates the financial and the clinical care delivery functions of health care into a single organized system by contracting to be responsible for the clinical outcomes of an enrolled population for a capitated (fixed) fee. Managed care grew rapidly in the 1980s and 1990s and, according to the National Center for Health Statistics (1998), by 1997, 66.8 million Americans were enrolled in a nongovernment managed care program. An additional 5.2 million were covered by Medicare (Health Care Financing Administration, 1999a) and 15.3 million by Medicaid (Health Care Financing Administration, 1999b). Second, Chang, Price, and Pfoutz (2001) point out, managed care emphasizes delivery of a coordinated continuum of services across the care spectrum from wellness to death using financial incentives to achieve cost-efficiency.

It is important to note that managed care is the only health services delivery model generated from a market response rather than a formal federal government legislative initiative (Liberman & Rotarius, 2001). The first recorded managed care program in the United States was established for maritime workers in 1798 (Benedict, 1996). The mission and vision of managed care was to provide wellness care at a minimal cost to keep people healthy and thus avoid providing illness care at a higher, even astronomical, cost. A secondary mission was to standardize diagnostic and treatment decisions across the nation (Corrato & Barron, 1999).

Often, preapproval of care is required under managed care, and coverage is selective, effectively rationing care. Choice of physician or other provider and choice of site for care are restricted, which are additional methods of rationing care. An added incentive to rationing is a copayment for care that must be paid by the patient at the time that care is received. Despite industry assurances that care is not rationed, rationing is the under-girding concept of managed care. Managed care is not about providing health care (Corrato & Barron, 1999); it is about being a for-profit brokerage business in which the managed care company acts as an agent who negotiates the contract about how the provision of health care will be accomplished.

There are a variety of models of managed care companies. Included are staff, group, network, preferred provider organization (PPO), point of service (POS), mixed, and so on, each having its own unique structure and risk arrangements (Friedman, 2001). The most common form is the PPO. A PPO generally consists of a hospital and a number of physician providers. The PPO contracts with health care providers (both physicians and hospitals) and payers (self-insured employers, insurance companies, or managed care organizations) to provide health care services to a defined population for predetermined fixed fees. Discount rates may be negotiated with the providers in return for expedited claims payment and a somewhat predictable market share. In the PPO model, patients have a choice of using PPO or non-PPO providers; however, financial incentives are built in to encourage utilization of PPO providers (Finkler & Kovner, 2000). The default of risk to the provider and the patient, rather than to the managed care payer, has generated heated animosity toward managed care (Friedman, 2001). It is simply the raw reality of doing business made evident to the naive.

Nongovernmental health insurance is predominantly accessed through employment. Employers provide coverage to employees as a benefit for working for their company. Therefore, the employer chooses the coverage with cost in mind and negotiates an acceptable package of benefits on behalf of the employees. If the employer offers a selection of benefit packages, the employee may choose the package that is most suitable. The range of available packages has narrowed to being nearly exclusively HMOs (Corrato & Barron, 1999).

Examination of the percentage of the gross domestic product (gross national product statistics were used until 1991) spent on health care over the past few years shows that managed care has achieved the goal of controlling cost, as shown in Figure 2-1, despite the continued increase in dollars spent, shown in Figure 2-2. Regardless of that success, managed care has become the focus for the anger of many health care providers and much of American society. As the public became more knowledgeable, it also became more demanding.

To ease the pressure from physicians, patients, consumer advocates, and employers, many HMO programs recently dropped the requirement for managed care preapproval prior to hospitalization or consultation with a specialist. In response to the demand for greater choice of provider, care plans were adapted to permit those who can afford to pay higher premiums and copayments to have broader choices. Efforts to salvage the reputation of managed care have spawned a new name—*coordinated care* is replacing the term *managed care* to better describe a system of mutual decision making among insurers, providers, and patients. In 2001, a patient's bill of rights was introduced into Congress to, among other things, allow patients to sue their coordinated care providers.

Such changes diminished the insurer's clout and with it the ability to contain costs. Nationally renowned health care economist, Uwe Reinhardt of Princeton University, stated that "health plans can no longer bully and threaten the providers of care." Dr. David Lawrence, chief executive of the Kaiser Foundation Health Plan and Hospitals, noted, "When one uses financial tools to try to change the delivery of care, A, they are not very powerful, and B, they make people mad" (Freudenheim, 2001).

It may come as a surprise to note in Figure 2-3 that the 1999 statistics show that the federal government, through the Medicare and Medicaid programs, paid for 33.6% and other public sources paid for 12.7% of all health care costs in the United States that year. In addition to the Medicare and Medicaid programs, government tax funds pay for the health care of members of the military, eligible veterans, Native Americans, federal prisoners, selected vulnerable or at-risk populations, and developmentally

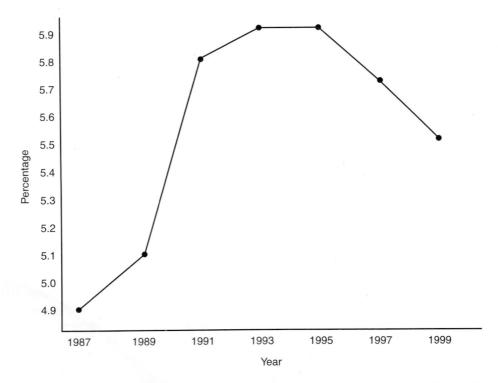

Figure 2-1 Health Care Costs As a Percentage of Gross Domestic Product, 1987–1999 (From "Industry Accounts Data. Gross Domestic Product by Industry," Bureau of Economic Analysis, 2000. Retrieved 6/16/01, from http://www.bea.doc.gov/bea/dn2/gposhr.htm#1987-99)

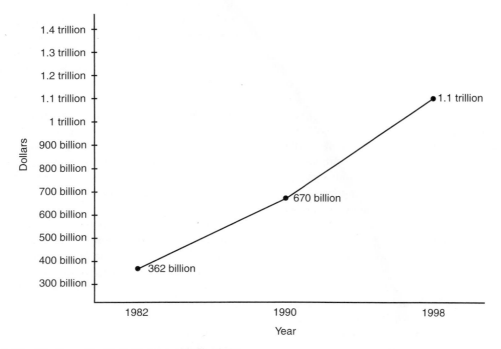

Figure 2-2 Health Care Costs in Dollars, 1982–1998

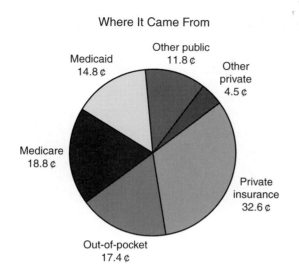

Where It Came From

Other public 11.8 ¢
Medicaid 14.8 ¢
Other private 4.5 ¢
Medicare 18.8 ¢
Private insurance 32.6 ¢
Out-of-pocket 17.4 ¢

Figure 2-3 The Nation's Health Dollar: 1999 (From "The Nation's Health Dollar: 1999," Health Care Financing Administration. Retrieved 12/17/01, from http://www.hcfa.gov/stats/nhe-oact/tables/chart.htm)

disabled and mentally ill patients who are institutionalized (Finkler & Kovner, 2000). Such funding bears some resemblance to the socialized medicine programs of other nations.

Socialized Medicine

Socialized systems of providing health care (socialized medicine) are in place around the world. Philosophically, under such systems, complete medical and hospital care is provided to all the citizens in a community, district, or nation (universal access). However, it is important to realize that the term *socialized medicine* refers to a variety of programs, each specific about what coverage is provided and how it is funded. Savage, Hoelscher, and Walker (1999) studied seven industrialized European countries and Canada for commonalities in coverage and funding. Their work reveals both centralized and decentralized compulsory single-payer systems with fee-for-service components, as well as some private insurance components.

Funding for the programs under study also varied. In general, care is funded through public taxation of citizens, who are then eligible for care but who may or may not use it. Programs in Canada, Sweden, and the United Kingdom are funded from income

taxes and selected other taxes. Germany and the Netherlands rely on payroll taxes for funding. Of the countries studied using 1996 statistics, Canada, the industrialized country most similar to the United States, spends 9.2% of its gross national product on health care. Germany spends the most at 10.5%, with the others spending as follows: Netherlands, 8.6%; Norway, 7.9%; Finland 7.5%; Sweden, 7.2%; United Kingdom, 6.9%; and Denmark, 6.4%.

The study also examined per capita spending and found that Canada spends $2,002; Germany, $2,222; and the United Kingdom, $1,304 per person. The study revealed life expectancy for males in Canada is 75.3 years, in Germany it is 73 years, and in the United Kingdom it is 74.3 years. Life expectancy for females in Canada, according to the study, is 81.3 years, in Germany it is 79.5 years, and in the United Kingdom it is 79.7 years. The authors of the study pointed out that the countries studied face similar challenges of aging populations with chronic disease, the need to ration costly technology, severe budget shortages, managed competition, decentralization, and vertical integration. Compare those study findings to the 13.6% of gross national product spent the same year by the United States (more than any other country in the world and nearly twice that of many of the European countries studied) and to the $3,759 spent per capita in the United States, as shown in Table 2-1. Still, there are approximately 44 million people in the United States without health insurance, and the United States continues to experience a stubbornly high infant mortality rate.

With U.S. life expectancy for males at 72.5 years and for females at 79.2 years, the benefits reaped in the U.S. health care system seem to be those of enhanced quality of life rather than enhanced longevity. Quality of life must be defined within the specific cultures and value systems of each country. In the United States, qualities of life highly valued by Americans include prompt access to diagnostic and treatment services, even when health problems are not life threatening; ready availability of cutting-edge technology and pharmaceuticals; the ability to choose among health care practitioners and sites for care; and participation in health care decisions. All these contribute to the cost of health care. Is that enough to justify spending more than any other country in the world (Pantel, 2001) and nearly twice as much as European countries with similar health and financial circumstances? Perhaps.

Country	% GNP	Per Capita Spending	Male Life Expectancy (years)	Female Life Expectancy (years)
United States	13.6	$3,759	72.5	79.2
Germany	10.5	$2,222	73.0	79.5
Canada	9.2	$2,002	75.3	81.3
United Kingdom	6.9	$1,304	74.3	79.7

TABLE 2-1 Comparison of Health Care Spending and Life Expectancy Across Four Industrialized Countries

FUTURE PERSPECTIVE ON COST OF HEALTH CARE

Futurists are in demand to guide health care to organize for success. Health care providers have been thrashing in chaos for nearly 20 years, reinventing their structures and processes, right-sizing their enterprises, outsourcing to better focus on their core business, and merging to share scarce or expensive resources. While there have been some short-term cost savings and the rise in health care spending has slowed, several evolving trends keep the overall cost growing.

Highly complex and expensive technology, including microsurgery, continues to develop. New diseases that require expensive or long-term treatment, such as AIDS and Ebola, continue to emerge. With the eradication or successful management of selected diseases, such as tuberculosis, populations are surviving longer. With that lengthened survival come debilitating diseases of aging.

We look to futurists to help us make decisions about what business we ought to be prepared to provide. Will the Veterans Affairs hospitals go out of business when all the veterans with illness or injuries related to their military service or who are indigent die? Will a few strategically located hospitals provide only an intensive level of care, while acute care is managed on an ambulatory basis without invasive procedures? Will preventive, primary, and restorative care be the purview of advanced nurse practitioners practicing in community sites? Will "duty" no longer be the basis for caring careers (Reverby, 2001)? Will nurses be "ordered to care" in a society that no

longer values caring (Reverby, 1987)? Will the United States adopt a health care delivery system similar to those in European countries and Canada?

THE COST EQUATION: MONEY = MISSION = MONEY

The mission statement of any health care business describes the purpose for existence of the business and the rationale that justifies that existence (Finkler & Kovner, 2000). The statement directs decision making about what is or is not within the purview of the business. The vision statement is a logical extension of the mission into the future that establishes long-range goals for the business. Once the vision is established and the business can articulate where it wants to go, a strategic plan for how to achieve the vision, or how to get to the goals, is developed. There must be cohesion and consistency across the mission, vision, and strategic plan for the business to successfully achieve its mission. There must also be money, for without it no mission can be accomplished.

Cohesion and Consistency of the Business

The question, then, is what is the cost of achieving the mission? Part of the cost may be in providing health care services that are not directly related to the mission, in the interest of political viability. Consider the Veterans Affairs (VA) health care system, established

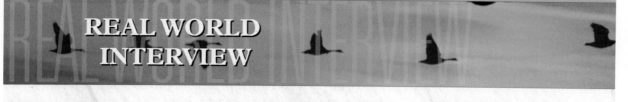

The age of "volume" as a measure of anything is long past. In health care, for so many years, the notion of unparalleled growth and expansion and anything for anyone was common. Subsequent introduction of broader concepts reflecting an understanding of value and sustainability now drive rational thinking about availability and delivery of health services. The issue of "value" now drives all elements of health service from access to delivery and, ultimately, to making a difference. Now we can more clearly enumerate the relationship between inputs and outcomes, process and product. Health services now must be able to establish the connection between what is done and what is achieved. Professions' addictions to what they do now gives way to tightening the connection between what is done and what difference it makes. The noise for both nurses and physicians is a closer look by everyone at the "value" of action in the light of the promise it holds. The issue: either deliver, or rethink why you're doing what you're doing. This critical examination and expectation will radically alter the economics and values of health care for the next two decades.

Tim Porter-O'Grady, EdD, PhD, RN, FAAN
Prolific Nurse Author and Speaker on New-Edge Health Care

to provide intensive, acute, and rehabilitative care to military veterans (not active or reserve duty personnel or family members) who meet complex care-eligibility criteria for service-related illness and injury and/or indigency. Among the 72 VA medical centers in the United States and Puerto Rico are five Blind Centers, which provide unique mechanical aids, training for activities of daily living, and job training. When a center still has beds available after admitting all veteran applicants who meet the VA eligibility criteria, it may admit others using more lenient standards. This practice may result in inconsistency with the core mission, but can maintain the program at capacity and better assure its ongoing viability. A great deal of soul-searching regularly occurs about whether the political obligation to provide this unique and valued health care service justifies the cost of existence—and its occasional extension beyond the VA mission—in a cost-sensitive health care environment.

A more familiar example of providing a costly service that is inconsistent with the mission of the health care business may be the small maternity service of a remote region that claims few women of childbearing age as inhabitants. Without the service, the women would need to relocate to a distant facility miles away for the duration of the pregnancy. A sense of commitment to the well-being of the surrounding community is viewed as justification for keeping the service open. Similarly, a commitment to charity as a component of their mission drives religious organizations that are otherwise astute businesses to provide free care to the poor. However, modern health care organizations have limited tolerance for diversification from their core business.

Refer to Chapter 9 in this text for more in-depth discussion of mission-vision-strategic plan cohesion.

Business Profit

Revenue (income) minus cost (expense) equals profit. Profit is not restricted to for-profit businesses. Profit is not a dirty word. All businesses must realize a profit to remain in business. In for-profit businesses, a portion of the profit is distributed to stockholders in appreciation for their investing in the business and the remainder is used to maintain and grow the organization. In nonprofit businesses, there are no stockholders to share the profit, so all of it is fed back into the business for maintenance and growth.

Not-for-profit organizations desiring a purer image than the term *profit* engenders refer to their profit as contribution to **margin**, with the rule of thumb being to secure 4% to 5% of the total budget as profit or margin. Mission and margin are strategically and operationally linked by the reality that resources are required to carry out the organization's strategic plan and achieve its mission. Without margin, or with limited margin, there would be a lack of money to replace worn-out equipment, to establish new services or enlarge existing services in response to changing community needs for health care, to purchase state-of-the-art technology, to maintain existing buildings or undertake new construction, to replace heating and lighting systems. Failure to maintain such infrastructure can impair the organization's ability to be competitive, resulting in failure to meet its mission and eventual organizational failure. Profit is the elasticity that accommodates improvements in patient and staff education, recruitment and hiring of expert staff, and special programming that yields personal professional growth. Profit is a critical requirement for doing business. A truism of business is, no margin, no mission.

Fundamental Costs

There are many ways to examine or classify the costs of care. One fundamental method is to view costs as direct or indirect. A **direct cost** is directly related to patient care within a manager's unit, such as the cost of nurses' wages and the cost of patient care supplies. An **indirect cost** is not explicitly related to care within a manager's unit but is necessary to support care. The

costs of electricity, heat, air conditioning, and of maintenance of the facility are all considered indirect.

Those same costs may also be considered either fixed or variable. These distinctions are somewhat artificial and are related to the volume of services that are provided. A **fixed cost** is one that exists irrespective of the number of patients for whom care is provided, as shown in Figure 2-4. Examples of this are the cost of the rent or the monthly mortgage for the space in which the care is provided and the cost of salaried (but not hourly) wage earners such as the nurse manager or nurse administrator. These costs would be the same whether 1 patient was served or 1,000 patients were served. A **variable cost**, on the other hand, varies with volume and will increase or decrease depending on the number of patients, as shown in Figure 2-5. The costs of medical supplies, laundry for the linens used in patient care, or patient meals are variable costs and increase or decrease in proportion to the number of patients served (McLean, 1997).

Some costs are step variable; that is, they vary with volume, but not smoothly. The key to step costs is that they are fixed over volume intervals but vary within the relevant range. For instance, a fixed number of nurses may be able to care for 11 to 21 patients. However, as depicted in Figure 2-6, when even one additional patient beyond 21 requires care, additional nurses are required (Finkler & Kovner, 2000; McLean, 1997).

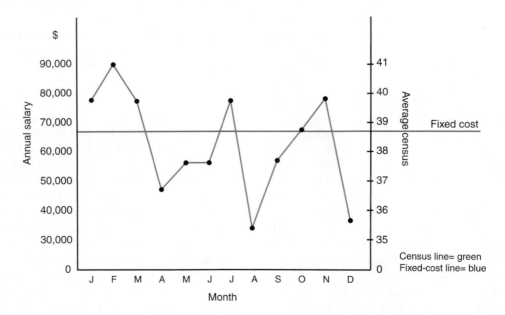

Figure 2-4 Fixed cost of a salaried employee does not vary by patient volume. (Salary is $70,000 annually regardless of census.)

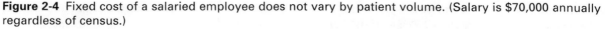

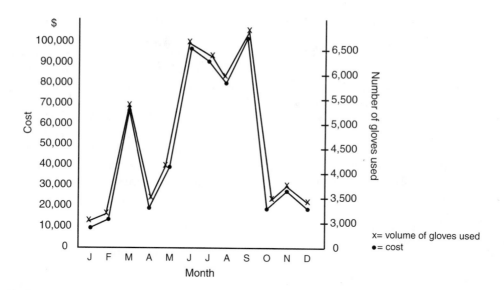

Figure 2-5 Variable cost of latex-free gloves varies by volume used.

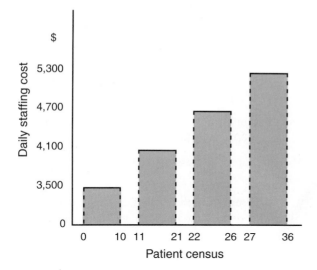

Figure 2-6 Step variable costs are fixed within a range and then increase when volume exceeds the upper end of the range.

Cost Analysis

There is an old saying that numbers don't lie. There is also an old saying that statistics can be manipulated to show whatever is desired. Both sayings are true, and therein lies the challenge, the frustration, and occasionally the glory of clinical cost management. Christman (2001) reminds us that the health care industry commonly accepts the belief that the past is prologue for forecasting its future. The ability to predict the behavior of cost in the future based on its past behavior, then, is considered requisite to successful cost management and thereby the achievement of mission and vision. A **budget** is a plan that provides formal quantitative expression for acquiring and distributing funds over the ensuing time period (generally 1 year). This budget is based on what is known about how much was spent in the past and how that will inevitably change in the coming year. A cost prediction is simply a tool for developing a budget. The three most common methods of cost prediction are high-low cost estimation, regression analysis, and break-even analysis.

High-Low Cost Estimation

This is not the tool to choose if a sophisticated, statistically rigorous prediction is needed, but it does surpass just guessing. Examining both fixed and variable cost information from the most recent 5 years for each category of expense provides a "good enough" cost projection for many items that remain relatively constant in volume of consumption and cost. Both fixed and variable dollars need to be adjusted upward to account for inflation, and the total projected cost needs to be adjusted upward to cover anticipated cost of living or other wage increases and to cover bad debt when services are rendered but payment does not occur (Finkler & Kovner, 2000).

Following is an example that clarifies the math:

> Highest wage cost = $500,000
> Lowest wage cost = $300,500
> Difference = $199,500
>
> Highest number of patient days = 9,000
> Lowest number of patient days = 7,500
> Difference = 1,500
>
> Difference in cost ($199,500)/Difference in volume (1,500) = $133 per patient day variable cost
>
> Variable cost ($133) × Lowest number of patient days (7,500) = $997,500 = Total annual variable cost

Total annual labor cost for the unit from this year's fiscal department records ($1,100,000) – Total annual variable cost ($997,500) = $102,500 Fixed cost

If 1,000 additional patient days are anticipated in the ensuing year, there would be an additional cost as follows:

> $133 per patient day variable
> cost × 1,000 additional days   = $133,000
>
> + Fixed cost (regardless of
> the number of patient days)   = $102,500
>
> Total additional cost   = $235,500

Thus, the total cost for this unit next year, using high-low cost estimation, will be this year's cost of $1,100,000 plus $235,500 in new costs, or $1,335,500.

Regression Analysis

A more precise prediction of cost can be realized using the statistical tool, regression analysis. Whereas the high-low method relies on only two data points—the highest and the lowest—for historical cost behavior, regression analysis examines all available past cost information over a specific time period. It assumes there is only one dependent variable—cost—with only one independent variable—volume—causing change in that dependent variable. It also assumes that mathematically, cost behavior can be shown in a linear fashion by drawing a straight line through a scatter diagram of all fixed and variable costs at all volumes of use. When all cost information is plotted on a vertical axis and all volume information is plotted on the horizontal axis, a scatter diagram results. The straight line through the scatter diagram that best approximates all the points is used to predict cost at a specific volume of use. Selecting a volume on the horizontal axis and examining where a vertical line from that point intersects the straight regression line, then moving horizontally to the vertical cost axis, provides the cost prediction for that specific volume as shown in the scatter diagram in Figure 2-7 (Finkler & Kovner, 2000). The analysis is carried out for each item for which cost needs to be predicted.

Break-Even Analysis

Because accruing profit to enhance the quality of services provided and to achieve optimal competitive market position is the business goal of health care organizations, projecting whether and when profitability will be achieved is necessary for both proposed and well-established programs and services. The third basic cost analysis tool is break-even analysis. It assists the provider to predict the volume of services that must be provided (and for which payment must be received) for the cost of providing the services to be equally matched by the payment received, yielding neither a profit nor loss. The formula for computing a break-even analysis (Finkler & Kovner, 2000) is as follows:

Volume of procedures = Fixed cost / Payment + Variable cost

A common application of the break-even analysis is the determination of how many procedures

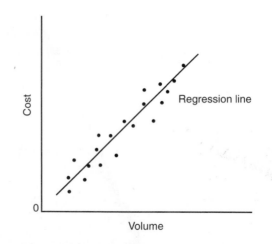

Figure 2-7 Regression Analysis

CRITICAL THINKING

Reducing costs and improving quality at the same time is a very realistic goal. Frequently, quality problems are very costly. Examples of this are found in Chassin and Galvin's (1998) article on improving health care quality. They cite underuse, overuse, and misuse of potentially effective interventions as a costly problem. Underuse—failing to use treatments that are known to be effective, such as thromboembolytics, beta blockers, aspirin, and angiotensin-converting enzyme inhibitors in myocardial infarctions—may account for as many as 18,000 preventable deaths each year. Overuse of drugs such as antibiotics is not only ineffective and expensive, but it is believed to lead to antibiotic resistance. Misuse is generally the failure to prevent complications of treatment and adds thousands of dollars to the costs of health care.

Identify some ways in which nurses can participate in reducing waste, influence best practices, and improve quality in these areas. Is keeping current with the literature in your specialty necessary to be effective in doing this?

CRITICAL THINKING

Nursing is a collaborative profession existing in a complex health care system. At one time it was influenced by three factors: cost, access, and quality. Today there are five influencing factors: cost, access, cost, quality, and cost.

(John M. Lantz, RN, PhD, Dean and Professor, School of Nursing, University of San Francisco, 2001)

Is this an accurate description of the things that influence contemporary nursing practice? What does this suggest may be an organization's focus as you interview for a staff nurse position?

You notice that a colleague frequently does not record patient charge items for elderly patients. When you inquire about it, you are told that your colleague feels sorry for those on fixed incomes and wants to save them money. Who pays when your colleague does this?

must be completed using a new piece of equipment before the payments for the procedure cover the cost of the equipment and other resources consumed doing the procedure (the **break-even point** at which income and expenses are equal), with all additional procedures generating profit. To make the use of the analysis more clear, consider that the purchase of a new piece of radiology equipment is proposed and the question has been posed, "Would this be a good investment?" The underlying question is, would the purchase generate a profit, a loss, or would the organization just break even?

If the new technology cost $50,000, the wages of the technician operating the equipment 1 hour for each use were $20/per use, and the payment for each procedure were $50, it would take 1,667 procedures to pay for the equipment and technician wages before a profit would begin to accrue.

Volume = $50,000 / ($50 − $20) = 1,667

If the payment for the procedure were $100, a profit would begin to accrue after only 625 procedures.

Volume = $50,000 / ($100 − $20) = 625

Thus, a projection can be made about how long it will take before the new equipment would be a profitable venture, guided by the decision about how much cost the purchaser of the procedure is likely to tolerate.

DIAGNOSTIC, THERAPEUTIC, AND INFORMATION TECHNOLOGY COST

A common perception held by both society and the health care industry is that payroll costs constitute the largest expense item in organizational budgets and that the most expensive health care personnel are registered nurses (RNs). Therein lies the rush to downsize RNs when a determination is made that costs need to be cut and better managed. Close examination of the entire budget, however, is likely to reveal that although the nursing payroll is the most expensive payroll item and the most expensive operating budget item, the most expensive item on the total budget is diagnostic, therapeutic, and information technology. This technology is required to meet society's demand for state-of-the-art care; professionals' demand for quicker, keener ways to work; and the organization's need to maintain a competitive business edge. Such items characteristically appear on the capital budget because of their considerable cost. With cost management generally focused on the operating budget, the cost of diagnostic, therapeutic, and information technology is often conveniently overlooked because it is deemed "strategic" and therefore untouchable during cost-cutting initiatives. Moreover, despite a rise in nursing payroll costs over the past 20 years, proportionately that rise has been considerably more gradual than the rise in diagnostic, therapeutic, information technology, and total hospital costs,

resulting in a widening gap in costs that suggests that nursing is a cost bargain. A hypothetical example of the proportional broadening of total hospital costs (including technology) and nursing payroll costs is shown in Figure 2-8.

Yet, the high cost of technology in particular has been recognized by regulatory agencies for many years. In pursuit of cost control in hospitals, the states independently established laws more than 30 years ago creating Certificate of Need (CON) agencies to oversee, regulate, and approve major technology and construction expenditures (Chang, Price, & Pfoutz, 2001). A secondary goal was to ensure equitable distribution of and access to high-end technology across the state. The CON approach was not successful because it focused only on hospitals and provided no incentives to change either physician or patient behavior (Chang, Price, & Pfoutz, 2001). Hospitals were given spending limits, but there was no incentive for physicians to change their practice, so they didn't. Without incentives, patients' expectations and demands for care also remained unchanged.

More recently, managed care programs have exerted oversight of the use of complex, expensive technology by requiring justification and approval prior to its use for payment to occur. Only when less costly approaches had been exhausted would the possibility of using highly specialized technology be considered. Diagnostically, movement has been away

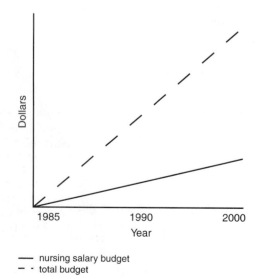

Figure 2-8 Comparison of Nursing Pay to Total Budget

from "fishing expeditions" such as ordering the comprehensive metabolic panel (CMP) and routine chest x-ray on all patients and toward completing only that which is minimally required to reach a reasonable diagnosis based on overt signs and symptoms. Exploration of subtle or subclinical signs or symptoms—the heart of the art of medical care—has, as a result, largely gone begging. The question that arises is whether assurance of correct diagnosis has been critically compromised or whether sharper clinical skill has resulted.

Therapeutically, there has been a movement toward rationing the most expensive technology to those with the ability and willingness to pay for it over and above their health insurance coverage. Underscoring public and professional concern about rationing was the best-selling book by John Kilner (1992), *Who Lives? Who Dies? Ethical Criteria in Patient Selection.* We have begun to see managed care programs become more lenient in response to a public and professional outcry about who possesses the appropriate expertise to make clinical decisions.

NURSING COST

Fiscally, most organizations view nursing as a cost center that does not independently generate revenue.

Although some deviation from that fiscal philosophy may occur when selected nursing practitioners are permitted by law to bill directly for their unique professional services, the cost of providing nursing care (wages, benefits, selected supplies and equipment, overhead) is commonly bundled into a catchall, room, or per diem, cost that assumes that every patient consumes identical nursing resources each day. Such a view is not only antiquated, it is incorrect. Nursing care is not an identical product delivered in assembly-line fashion. It varies remarkably in intensity, in depth, and in breadth across patients, consistent with their unique, individual dependency needs.

Those unique needs have contributed to nursing care being more broadly available than ever before across a variety of sites. Access to a high degree of nursing care is still accepted as second only in importance to access to medical technology as a reason for hospitalization. When access to both nursing care and such medical technology is needed, hospitalization is unquestionably appropriate. Consequently, the revenue generated from hospitalization is, in fact, payment, primarily, for consumption of medical technology and nursing services and should be recognized as such. The revenue generated from consumption of nursing resources also should be accurately quantified to each patient and charged at a rate consistent with the level and intensity of care consumed.

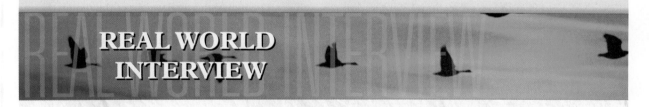

REAL WORLD INTERVIEW

The rapidly evolving shortage of nurses and other health care professionals will be an issue for the first quarter of the 21st century. There must be valid and reliable mechanisms for calculating the demand for nursing care time and intensity. Models of care delivery that maximize the use of assistive personnel and provide for sufficient professional nursing expertise and time for both care delivery and supervision are a necessity. Hours per patient day provide insufficient information for planning and staffing decisions to ensure quality patient outcomes. Mechanisms used to predict or track nursing workload must be able to differentiate the demand for professional care dimensions from the demand for dimensions of care that can be done by assistive personnel. Definitions and measurement of nursing workload must be standardized so that comparative data can be collected and analyzed.

Sheila Haas, PhD, RN
Dean and Professor

Ongoing efforts to measure and establish the cost of the diverse, yet related, components of nursing care are disappointing. That care includes direct hands-on care, teaching, and coordinating discharge, as well as indirect documentation, consultation, critical problem solving and decision making, and supervision of multiple levels of workers. These same components contribute to the long-established cost of physician and therapist services, yet the value, and thus the cost, of nursing care eludes measurement and agreement. Perhaps reluctance to legitimize the independent professional practice of the largest unit of health care providers (more than 2.2 million RNs are employed in nursing in the United States) contributes to the inability to reach agreement about how to cost out nursing.

Consequently, nursing cost is narrowly associated with budgeted and actual nursing care hours per patient day, a measure of time rather than a measure of type or level of care. Guiding the budgeted hours are historical consumption and projected changes in future demand for nursing care in response to market competition and projected changes in community demographics or consumer demands. Volume, acuity, and complexity of required care comprise workload and drive the actual nursing hours consumed.

While volume and acuity are relatively straightforward concepts that lend themselves to measurement, measuring complexity is multifaceted. Various federal, state, and local laws regulate who can accomplish what work based on educational preparation and ability to demonstrate command of a minimum body of knowledge on a standardized examination. These laws affect workload. The efficiency and effectiveness of work flow, the way work is accomplished, affect workload. This may involve something as simple as the nurse making multiple trips back and forth to access supplies in an awkward physical configuration of the work environment. It may also involve something as complex as making innovative adjustments to a familiar work pattern to accommodate physical, cognitive, behavioral, or sociocultural challenges presented by a "difficult" patient.

Patient Classification System (PCS)

The tool most broadly used to identify nursing cost is the patient classification system (PCS), a system for distinguishing among different patients based on their acuity, functional ability, or resource needs. Originally developed to predict staffing, it is used across diverse settings as a moderately robust measure of cost, as well as to predict staffing. Patients with similar requirements for care are assigned to one of five progressively weighted categories of acuity from minimal to maximal. The weights are the average number of hours of nursing care deemed required by all of the patients in each respective category; some patients within the category will actually require more hours, while others will require fewer hours (Finkler & Kovner, 2000).

Most PCSs are designed commercially and tailored to the descriptive data and information provided by the actual work group that will be using the PCS. The users describe the acuity and complexity of their typical workload and the volume and mix of nursing resources typically needed to do the work. Changes to the profile of the work or to the profile of the workers are expensive, so it is important not to minimize or exaggerate either description when working with the vendor. To protect the business interest of the PCS vendor, the specific formula used to compute the nursing hours needed for each category is not revealed to the organization in which the PCS will be used.

Each work shift, on-site nurses who are providing direct care and can therefore best judge the actual patient acuity select the category of care each patient requires from a standard weighted menu of procedures. The higher the total weight of the required care, the higher the acuity. The higher the total acuity for all the patients assessed, the more nursing resources the PCS assigns. The more resources assigned, the higher the cost. Perfect logic? Not quite.

There are several shortcomings to a formula that measures only time. First, it cannot account for the presence, or absence, of knowledge, skill, or experience in the nurses providing the hours of care. Even the gross categories of RN and LPN cannot be taken into account. It cannot, therefore, account for the richness in clinical assessment and decision making that occurs when the same procedure or care is provided by an RN versus an LPN. Second, there is no ability to account for the atypical physical, cognitive, behavioral, or sociocultural challenges that consume above-average hours. Similarly, the way one patient manages pain, fear, or anxiety is seldom identical to the way another patient copes, and supporting one may require very different resources than supporting the other, identical acuity notwithstanding. In other words, a category 4 patient is not a category 4 patient is not a category 4 patient. Innumerable nursing hours are spent attempting to justify the actual nursing hours consumed when that number slides above the number of hours assigned by the PCS.

Relative Value Unit (RVU)

A relative value unit (RVU) is an index number assigned to various health care services based on the relative amount of resources (labor and capital) used to produce the service. The actual consumption of nursing resources is not linear; that is, caring for an acuity level 2 patient does not consume twice as many nursing resources as caring for an acuity level 1 patient. RVUs provide a proportional comparison between the resources required by level 1 acuity (always a value of 1) and any other level. For example, only 20% (1.2 RVUs) more resources may be consumed by a level 2 acuity patient than a level 1, but twice as many resources may be consumed by a level 3 acuity (2.0 RVUs) and more than three times as much by a level 4 acuity (3.33 RVUs) and so forth, as shown in Table 2-2.

The RVUs can be used to calculate the relative costs of nursing care using the following reasoning:

For the time period of interest, the total cost of nursing wages = $1,250,000.

For the time period of interest, the total RVUs by acuity level and patient days are as follows:

Acuity	Days		RVU weight		Total RVUs
1	125	×	1.00	=	125.00
2	200	×	1.20	=	240.00
3	500	×	2.00	=	1,000.00
4	550	×	3.33	=	1,831.50
5	400	×	5.00	=	2,000.00
Total	1775				5,196.50

Dividing the total nursing costs by the total RVUs yields the cost per RVU.

$1,250,000 / 5,196.50 = $240.55 per RVU

The cost for one level 5 acuity patient for 1 day, then, is $240.55 × 5 (the RVU weight for acuity level 5), or $1,202.75.

Patients acuity varies, even within the same day, as they experience invasive procedures, intensive treatments and medication, complications, or progress toward wellness. As acuity varies, consumption of nursing resources varies. It follows that the cost for direct nursing care would be consistent with nursing resource consumption and could be determined using RVU calculations.

This approach provides a reasonably accurate per-patient costing approach (Finkler & Kovner, 2000). It does not account for the difference in cost based on the category of worker providing the care. Indirect fixed costs that do not vary dependent on patient classification such as salaried wages, overhead, service contracts, and noncapital equipment purchases must be added to arrive at the full cost of nursing care. Both administrators and clinicians recognize the serious shortcomings of the current methods available to calculate the cost of nursing care and

TABLE 2-2	Comparative Values of Acuity, Care Hours, and Relative Value Units	
PCS Acuity	**Care Hours**	**Relative Value Weight**
1	3.00	1.00
2	3.60	1.20
3	6.00	2.00
4	9.99	3.33
5	15.00	5.00

CRITICAL THINKING

Securing a profit might suggest that high quality is also secured because it facilitates purchase of state-of-the-art equipment and expert practitioners. Quality and profit do not necessarily go together. The Nosek-Androwich Profit:Quality (NAPQ) Matrix shown in Figure 2-9 models four possible relationships between profit and quality that may exist in a health care organization. Any organization can fit into any quadrant and a single organization may shift among quadrants from time to time in response to market forces. The challenge for the organization is to maintain existence in the high-profit, high-quality quadrant to be best positioned for clinical success and for business success, the mission of the organ-

ization. A common mission, consistent vision, collaboration, and constant vigilance to the elements of quality and profit by all employees and stakeholders together are keys to maintaining organizational positioning and achieving economic and quality success.

Into which quadrant of the NAPQ Matrix does a health care organization with which you are familiar fit? What kind of fiscal practices would you expect to find in each quadrant? What kind of clinical practices would you expect to find in each quadrant? How does patient choice influence the quadrant an organization occupies?

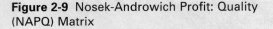

Figure 2-9 Nosek-Androwich Profit: Quality (NAPQ) Matrix

the critical need for something more accurate. But the current tools offer at least a rudimentary method for capturing nursing cost.

QUALITY MEASUREMENT

An evidence-based concept of quality is grounded on scientific evidence that a diagnostic or therapeutic approach improves patient outcomes. This concept exploded into the health care industry in the early 1990s with evidence-based clinical practices. The four core components are (1) a mechanism that establishes local or regional consensus about what constitutes the best practices based on scientific research findings, (2) strong feasible processes to accomplish such practices, (3) a deliberate program of outreach to the community on disease prevention and health promotion, and (4) a rigorous system to review actual performance and clinical outcomes, as

well as identification and implementation of improvement methodologies that achieve a dynamic balance between economy and quality (Griffith, 1999). The essence of that dynamic balance may be the "value" Dr. Tim Porter-O'Grady projects as the future focus of health care (see interview within this chapter).

Regardless of its particular size or mission, every contemporary health care enterprise (an organization of any size established as a business venture) must commit to cost improvement and quality improvement as core goals for strategic business success and for strategic clinical success. Clearly, this is not a new notion, but the recent intensification of the focus on cost and quality improvement and its expansion from hospitals to diverse ambulatory and home care sites is startling. The more critical cost containment and cost management become, the more critical attention to quality management becomes. Quality and cost are inextricably linked.

Logic suggests that higher quality could lead to a higher volume of use of the organization by patients and providers who have the flexibility to make choices about where they seek health care. Higher volume generally leads to higher profits, which, in turn, may be directed toward improving programs and services, thus achieving higher quality, a very positive spiral that can result in the organization's thriving.

Increased quality > Increased volume > Increased profit > Enhanced programs/services > Increased quality

The obverse spiral is more likely when quality is shoddy, a very negative and potentially fatal spiral.

Decreased quality > Decreased volume > Decreased profit > Cutting corners > Decreased quality

Regulatory Oversight

The quality industry measures and tracks organizational performance to ensure that organizations' structures and processes are designed, monitored, and constantly ratcheted toward improved performance and improved patient outcomes (Joint Commission on Accreditation of Healthcare Organizations, 2000). The Joint Commission on Accreditation of Healthcare Organizations (JCAHO) is the preeminent regulatory body overseeing health care quality. Its review processes are extensive, and payments to an organization by government insurers of health care (Medicare and Medicaid) are dependent on the organization's ability to meet JCAHO standards with a high degree of compliance. In addition, other federal, state, local, and voluntary regulatory agencies oversee the quality of specific organizational components such as pharmacy, laboratory, long-term care, rehabilitative care, dietary, behavioral health, and fire safety. Accreditation, which signifies that the organization meets the standards for practice of these oversight agencies, influences market perception about the quality of health care that the organization provides and engenders trust and confidence in the organization. Accreditation also ensures payment from both governmental and nongovernmental insurers.

Sally Sample was the first nurse appointed by the JCAHO to the at-large seat created on the board of commissioners. She was appointed to the board in 1992 and has witnessed firsthand the tumultuous changes in the perspective on health care quality and

in the operations of the commission. She characterizes the mission and the work of JCAHO in the following interview.

Customer Satisfaction

Regardless of how superior providers may perceive their own product or service to be, if customers fail to perceive it to be the needed or wanted service provided conveniently by skilled and knowledgeable people in a caring manner at a reasonable cost and consistent with their own culture and value system, the organization may fail. Perception, accurate or not, is the key. Therefore, organizations use a variety of indices to measure both internal and external customer satisfaction.

Commercial surveys measure how satisfied the patients are with their care, food, physical environment, emotional ambiance, and their interactions with various health care workers, then provide comparison rankings across similar organizations and populations nationally. The Veterans Affairs system of hospitals conducts its own unique survey after patient discharge. Many organizations use instruments developed internally to measure attributes of unique interest to that organization. Research protocols use a variety of statistical methods to test satisfaction. Results of such surveys are analyzed as part of the organization's quality management program.

HEALTH CARE SITE ECONOMICS

The study of economics focuses on how choices are made to overcome a scarcity of resources. Christensen, Bohmer, and Kenagy (2000) rate health care as possibly the most entrenched, change-aversive industry in the United States. Their thesis is that the three Rs, redesigning, restructuring, and **reengineering** (despite the latter's claim to turn organizations upside down and inside out through fundamental rethinking and radical redesign of processes to achieve dramatic improvements in critical performance), simply tweak the existing health care structure and processes. They believe that changes that offer cheaper, simpler, more convenient products or services aimed at the lower end of the market are key to the survival of the industry. They further believe that only a whole host of large and small changes—"disruptive innovations"—in technologies and business models that "sneak up from

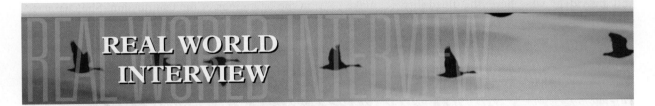

The Joint Commission on Accreditation of Healthcare Organizations is a nonprofit organization that is committed to continuously improve the safety and quality of care provided to the public through the provision of health care accreditation and related services that support performance improvement in health care organizations. JCAHO currently evaluates and accredits nearly 19,000 health care organizations in the United States, including burn hospitals and home care organizations, more than 8,000 organizations that provide long term care, behavioral health care, laboratory and ambulatory services, as well as health plans and integrated delivery networks.

The JCAHO is a voluntary accreditation service with organizations surveyed on site every 3 years. The status of accreditation is reported to the public and to the payers who require a JCAHO quality evaluation or a federal inspection prior to paying for services provided under Medicare. The cost of this accreditation is borne by the organization on a sliding scale, dependent upon its size and the extent of its services.

Health care organizations commit a great deal of time and energy to preparing for the on-site survey to successfully comply with the standards and receive a favorable accreditation status. The JCAHO standards are developed through a definitive process of input from the field, expert consultation, and research to validate the standard as a measure of quality.

Sally A. Sample, RN, MN, ND, DSc, FAAN
Nurse at Large, Board of Governors, Joint Commission on Accreditation of Healthcare Organizations

the bottom" can end the health care crisis. These disruptive innovations should come from workers in the trenches who know what would work better. Disruptive innovations in the usual setting for health care may already be under way as more care moves away from the hospital site.

HEALTH CARE PROVIDER ECONOMICS

Economic risk is borne by individuals, as well as by organizations. Both individuals and organizations may experience actual, or perceived, pressure to provide less health care service than is optimal in order to contain costs. Individual professionals risk what can be referred to as "dumbing down" of their respective professions. Dumbing down occurs when cost-saving strategies include using individuals with less knowledge to perform health care services usually performed by people with advanced knowledge. When this happens, the quality of the services delivered may decrease without actual harm occurring to

patients and without patient recognition that the services are not optimal. If the enterprise is willing to provide less-than-optimal services to save money, those with the advanced knowledge may face loss of job security. Eventually, if care is judged to be inadequate or inappropriate, there may be risk of expensive litigation that can threaten both individuals and the organization with loss of licensure and livelihood.

Organizations' attempts to provide more economical care by changing the mix of caregivers is ultimately regulated by the respective state's practice acts (laws) with their accompanying rules. Medical practice acts define the scope of physician practice. Nurse practice acts define the scope of nursing practice. Both types of acts regulate the practice components that can be delegated and the accountability that follows delegation of care. The law determines the extent to which an organization can stipulate that medical care or nursing care will be managed by delegation of that care in order to capture fiscal economies.

Individual providers such as physicians and therapists receiving direct payment from insurers bear risk when they must lower their usual fees to a

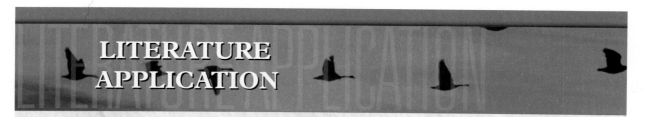

LITERATURE APPLICATION

Citation: Brooten, D., Kumar, S., Brown, L., Butts, P., Finkler, S., Bakewell-Sachs, S., Gibbons, A., & Delivoria-Papadopoulos, M. (1986). A randomized clinical trial of early hospital discharge and home follow-up of very-low-birth-weight infants. *New England Journal of Medicine, 315*(15), 934–939.

Discussion: This study marks the first nursing research accepted for publication in the prestigious *New England Journal of Medicine*. Lending credence to the rigor and importance of the investigation is the collaboration, under a Robert Wood Johnson Foundation grant, of the Division of Women's Health and Childbearing, University of Pennsylvania School of Nursing; the Division of Neonatology, Department of Pediatrics, University of Pennsylvania School of Medicine; and a nationally recognized New York University expert in management of nursing costs. The focus of the study is the interdependence of the quality and cost of health care for an at-risk population.

To determine the safety, efficacy, and cost savings of early hospital discharge of very-low-birth-weight infants, the early-discharge group (n = 39) received instruction, counseling, home visits by nurses with master's preparation, and daily on-call availability of a hospital nurse specialist for 18 months. The control group (n = 40) of infants was discharged according to the routine nursery criteria. Discharged a mean of 11 days earlier, the early-discharge group showed a 27% savings for hospital charges and 22% savings for the physician charge, a net savings of $18,560. The two groups demonstrated no difference in numbers of rehospitalizations or acute care visits or in physical and mental growth, suggesting that early discharge can enhance quality through improved and extended service and simultaneously be cost-effective.

This study epitomizes the potential for win-win-win quality and cost management program improvement. Clearly, the families win by decreasing the time, travel, and personal expense of caring for their newborn in a hospital rather than at home. Improved and extended service is also a plus for the family. The hospital wins when the cost of providing care is decreased by the shortened stay. And the nursing profession wins big when the efficacy and cost-effectiveness of nursing care is demonstrated so unequivocally.

Implications for Practice: The findings of this study are consistent with Henderson's definition of nursing and its goals, that is, to assist the patient to be independent from nursing care as quickly as possible. In addition, the findings demonstrate that scientifically based nursing practice and logical, timely nursing care can achieve superior clinical and business outcomes—healthy very-low-birth-weight infants, less-stressed families, and lower health care costs.

flat rate in order to be included for payment by the HMO. A catch-22 exists for individual providers. If the provider agrees to participate in an HMO as a preferred provider, a lower payment rate may be part of the agreement. If the provider chooses not to participate in an HMO as a preferred provider, there is risk of attracting only the limited number of patients willing and able to pay out-of-pocket fee-for-service rates. To minimize their own expenses for providing services, individual providers regulate the amount and selection of services they provide, as well as the time spent with each patient. As a result, patients may be dissatisfied with the services and choose an alternate provider.

Patients bear the risk of being unable to access services they regard as optimal, or that they perceive as bearing the least risk of harm. Clearly, frivolous services are not available under the managed care philosophy, but patients may find themselves co-opted from their demands for health care services by incentives to accept less expensive levels of service. Their out-of-pocket expense, or copayment, is usually considerably lower if they accept care from a member of the PPO than it would be if they choose to obtain care from a provider that is not a member of the PPO. Employers who provide health insurance as part of an employee's compensation package choose the insurance plan most economical for the

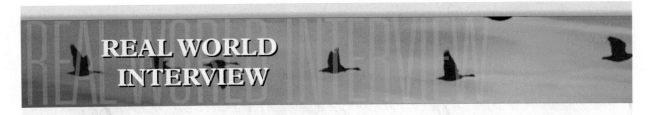

REAL WORLD INTERVIEW

One generally does not associate nurse practice acts with nursing economics. However, a connection can be formulated. Nurse practice acts delineate scope of practice and define the educational preparation necessary to perform nursing acts. These laws restrict the health care agencies from unilaterally determining that a registered nurse, practical nurse, or nursing assistant may work beyond their scope of practice. The agencies must conform to the law and employ qualified nurses, which invariably may impact health care costs.

Anita Ristau, RN, MS
Executive Director, Vermont State Board of Nursing

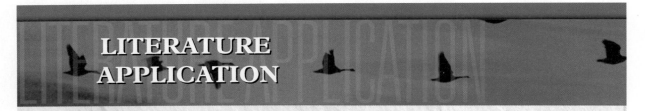

LITERATURE APPLICATION

Citation: Nosek, L. (1986). Explanation of hospital stay by nursing diagnoses, medical diagnoses, and social position. (Doctoral dissertation, Case Western Reserve University, 1986). *Dissertation Abstracts International, 47*(07B), 00215. (University Microfilms No. AAG8622844).

Discussion: This study described the amount of variation in length of stay explained by 127 nursing diagnoses, 288 diagnosis-related groups of medical diagnoses, and 8 demographic descriptors of social and economic status. These three elements explained a very high proportion of the total variation, 71.48%. Of that, 59.98% of the variation was attributed to nursing diagnoses, an additional 11.12% to medical diagnoses, and merely 0.38% was attributed to social position descriptors. The decision about when a patient is able to be discharged, then, is based on that patient's progress toward independence from nursing care, a concept consistent with Henderson's 1978 definition of nursing. The proposal that emerged from the findings was that while physicians may be best able to determine the need for hospital admission, decisions about when hospital discharge could best occur and the appropriate sequential site for the patient's health care could best be managed by nurses.

Implications for Practice: The findings of this study suggest that the most appropriate clinician to make the discharge decision is the registered nurse responsible for the patient's discharge planning because that is the person most knowledgeable about the patient's needs for ongoing nursing care.

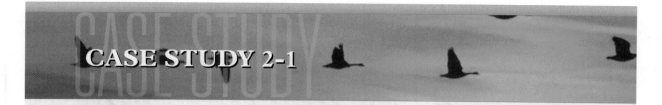

CASE STUDY 2-1

You have just been hired as a nurse in a home care agency. One of the first things you notice is that equipment and medical supplies are stacked all over the supply room. Nurses are often not aware of what is available and what needs to be ordered. Your head nurse calls a meeting to discuss the situation. Staff identifies the following problems:

- There are many outdated, damaged, or obsolete supplies.

- Staff often order items that are already in stock, as no one knows the current inventory.

- There is no system to document which patient used which supplies and equipment; consequently, the agency cannot bill patients for these items.

- No one has tried to establish any type of inventory management program.

The head nurse asks for help in assessing the situation and appoints a task force, including you, to review the situation and report your findings at the next staff meeting. At that time, your task force reports that the cost of storing an item for a year is about 30% of its original cost. Your task force has sorted all stock items into four categories: current and needed; useful but overstocked; soon to be outdated; and outdated, to be discarded. You recommend that an inventory software system be purchased to track inventory in the future, provide monthly reports, and assist with billing.

Do you think that you and the task force have solved the problem? What method was used to identify the problem? Is there anything else that should be done in this case to improve inventory management?

employer, not necessarily the plan providing the best quality (Finkler, 2001).

Authors of the two seminal magnet hospital studies (McClure, Poulin, Sovie, & Wandelt, 1983; Kramer, 1990) eloquently concluded that a high level of performance by registered nurses is inseparable from high-quality patient care. Christensen, Bohmer, and Kenagy (2000), protagonists of disruptive innovation as the answer to the health care crisis, believe that most ailments are relatively straightforward disorders whose diagnosis and treatment tap but a small fraction of what physicians are educated to do and what nurse practitioners do so capably. They point out that most of the powerful innovations that disrupted other industries did so by enabling a larger population of less-skilled people to do, in a more convenient and less expensive way, things that historically were carried out only by a defined group of "experts." The findings of the cited study are consistent with the magnet hospital findings and with disruptive innovation as an appropriate tool for change.

KEY CONCEPTS

- Health care economics is grounded in past values and culture. Nearly 150 years ago, Florence Nightingale recognized that the resources being used to care for sick people ought to be tracked and analyzed to improve clinical and business outcomes.

- Contemporary health care is characterized as a business struggling to balance cost and quality. Patients are fearful that health care is rapidly becoming unaffordable and are demanding care at a reasonable cost.

- In the United States, multiple programs exist to pay for health care. Managed care is the most common nongovernmental structure, with a variety of health maintenance organizations, operating independently, offering a plethora of health insurance packages mainly through employment benefits. Government programs for eligible individuals are tax supported. Other industrialized countries around the world offer tax-supported socialized medicine to every citizen through centralized or decentralized programs at about half of the U.S. per capita cost.

- Futurists agree that significant change will occur in the health care industry and predict that the mechanism of change will be tumultuous. They believe the focus on value received for dollars spent—the inextricable link of cost and quality—will grow.

- The ability to track and manage both cost and quality is critical. To achieve the organization's economic and quality goals, administrators and clinicians at all levels and in diverse health care enterprises must focus on a common mission and consistent vision.

- Accounting for the cost of nursing care must be simplified and standardized. Regression analyses, PCSs, and RVU computations are complex, time consuming, and lack the support of both administrators and clinicians.

- Quality measurement in organizations is supplemented by external regulatory bodies that oversee safety and quality on behalf of society. Satisfaction indices may be measured both internally and externally, then compared to the performance of similar organizations.

KEY TERMS

altruism	margin
break-even point	patient classification system
budget	(PCS)
direct cost	payer
economics	preferred provider
egoism	organization (PPO)
enterprise	reengineering
ethics	relative value unit (RVU)
fixed cost	stakeholder
indirect cost	variable cost

REVIEW QUESTIONS

1. Which of the following documents articulates the purpose for which a health care organization is in business?
   A. Strategic plan
   B. Mission statement
   C. Vision statement
   D. Corporate philosophy

2. Economics is the study of
   A. the cost:quality interface.
   B. cost accounting.
   C. the cost of doing business.
   D. how to manage scarcity of resources.

3. Which of the following nurse leaders was not mentioned in this chapter as having a perspective on economics?
   A. Abdellah
   B. Chang
   C. Barton
   D. Henderson

4. Profit is synonymous with
   A. dividends.
   B. billing privileges.
   C. contribution to margin.
   D. certificate of Need.

REVIEW ACTIVITIES

1. Interview the chief financial officer of a health care organization to gain an understanding of how various costs are managed. Use the following questions to guide the interview:
   What method is used to measure nursing cost?
   What level of confidence does Fiscal Services have in its accuracy and why?
   How are contracts with various insurers such as Medicare, Medicaid, PPOs, and Blue Cross discounted?
   What percentage of profit did the organization make last year and how was it allocated? How typical was this?
   Which therapists' services are billed directly?

2. Consult a seasoned member of the medical staff for a personal perspective on the adjustments in practice that person made, if any, related to cost and quality issues in the practice as his or her career unfolded. Compare and contrast what you discover to the experiences of a second person you consult who has been in practice for only the past 10 years. What level of passion about the discussion was demonstrated by each interviewee? What did they view as their greatest challenge?

3. Explore with the chief nursing officer what the most challenging clinical economic issue currently is for nursing in the organization and how it is being addressed.

4. Using the formulas provided in this chapter, determine the cost of nursing care for the past 24 hours for your work unit or for any manageable unit to which you have access.

EXPLORING THE WEB

- What sites could you recommend to a colleague interested in tracking health care cost trends over time?

- Go to the site for the Health Care Financing Administration: *http://www.hcfa.gov/stats/ nhe-oact/tables/chart.htm*
  How do the data on alternative Health Care Financing Administration sites such as *http://www.hcfa.gov/facts/f970128.htm* differ from the first site?

- Search an alternate government bureau site. What does the Bureau of Labor Statistics offer at *http://www.stats.bls.gov/news.release/cpi.toc. htm*?

- Go to a site designed for nurses such as *http:// www.nursingworld.org/readroom/usworder.htm* What type of information is available on the site?
  Is it relevant to cost or quality issues?

- Search the following web sites for information of interest to nurses:
  http://www.florence-nightingale.co.uk/
  http://www.aahn.org
  http://www.gnv.fdt.net/~dforest/hxindex.htm
  http://www.onhealth.com
  http://www.medexplorer.com
  http://www.selfcare.com
  http://www.healthology.juno.com
  http://www.medicarerights.org

REFERENCES

Abdellah, F., Beland, I., Martin, A., & Matheney, R. (1960). *Patient centered approaches to nursing.* New York: Macmillan.

Agnes, M. (2000). (Ed). *Webster's new world collegiate dictionary* (4th ed.). Foster City, CA: IDG Books Worldwide.

Benedict, G. (1996). *The development and management of medical groups.* Englewood, CO: Medical Group Management Press.

Brooten, D., Kumar, S., Brown, L., Butts, P., Finkler, S., Bakewell-Sachs, S., Gibbons, A., & Delivoria-Papadopoulos, M. (1986). A randomized clinical trial of early hospital discharge and home follow-up of very-low-birth-weight infants. *New England Journal of Medicine, 315*(15), 934–939.

Bureau of Economic Analysis. (2000). *Industry accounts data: Gross domestic product by industry.* Retrieved June 16, 2001, from http://www.bea.doc.gov/bea/ dn2/gposhr.htm#1987-99

Chang, C., Price, S., & Pfoutz, S. (2001). *Economics and nursing: Critical professional issues.* Philadelphia: F. A. Davis.

Chassin, M. R., & Galvin, R. W. (1998). The urgent need to improve health care quality. Institute of Medicine National Roundtable on Health Care Quality. *Journal of the American Medical Association, 280*(11), 1000–1005.

Christensen, C., Bohmer, R., & Kenagy, J. (2000, September/October). Will disruptive innovations cure health care? *Harvard Business Review*, 102–112, 199.

Christman, L. (2001). The future of the nursing profession. In E. Hein (Ed.), Nursing issues in the 21st century: Perspectives from the literature. Philadelphia: Lippincott.

Corrato, R., & Barron, B. (1999). *Getting the most out of managed care.* Retrieved 6/25/01, from the Healthology web site: http://www.healthology.com/webcast_ transcript.asp?f=healthcare&c=healthcare_manage

Finkler, S. (2001). *Budgeting concepts for nurse managers* (3rd ed.). Philadelphia: Saunders.

Finkler, S., & Kovner, C. (2000). *Financial management for nurse managers and executives* (2nd ed.). Philadelphia: Saunders.

Friedman, E. (2001). Managed care devils, angels, and the truth in between. In E. Hein (Ed.), *Nursing issues in the 21st century: Perspectives from the literature.* Philadelphia: Lippincott.

Freudenheim, M. (2001, July 2). Health care plans adapt; costs go up. *Plain Dealer* (Cleveland, Ohio), p. 2.

Griffith, J. (1999). *The well-managed health care organization* (4th ed.). Chicago: Health Administration Press.

Health Care Financing Administration. (1999a). *Medicare and managed care.* Retrieved 6/16/01, from http://www.hcfa.gov/medicare/mgdcar.htm

Health Care Financing Administration. (1999b). *National summary of state Medicaid managed care programs*. Retrieved 6/16/01, from http://www.hcfa. gov/medicaid/omc1998.htm

Health Care Financing Administration. (1999c). *The nation's health dollar: 1999*. Retrieved January 17, 2001, from http://www.hcfa.gov/stats/nhe=oact/ tables/chart.htm

Hein, E. (2001). Nursing issues in the 21st century: Perspectives from the literature. Philadelphia: Lippincott.

Henderson, V., & Nite, G. (1978). *Principles and practice of nursing* (6th ed.). New York: Macmillan.

Joint Commission on Accreditation of Healthcare Organizations. (2000). *Comprehensive accreditation manual for hospitals: The official handbook*. Chicago: Author.

Kilner, J. (1992). *Who lives? Who dies? Ethical criteria in patient selection*. New Haven, CT: Yale University Press.

Kramer, M. (1990, June). Trends to watch at the magnet hospitals. *Nursing90*, 67–74.

Liberman, A., & Rotarius, T. (2001). Managed care evolution—where did it come from and where is it going? In E. Hein (Ed.), *Nursing Issues in the 21st century: Perspectives from the literature*. Philadelphia: Lippincott.

McClure, M., Poulin, M., Sovie, M., & Wandelt, M. (1983). *Magnet hospitals. Attraction and retention of professional nurses*. Kansas City, MO: American Academy of Nursing.

McLean, R. (1997). *Financial management in health care*. Clifton Park, NY: Delmar Learning.

National Center for Health Statistics. (1998). *Health, United States, 1998*. Hyattsville, MD: U.S. Public Health Service.

Nightingale, F. (1859). *Notes on hospitals; being two papers read before the National Association for the Promotion of Social Science, at Liverpool in October, 1858. With evidence given to the Royal Commissioners on the State of the Army in 1857* (2nd ed.). London: Parker.

Nosek, L. (1986). Explanation of hospital stay by nursing diagnoses, medical diagnoses, and social position. (Doctoral dissertation, Case Western Reserve University, 1986). *Dissertation Abstracts International, 47*(07B), 00215. (University Microfilms No. AAG8622844).

Pantel, E. (2001). Why does healthcare cost so much?. Retrieved April 2, 2002, from the Healthology web site: http://www.healthology.com/focus_article.asp? f=healthcare&c=healthcare_cost

Reverby, S. (1987). *Ordered to care: The Dilemma of American nursing*, 1850–1945. New York: Cambridge.

Reverby, S. (2001). A caring dilemma: Womanhood and nursing in historical perspective. In E. Hein (Ed.), *Nursing issues in the 21st century: Perspectives from the literature*. Philadelphia: Lippincott.

Savage, G., Hoelscher, M., & Walker, E. (1999). International health care: A comparison of the United States, Canada, and Western Europe. In L. Wolper (Ed.), *Health care administration: Planning, implementing, and managing organized delivery systems* (3rd ed). Gaithersburg, MD: Aspen.

vos Savant, M. (2001, May 6). Ask Marilyn. *Parade*, 26.

Wolper, L. (1999). *Health care administration planning, implementing, and managing organized delivery systems* (3rd ed.). Gaithersburg, MD: Aspen.

SUGGESTED READINGS

Copeland, T. (2001, September/October). Cutting costs without drawing blood. *Harvard Business Review*, 155–156, 159–160, 162, 164.

Feldstein, P. (1993). *Health care economics* (5th ed.). Clifton Park, NY: Delmar Learning.

Hoppszallern, S. (2001, January). 2001 benchmarking guide. *Hospitals and health networks*, 43–50.

Institute of Medicine. (1990). *Medicare: A strategy for quality assurance*. K. N. Lohr (Ed.). Washington, DC: National Academy Press.

McCullough, C. (2001). *Creating responsive solutions to healthcare change*. Indianapolis, IN: Sigma Theta Tau International.

Rowland, H., & Rowland, B. (1997). *Nursing administration handbook* (4th ed.). Gaithersburg, MD: Aspen.

Senge, P. (1990). *The fifth discipline*. New York: Doubleday.

Shamian, J., & Lightstone, E. (1997). Hospital restructuring initiatives in Canada. *Medical Care, 35*(10), 0S62–0S69.

Shortell, S. (1996). *Remaking health care in America: Building organized delivery systems*. San Francisco: Jossey-Bass.

CHAPTER 3

Evidence-Based Health Care

Rinda Alexander, PhD, RN, CS

Evidence-based practice is about clinical competence in the individual care of patients, decision analysis, human values, use of information technology for best available clinical evidence from systematic research, and stewardship of resources.

(Sister Maurita Soukup, 2000)

OBJECTIVES

Upon completion of this chapter, the reader should be able to:

1. Know the history of evidence-based care (EBC) in nursing.
2. Discuss the importance of EBC.
3. Identify terminology used in research and EBC.
4. Understand the issues that stimulate the development of an EBC model for health care delivery.
5. Assess the types of evidence used in EBC processes.
6. Understand the role of the Agency for Healthcare Research and Quality (AHRQ) in the development of EBC.

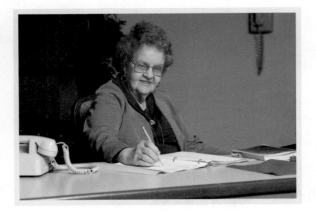

You are at the annual Appreciation of Nurses luncheon at your institution, and the nursing manager of both your unit and three other units stops to chat. She says she is concerned because she has noticed much variability in nursing interventions on the units. This variability is affecting patient outcomes in the institution. She has heard about evidence-based care (EBC) and wants to appoint you to a task force to consider using evidence-based care as a means of reducing variability and improving patient outcomes. This scenario is becoming more and more common in health care institutions as managers of care explore new ways to improve the quality of care.

What do you know about EBC?

What are some things you need to know before you can accept the appointment to the task force?

How will you prepare yourself for the task?

Many professionals and society in general accept the position that nurses are the coordinators of care within institutions. However, as the new health care system continues to evolve, nurses must consider new ways to deliver more effective and efficient interventions. In fact, there is probably no greater challenge for nursing than to ensure that we have the competencies needed in the 21st century for health care delivery. Nursing leaders and managers are particularly well positioned to see that health care institutions have processes in place that provide professional nurses with support to meet new challenges in the clinical delivery of care. Significantly, the Pew Health Professions Commission lists 21 competencies required for future health care providers (Bellack & O'Neil, 1999). The third competency listed is that of providing evidence-based, clinically competent care. This **evidence-based care** (EBC) is clinically competent care based on the best scientific evidence available. Individual nurses have responsibility for evaluating and promoting the use of patient care based on the best scientific evidence available.

The purpose of this chapter is to define what constitutes evidence for clinical practice and discuss the importance of EBC to patients and nursing. EBC decision making is the trend of the future. Future trends in health care will require the use of sophisticated evidence-based tools to deliver care and measure outcomes of care. This suggests that nursing must become more comfortable using a scientific process driven by evidence-based standards and practice guidelines while also emphasizing continuing quality improvement. Refer to Table 3-1 for an overview of research terminology useful in developing skill in EBC.

HISTORY OF EBC

Initially, the movement into evidence-based clinical application began with medicine. The term **evidence-based medicine** (EBM) was coined at McMaster Medical School in Canada during the 1980s. It referred to a clinical learning strategy that had been in use at McMaster since the 1970s (Rosen & Donald, 1995). D. L. Sackett, well known in the EBM and EBC movement, along with his Oxford colleagues, encouraged EBM as a way to integrate individual clinical medical experience with external clinical evidence using a systematic research approach (Sackett, Rosenberg, Gray, Haynes, & Richardson, 1996). Sackett et al. define evidence-based medicine (EBM) as the "conscientious, explicit, and judicious use of current best evidence in making decisions about the care of individual patients" (1996, p. 71). Evidence-based medicine integrates the clinical expertise of individual clinicians with the best available external clinical evidence from systematic research into the accuracy and precision of diagnostic tests; the clinical examination; and other elements of the therapeutic, rehabilitative, and preventive regimens prescribed for patients.

EBC is a newer term and has broadened the EBM methods to include other clinical health care providers. Nursing-oriented sources include the *Online Journal of Knowledge Synthesis for Nursing* from Sigma Theta Tau International, a journal from the United Kingdom called *Evidence-Based Nursing:*

TABLE 3-1	*Research Terminology*
Case control study	A research method that involves identifying patients who have an outcome of interest (cases) and then identifying patients without the same outcome and looking back to see whether they had the exposure of interest
Cohort study	A study that identifies two groups (cohorts) of patients; one group received the exposure of interest and one group did not receive the exposure; the cohort study follows the two groups forward for the outcome of interest
Comparative research	In designing comparison research, the researcher specifies the type of comparison; there are several ways comparisons are used in research; examples are comparison between two or more groups, comparison of a single group at two or more points in time, or comparison of a single group under different circumstances or experiences
Control group	Subjects in an experiment who do not receive the experimental treatment and whose performance provides a baseline against which the effects of the treatment can be measured
Correlational research	Investigations that explore the interrelationships among variables of interest without any active intervention on the part of the researcher
Dependent variable	The outcome variable of interest; the variable that is hypothesized or thought to depend on or be caused by another variable, called the independent variable
Descriptive research	Research studies that have as their main objective the accurate portrayal of the characteristics of people, situations, or groups, and the frequency with which certain phenomena occur
Follow-up study	A study undertaken to determine the subsequent development of individuals with a specified condition or a study of people who have received a specified treatment
Independent variable	The variable that is believed to cause or influence the dependent variable; in experimental research, the independent variable is the variable that is manipulated
Longitudinal study	A study designed to collect data at more than one point in time, in contrast to a cross-sectional study
Matched case-controlled study	A research technique that uses select sample characteristics to match experimental subjects with a control group (matched sample)
Meta-analysis	A technique for combining study results and thus integrating the results of multiple studies on a given topic
Nonexperimental study	A study in which the researcher collects data without introducing any new treatments or changes

(continues)

Table 3-1 *(continued)*

Outcomes study	Observation of a defined population at a single point in time or at time intervals
Program evaluation	Research investigating how well a program, practice, or policy is working
Prospective study	A study that begins with an examination of presumed causes (e.g., cigarette smoking) and then goes forward in time to observe presumed effects (e.g., lung cancer)
Qualitative analysis	The nonnumeric organization and interpretation of observations for the purpose of discovering important underlying dimensions and patterns of relationships
Quality improvement project	Selection of a particular diagnostic group, unit, or other measurement that needs scientific investigation to identify needed improvement
Quantitative analysis	The manipulation of numerical data through statistical procedures for the purpose of describing phenomena or assessing the magnitude and reliability of relationships among them
Quasi-experiment	A study in which subjects cannot be randomly assigned to treatment conditions, although the researcher does manipulate the independent variable and exercises certain controls to enhance the internal validity of the results
Quasi-experimental pre-post study	Same as quasi-experiment but uses a pretest-posttest research design
Randomized controlled trials	An application of a research design that always involves testing of a clinical treatment with random assignment of research subjects to either the experimental group (which receives the intervention under study) or to the control group (which receives standard treatment or a placebo); these two groups are then studied for the variable of interest
Research utilization	The use of some aspect of a research or scientific investigation in an application unrelated to the original research
Retrospective study	A study that begins with the manifestation of the dependent variable in the present (e.g., lung cancer) and then links this effect to some presumed cause occurring in the past (e.g., cigarette smoking)
Time series design	A quasi-experimental design that involves the collection of information over an extended period of time, with multiple data collection points both prior to and after the introduction of a treatment
Variable	A characteristic or attribute of a person or object that varies (i.e., takes on different values) within the population under study (e.g., body temperature, heart rate)

Adapted from *Nursing Research Principles and Methods* (6th ed., pp. 425–438), by D. Polit and B. Hungler, 1998, Philadelphia: Lippincott-Raven.

Linking Research to Practice, Evidence Based Nursing, Clinical Effectiveness in Nursing, Internet Journal of Advanced Nursing Practice, Journal of American Academy of Nurse Practitioners, and the *Journal of Evidence-Based Nursing*, to name just a few. Since the early work of the McMaster group, methods for review and summarization of evidence have undergone dramatic advances. A. Cochrane of the Cochrane Library group was a pioneer in the movement and preparation of high-quality reviews. In 1978, Cochrane suggested that only 15% to 20% of physician interventions were supported by objective evidence. This led to much variation in patient care delivery and patient care outcomes.

IMPORTANCE OF EBC

There is nothing more important to patients and professional nursing than evidence-based clinical interventions that can be linked to clinical outcomes and used as a basis for care within the institution. However, there has been a lack of generally agreed-upon standards or processes that are based on evidence. This lack of standards has been addressed of late with the development of EBC.

Generally speaking, nursing, medicine, health care institutions and health policy makers recognize evidence-based care as care based on state-of-the-art science reports. It is a process approach to collecting, reviewing, interpreting, critiquing, and evaluating research and other relevant literature for direct application to patient care. EBC uses evidence from research; performance data; and quality improvement studies such as hospital or nursing report cards, program evaluations, surveys, national and local consensus recommendations of experts, and clinical experience (Stetler et al., 1998a).

The EBC process further involves the integrating of both clinician-observed evidence and research-directed evidence. This then leads to state-of-the-art integration of available knowledge and evidence in a particular area of clinical concern that can be evaluated and measured through outcomes of care.

Applying the best available evidence does not guarantee good decisions, but it is one of the keys to improving outcomes affecting health. EBC should be viewed as the highest standard of care so long as critical thinking and sound clinical judgment support it. Nurses and doctors will always need to search for the best evidence available to support their clinical decisions. Sometimes, there is little research backing for

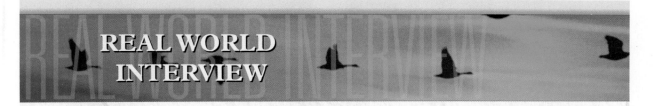

REAL WORLD INTERVIEW

With over 20 years in nursing and hospice care, I have increasingly realized that a large part of the health care system, both doctors and nurses, do not understand the need for adequate pain control. One of my patients was a young man with cancer of the throat. He had received a radical laryngectomy and had had his tongue removed. He was left with a tracheotomy and was rendered speechless. His doctors at a top-rated university hospital seemed amazed that he was in as much pain as he was. It was not until he entered hospice care, where we emphasized an evidence-based holistic pain protocol, that he received some degree of comfort. This man was an exceptional person who never complained. He also had exceptionally strong support from his wife and family.

As nurses, please advocate for adequate pain relief for your patient. I have seen over and over that patients do not abuse the medications or the system. Our hospice saying is, "Meet the patients where they are, not where you think they should be!" When our patients are comfortable, there is peace for everyone.

Sylvia Komyatte, RN, MPS
Chaplain, Hospice

clinical actions. In that case, nurse and physician clinicians should use their critical thinking skills and apply the consensus of experts. Institutions of care have a responsibility to provide nurses and others in health care with an environment supportive of EBC.

Demonstrating that outcomes of health care are effective, efficient, and safe is a major responsibility for nursing. It is evident as we consider the art and science of nursing that recognizing the importance of EBC and stimulating an environment within institutions in which evidence-based models of care can flourish will result in improved outcomes of clinical care. Table 3-2 summarizes trends driving the development of EBC in nursing.

Nursing and EBC

It was inevitable that nursing would move to EBC. One of the earlier proponents for EBC in nursing was the Joanna Briggs Institute for Evidence Based Nursing & Midwifery (JBIEBN), established in 1996. Significant work has been done worldwide to implement EBC into Australian, New Zealand, and Hong Kong institutions of care.

In the United States, the Agency for Healthcare Research and Quality (AHRQ) has provided stimulus for the EBC movement through recognition of a need for evidence to guide practice throughout the health care system. In 1997, the AHRQ launched its initiative establishing 12 evidence-based practice centers. This initiative partnered AHRQ with other private and public organizations in an effort to improve the quality, effectiveness, and appropriateness of care. The initiative facilitates the translation of evidence-based research findings into clinical practice.

Attributes of EBC

A new culture that can support EBC needs to evolve in institutions. Stetler et al. (1998a) identify three specific attributes of establishing an evidence-based environment within an institution: (1) establishing

TABLE 3-2	Current Trends Driving Development of EBC in Nursing

- Increased numbers of well-designed, randomized controlled trials (RCTs)
- Need for decreased variability in implementation of practice
- Need for implementation of research in practice to improve effectiveness and efficiency
- Demands of Pew Health Professions Commission report for evidence-based, clinically competent care (Bellack & O'Neil, 1999)
- Growth of advanced practice roles with development of prescriptive power and evidence-based diagnostic decision making
- Increased experience in clinical pathways, standards, protocols, and algorithms
- Increase in integrated systematic reviews of research studies found in the nursing, medical, and health care literature
- Need for outcome data to guide patient care
- Explosion in information technology with better-organized, rapidly retrievable information in the literature and on the Internet
- Improved knowledge base facilitating research capable of supporting EBC models
- Need to collaborate in complex decision making with patients and other members of the health care team
- Requirement for evidence-based standards of care implemented by the Joint Commission on Accreditation of Healthcare Organizations (JCAHO)

REAL WORLD INTERVIEW

I have been a nurse for 39 years and have seen many changes in health care during that time. About 5 years ago, I had a ruptured brain aneurysm, which occurred after having an angiogram. I was airlifted to a nearby university hospital. The knowledge and competence of the air transport team was impeccable. I was glad to be in the hands of people who were up to date on the best way to care for me. They were definitely in control—a nice thing to have when you're not.

Before the surgery, I was unconscious, and my family was informed of the dangers and the necessity to either coil or clip the aneurysm. During the 14-hour operation, the neurosurgeon's nurse updated them periodically on my progress. During my entire hospital stay, she visited me daily and was available by pager if my husband had any questions, doubts, or fears. While I was in the ICU, I was the only patient cared for by one nurse for 3 days. Although I had short-term memory loss at the time, I do remember that I did not have any concerns about my needs not being met. In fact, I felt the nurses predicted the problems I had before I even vocalized them. I was given quality patient care, and as an RN, I am very proud to say that. I am back working as a nurse now, and my experience has given me a whole new level of understanding for patients. I am glad that the people who cared for me were up to date on the latest!

Janice Klepitch, RN
Office Nurse

the culture, (2) creating a capacity for change, and (3) using the organizational infrastructure to sustain and reinforce change. They highlight the need to do such things as define the meaning of evidence in each agency, begin to use the term *evidence* in daily practice, and look for the best evidence when evaluating new goals and new programs. They encourage the use of visible, formal supports for EBC and the development of systems in the health care agency that support EBC on an ongoing basis. They suggest that the development of such attributes as these will help make EBC the usual method of care delivery.

EVIDENCE: HOW IT IS DEVELOPED AND EVALUATED

The literature available to both nursing and medicine is immense, but only a small portion is immediately useful for answering clinical questions. To recognize that the available evidence in the literature for any clinical question exists at various levels can help

nurses retrieve the highest level of evidence available for use in providing care. There are up to six levels of evidence included in the various EBC models. Following is an overview of two models used to judge acceptability of available evidence to be used in EBC. The first model is called Level and Type of Evidence for Nursing Intervention and is based on the work of Stetler et al. (1998b). It is an excellent guide for nurses to use in applying EBC to their clinical practice and shows the type and level of evidence as well as a description of the process for each level (Table 3-3).

A second model for determining the level of evidence, shown in Figure 3-1, is from the 1999 Consensus Recommendations of the American College of Cardiology/American Heart Association (ACC/AHA) Task Force on Practice Guidelines.

Conducting Evidence Reports in Nursing

A practical approach to evidence grading has been identified by Greer, Mosser, Logan, and Halaas (2000). For the new nurse, understanding how evi-

| TABLE 3-3 | *Level and Type of Evidence for Nursing Intervention* |

Type of Evidence	Description of Process/Level of Evidence (I to VI)
I. Meta-analysis of multiple controlled studies	I. Merging of findings from several controlled research studies on a topic to determine what is known about a particular phenomenon. This is the highest level of evidence.
II. Individual experimental studies	II. This second level of evidence includes findings from an individual controlled, experimental research study. This study provides the greatest amount of control possible to examine the probability and causality of research variables. This evidence provides even stronger recommendations when there are consistent findings from multiple level II studies.
III. Quasi-experimental studies, such as single group pre-post, cohort, time series, or matched case-controlled studies	III. This third level of evidence—quasi-experimental research studies—has less control over the research variables than the experimental designs just described. These are alternative, less desirable means for completing a research study when the experimental designs just described cannot be used, as, for example, when the research subjects cannot be randomly assigned to treatment conditions. This level of study usually leads to moderate recommendations for action.
IV. Nonexperimental studies, such as comparative and correlational studies, descriptive research, and qualitative studies	IV. This fourth level of evidence—non-experimental research studies—does not have the degree of control of the experimental or quasi-experimental research studies. The researcher collects data without using controls and merely describes the negative or positive relationships of variables in the research study. This level of study also usually leads to moderate recommendations for action.
V. Program evaluation, research utilization, quality improvement projects or case reports	V. This fifth level of evidence includes literature reviews. Much of the evidence in this limited evidence level can come from within the institution and from benchmarking or comparing an institution's data with data from another institution.
VI. Opinions of respected authorities, or the opinions of expert committees, including their interpretation of nonresearch-based information	VI. This lowest, sixth, level of evidence includes opinions from an institutional research committee group, the continuous quality improvement group, or an individual known to have expertise in a particular or specific area. These recommendations are made in light of little or no evidence other than consensus opinions of experts.

Revised model compiled with information from "Utilization-Focused Integrative Reviews in a Nursing Service," by C. B. Stetler, D. Morsi, S. Rucki, S. Broughton, B. Corrigan, J. Fitzgerald, K. Guiliano, P. Havener, and E. A. Sheridan, 1998, *Applied Nursing Research, 11*(4), 195–206.

Evidence Level	Definition
1. Positive RCTs (*P*<0.05)	A prospective, randomized, controlled trial, RCT; conclusions: new treatment significantly better (or worse) than control treatment.
2. Negative RCTs (NS)	An RCT, conclusions: new treatment no better than control treatment.
3. Prospective, nonrandom	Nonrandomized, prospective, observational study: 1 group used new treatment; must have a control group for comparison.
4. Retrospective, nonrandom	Nonrandomized, retrospective, observational study: 1 group used new treatment; must have a control group for comparison.
5. Case series	Series of patients received new treatment in past or will receive in future: watch to see what outcomes occur; no control group.
6. Animal studies (A and B)	Studies using animals or mechanical models: A-level animal studies are higher quality than B-level studies.
7. Extrapolations	Reasonable extrapolations from existing data or data gathered for other purposes: quasi-experimental designs.
8. Rational conjecture, common sense	Fits with common sense: has face validity: applies to many non–evidence-based guidelines that "made sense." No evidence of harm.

Integration of many articles across all evidence levels with
- Critical appraisal
- Experts' consensus discussions
- Input from Evidence Evaluation Conference
- Input from Guidelines 2000 Conference

Class of Recommendation	Criteria for Class	Clinical Definition
Class I Definitely recommended	Supported by **excellent** evidence with at least 1 **prospective, randomized, controlled trial.**	**Class I** interventions are always acceptable, safe and effective. Considered definitive care, standard of care.
Class IIa Acceptable and useful	Supported by **good** to **very good** evidence. Weight of evidence and expert opinion strongly in favor.	**Class IIa** interventions are acceptable, safe, and useful. Considered *intervention of choice* by majority of experts.
Class IIb Acceptable and useful	Supported by **fair** to **good** evidence. Weight of evidence and expert opinion not strongly in favor.	**Class IIb** interventions are also acceptable, safe, and useful. Considered *optional* or *alternative interventions* by majority of experts.
Indeterminate Promising, evidence lacking, immature	Preliminary research stage. Evidence: no harm but no benefit. Evidence insufficient to support a final class decision.	**Indeterminate:** describes treatments of promise but limited evidence. AHA-ILCOR accepts some indeterminates but only by expert consensus.
Class III May be harmful: no benefit documented	Not acceptable, not useful, **may be harmful.**	**Class III** refers to interventions with no evidence of any benefit: often some evidence of harm.

Figure 3-1 ACC/AHA Evidence-Based Levels (From "1999 Consensus Recommendations of the American College of Cardiology/American Heart Association Task Force on Practice Guidelines," *American Heart Association 2000 Handbook of Emergency Cardiovascular Care for Healthcare Providers*, 2000, Dallas, TX: American Heart Association.)

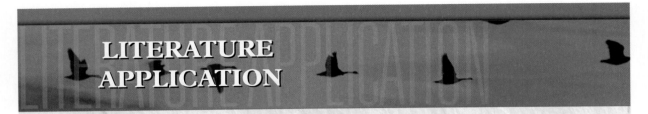

LITERATURE APPLICATION

Citation: Sheaffer, C. M., Phillips, C. Y., Donlevy, J. A., & Pietruch, B. L. (1998). Continuing education as a facilitator of change: Implementing a new nursing delivery model. *The Journal of Continuing Education in Nursing, 29*(1), 35–39.

Discussion: The authors report that an educational program geared at keeping staff nurses well informed and accepting of a new care model was implemented in four hour-long sessions. This program resulted in nurses having a better understanding of the need for health care reform and more willingness to work for needed change in the health care delivery system.

Implications for Practice: This approach can be useful in establishing EBC as a means of improving consistency and outcomes of care.

CRITICAL THINKING

You work on a unit delivering care to patients. You want to be sure your care delivery is state of the art.

How will EBC be important to you as a new nurse? What contributions can you make to EBC? How can nurses help overcome potential resistance to EBC?

dence is judged can seem to be a very complex task. However, experience in reviewing and critiquing research and using research in clinical activities can be very rewarding. A framework to guide you in the process, such as that shown in Table 3-4, can be useful.

Using EBC References

Several evidence-based sources are listed in the Exploring the Web section of this chapter.

EBC CENTERS IN THE UNITED STATES

For many years, clinicians have coped with accusations that only 10% to 20% of treatments provided have scientific foundations. Many within the health care system have supported this accusation. For example, Dr. Robert Califf, director of the Duke University Clinical Research Institute, reported in *Time* magazine (Thompson, 1998) that he estimates that currently less than 15% of U.S. health care clinical applications are evidence based. In response to this ongoing lack of evidence to make clinical decisions, as previously mentioned, the AHRQ has undertaken the development and funding of 12 evidence-based centers to carry out development and dissemination of best practice models based on available scientific information and data. Development of these special centers has been a driving force for state-of-the-art evaluations of current knowledge used in EBC in the United States.

TABLE 3-4	*Method for Conducting Evidence Reports in Nursing*
• Select topic or identified problem.	The nurses and doctors on your unit have reported that falls in the evening seem excessive and want to try to reduce falls on the unit using principles of evidence-based care.
• Report the evidence.	Evidence is reviewed and ranked by using either Table 3-3 or Figure 3-1.
• Identify methods for assigning level of evidence.	Research articles are reviewed from evidence levels I, II, III, and IV (refer to Table 3-3).
• Report findings, including statistical summary if appropriate.	Statistical information is reviewed from research articles that report less than 0.05 levels of significance between falls and nighttime environment in institutions; data from the unit found most falls were a result of patients getting up to go to bathroom in evening, slipping, not using the light, and so on.
• Give summary of evidence review.	As above. Include specific research articles with levels of significance of findings, and so on.
• Make recommendations for level of evidence to be assigned and potential for clinical application.	Review on falls shows that level III evidence supported by level V and VI evidence can be used. Document major reasons for this recommendation.

Adapted from *Nursing Leadership: Implications for Practice*, by R. Alexander, 2000 Unpublished manuscript.

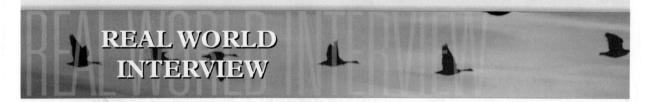

REAL WORLD INTERVIEW

I entered the hospital last year for a complete knee replacement. I was confident that I had the best orthopedic surgeon. He had told me of the pain that would follow the surgery and accompany the therapy. He told me that the hospital followed a clinical protocol for pain management that had been developed from the best research possible, and so I approached surgery confidently. The anesthetist administered the epidural and enough anesthesia to keep me semiawake during surgery. I relaxed and slept until I was moved to my room. When I was awake, I experienced the most excruciating pain I had ever experienced. My family was in the room, and when I asked for the nurse, she came in and told me I was going to have pain. She also said I would be able to press the button and receive measured doses of the epidural and be relieved. Each time she checked on me, she asked what number between 1 and 10 was my pain. I told her for 7 hours that the pain was unbearable. My family pleaded for the nurse to get help. She said she had called the anesthetist, who finally appeared and checked the epidural. He said it was not working, but he would be happy to insert a new tube, and if he did it, it would work. That means for 7 solid hours I had no working treatment to manage postsurgery bone pain. What's the use of having well-researched pain protocols if they are not used properly?

(continues)

Real World Interview (continued)

Instead of having another epidural inserted, I asked for the morphine, which I was not able to tolerate. The next day, they gave me Demerol, which made my therapy bearable. I did not fill out the patient satisfaction survey they sent following my dismissal because I was disgusted and I did not feel they would ever take any action anyway. Something was definitely wrong with their pain management system. So much for the best research possible! It only works if it is administered properly. I want to add that caring and compassion should be the most important qualities a health caregiver should be taught. I did have one nurse who was very considerate and informative. I wish she were working the day I went to surgery. Maybe she would have gotten help for my pain.

Patricia A. Murry Kelly
Patient

PROMOTING EVIDENCE-BASED BEST PRACTICES

The U.S. health care system is a $1 trillion industry and yet it is difficult to get all clinical health care providers to carefully consider the findings of both nursing and medical research and then deliver quality outcomes. Clinicians, nursing leaders, and nursing managers must promote the use of EBC to develop best practices at all levels of care. Research can be facilitated within the institution and then the findings can be reviewed and implemented. A change in practice can be facilitated through the collaboration of nursing and medicine working closely with quality improvement teams to deliver quality outcomes.

KEY CONCEPTS

- The focus on EBC can be expected to remain a driving force in the health care arena in the foreseeable future.
- Nursing can make significant contributions to the advancement of evidence-based care.
- Nursing leaders and managers can promote a culture receptive to the practice of evidence-based care, and all nurses can support this.
- Ultimately, evidence-based care is the gold standard in clinical care.
- By accepting the challenge to provide EBC, nursing can pursue its future confident of its ability to contribute to an increasingly complex health care system.

KEY TERMS

evidence-based care
evidence-based medicine

REVIEW QUESTIONS

1. What is the major purpose of evidence-based care (EBC)?
   A. To increase variability of care
   B. To cause a link to be missing in clinical care
   C. To determine what medical models can be applied by nursing
   D. To provide evidence-based care supporting clinical competency

2. Concerning EBC, which of the following is an accurate statement at this time?
   A. EBC takes the place of continuous quality improvement.
   B. Because we can already demonstrate effective and efficient care, EBC is redundant.
   C. Leaders and managers in nursing are not clinicians, generally speaking, and so do not have a part in EBC processes.
   D. Generally speaking, EBC is recognized by nursing, medicine, and health policy makers as state-of-the-art science reports.

3. Which of the following organizations develops clinical practice guidelines?
   A. American Heart Association
   B. Agency for Healthcare Research and Quality (AHRQ)

C. Pew Health Professions Commission

D. Joint Commission on Accreditation of Healthcare Organizations (JCAHO)

4. Which of the following is a research design that always involves testing of a clinical treatment with assignments of research subjects to either experimental or control conditions?
A. Lonitudinal study
B. Randomized controlled trial
C. Meta-analysis
D. Time series design

REVIEW ACTIVITIES

1. Review Table 3-3 and Figure 3-1. Are the evidence levels clear to you? Look at a patient's condition that you encounter in your clinical lab experience. Which level of evidence supports the care delivery approaches to this patient? Are any clinical pathways or standards in use in caring for this patient?

2. To understand some of the studies used in evidence-based care, it is necessary to understand some of the research terminology. Review the research terminology in Table 3-1. Check the library and see whether you can find an example of one of the studies.

3. Using Table 3-4 on conducting evidence reports in nursing, study the treatment of depression.

EXPLORING THE WEB

- Go to the site for the Joanna Briggs Institute for Evidence Based Nursing & Midwifery. http://www.joannabriggs.edu.au/

- Go to Health Care Information Resources— Nurses Links. http://www-hsl.mcmaster.ca/tomflem/nurses.html

- Go to the site for the *Online Journal of Knowledge Synthesis for Nursing*, sponsored by Sigma Theta Tau International. http://www.stti.iupui.edu/library/ojksn

- Go to the Core List for Evidence-based Practice at the University of Sheffield in England

and note the references you see there. http://www.shef.ac.uk/uni/academic/R-Z/scharr/ir/corelist.html

- Go to a site for a journal called *Evidence-based Healthcare*. http://www.harcourt-international.com/journals/ebhc/

- Go to the University of Rochester Medical Center site for evidence-based health care resources. http://www.urmc.rochester.edu/miner/links/ebmlinks.html

- Visit the site of the Oncology Nursing Society Evidence-Based Practice Online Resource Center. http://www.ons.org

REFERENCES

Alexander, R. (2000). *Nursing leadership: implications for practice*. Unpublished manuscript.

American Heart Association. (2000). 1999 consensus recommendations of the American College of Cardiology/American Heart Association Task Force on Practice Guidelines. In *American Heart Association 2000 Handbook of Emergency Cardiovascular Care for Healthcare Providers*. Dallas, TX: Author.

Bellack, J. P., & O'Neil, E. H. (1999). Recreating nursing practice for a new century: Recommendations and implications of the Pew Health Professions Commission's final report. *Nursing and Health Care Perspectives, 21*(1), 14–21.

Cochrane Library at McMaster University. (2000, March). *Using Medline to search for evidence*. Retrieved from http://www.londonlinks.ac.uk./evidence_strategies/coch_search.htm

Greer, N., Mosser, G., Logan, G., & Halaas, G. W. (2000). A practical approach to evidence grading. *Joint Commission Journal on Quality Improvement, 26*, 700–712.

Joanna Briggs Institute for Evidence Based Nursing & Midwifery. (2000). http://www.joannabriggs.edu.au/about.html

Polit, D., & Hungler, B. (1998). Nursing research principles and methods (6th ed.). Philadelphia: Lippincott-Raven.

Rosen, W., & Donald, A. (1995). Evidence based medicine: An approach to clinical problem solving. *British Medical Journal, 310*, 1122–1125.

Sackett, D. L., Rosenberg, W. M. C., Gray, J. A. M., Haynes, R. B., & Richardson, W. S. (1996). Evidence-based medicine: What it is and what it isn't. *British Medical Journal, 312*, 71–72.

Sheaffer, C. M., Phillips, C. Y., Donlevy, J. A., & Pietruch, B. L. (1998). Continuing education as a facilitator of change: Implementing a new nursing delivery model. *Journal of Continuing Education in Nursing, 29*(1), 35–39.

Soukup, M. (2000). Evidence-based nursing practice [Preface]. *Nursing Clinics of North America, 35,* xvii–xviii.

Stetler, C. B., Brunell, M., Giuliano, K., Morsi, D., Prince, L., & Newell-Stokes, V. (1998a). Evidence-based practice and the role of nursing leadership. *Journal of Nursing Administration, 28*(7/8), 45–53.

Stetler, C. B., Morsi, D., Rucki, S., Broughton, S., Corrigan, B., Fitzgerald, J., Giuliano, K., Havener, P., & Sheridan, E. A. (1998b). Utilization-focused integrative reviews in a nursing service. *Applied Nursing Research, 11*(4). 195–206.

Thompson, D. (1998). A week in the life of a hospital, "More science...and much more money" [Special report]. *Time, 152*(15).

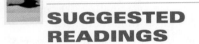

SUGGESTED READINGS

Anderson, C. A. (1998). Does evidence-based practice equal quality nursing care? *Nursing Outlook, 46,* 257–258.

Angel, B. F., Duffey, M., & Belyea, M. (2000). An evidence-based project for evaluating strategies to improve knowledge acquisition and critical-thinking performance in nursing students. *Journal of Nursing Education, 39,* 219–228.

Bakken, S., & McArthur, J. (2001). Evidence-based nursing practice: A call to action for nursing informatics. *Journal of the American Medical Informatics Association, 8,* 289–290.

Beason, C. (2000). Creating an innovative organization. *Nursing Clinics of North America, 35,* 443–452.

Bonell, C. (1999). Evidence-based nursing: A stereotyped view of quantitative and experimental research could work against professional autonomy and authority. *Journal of Advanced Nursing, 30*(1), 18–23.

Bradham, D., Mangan, M., Warrick, A., Geiger-Brown, J., Reiner, J. I., & Saunders, H. J. (2000). Linking innovative nursing practice to health services research. *Nursing Clinics of North America, 35,* 557–568.

Chalmers, T. C. (1994). Implications of meta-analysis: Need for a new generation of randomized control trials. In K. A. McCormick, S. R. Moore, & R. A. Siegel (Eds.), *Clinical practice guideline development: Methodology perspectives* (AHCPR Publication No. 95-0009, pp. 1–3). Washington, DC: U.S. Department of Health and Human Services.

Closs, S., & Cheater, F. (1999). Evidence for nursing practice: A clarification of the issues. *Journal of Advanced Nursing, 30*(1), 10–17.

Cohen, P. A. & Dacanay, L. S. (1994). A meta-analysis of computer-based instruction in nursing education. *Computers in Nursing, 12* (2), 89–97.

Colyer, H., & Kamath, P. (1999). Evidence-based practice. A philosophical and political analysis: Some matters for consideration by professional practitioners. *Journal of Advanced Nursing, 29*(1), 188–193.

Cook, D. (1998). Evidenced-based medicine. *Critical Care Clinic, 14,* 353–358.

Cullum, N. (2000). Users' guides to the nursing literature: An introduction. *Evidence Based Nursing, 3,* 71–72.

Deaton, C. (2001). Outcomes measurement and evidence-based nursing practice. *Journal of Cardiovascular Nursing, 15*(2), 83–86.

Ellis, J., Mulligan, I., Rowe, J., & Sackett, D. L. (1995). Inpatient general medicine is evidence based. *Lancet, 346,* 407–410.

Eysenck, H. (1995). Meta-analysis of best-evidence synthesis? *Journal of Evaluating Clinical Practice, 1*(1), 29–36.

French, P. (1999). The development of evidence-based nursing. *Journal of Advanced Nursing, 29*(1), 72–78.

Funk, S. G., Tornquist, E. M., & Champagne, M. T. (1995). Barriers and facilitators of research utilization: An integrative review. *Nursing Clinics of North America, 30,* 395–407.

Goode, C. J. (2000). What constitutes the "evidence" in evidence-based practice? *Applied Nursing Research, 13,* 222–225.

Goode, C. J., & Titler, M. G. (1996). Moving research-based practice throughout the health care system. *MEDSURG Nursing, 5,* 380–383.

Graves, J. R. (1998). The Sigma Theta Tau International nursing research classification system. In J. J. Fitzpatrick (Ed.), *Encyclopedia of nursing research.* New York: Springer.

Guyatt, G. H., Haynes, R. B., Jaeschke, R. Z., Cook, D. J., Green, L., Naylor, C. D., Wilson, M. C., & Richardson, W. S. (2000). Users' guides to the medical literature: XXV, Evidence-based medicine: Principles for applying the users guides to patient care. *Journal of the American Medical Association, 284,* 1290–1296.

Guyatt, G. H., Sackett, D. L., Sinclair, J. C., Hayward, R., Cook, D. J., & Cook, R. J. (1995). Users' guides to the medical literature: IX. A method for grading health care recommendations. *Journal of the American Medical Association, 274,* 1800–1804.

Haynes, E. (2000). Research as a key to promoting and sustaining innovative practice. *Nursing Clinics of North America, 35,* 453–463.

Hewison, A. (1997). Evidence-based medicine: What about evidence-based management? *Journal of Nursing Management, 5*, 195–198.

Hicks, C. (1998). Barriers to evidence-based care in nursing: Historical legacies and conflicting cultures. *Health Services Management Research, 11*, 137–147.

Huber, D., Schumacher, L., & Delaney, C. (1997). Nursing management minimum data set (NMMDS). *Journal of Nursing Administration, 27*(4), 42–48.

Ingersoll, G. L. (2000). Evidence-based nursing: What it is and what it isn't. *Nursing Outlook, 48*, 151–152.

Kavale, K. A. (1995). Meta-analysis at 20: A retrospect and prospect. *Evaluation and the Health Professions, 18*(4), 349–369.

Kessenich, C. R., Guyatt, G. H., & DiCenso, A. (1997). Teaching nursing students evidence-based nursing. *Nurse Educator, 22*(6), 25–29.

Kitson, A. (2000). Towards evidence-based quality improvement: Perspectives from nursing practice. *International Journal for Quality in Health Care, 12*, 459–464.

Kizer, K. (2000). Promoting innovative nursing practice during radical health system change. *Nursing Clinics of North America, 35*, 430–449.

Lang, N. M. (1999). Discipline-based approaches to evidence-based practice: A view from nursing. *Joint Commission Journal on Quality Improvement, 25*, 539–544.

Mark, B. A., & Salyer, J. (1999). Methodological issues in treatment effectiveness and outcomes research. *Outcomes Management for Nursing Practice, 3*, 12–18.

McPheeters, M., & Lohr, K. N. (1999). Evidence-based practice and nursing: Commentary. *Outcomes Management for Nursing Practice. 3*, 99–101.

Mehta, N., & Jain, A. (2001). Finding evidence-based answers to clinical questions online. *Cleveland Clinic Journal of Medicine, 68*, 307–317.

National Institute of Nursing Research. (1993). *National nursing research agenda: Setting nursing research priorities*. Bethesda, MD: National Institutes of Health.

NHS Centre for Reviews and Dissemination. (1996). *Undertaking systematic reviews of research on effectiveness. CRD guidelines*. York, England: Author.

Parson, E. (1999). Evidence-based clinical outcome management in interventional cardiology. *Critical Care Nursing Clinics of North America, 11*, 143.

Rambur, B. (1999). Fostering evidence-based practice in nursing education. *Journal of Professional Nursing, 15*, 270–274.

Rosenfeld, P., Duthie, E., Bier, J., Bowar-Ferres, S., Fulmer, T., Iervolino, L., McClure, M. L., McGivern, D. O., & Roncoli, M. (2000). Engaging staff nurses in evidence-based research to identify nursing practice problems and solutions. *Applied Nursing Research, 13*(4), 197–203.

Rosswurm, M. A., & Larrabee, J. H. (1999). A model for change to evidence-based practice. *Image: Journal of Nursing Scholarship, 31*, 317–322.

Shorten, A., Wallace, M. C., & Crookes, P. A. (2001). Developing information literacy: A key to evidence-based nursing. *International Nursing Review, 48*, 86–92.

Simpson, K. R., & Knox, G. E. (1999). Strategies for developing an evidence-based approach to perinatal care. *MCN American Journal of Maternal Child Nursing, 24*, 122–131.

Soukup, S. M. (2000). The Center for Advanced Nursing Practice evidence-based practice model: Promoting the scholarship of practice. *Nursing Clinics of North America, 35*, 301–310.

Stetler, C. B., Corrigan, B., Sander-Buscemi, K., & Burns, M. (1999). Integration of evidence into practice and the change process: Fall prevention program as a model. *Outcomes Management for Nursing Practice, 3*, 102–111.

Stevens, K. R. (1997, October 23). *Knowledge for clinical practice*. Paper presented to Sigma Theta Tau Kappa Epsilon Chapter-at-Large, Grand Rapids, MI.

Stevens, K. R. & Cassidy, V. R. (1999). Evidence-based teaching/current research in nursing education. Boston: Jones and Bartlett.

Swanson, E. A., McCloskey, J. C., & Bodensteiner, A. (1991). Publishing opportunities for nurses: A comparison of 92 U.S. journals. *Image: Journal of Nursing Scholarship, 23*(1), 33–38.

Taylor-Piliae, R. (1998). Establishing evidence-based practice: Issues and implications in critical care nursing. *Intensive and Critical Care Nursing, 14,* 30–37.

Titler, M. G., Kleiber, C., Steelman, V., Goode, C., Rakel, B., Barry-Walker, J., Small, S., & Buckwalter, K. (1994). Infusing research into practice to promote quality care. *Nursing Research, 43*, 307–313.

Titler, M. G., & Mentes, J. C. (1999). Research utilization in gerontological nursing practice. *Journal of Gerontological Nursing, 25*(6), 6–9.

Titler, M. G., Mentes, J. C., Rakel, B. A., Abbott, L., & Baumler, S. (1999). From book to bedside: Putting evidence to use in the care of the elderly. *Joint Commission Journal on Quality Improvement, 25*, 545–556.

Tranmer, J. E., Coulson, K., Holtom, D., Lively, T., & Maloney, R. (1998). The emergence of a culture that promotes evidence based decision making within an acute care setting. *Canadian Journal of Nursing Administration, 11*(2), 36–58.

Urbshott, G. B., Kennedy, G., & Rutherford, G. (2001). The Cochrane HIV/AIDS review group and evidence-based practice in nursing. *Journal of the Association of Nurses in AIDS Care, 12*(6), 94–101.

White, S. J. (1997). Evidence-based practice and nursing: The new panacea? *British Journal of Nursing, 6*(3), 175–178.

CHAPTER 4

Nursing and Health Care Informatics

Leslie H. Nicoll, PhD, MBA, RN

From then on, when anything went wrong with a computer, we said it had bugs in it. (Admiral Grace Murray Hopper, on the removal of a 2-inch-long moth from an experimental computer at Harvard University, September 9, 1945)

OBJECTIVES

Upon completion of this chapter, the reader should be able to:

1. List the components that define a nursing specialty and discuss how nursing informatics meets these requirements.
2. Discuss educational opportunities for nurses interested in pursuing a career in nursing informatics.
3. Describe highlights in the history of modern computing.
4. Discuss how ubiquitous computing and virtual reality have the potential to influence nursing education and practice.
5. Use established criteria to evaluate the content of health-related sites found on the World Wide Web.

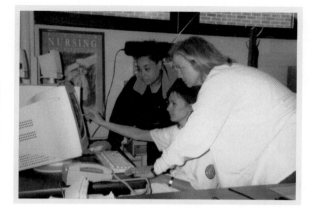

What is the most important card in your wallet? Your driver's license? Your nursing license? Your library card? In a few years, it might be your "personal health database." This card would be encoded with your personal health history, information from encounters with health care providers, payer information, and more. A swipe of the card in a bar-code reader would bring up the information on a screen, making a complete health history available, no matter where you are or the nature of your complaint. At each encounter, the card would be updated, ensuring that every health care provider you come in contact with has the most complete and current health information available for your care.

Does this sound like science fiction or is it the possible reality within the coming years?

What would be some advantages to a portable personal health database? Possible disadvantages?

Like it or not, computers are here to stay. Computers have changed the way we communicate, obtain information, work, and, most recently, shop. As evidence, during the 2000 holiday shopping season, 25 million people spent $6.2 billion on-line, up from $3.2 billion in 1999 (Shop.org, 1999, 2000). Recent statistics indicate that in the United States, more than half (51%) of the households in the country have at least one personal computer, and 61% (168 million) of the U.S. population has an Internet connection at home or work (CyberAtlas, 2000). Throughout the world, computer use is becoming pervasive, too. Statistics from the first quarter of 2001 indicate that 420 million people from 27 countries have Internet access (CyberAtlas, 2001).

Consumers are also going on-line for health content. In 1999, 31.1 million people went on-line to obtain health information, shop for health products, or interact with a health provider or payer. While most people are on-line to search for health information, industry experts predict other forms of "e-health"—connecting with providers or receiving case management on-line—will continue to experience rapid development (Bard, 2000).

Computers and the Internet are changing health care delivery, too. For example, during a 3-year study, investigators found that a computer reminder to physicians doubled the likelihood that they would administer flu vaccine to high-risk patients. This increased vaccination level resulted in 10% to 30% fewer winter hospitalizations, emergency room visits, and tests for respiratory problems (Agency for Health Care Policy and Research, 1996). In another study, a computer-based clinical information and decision system detected 60 times more adverse drug reactions in patients than the traditional system. The computer-detected reactions—95% of which were moderate to severe—occurred in 648 patients during an 18-month period (Agency for Health Care Policy and Research, 1996).

Nurses are not immune to the changes that computers are bringing to both everyday life and nursing practice. Computer technology can help nurses to achieve the goals of quality patient care and positive patient outcomes. Whether you are a student learning a clinical procedure using a computer-based instruction program or an administrator using a spreadsheet and database to plan a budget, it is evident that computer technology is an essential part of professional nursing practice, both on the individual and institutional level.

Although everyone is involved with computers to some degree today, there are some who have chosen to specialize within the field of computer science, information, and technology. Within nursing, this specialty area is known as nursing informatics. Nurses in informatics have taken on a wide variety of roles and are involved in a myriad of activities, ranging from the design and implementation of clinical information systems to research on the use of technology to improve patient outcomes. Although this is a fairly new specialty within the profession, it is clear that informatics nurses are having a major impact on the way care is planned and delivered in the current health care environment.

This chapter will introduce you to both dimensions of computing in professional nursing: the world of nursing informatics as well as the world of computing "for the rest of us." While it may not be your career choice to become an informaticist, the professional registered nurse of the 21st century will not be effective in the role without a solid base of knowledge related to computers and technology and their impact on nursing practice, patient care, and patient outcomes.

WHAT IS NURSING INFORMATICS?

The term *informatics* was derived from the French word *informatique*. Gorn (1983) first defined the term as computer science plus information science. Informatics involves more than just computers—it includes all aspects of technology and science, from the theoretical to the applied. Another important part of the field of informatics concerns learning how to use new tools and maximizing the capabilities provided by computers and related information technologies (Ball, Hannah, & Douglas, 2000).

Nursing informatics refers to that component of informatics designed for and relevant to nurses. The first definition of nursing informatics was developed by Ball and Hannah in 1984. Various authors modified and embellished the definition during the ensuing decade (Figure 4-1). The definition set forth by the American Nurses Association (ANA) in 1994 has been generally accepted by the community of informaticists and is considered the standard. Note that this definition includes many components of nursing informatics: information management, knowledge from sciences other than nursing, and the importance of informatics within all areas of nursing practice. For nurses studying to become informatics specialists and for those developing curricula for education in nursing informatics, the definition also provides guidance (Gassert, 2000).

The Specialty of Nursing Informatics

There are many specialties in nursing that cover a range of interests and clinical domains, such as critical care nursing, community health, or administration. Key attributes of a specialty were identified by Styles (1989) as follows:

- Differentiated practice
- A research program
- Representation of the specialty by at least one organized body
- A mechanism for credentialing nurses in the specialty
- Educational programs for preparing nurses to practice in the specialty

In 1992, the ANA acknowledged that nursing informatics possessed these attributes and designated nursing informatics as an area of specialty practice.

Education in Informatics

There are both formal and informal opportunities for education in nursing informatics. The first formal programs that offered specific degrees in nursing informatics were established within the past 15 years, and the number of programs has been increasing steadily. However, because educational options were limited, there are many nurses practicing in informatics that have been prepared for their role through on-the-job training or by receiving education outside of nursing. For example, a nurse may have a bachelor of science in nursing (BSN) plus a second degree in computer science or information technology. Nurses have been successful in educating themselves using formal and informal resources. Nurses considering a career in informatics need to carefully consider options that are available and plan their educational program accordingly.

Formal Programs. The Nursing Working Informatics Group of the American Medical Informatics Association (NWIG-AMIA) describes formal educational programs in nursing informatics as Category I, Category II, and Category III. Category I programs are those graduate programs with a specialist nursing informatics focus. There are currently five Category I programs, based at the following institutions of higher learning: Excelsior College (formerly Regents College), Albany, NY; New York University, New York, NY; St. Louis University, St. Louis, MO; University of Colorado Health Sciences Center, Denver, CO; University of Maryland, Baltimore, MD; and University of Utah, Salt Lake City, UT. Although each program is unique, there are similarities. For example, students pursing an education at the master's level will take approximately 42 semester credit hours of course work, which are

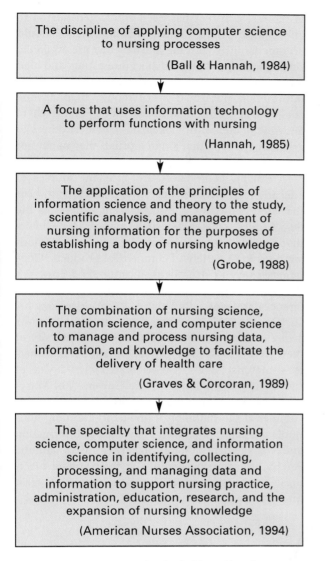

The discipline of applying computer science to nursing processes

(Ball & Hannah, 1984)

↓

A focus that uses information technology to perform functions with nursing

(Hannah, 1985)

↓

The application of the principles of information science and theory to the study, scientific analysis, and management of nursing information for the purposes of establishing a body of nursing knowledge

(Grobe, 1988)

↓

The combination of nursing science, information science, and computer science to manage and process nursing data, information, and knowledge to facilitate the delivery of health care

(Graves & Corcoran, 1989)

↓

The specialty that integrates nursing science, computer science, and information science in identifying, collecting, processing, and managing data and information to support nursing practice, administration, education, research, and the expansion of nursing knowledge

(American Nurses Association, 1994)

Figure 4-1 Evolution of a Definition: Nursing Informatics

divided among core courses (such as theory, research, policy, and advanced nursing), courses in nursing informatics (such as programming, database design, systems analysis and design, clinical decision making, informatics models, and practice activities), and support courses. Similarly, students at the University of Utah and the University of Maryland may pursue doctoral study with substantive course work in nursing informatics. Again, courses are taken in nursing theory, research, statistics, and nursing informatics. As with any doctoral degree, a dissertation is required.

Category II programs are graduate and under-graduate programs and courses that allow a student to pursue a concentration (or minor) in nursing informatics. In these programs, students take 6 to 12 credits of course work in informatics. Category II programs are available at Case Western Reserve University, Cleveland, OH; Duke School of Nursing, Durham, NC; Loyola of Chicago, Chicago, IL; Northeastern University, Boston, MA; Slippery Rock University, Slippery Rock, PA; and the Universities of Arizona, Tucson, AZ; Iowa, Iowa City, IA; Pennsylvania, Philadelphia, PA; and Phoenix (Phoenix Online), Phoenix, AZ.

Category III programs offer individual courses in nursing informatics at both the graduate and undergraduate level. The NWIG-AMIA has identified six such programs (Georgia College and State University, Milledgeville, GA; Lewis College, Romeoville, IL; Oregon Health Sciences University, Portland, OR; Western Michigan University, Kalamazoo, MI; Wichita State University, Wichita, KS; University of North Carolina, Chapel Hill, NC; and University of Vermont, Burlington, VT), although it is likely that this list is incomplete. If you are interested in formal study in informatics, check with schools and colleges of nursing in your locale to see what is available.

While these are the only formal programs available at this time, many universities have courses in computer science and information technology. Interested students are able to self-design programs that meet their individual learning needs. Programs at the University of Texas at Austin, University of California San Francisco, and the University of Wisconsin at Madison have been identified as having particularly strong concentrations of courses available in informatics (Gassert, 2000).

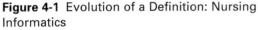**Informal Education.** For many nurses, graduate education is not an option or personal choice, but they still desire to become more knowledgeable about informatics. In this case, many informal opportunities exist, including networking through professional organizations, keeping abreast of the literature by reading journals, and attending professional conferences.

Organizations vary in the scope of services offered to members and the types of educational programs offered. Nelson and Joos (1992) describe five types of organizations:

- *Special interest groups* such as the councils of the ANA and the National League for Nursing

(NLN). Nonnursing organizations that have special interest groups of interest to nurses include the American Hospital Association and the Healthcare Financial Management Association.

- *Information science and computer organizations* such as the Association for Computing Machinery. There also are specialty organizations within this category, such as the Health Sciences Communications Association.
- *Health computing organizations* such as the AMIA and the International Medical Informatics Association. Other organizations in this category include the Medical Records Institute (MRI) and the Computer-based Patient Record Institute (CPRI).
- *User groups,* which consist of individuals working with a specific language, software, or vendor. One such group of interest to nurses is the Microsoft Healthcare Users Group (MS-HUG), which focuses on applications of Microsoft products in health care environments.
- *Local groups* such as the Capital Area Roundtable on Informatics in Nursing (CARING), located in Washington, D.C., or the Tri-State Nursing Computer Network, located in Pittsburgh, Pennsylvania. These groups provide local contacts, opportunities for networking, and education. CARING, for example, offers a popular review course for people preparing to take the nursing informatics certification examination.

Anyone interested in learning more about informatics should become active in at least one related organization. As a member, a nurse has access to the meetings, publications, and educational offerings that the organization provides. Getting on mailing lists or visiting organizational sites on the World Wide Web also allows a nurse to keep abreast of different opportunities available through each organization.

Reading journals and newsletters is another way to become more knowledgeable about informatics. Offerings include trade magazines that are not related to health but are important sources of information, such as *PC Magazine* or *Byte,* and specialized nursing journals, such as *Computers in Nursing.* Since 1995, *Computers in Nursing* has offered continuing education credit for articles published in the journal. AMIA publishes the *Journal of the American Medical Informatics Association,* a publication source for much

of the research that has been conducted related to informatics. A nurse interested in informatics should become familiar with the journals that are available, subscribe to those that are most interesting, and read others in the library. Unfortunately, there is more information published every month than anyone could possibly hope to keep abreast of—that is where networking comes in! Colleagues can alert others to articles of interest that are in journals they might not regularly read.

Finally, conferences are excellent sources of education. At a conference the nurse is able to hear the latest information directly from experts in the field. Larger conferences usually have vendor exhibits that provide the opportunity for hands-on demonstrations for a variety of commercial products. Conferences vary in size, focus, location, and cost. For those interested in nursing informatics, nursing conferences are especially helpful. Local organizations, such as CARING, sponsor a variety of half-day or 1-day conferences. Rutgers, the State University of New Jersey, in Newark, NJ, has an annual informatics conference; in 2001, it celebrated its 19th year of successful implementation. The University of Maryland hosts a weeklong institute on informatics every summer at the Baltimore campus. In addition, nonnursing organizations such as the Health Information and Management Systems Society (HIMSS) and the AMIA have nursing sessions at their annual meetings. Nonnursing sessions also are often of great interest to nurse attendees.

Certification

Whether a nurse has pursued a formal or informal educational path in nursing informatics, many practicing in the specialty choose to become certified. Certification in a specialty is a formal, systematic mechanism whereby nurses can voluntarily seek a credential that recognizes their quality and excellence in professional practice and continuing education (American Nurses Credentialing Center, 1993). For many nurses, becoming certified is a professional milestone and validation of their qualifications, knowledge, and skills in a defined area of nursing practice. The American Nurses Credentialing Center (ANCC) offers certification examinations for a variety of specialties in nursing, including informatics.

To be eligible for the nursing informatics examination, which was first offered in 1995, a nurse must meet the following requirements:

- Possess an active registered nursing license in the United States or its territories
- Have earned a baccalaureate or higher nursing degree
- Have practiced actively as a registered nurse for at least 2 years
- Have practiced at least 2,000 hours in the field of nursing informatics within the past 5 years or completed at least 12 semester hours of academic credits in informatics in a graduate program in nursing and have practiced a minimum of 1,000 hours in informatics within the past 5 years
- Have earned 20 contact hours of continuing education credit applicable to the specialty area within the past 2 years (American Nurses Credentialing Center, 2001b)

The nurse who successfully passes the examination is certified as a generalist in informatics nursing. The ANCC is planning to offer an examination for a specialist in informatics nursing in the future. Once certified, the nurse must be recertified every 5 years. In the first year the examination was offered, 83 nurses became certified in informatics (Newbold, 1996). Currently, there are more than 400 nurses who are certified in the specialty (American Nurses Credentialing Center, 2001a).

Career Opportunities

Career opportunities in the fields of computer science and information technology are growing at an exponential rate, and nursing is no exception. Nurses working in informatics can look forward to multiple job opportunities, with new roles continuously being developed as technology changes and matures. Changes in health care delivery, particularly managed care, have caused shifts in computer systems to care management, clinical systems, clinical data repositories, care mapping, and outcomes measures (Hersher, 2000).

Career opportunities for nurses in informatics exist in a number of different types of industries. Health care institutions, such as hospitals, are an obvious choice, but nurses also work for vendors of clinical information systems, insurance companies, managed care organizations, and consulting firms.

CLINICAL INFORMATION

Clinical information systems are changing the way health care is delivered, whether in the hospital, the clinic, the provider's office, or the patient's home. With capabilities ranging from advanced instrumentation to high-level decision support, a **clinical information system** (CIS) offers nurses and other clinicians information when, where, and how they need it. Increasingly, CIS applications function as the mechanisms for delivering patient-centered care and for supporting the move toward the computer-based patient record (CPR).

What exactly is a CIS? Definitions vary, often from organization to organization. Semancik (1997) describes a CIS as a collection of software programs and associated hardware that supports the entry, retrieval, update, and analysis of patient care information and associated clinical information related to patient care. The CIS is primarily a computer system

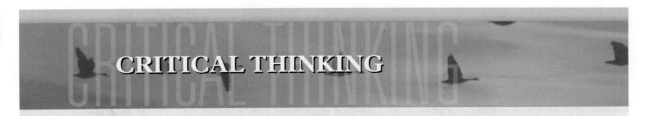

CRITICAL THINKING

Visit the American Nurses Credentialing Center at *http://www.nursingworld.org/ancc/*. Choose another specialty in which a nurse can be certified and compare it to the certification in informatics.

How are they similar? How are they different?

used to provide clinical information for the care of a patient.

Clinical Information Systems

A CIS can be patient-focused or departmental. In patient-focused systems, automation supports patient care processes. Typical applications found in a **patient-focused clinical information system** include order entry, results reporting, clinical documentation, care planning, and clinical pathways. As data are entered into the system, data repositories are established that can be accessed to look for trends in patient care. The **departmental clinical information system** evolved to meet the operational needs of a particular department, such as the laboratory, radiology, pharmacy, medical records, or billing department. Early systems often were stand-alone systems designed for an individual department. A major challenge facing CIS developers is to integrate these stand-alone systems to work with each other and with the newer patient-focused systems.

Computerized Patient Records

A CIS is not the same as a **computerized patient record** (CPR) or electronic patient record. Ideally, the CPR will include all information about an individual's lifetime health status and health care. The

CPR is a replacement for the paper medical record as the primary source of information for health care, meeting all clinical, legal, and administrative requirements. However, the CPR is more than today's medical record. Information technology permits much more data to be captured, processed, and integrated, which results in information that is broader than that found in a linear paper record.

The CPR is not a record in the traditional sense of the term. *Record* connotes a repository with limitations of size, content, and location. The term traditionally has suggested that the sole purpose for maintaining health data is to document events. Although this is an important purpose, the CPR permits health information to be used to support the generation and communication of knowledge.

The health care delivery system is dramatically changing, with a strong emphasis on improving outcomes of care and maintaining health. The CPR needs to be considered in a broader context and is not applicable only to patients, that is, individuals with the presence of an illness or disease. Rather, in the CPR, the focus is on the individuals' health, encompassing both wellness and illness.

As a result of this focus on the individual, the CPR is a virtual compilation of nonredundant health data about the person across her lifetime, including facts, observations, interpretations, plans, actions, and outcomes. Health data include information on allergies, history of illness and injury, functional status, diagnostic studies, assessments, orders, consultation reports, and treatment records. Health data

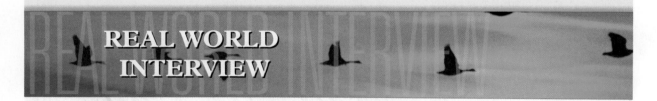

To me, the greatest contribution of health care information technology and systems is its power to support clinician decision making. Far too often we focus on the technical aspects of hardware and software design while minimizing the real intent of this powerful technology, which is to support clinicians in their practice endeavors. We need to make clinicians' knowledge paramount as we transform our clinical practice environments through the design and implementation of new health care information technology and systems.

Rita Snyder-Halpern, PhD, RN, CNAA
Associate Professor

also include wellness information such as immunization history, behavioral data, environmental information, demographics, health insurance, administrative data for care delivery processes, and legal data such as consents. The who, what, when, and where of data capture also are identified. The structure of the data includes text, numbers, sounds, images, and full-motion video. These are thoroughly integrated so that any given view of health data may incorporate one or more structural elements.

Within a CPR, an individual's health data are maintained and distributed over different systems in different locations, such as a hospital, clinic, physician's office, and pharmacy. Intelligent software agents with appropriate security measures are necessary to access data across these distributed systems. The nurse or other user who is retrieving these data must be able to assemble the data in such a way as to provide a chronology of health information about the individual.

The CPR is maintained in a system that captures, processes, communicates, secures, and presents the data about the patient. This system may include the CIS. Other components of the CPR system include clinical rules, literature for patient education, expert opinions, and payer rules related to reimbursement. When these elements work together in an integrated fashion, the CPR becomes much more than a patient record—it becomes a knowledge tool. The system is able to integrate information from multiple sources and provides decision support; thus, the CPR serves as the primary source of information for patient care.

A fully functional CPR is a complex system. Consider a single data element (datum), such as a person's weight. The system must be able to record the weight; store it; process it; communicate it to others; and present it in a different format, such as a bar graph or chart. It may also be necessary to convert a weight in pounds to kilograms or vice versa. All of this must be done in a secure environment that protects the patient's confidentiality and privacy. The complexity of these issues and the development of the necessary systems help to explain why few fully functional CPR systems are in place today.

Data Capture

Data capture refers to the collection and entry of data into a computer system. The origin of the data may be local or remote, with the data coming from patient-monitoring devices, from telemedicine applications, directly from the individual recipient of health care, and even from others who have information about the recipient's health or environment, such as relatives and friends and public health agencies. Data may be captured by multiple means, including key entry, pattern recognition (voice, handwriting, or biological characteristics), and medical device transmission.

All data entered into a computer are not necessarily structured for subsequent processing. Document imaging systems, for example, provide for creation of electronically stored text but have limitations on the ability to process that text. Data capture includes the use of controlled vocabularies and code systems to ensure common meaning for terminology and the ability to process units of information. As noted earlier, great strides have been made in the development of standardized nursing languages. These languages provide structured data entry and text processing that result in common meaning and processing.

Data capture also encompasses authentication to identify the author of an entry and to ensure that the author has been granted permission to access the system and change the CPR.

Storage

Storage refers to the physical location of data. In CPR systems, health data are distributed across multiple systems at different sites. For this reason, there need to be common access protocols, retention schedules, and universal identification.

Access protocols permit only authorized users to obtain data for legitimate uses. The systems must have backup and recovery mechanisms in the event of failure. Retention schedules address the maintenance of the data in active and inactive form and the permanence of the storage medium.

A person's identity can be determined by many types of data in addition to common identifiers such as name and number. Universal identifiers or other methods are required for integrating health data of an individual distributed across multiple systems at different sites.

Information Processing

Computer processing functions provide for effective retrieval and processing of data into useful information.

These include decision support tools such as alerts and alarms for drug interactions, allergies, and abnormal laboratory results. Reminders can be provided for appointments, critical path actions, medication administration, and other activities. The systems also may provide access to consensus- and evidence-driven diagnostic and treatment guidelines and protocols. The nurse could integrate a standard guideline, protocol, or critical path into a specific individual's CPR, modify it to meet unique circumstances, and use it as a basis for managing and documenting care. Outcome data communicated from various caregivers and health care recipients themselves also may be analyzed and used for continuous improvement of the guidelines and protocols.

Information Communication

Information communication refers to the interoperability of systems and linkages for exchange of data across disparate systems. To integrate health data across multiple systems at different sites, identifier systems (unique numbers or other methodology) for health care recipients, caregivers, providers, payers, and sites are essential. Local, regional, and national health information infrastructures that tie all participants together using standard data communication protocols are key to the linkage function. There are hundreds of types of transactions or messages that must be defined and agreed to by the participating stakeholders. Vocabulary and code systems must permit the exchange and processing of data into meaningful information. CPR systems must provide

access to point-of-care information databases and knowledge sources, such as pharmaceutical formularies, referral databases, and reference literature.

Security

Computer-based patient record systems provide better protection of confidential health information than paper-based systems because they support controls that ensure that only authorized users with legitimate uses have access to health information. Security functions address the confidentiality of private health information and the integrity of the data. Security functions must be designed to ensure compliance with applicable laws, regulations, and standards. Security systems must ensure that access to data is provided only to those who are authorized and have a legitimate purpose for using the data. Security functions also must provide a means to audit for inappropriate access.

There are three important terms that are used when discussing security: privacy, confidentiality, and security. It is important to understand the differences between these concepts.

- *Privacy* refers to the right of individuals to keep information about themselves from being disclosed to anyone. If a patient had had an abortion and chose not to tell a health care provider this fact, the patient would be keeping that information private.
- *Confidentiality* refers to the act of limiting disclosure of private matters. Once a patient has

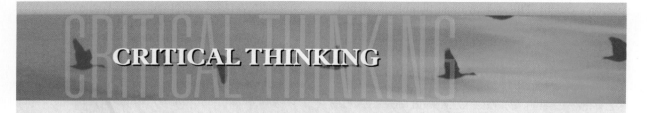

CRITICAL THINKING

In your clinical practice, you have likely interacted with a clinical information system to both enter and access data for the patient you were caring for.

What security systems were in place to maintain the confidentiality of patient data, for example, passwords, identification cards, and so on? Do you believe the security system was effective? Was it updated on a regular basis? Did the security system present any barriers to your obtaining necessary information for providing quality patient care—for example, were the results of certain tests or past history restricted in any way?

REAL WORLD INTERVIEW

Several thoughts immediately come to mind about the marriage between nursing and trends in computing. First, nursing leadership within organizational informatics is pivotal especially within the next few years. Without strong nursing informatics leadership, nursing requirements stand to be overlooked or ignored during large systems installation. Nursing is at the heart of information integration at the patient level, and systems need to support this kind of patient-centered design, including functions needed by nurses. Having an educated informatics nurse specialist reporting directly to the executive staff is the beginning to solving this problem. Second, chief financial officers (CFOs) can balk at the cost of electronic patient records and the other resources required to install these large-scale informatics projects. However, clinical care can no longer exist efficiently and effectively without electronic tools like the electronic patient record, decision support, and Internet access. Additionally, the external impetus to install electronic patient records is great. For example, the Leapfrog group set standards for hospitals to meet in order to obtain business from large corporations such as General Motors, Ford Motor Company, IBM, and 75 other companies. One of those standards is computerized physician order entry, which is projected to reduce prescribing errors by more than 50%. CFOs need to realize that their institutions will not be competitive in the health industry without electronic access for patients, computerized orders, and protections for patients like decision support. It is no longer a question of whether to install these computerized functions but when.

Nancy Staggers, PhD, RN, FAAN
Associate CIO

disclosed private information to a health care provider, that provider has a responsibility to maintain the confidentiality of that information.

- *Security* refers to the means to control access and protect information from accidental or intentional disclosure to unauthorized persons and from alteration, destruction, or loss. When private information is placed in a confidential CPR, the system must have controls in place to maintain the security of the system and not allow unauthorized persons access to the data (CPRI Work Group on Confidentiality, Privacy & Security, 1995).

Information Presentation

The wealth of information available through CPR systems must be managed to ensure that authorized caregivers, including nurses, and others with legitimate uses have the information they need in their preferred presentation form. A nurse, for example, may like to see data organized by source, caregiver,

encounter, problem, or date. Data can be presented in detail or summary form. Tables, graphs, narrative, and other forms of information presentation must be accommodated. Some users may need to know only of the presence or absence of certain data, not the nature of the data itself. For example, blood donation centers test blood for HIV, hepatitis, and other conditions. If a donor has a positive test result, the center may not be given the specific information regarding the test but just general information that a test result was abnormal and that the patient should be referred to an appropriate health care provider.

INTERFACE BETWEEN THE INFORMATICS NURSE AND THE CLINICAL INFORMATION SYSTEM

Information demands in health care systems are pushing the development of CISs and CPRs. The ongoing development of computer technology—smaller, faster machines with extensive storage capabilities and the ability for cross-platform communication—is making the goal of an integrated electronic system a realistic option, not just a long-term dream. As these systems evolve, informatics nurses will play an important role in their development, implementation, and evaluation.

Informatics nurses, because of their expertise, are in an ideal position to assist with the development, implementation, and evaluation of CISs. Their knowledge of policies, procedures, and clinical care is essential as work-flow systems are redesigned within a CIS. It is not unusual for nurses within an institution to have more hands-on interaction with and knowledge of different departments than any other group of employees in an institution. Jenkins (2000) suggests that the process model of nursing (assessment, planning, implementation, and evaluation) works well during a CIS implementation, thus nurses have a familiar framework from which to understand the complexity of a major system change.

TRENDS IN COMPUTING

As noted earlier, computers have moved from the realm of a "nice to know" luxury item to a "need to know" essential resource for professional practice. Nurses are knowledge workers who require accurate and up-to-date information for their professional work. The explosion in information—some estimate that all information is replaced every 9 to 12 months—requires nurses to be on the cutting edge of knowledge to practice ethically and safely. Trends in computing will also affect the work of professional nurses and not just through the development of CISs and CPRs. Research advances, new devices, monitoring equipment, sensors, and "smart body parts" will all change the way that health care is conceptualized, practiced, and delivered.

Within this context, not every nurse will need to be an informatics specialist, but every nurse must be computer literate. **Computer literacy** is defined as the knowledge and understanding of computers combined with the ability to use them effectively (Joos, Whitman, Smith & Nelson, 1996). Computer literacy may be interpreted as different levels of

expertise for different people in various roles. On the least specialized level, computer literacy involves knowing how to turn on a computer, start and stop simple application programs, and save and print information. For health care professionals, computer literacy requires having an understanding of systems used in clinical practice, education, and research settings. In clinical practice, for example, electronic patient records and clinical information systems are becoming more widely used. The computer literate nurse is able to use these systems effectively and can address issues discussed earlier, such as confidentiality, security, and privacy. At the same time, the nurse must be able to effectively use applications typically found on personal computers (PCs), such as word processing software, spreadsheets, presentation graphics, and statistics for research. Finally, the computer literate nurse must know how to access information from a variety of electronic sources and how to evaluate the appropriateness of the information at both the professional and patient level. The remainder of this chapter is designed to help you gain a broader understanding of computer literacy and the computing environment of PCs and the on-line world, and includes a discussion of future trends.

Development of Modern Computing

Weiser and Brown (1996) have characterized the history and future of computing as having three phases. The first phase is known as the "mainframe era" in which many people share one computer. Computers were found behind closed doors and run by experts with specialized knowledge and skills. Although we have mostly moved beyond the mainframe era, it still exists in CISs (hence, some of the problems discussed previously) or other situations with large mainframe systems, such as banking, weather forecasting, and academic institutions.

The archetypal computer of the mainframe era must be the ENIAC, developed at the University of Pennsylvania in 1945. The Electronic Numerical Integrator and Computer (ENIAC) was conceived by John Mauchly, an American physicist, and built at the Moore School of Engineering by Mauchly and J. Presper Eckert, an engineer. It is regarded as the first successful digital computer. It weighed more than 60,000 pounds and contained more than 18,000 vacuum tubes. About 2,000 of the computer's vacuum tubes were replaced each month by a team of six technicians. Even though one vacuum tube blew approximately every 15 minutes, the functioning of the ENIAC was still considered to be reliable! Many of the ENIAC's first tasks were for military purposes, such as calculating ballistic firing tables and designing atomic weapons. Because the ENIAC was initially not a stored program machine, it had to be reprogrammed for each task.

Phase II in modern computing is the "PC era," which is characterized by one person to one computer. In this era, the personal computing relationship is personal and intimate. Similar to a car, the computer is seen as a special, relatively expensive item, which requires attention but provides a very valuable service in one's life.

The first harbinger of the PC era was in 1948 with the development of the transistor at Bell Telephone Laboratories. The transistor, which could act as an electric switch, replaced the costly, energy-inefficient, and unreliable vacuum tubes in computers and other devices, including televisions. By the late 1960s, integrated circuits, tiny transistors, and other electrical components arranged on a single chip of silicon replaced individual transistors in computers. Integrated circuits became miniaturized, enabling more components to be designed into a single computer circuit. In the 1970s, refinements in integrated circuit technology led to the development of the modern microprocessor, integrated circuits that contained thousands of transistors. Weiser and Brown (1996) date the true start of the second phase as 1984, when the number of people using personal computers surpassed the number of people using shared computers.

Manufacturers used integrated circuit technology to build smaller and cheaper computers. The first PCs were sold by Instrumentation Telemetry Systems. The Altair 8800 appeared in 1975. Graphical user interfaces were first designed by the Xerox Corporation in a prototype computer, the Alto, developed in 1974. This prototype computer incorporated many of the features found on computers today, including a mouse, a graphical user interface, and a "user friendly" operating system. However, the Xerox Corporation made a corporate decision to not pursue commercial development of the PC, the rationale being that the core business strategy of Xerox was copiers, not computers. One only has to look at how PCs have proliferated throughout the world to realize that this may not have been the smartest business decision ever made. In fact, this whole episode has become a bit of a computer history legend (Hiltzik, 2000; Smith & Alexander, 1988). Continuing development of sophisticated operating systems and miniaturization of components (modern microprocessors contain as many as 10 million transistors) have enabled computers to be developed that can run programs and manipulate data in ways that were unimaginable in the era of the ENIAC.

Ubiquitous Computing

Phase III has been dubbed the era of **ubiquitous computing** (UC), in which there will be many computers to each person. Weiser and Brown (1996) estimate that the crossover with the PC era will be between 2005 and 2020. In this phase, computers will be everywhere—in walls, chairs, clothing, light switches, cars, appliances, and so on. Computers will become so fundamental to our human experience that they will "disappear" and we will cease to be aware of them. The result will be "calm technology," in which computers do not cause stress and anxiety for the user but, rather, recede into the background of life. For those who are skeptical that this will come to pass, consider two other ubiquitous technologies: writing and electricity (Weiser, 1991). In Egyptian times, writing was a secret art, known and performed only by specially trained scribes who lived on a level close to royalty. Clay tablets and later papyrus were precious commodities. Many people died without ever having seen a piece of paper in their lives! Now, paper and writing are everywhere. Within the course of an average day, most people use and discard hundreds of pieces of paper, never giving them a second thought. Electricity has a similar history. When electricity was first invented in the 19th century, entire factories were designed to accommodate the presence of light bulbs and bulky motors. The placement of workers, machines, and parts was designed around the need of electricity and motors. Today, electricity is everywhere. It is hidden in the walls and stored in tiny batteries. The average car has more than 22 motors and 25 solenoids.

One only has to look around a typical house to see how UC is becoming part of our lives. Microprocessors exist in every room: appliances in the kitchen, remote controls for the TV and stereo in the den, and clock radios and cordless phones in the bedroom. And the bathroom? Matsushita of Japan has developed a prototype toilet (dubbed the "smart toilet") that includes an on-line, real-time health monitoring system. It measures the user's weight, fat content, and urine sugar level; plots the recorded data on a graph; and sends the data instantaneously to a health care provider for monitoring (Watts, 1999).

Another dimension of UC is the Internet. Each time you connect to the Internet, you are connecting with millions of information resources and hundreds of information delivery systems. A person truly does become one person to hundreds of computers. It is ironic that the interface to the UC world of the Internet is still through a PC. But this is changing. Wireless, infrared connections will eliminate wires; handheld devices will eliminate the bulky PC. Once we become wireless and mobile, UC will become a reality.

Virtual Reality

According to Weiser (1991), virtual reality (VR) is roughly the opposite of ubiquitous computing. Virtual reality puts people inside a computer-generated world while UC puts the computer out in the world with people. Virtual reality, while still somewhat limited in its development, does have enormous potential in health care applications.

Virtual reality, despite recent popularization, is not new. Just like the Internet, it had its beginnings within the Department of Defense and innovations developed during the 1960s. A brief review of history: during the time of the Cold War, there was great fear of a nuclear attack. Military leaders sought to develop systems that would remain intact in the face of great destruction. The Internet, which is a worldwide network of computers (there is not one large "Internet

computer") was developed so that the electronic communication infrastructure could not be destroyed. Electronic mail (e-mail) was created to ensure rapid and secure communication in the event the wire-based telephone system was destroyed. Virtual reality simulations were developed so that jet pilots could have training that would mimic a world turned upside down: flying through fire, mushroom clouds, and poisonous gases in planes that might lack air-to-ground control systems.

Current virtual reality systems have developed from these early applications. With VR, a person can see, move through, and react to computer-simulated items or environments. Using certain tools such as a head-mounted computer display and a handheld input device, the user feels immersed in and can interact with this world. The virtual world can represent the current world or a world that is difficult or impossible to experience firsthand—for example, the world of molecules, the interior of the human body, or the surface of Pluto. By putting the sensors on the person (head-mounted computer display, sensors in gloves, shoes, and glasses), the person can move and experience the world in a typical way—by walking, moving, and using the senses of touch, sight, smell, and hearing.

To date, VR applications have been more developed in medicine and other fields, but there is interest in nursing. Within medicine, VR has allowed physicians to develop minimally invasive surgical techniques. Traditionally, surgery is performed by making incisions and directly interacting with the organs and tissues. Recent innovations in video technology allow direct viewing of internal body cavities

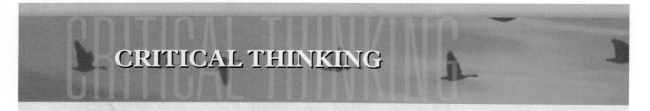

CRITICAL THINKING

Think of the freedom of going wireless. Modern wireless phones allow one to walk around the house, fold laundry, make the bed, straighten up a room, and yes, even go to the bathroom, all while talking on the phone. Remember being tethered by a phone cord?

Many businesses still do not provide their workers with wireless technology. Think of possible reasons why. Would wireless applications in health care settings improve the efficiency of care delivery systems? Why or why not?

through natural orifices or small incisions. The surgeon operates on a virtual image. The manipulation of instruments by the surgeon or assistants can be direct or via virtual environments. In the latter case, a robot reproduces the movements of humans using virtual instruments. The precision of the operation may be augmented by data or images superimposed on the virtual patient (Satava, 1995).

Applications in medical education also exist. Virtual reality allows information visualization through the display of enormous amounts of information contained in large databases. Through 3-D visualization, students can understand important physiological principles or basic anatomy. Students can go "inside" the body to visualize structures and see how they work. It is also possible to observe changes in physiologic functioning. For example, a student can visualize the vascular system of a patient going into shock (Satava, 1993, 1995).

A popular use in psychology has been in exposure therapy for patients with specific phobias. Hodges and colleagues (1995) used a VR reality simulation to treat patients with a fear of flying. Other researchers have found significant improvements in patients with agoraphobia using exposure therapy and VR (North, North, & Coble 1996).

At the University of Dayton Research Institute, Dayton, OH, researchers collaborated with the Miami Valley Transit Authority to assist disabled students to learn to ride the bus. Using a simulation of a public bus, students were able to learn how to get on, get off, and negotiate the interior, which gave them increased confidence and skills when faced with a real bus for the first time (Buckert-Donelson, 1995).

Applications in nursing will be similar. For students learning clinical procedures, VR will give them the opportunity to practice invasive and less commonly occurring procedures in the lab so they will have both the skill and confidence necessary when encountering a patient requiring the procedure for the first time. Likewise, VR will enhance patient education materials. Diabetic patients needing to understand the physiologic processes of the pancreas could visualize the organ to more fully understand their disease and treatment. Patients requiring painful or unusual procedures could experience a VR simulation as a means of preparation. By providing an alternate environment, VR also has the potential to mitigate or minimize the side effects of certain procedures such as chemotherapy in patients with cancer.

THE INTERNET

The Internet will continue to change the way we communicate and obtain information. Many mistakenly believe that the Internet is a recent development. But, like VR, it has been around for more than three decades. The modern Internet started out in 1969 as a U.S. Defense Department network called ARPAnet. Scientists built ARPAnet with the intention of creating a network that would still be able to function efficiently if part of the network were damaged. Since then, the Internet has grown, changed, matured, and mutated, but the essential structure of interconnected domains randomly distributed throughout the world has remained the same. ARPAnet no longer exists, but many of the standards established for that first network still govern the communication and structure of the modern Internet.

In 1989, English computer scientist Timothy Berners-Lee introduced the World Wide Web (WWW). Berners-Lee initially designed the WWW to aid communication between physicists who were working in different parts of the world for the European Laboratory for Particle Physics (CERN). As it grew, however, the WWW revolutionized the use of the Internet. During the early 1990s, increasingly large numbers of users who were not part of the scientific or academic communities began to use the Internet, in large part because of the ability of the WWW to easily handle multimedia documents. Other changes have also influenced the growth of the Internet, such as the High-Performance Computing Act of 1991; the decision to allow computers other than those used for research and military purposes to connect to the network; and the development of "user-friendly" software and tools that allowed less experienced computer users to obtain information quickly and easily.

Using the Internet for Clinical Practice

A major use of the Internet is to obtain information. In clinical practice, this dimension of the Internet is becoming essential to ensure that you have accurate and up-to-date information for your nursing work. To use information that exists on the Internet, it is important to develop skills for searching quickly and efficiently. There are a variety of strategies you can use for searching, including quick and dirty searching, links, and brute force. Keep in mind that you must be persistent: no one search strategy is going to work all the time, nor is any one search engine more effective than any other. A study published in *Science* (Lawrence & Giles, 1998) revealed that the best search engines found approximately 33% of the information available on the Web. That means, of course, that 67% of useful information is being missed. Search engines are good starting points, but you can augment their effectiveness by adding a few other strategies to your Web exploration tool kit.

The P-F-A Assessment

One strategy to develop your search is to conduct a "purpose-focus-approach" (P-F-A) assessment. To determine your purpose, ask yourself why you are doing the search and why you need the information. Consider questions such as the following:

- Is it for personal interest?
- Do you want to obtain information to share with coworkers or a client?
- Are you verifying information given to you by someone else?
- Are you preparing a report or writing a paper for a class or project?

Based on your purpose, your focus may be as follows:

- Broad and general (basic information for yourself)
- Lay oriented (to give information to a patient) or professionally oriented (for colleagues)
- Narrow and technical with a research orientation

Purpose combined with focus determines your approach. For example, information that is broad and general can be found using brute force methods or quick and dirty searching. Lay information can be quickly accessed at a few key sites, including MEDLINE*plus* and consumer health organizations. Similarly, professional associations and societies are a good starting point for professionally oriented information. Scientific and research information usually requires literature resources that can be found in databases such as MEDLINE or CINAHL (Cumulative Index to Nursing and Allied Health Literature).

Quick and Dirty Searching

Quick and dirty searching is a very simple but surprisingly effective search strategy. First, start with a search engine, such as AltaVista (*www.altavista.com*). Next, type in the term of interest. At this point, do not worry about being overly broad or general. You will retrieve an enormous number of found references (called "hits"), but you are interested only in the first 10 to 20. Look at the universal resource locators (URLs), that is, the addresses of the sites that are returned by your search, and try to decipher what they mean. Pay attention to the domains: .com is commercial; .edu is an educational institution; .gov is the government. Quickly visit a few sites. Look for the information you need, or useful links. If a site is not relevant, use the back button on your browser to return to your search results and go to the next site. Once you find a site that appears to be useful, begin to explore the site. Many sites will connect you to other sites, using links, or hot buttons. If you click on a link, it will take you to a related site. If the site you are looking at has links (most do), use them to connect to other relevant sites. This process—quick search, quick review, clicking, and linking—can provide a starting point for finding useful information in a relatively short period of time.

Brute Force

Brute force searching is another alternative. To do this, type in an address in the URL box (the address box at the top of the browser window) and see what happens. The worst outcome is an annoying error message, but you may land on a site that is exactly what you want. To be effective, think how URLs work: they usually start with www (for World Wide Web). Then there is the "thing in the middle" followed by a domain. Perhaps you are trying to find a school of nursing at a certain university. What is the common name for the university? *WWW.unh.edu* is the very logical URL for the University of New Hampshire. Organizations are also quite logical in their URLs: *www.aorn.org* is the Association of periOperative Registered Nurses (AORN); *www.aone.org* is the American Organization of Nurse Executives (AONE).

Links and Bookmarks

As noted earlier, just about every single web site has links to other web sites of related interest. Take advantage of these links because the site developer has already done some of the work of finding other useful resources. Combine quick and dirty searching or brute force with links to get the information you need. Each site you visit will have more links, and in this way, the resources keep building. Visiting a variety of sites will open up the vistas of information that are available. When you find a site of interest, "bookmark" it or add it to your list of favorites. A bookmark list, or list of favorites, is like a personal address book. Each time you find a site that is particularly useful, you can add it to your list of favorites, using the appropriate feature in your browser. Eventually, you will have a comprehensive list of sites that are relevant to your work and interests. By having this list, you will be able to quickly return to sites during future Internet sessions.

Resources for Professionals and Consumers

The preceding discussion has focused on strategies to use when you are faced with a "needle in a haystack" searching situation—just dive in and see what you find. The advantage of this method is that it is fast and easy. There are disadvantages though: sites of dubious quality may be obtained, and the process, while fast, is not terribly efficient.

Another approach is to develop a "short list" of well-known, well-researched sites that can be used as starting points for further exploration. Such a list is useful to share with others so that they can begin their own exploration. These should be sites that you have determined are trustworthy and reliable. Examples of such sites include organizations and associations with which we are all familiar, such as the American Cancer Society (ACS). The ACS has patient education and consumer information materials that can be obtained by a virtual, Internet visit to *www.cancer.org*. In addition to the traditional types of resources available from the ACS, at the web site it is also possible to send an e-mail requesting more information, sign up for regular updates and news, read news items, and obtain updated statistical information. The web site is truly a "value-added" version of the ACS. Practically any health organization you can think of has created a virtual storefront on the Web. Professional associations, in nursing, medicine, and other disciplines, are also becoming comprehensive resource sites on the Web. NursingCenter.com

(*www.nursingcenter.com*) has a handy list of associations in nursing and related disciplines. Use the AssociationLink button on the home page of this site to go to the complete listing.

Other resources include U.S. government agencies, such as the Agency for Healthcare Research and Quality (*www.ahrq.gov*) and the National Institutes of Health (*www.nih.gov*). Once again, all these agencies have been busy creating virtual institutes on the Web. A useful resource is Healthfinder (*www.healthfinder.gov*), which can point you to news, information, tools, and databases.

While these resources are the web versions of known and useful organizations, there are also virtual resources that exist only on the Web. One such site that is particularly impressive is MEDLINE*plus* (*http://medlineplus.gov*), developed by the National Library of Medicine. A similar resource, specific to oncology, is OncoLink at the University of Pennsylvania (*www.oncolink.org*). OncoLink was created in 1994 and was the first multimedia oncology information resource placed on the Internet. It continues to be true to its original mission to "help cancer patients, families, health care professionals and the general public get accurate cancer-related information at no charge" (About Oncolink, 2001).

Literature Resources

Thinking back to P-F-A, if you are searching for scientific, technical, or research-oriented information, then you must search literature databases. In this case, the first place to turn to is the National Library of Medicine, which is the home of the **MEDLARS** (Medical Literature Analysis and Retrieval System), a computerized system of databases and databanks offered by the National Library of Medicine (NLM). A person may search the computer files either to produce a list of publications (bibliographic citations) or to retrieve factual information on a specific question. The most well-known of all the databases in the MEDLARS system is MEDLINE, NLM's premier bibliographic database covering the fields of medicine, nursing, dentistry, veterinary medicine, and the preclinical sciences. Journal articles are indexed for MEDLINE, and their citations are searchable using NLM's controlled vocabulary, called MeSH (Medical Subject Headings). MEDLINE contains all citations published in *Index Medicus* and corresponds in part to the International Nursing Index and the

Index to Dental Literature. Citations include the English abstract when it is published with the article (approximately 76% of the current file). MEDLINE contains more than 11 million records from 4,000 health science journals. The file is updated weekly. An individual can search MEDLINE for free, using PubMed, a specially designed search engine (*http://www.ncbi.nlm.nih.gov/entrez/query.fcgi*). With this search engine, there are no fees to the user to access the MEDLINE database.

Another literature resource to investigate is the National Guideline Clearinghouse (NGC) (*www.ngc.gov*). While MEDLINE includes citations to articles in professional journals, the NGC is a comprehensive database of evidence-based clinical practice guidelines and related documents produced by the Agency for Healthcare Research and Quality (AHRQ) in partnership with the American Medical Association (AMA) and the American Association of Health Plans (AAHP). The NGC mission is to provide physicians, nurses, and other health professionals and health care providers; health plans; integrated delivery systems; purchasers; and others an accessible mechanism for obtaining objective, detailed information on clinical practice guidelines and to further their dissemination, implementation, and use.

There are also a variety of other literature resources available on the Web, some of which have fees attached. However, do not automatically assume that you must pay the fee. Your workplace or school may have licensing agreements in place with different vendors, and as an employee or student you may have access to the literature resources. Check with your library or information services department to see if this applies to you.

The final element of searching for literature on-line is finding full-text articles. The databases so far discussed (MEDLINE and so on) do not contain full text—they include only literature citations. Finding full-text on-line at the present time is an unorganized situation. Options include journals that have full-text available either for free or for a fee, or you can do things the old-fashioned way, that is, take a trip to the library and photocopy articles by hand. Given the state of confusion that exists, your best approach is to begin exploring, using quick and dirty or brute force methods. You can also visit the publisher's web site to see whether access to the journal is available. A final option is to use a document delivery service,

such as UnCover (*http://uncweb.carl.org/*). This resource allows you to conduct a search. It identifies which articles can be sent to you, and what the fees will be (including article fees, service charges, and copyright fees). If you elect to order the article, you can identify how you want to have it sent to you (mail, fax, or other).

Evaluation of Information Found on the Internet

Traveling through the Internet, one must always use critical thinking skills to evaluate the information that is found. The "wide open" nature of the Internet means that just about anyone with a computer and on-line access can create a home page and post it for the world to see. Although there are many excellent health- and nursing-related sites, there are others that just do not measure up in terms of accuracy, content, or currency.

In recent years, criteria for web site evaluation have proliferated. They range from the simple and cursory to the elaborate and expansive. I have found a simple mnemonic, "Are you PLEASED with the site?" to be very helpful (Table 4-1).

The mnemonic makes the seven criteria very easy to remember, but I have found, in hundreds of hours of surfing and evaluating, they are extremely comprehensive (Nicoll, 2000, 2001). To determine whether you are PLEASED, consider the following:

- *P—Purpose.* What is the author's purpose in developing the site? Are the author's objectives clear? Many people will develop a web site as a hobby or way of sharing information they have gathered. It should be immediately evident to you what the true purpose of the site is. At the same time, consider your purpose; that is, think back to your P-F-A assessment. There should be congruence between the author's purpose and yours.
- *L—Links.* Evaluate the links at the site. Are they working? Links that do not take you anywhere are called "dead links." Do they link to reliable sites? It is important to critically evaluate the links at sites hosted by organizations, businesses, or institutions because these entities are usually presenting themselves as authorities on the subject at hand. Some pages,

TABLE 4-1	*Website Evaluation: Ask Yourself, "Am I PLEASED with the Site?"*
P	Purpose
L	Links
E	Editorial (site content)
A	Author
S	Site navigation
E	Ethical disclosure
D	Date site last updated

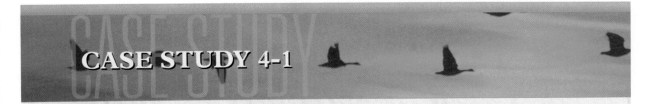

CRITICAL THINKING

PubMed has made the vast resources of the NLM available, for free, to anyone with a computer and Internet hookup. Some argue that scientific publications, such as the *New England Journal of Medicine,* are too technical and sophisticated for laypeople. Others contend that the resources of the NLM are maintained with taxpayer dollars and, therefore, should be available to all taxpayers.

Which point of view do you support? Why? As a health care professional, what resources for understanding and clarification would you suggest to your patients who are accessing abstracts and article citations from the professional health care literature?

CASE STUDY 4-1

You are working in a women's health clinic with a number of nurse practitioners and family physicians. The clinic receives at least two to three telephone calls a day from women with a urinary tract infection (UTI). The question comes up: do all these women need to be seen by a practitioner or is there a way to manage some of the cases by telephone? You are asked to be on a committee to explore this issue and possibly come up with a protocol. Where do you begin? Is a protocol for telephone management of UTI realistic?

such as those created by individuals, are really nothing more than a collection of links. These can be useful as a starting point for a search, but it is still important to evaluate the links that are provided at the site.

- *E—Editorial (site content).* Is the information contained in the site accurate, comprehensive, and current? Is there a particular bias, or is the information presented in an objective way? Who is the consumer of the site: is it designed for health professionals, patients, consumers, or other audiences? Is the information presented in an appropriate format for the intended audience? Look at details, too. Are there misspellings and grammatical errors? "Under construction" banners that have been there forever? These types of errors can be very telling about the overall quality of the site.
- *A—Author.* Who is the author of the site? Does that person or group of people have the

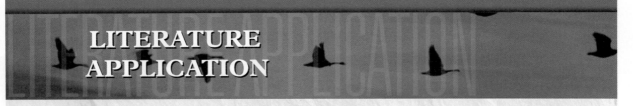

LITERATURE APPLICATION

Citation: Ward, B. O. (1999). "Internet-positive patients" driving you crazy? Find out how to get online and cope. *Internet Medicine, 4*(7), 1, 6.

Discussion: One of the major reasons that people go on-line is to search for health information on the Internet. In fact, since 1996, the number of people who use the Internet for health information climbed from 7.8 million to 31.1 million in the second quarter of 1999. Ready availability of electronic resources to patients is providing health care providers with unique challenges. Patients may arrive in an office or clinic with information that is more up to date and comprehensive than information the provider currently possesses.

What is the best approach to such Internet-positive patients? Keep in mind that your professional education has provided you with skills to critically analyze the information presented, something the patient may not be able to do. Use this as an opportunity to teach; empower the patient for taking the time to research and learn more about his health condition. In addition, you can take the following actions:

- React in a positive manner about information from the Internet, but remind the patient that its quality and reliability are unknown.

- Inform patients that time constraints will not permit you to read the information on the spot; ask them to send it to you (via e-mail, perhaps) before a scheduled appointment.

- Accept patients' contributions and acknowledge that they may have valuable information that you may not have come across yet.

Things you should *not* do include the following:

- Be dismissive or paternalistic
- Be derogatory about others' comments on the Internet
- Refuse Internet material
- Try to "one-up" the patient or family members regarding the information
- Break normal rules of patient confidentiality

Implications for Practice: Clinicians may improve their care delivery by acknowledging Internet information gathered by patients.

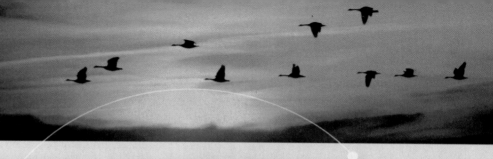

CHAPTER 5

The selection of groups for care should be based on the questions: What difference might nursing care be expected to make in this situation? Is it more or less than would be expected in other groups? (Ruth B. Freeman, 1957)

Population-Based Health Care Practice

Patricia M. Lentsch Schoon, MPH, RN

OBJECTIVES

Upon completion of this chapter, the reader should be able to:

1. Discuss the social mandate to provide population-based health care at the global, national, state, and local levels.

2. Describe how population-based nursing is practiced within the community and the health care system.

3. Identify vulnerable and high-risk population groups for whom specific health promotion and disease prevention services are indicated.

4. Outline a multidisciplinary population-based planning and evaluation process that includes partnerships with the community and health care consumers.

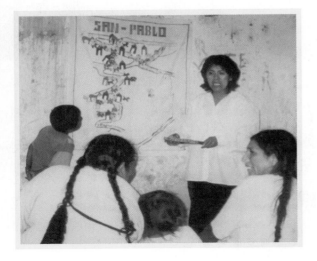

You are completing a clinical experience in an elementary school located in a large metropolitan area. This school has 600 students from kindergarten through sixth grade; 95% of them are from families living at or below the poverty level. Seventy-five percent of the student body transfers in or out of the school during each school year. Of these children, 40% are Southeast Asian, 25% are Hispanic, 10% are African-American, 10% are white, 10% are Somali refugees, and 5% are Native Americans. Sixty percent of the students speak English as a second language. While 95% of the students are eligible for state-sponsored health insurance, only 30% of the children have health insurance, and only 10% have dental insurance. You observe that many children have significant dental problems and many are below the 5th percentile in height and weight on the standardized growth grid. The school nurse encourages you to think about what nursing actions you might take with these two groups of children.

What health problems can you identify in this group of schoolchildren?

What social and environmental factors might contribute to these health problems?

What nursing actions directed at groups of children, rather than individuals, could you take to help these children?

Nurses have acted to improve the health of populations and communities since the time of Florence Nightingale. Nightingale's actions to improve the health care of soldiers on the battlefields of the Crimean War and of the poor and infirm in London were directed at vulnerable population groups. Nightingale's actions were based on the recognition that vulnerable population groups

were not able to advocate effectively for themselves. She became their advocate. Nightingale was able to intervene to improve the health status of disenfranchised groups of people by influencing the health policies of the English government and changing the health care delivery systems in London and on the battlefield. That same spirit of advocacy and call to action is alive today among nurses throughout the world.

The primary thrust of this advocacy is directed at population groups that are at greatest risk for a decrease in health status and those groups that are most vulnerable to the socioeconomic forces that interfere with access to affordable quality health care. Nurses are united in partnership with other health care disciplines, the community, and health care consumers to achieve population-based global, national, state, and local health care goals related to access, cost, and quality. This chapter provides readers with an understanding of how population-based health care is practiced in the public and private health care sectors.

Population-based care requires active partnership of both providers and recipients of care. The phrase *health care consumers* includes current recipients of care, potential or past recipients of care, and other interested parties within the community.

POPULATION-BASED HEALTH CARE PRACTICE

Population-based health care practice is the development, provision, and evaluation of multidisciplinary health care services to population groups experiencing increased health risks or disparities, in partnership with health care consumers and the community in order to improve the health of the community and its diverse population groups. **Vulnerable population groups** are subgroups of a community that are powerless, marginalized, or disenfranchised and are experiencing health disparities.

Health risk factors are variables that increase or decrease the probability of illness or death. Health risk factors may be modifiable (i.e., they can be changed), for example, health care prevention practices, or nonmodifiable (i.e., cannot be changed), for example, age, sex, race, or other inherent physical characteristic. **Health determinants**, a synonym for health risk factors, are variables that include biological, psychosocial, environmental (physical and social), and health system factors or etiologies that may cause changes in the health status of individuals, families, groups, populations, and communities.

The goals of population-based health care include (1) improvement of access to health care services, (2) improvement of quality of health care services, (3) reduction of health disparities among different population groups, and (4) reduction of health care delivery costs. Population-based interventions are provided at three levels: (1) individuals, families, and groups; (2) systems within the community such as health care systems; and, (3) community systems. Outcomes of these interventions are measured in three domains: population health status, quality of life, and functional health status.

Health status is the level of health of an individual, family, group, population, or community. It is the sum of existing health risk factors, level of wellness, existing diseases, functional health status, and quality of life. **Quality of life** is the level of satisfaction one has with the actual conditions of one's life, including satisfaction with socioeconomic status, education, occupation, home, family life, recreation, and the ability to enjoy life, freedom, and independence. Quality of life assessment reviews the perceived and actual ability to be autonomous and independent in making life choices; one's sense of happiness, satisfaction, and security; and the ongoing ability to strive to reach one's potential. **Health-related quality of life** refers to one's level of satisfaction with those aspects of life that are influenced either positively or negatively by one's health status and health risk factors.

Functional health status is the ability to care for oneself and meet one's human needs. Functional abilities are the combined abilities to be independent in both activities of daily life and in the instrumental activities of daily living. **Activities of daily living** are activities related to toileting, bathing, grooming, dressing, feeding, mobility, and verbal and written personal communication. **Instrumental activities of daily living** (IADLs) are activities related to food preparation and shopping; cleaning; laundry; home maintenance; verbal, written, and electronic communications; financial management; and transportation, as well as activities to meet social and support needs, manage health care needs, access community services and resources, and meet spiritual needs. Functional health status affects health-related quality of life.

Addressing the priority health needs of the most vulnerable population groups at the population level rather than the individual level challenges

nurses to target finite health care resources more effectively. Vulnerable population groups are often underserved. The term *underserved* traditionally refers to those who have not received adequate medical care services (Mundt, 1998). These vulnerable groups may have decreased health status and increased risk for morbidity and mortality because of multiple and complex medical and social problems. They may be marginalized, meaning they exist at the margins of mainstream society without access to the majority of community resources and networks. They may be disenfranchised, meaning they do not have the ability to participate in or influence decisions that affect their health care status.

Marginalized groups are often of a different color or ethnic origin than the dominant culture, may speak a different language, may be recent immigrants, and may live in poverty. Partnerships between providers and consumers of health care within diverse communities at any of these levels require cultural sensitivity and competence (Holland & Courtney, 1998). Population-based health care initiatives to help these groups exist at the global, national, regional, and state level. Table 5-1 contains examples of population-based health care initiatives.

HEALTH DETERMINANT MODELS

Health determinant models provide conceptual tools to use in assessing and addressing the priority health needs of at-risk population groups. Recent assessment and intervention models take into account the importance of community systems such as health, social service, government, and economics in influencing the health outcomes in population groups as well as individuals (U.S. Department of Health and Human Services [USDHHS], 2000; Kindig, 1999; Keller, Schaffer, Lia-Hoagberg, & Strohschein, in press). Kindig refers to these influences as mediating variables (Kindig, 1999).

An analysis every 10 years of U.S. health statistics provides the direction for national priorities (USDHHS, 2000). The Healthy People in Healthy Communities 2010 model in Figure 5-1 emphasizes the use of four key elements to achieve health improvement: goals, objectives, determinants of health, and health status. This model lends itself to a partnership approach between health consumers, the community, and health care providers in addressing health needs.

TABLE 5-1	Population-Based Health Care Initiatives

Global Group	Initiatives
World Health Organization	Health for All by the Year 2000. Principles delineated in the Health for All by the Year 2000 plan include (1) the right to health, (2) equity in health, (3) community participation, (4) intersectoral collaboration, (5) health promotion, (6) primary health care, and (7) international cooperation (Bastian, 1989, p. 15).
United Nations	Cairo Action Plan for Women's Health. This plan illustrates the clear link between education, poverty, gender equality, culture, national politics and economies, population growth, and the health status of women (Nelson, Proctor, Regev, Barnes, Sawyer, Messias, Yoder, & Meleis, 1996).

National and Regional Group	Initiatives
Great Britain	Saving Lives: Our Healthier Nation. This initiative focused on the prevention of 300,000 deaths in a 10-year period (Mitchell, 1999).
United States	Healthy People 2010. This initiative highlights health indicators related to the leading causes of death, including health behaviors, physical and social and environmental factors, and health systems factors. (Healthy People, n. d.).
American Public Association (APHA)	Recommends the development of a universal health care system to Health provide for the uninsured and disenfranchised of the country. Commentary on the State of the Public's Health (American Public Health Association, 2001)

State	Initiatives
Arizona	Tobacco Education and Prevention Program (TEPP).Centers for Disease Control. (2001). Tobacco use among adults—Arizona, 1996 and 1999. *Morbidity and Mortality Weekly Report May 25, 2001, 50:20; 402-406.* Retrieved from http://www.cdc.gov/mmwr/preview/mmwrhtml/mm5020a2.htm on 3/27/02.
Arkansas	Community-oriented primary care (COPC) model utilizing family nurse practitioners (Hartwig & Landis, 1999).
New Hampshire	The New Hampshire Coalition against Domestic and Sexual Violence (Hastings, 2001).
New Mexico	"Roll up Your Sleeves" campaign to combat the high incidence of hepatitis B in the state's population. (Harris, Kerr, & Steffen, 1997).
Tennessee	Tenncare, a program to extend health care benefits to the uninsured and to slow down the rapid growth of Medicaid spending (Lyons & Scheb, 1998).

POPULATION-FOCUSED AND POPULATION-BASED NURSING PRACTICE

Population-focused nursing practice and *population-based nursing practice* are terms that are used inter-changeably in contemporary community health nursing literature. Population-focused practice has been an integral part of nursing since the profession began. Florence Nightingale's use of aggregated statistics as population-based indices and outcome measures demonstrates her population-focused practice. Lillian Wald established population-

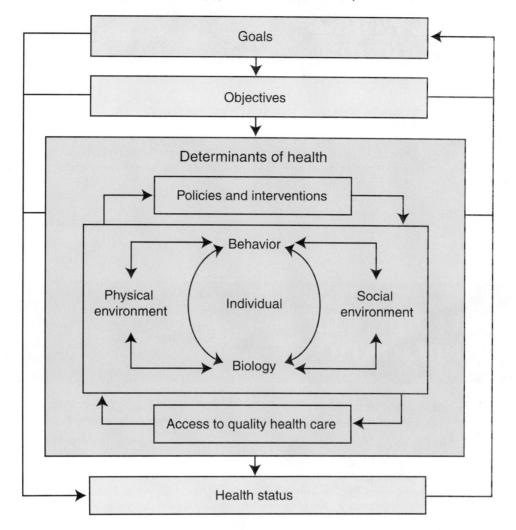

A Systematic Approach to Health Improvement

Figure 5-1 Healthy People 2010. Retrieved January 20, 2002, from
http://www.health.gov/healthypeople/document/pdf/uih/2010uih.pdf.

focused nursing practice in the United States in
the early 1900s. Her population-focused efforts
included founding the Henry Street Nurses' Settle-
ment; helping to establish the Children's Bureau;
and advocating for the rights of children, the mentally ill, the indigent, and immigrants. Wald's vision
of nurses was that they would be "carriers of health"
(Peters, 1995). According to Wald (1915), nurses
were "part of the community plan for the attainment
of communal health" (p. 60). As nursing in the
community became more organized, particularly
in public health agencies, nursing leaders like

Ruth Freeman encouraged nurses to consider the
health needs of the total community as their mission
(Freeman, 1957).

Major societal forces at the beginning of the
21st century are driving transformations in nursing
education and practice. Recommendations from the
Pew Health Professions Commission and others
address the need for nurses to become competent in
population-based practice (Bellack & O'Neil, 2000;
Heller, Oros, & Durney-Crowley, 2000). Paradigm
shifts in health care (McBride, 1999) require an
expansion of the traditional scope of nursing

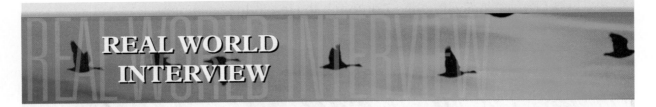

REAL WORLD INTERVIEW

It is amazing what some people have gone through. I work at a free clinic and I couldn't believe some of the things I ran into such as the torture experienced by Mexicans trying to cross the border. We work with illegal immigrants who need us to provide everything they need, including free health visits and free medications. If we set up a free referral to a specialty, they need us to provide transportation and an interpreter. For the most part, the immigrants I have met are grateful for what we do for them.

Anita M. Matos, RN
Degree Completion Nursing Student

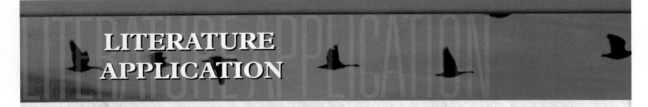

LITERATURE APPLICATION

Citation: Bauer, H. M., Rodriguez, M. A., Quiroga, S. S., & Flores-Ortiz, Y. G. (2000). Barriers to health care for abused Latina and Asian immigrant women. *Journal of Health Care for the Poor and Underserved, 11*(1), 33–44.

Discussion: This qualitative study included 28 abused Latina and Asian immigrant women. Data were collected using four semistructured, ethnic-specific focus group interviews. Many sociopolitical and sociocultural factors were identified as barriers to seeking help and patient-provider communication. Sociopolitical barriers included social isolation, language barriers, discrimination, and fear of deportation. Sociocultural barriers included dedication to children and family unity, shame related to the abuse, and the cultural stigma of abuse.

Implications for Practice: Nurses must be aware not only of those who seek care but also those who do not. Culturally competent outreach and case finding programs are needed to identify and serve hidden underserved populations. Nurses can play a strong advocacy role in the process.

practice as well as changes in how nursing education is provided. In the future, both nursing education and nursing practice will place a greater emphasis on use of population-based mortality and morbidity statistics for assessment of community health needs. They will focus on maximizing health status, functional abilities, and improving the quality of life of groups of health care consumers.

Population-Focused Nursing Practice

The American Nurses Association (1995) states that population-focused nursing practice is "defined by nursing activities that focus on all of the people and reflects responsibility to and for the people." Furthermore, "provision of services to those who appear for service are not population focused without actions to gain participation of the entire population who might benefit from that service."

Baldwin and colleagues describe population-focused nursing "as the nursing specialty arena that concentrates upon specific groups of well or sick people, focusing on health promotion and disease prevention regardless of geographic location" (Baldwin, Conger, Abegglen, & Hill, 1998, p. 17). In population-focused nursing practice, the nurse assesses the health of the community, arrives at a nursing diagnosis, and identifies population groups most in need of health care services. This process involves the investigation of major health and environmental problems, health surveillance, and monitoring and evaluation of community and population health status (Williams, 2000).

Williams (2000) describes population-focused practice as nursing practice that is based on public health philosophy, grounded in basic clinical nursing practice, and involving the identification of problems (assessment and diagnosis) and solutions (interventions) that are implemented with a defined population, subpopulation, or aggregate (group of people with shared risk factor). Williams' concept extends the practice of community health nursing and the specialty area of population-based nursing practice into noncommunity health clinical practice settings (Figure 5-2).

Population-Based Nursing Practice

Population-based nursing practice is defined as the practice of nursing in which the focus of care is to improve the health status of vulnerable or at-risk population groups within the community by employing health promotion and disease prevention interventions across the health continuum. Health care consumers are involved as full partners in the planning and evaluation of the nursing services provided. Population-based nursing practice is holistic in nature, taking into account cultural and ethnic diversity, religious and spiritual uniqueness, economic disparities, and geographic and regional differences. It seeks to empower population groups by enhancing their protective factors and resiliency. **Protective factors** are client strengths and resources that clients can use to combat health threats that compromise core human functions. Resilience includes complex psychological mechanisms such as, risk taking, coping, protective factors, capacity to change and persevere, ability to attach meaning to events, and self-reliance (Rew, Taylor-Seehafer, Thomas, & Yockey, 2001). **Resilience** is the

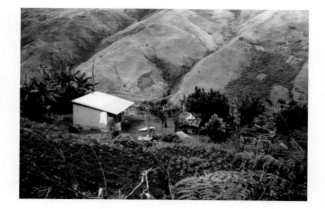

Figure 5-2a Bolivian mountain homestead where nursing students help Indian women plant and harvest their vegetable gardens, so their children will have nutritious food.

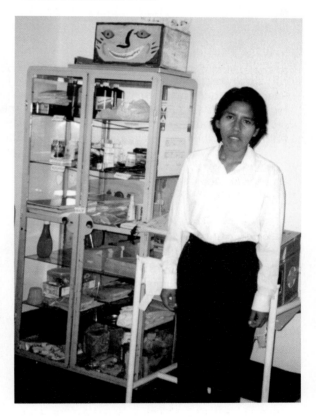

Figure 5-2b Public health nursing instructor holds clinic hours in Andes mountain village in Bolivia. The clinic was built by student workers and villagers.

social and psychosocial capacity of individuals and groups to adapt, succeed, and persevere over time in the face of recurring threats to psychosocial and physiologic integrity. For purposes of simplicity, the

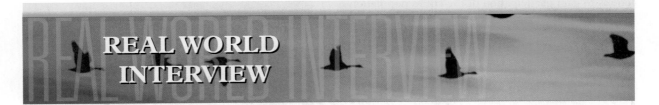

A collaborative partnership between two colleges a continent apart took me to Unidad Academica Campesina, a satellite of the Catholic University of Bolivia, in Carmen Panpa, Bolivia. Students from this rural area attend the college to study nursing, agronomy, education, and veterinary science. Community service in each program provides assistance, including nursing care, to at least 13 surrounding villages in the highlands of the Andes Mountains.

The Aymaran and Quechuan Indians, agrarian people who live in these villages, have a per capita annual income of $200. Transportation to their villages is very difficult. Primary health concerns are malnutrition, parasitic diseases, diarrhea and dehydration, skin infections, pneumonia, and tuberculosis. Nursing education and practice have been modified to fit the primary health needs of these natives. Nursing students, carrying supplies in their backpacks, often walk 2 to 4 hours each way to provide health care to people who have no other access to health care. Student nurses and faculty often leave the college at 4:00 A.M. in order to reach rural homes before mothers leave for the fields to work. Students work with women to improve family nutrition by helping them plant gardens and teaching women to cook using nutritious foods. They work to empower these illiterate, impoverished women.

Each village has built a small clinic from which students provide health services such as prenatal screening and treatments for various diseases, using medications made from many indigenous plants. People too ill to come to the clinic receive home visits. Nursing students also provide health education on nutrition, hygiene, and parasitic diseases to children and their families in the village schools.

Carol Pavlish
Associate Professor, College of St. Catherine

term *population-based nursing practice* will refer to both population-focused nursing practice and population-based nursing practice for the rest of the chapter.

The goals of population-based nursing practice are consistent with the health goals identified by the World Health Organization (WHO), Healthy People 2010, and the American Nurses Association (ANA). Population-based nursing practice goals address the health needs of individuals, families, communities, and population groups and focus on the goals of health care access, quality, cost, and equity.

POPULATION-BASED NURSING PRACTICE APPLICATIONS

A population-based public health interventions, applications for public health nursing practice model developed by the Minnesota Department of Health

(2001) is in concert with the public mandate that directs public health agencies to protect the health of the public they serve. A primary principle of population-based nursing practice is that it is initiated with a community health assessment. Multidisciplinary interventions are developed based on the community health priorities identified in the assessment process.

Population-based interventions encompass three levels: the community; systems within the community; and individuals, families, and groups. Population-based community-focused practice changes community norms, attitudes, practices, and behaviors. Population-based systems-focused practice changes laws, power structures, policies, and organizations. Population-based individual-focused practice changes the knowledge, attitudes, beliefs, practices, and behaviors of individuals, families, and groups (Keller, Strohschein, Lia-Hoagberg, & Schaffer, 1998; Keller, Schaffer, Lia-Hoagberg, & Strohschein, in press). Figure 5-3 depicts the Minnesota Depart-

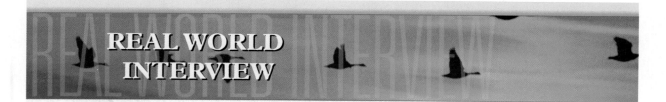

REAL WORLD INTERVIEW

The Hmong Health Care Professionals Coalition received a grant to do community education to the elderly Hmong population regarding depression. Depression was considered a risk for Hmong elders because there had been several suicides in that population. Many Hmong elders were isolated and did not view depression as a disease. In addition, other agencies serving this population had also identified depression as an issue for the elders.

In doing outreach to the target population, several adaptations specific to the Hmong culture were made. One was in regard to eligibility criteria. Even though the program targeted persons over 50, people were allowed to determine their own eligibility. That is, if they "felt old," they qualified. Second, although the coalition had a booth at the annual Hmong Health Fair, the coalition members considered it unlikely that the elders would come to the booth. Therefore, the interviewers decided to walk around and talk with elders in a more relaxed setting. They approached elders while sitting under shade trees, selling products at the market booth, and the like. Third, interviews were done entirely in the Hmong language. Elderly persons were screened, provided information about depression, and given a list of community resources.

Ma Her, PHN
St. Paul-Ramsey County Department of Public Health

From Her, M. (2001) "Outreach" in Getting Behind the Wheel, *Public Health Nursing Online Newsletter*, 15. Section of Public Health Nursing, Minnesota Department of Health. Retrieved from http://www.health.state. mn.us/divs/chs/phn/phnnews15.html on 7/13/01.

ment of Health Public Health Interventions II Wheel developed by the section of public health nursing.

These interventions have a logical sequence. For example, to provide health services to underserved and vulnerable population groups, outreach (finding the people at risk in the community) and screening must precede referral, teaching, counseling, and consultation.

Nursing interventions need to be provided in a culturally proficient manner to be effective with culturally diverse population groups. Cultural proficiency involves the integration of cultural competence into all areas of nursing practice and health care organizational culture (Wells, 2000). Cultural incompetence is a barrier to access, quality, and equity in health care for populations of color and ethnic diversity. Cultural sensitivity and competence are necessary for the provision of health promotion interventions which result in improved health status of culturally diverse population groups. Populations of diversity cannot retain their autonomy in health care decision making and self-care if they do not have an under-standing of how the health care system works and how to access health services congruent with their cultural beliefs and practices (Crow, Matheson, & Steed, 2000).

Nontraditional Model

A nontraditional model of population-based nursing practice is emerging. This model is being developed by private for-profit and nonprofit health care organizations. In this model, the vulnerable or at-risk population group is identified before community assessment occurs, and the subsequent community assessment process focuses on health determinants related to the at-risk group. The organizations generally focus on the population groups within their service areas, their market niche, and current membership. The primary goal of these organizations is usually to contain or reduce health care costs. The secondary goal is to improve the quality of care provided to their membership to improve health outcomes. Generally, the population groups who have the highest health risks, the poorest health outcomes,

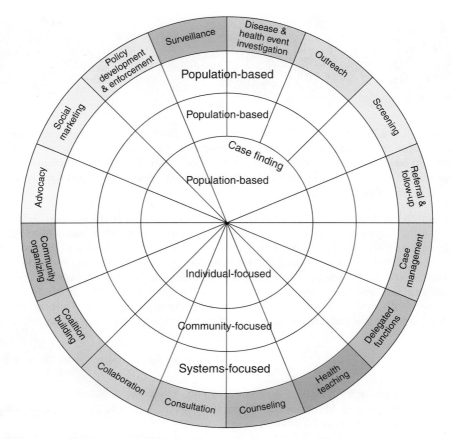

Figure 5-3 The Minnesota Department of Health Public Health Interventions II Wheel. Used with permission of the Section of Public Health Nursing, Minnesota Department of Health. Retrieved from http://www.health.state.mn.us/divs/chs/phn/manfrm.html on July 13, 2001.

and the highest service costs are the groups targeted for additional services. Population groups with multiple diagnoses, called comorbidities, as well as complex therapeutic treatment regimes and a pattern of noncompliance and missed visits are also targeted for services. Note the traditional and nontraditional models of population-based nursing practice outlined in Table 5-2.

USE OF THE NURSING PROCESS IN POPULATION-BASED NURSING PRACTICE

The nursing process is used in population-based nursing practice to assess, diagnose, plan, implement, and evaluate nursing practice.

Assessment

Population assessment is structured by using a model as a guide for data collection. Table 5-3 is an excerpt from a template for data collection based on the health determinants in the Healthy People in Healthy Communities model discussed previously. Table 5-4 lists data sources for population-based assessment.

Nursing Diagnosis

The first step in constructing a population-based nursing diagnosis is to identify the North American Nursing Diagnosis Association (NANDA) diagnostic category. The next step is to identify the etiology and list the key evidence that supports the diagnostic category. An example of a complete diagnosis is "ineffective community coping in Unity County related to

TABLE 5-2	*Population-Based Nursing Practice*

Traditional Model	**Nontraditional Model**
Total community is primary focus.	At-risk or high-risk population is primary focus.
⬇	⬇
Assess total community needs.	Assess health needs of at-risk or high-risk population group.
⬇	⬇
Identify at-risk or vulnerable population groups.	Assess service area/surrounding community to identify health determinants and resources.
⬇	⬇
Identify fit between nursing resources and at-risk population group health needs.	Identify fit between nursing resources and at-risk population group health needs.
⬇	⬇
Target resources and provide interventions.	Target resources and provide interventions.
⬇	⬇
Evaluate population outcomes.	Evaluate population outcomes.
⬇	⬇
Reassess total community health needs.	Reassess at-risk population group health.
⬇	⬇
Determine new priority: Health need of other at-risk groups within community.	Determine new priority: Health need of other at-risk groups within service area.

hunger and loss secondary to hurricane damage as evidenced by the number of people reporting stress and the lack of food for over 24 hours after the storm."

Planning and Implementation

The primary planning and implementation framework for population-based nursing practice is drawn from community health nursing. The Minnesota Department of Health (MDH), Section of Public Health Nursing, with an advisory group of public health nurses, developed a population-based nursing practice intervention model (Keller, Schaffer, Lia-Hoagberg, & Strohschein, 2002). Table 5-5 (page 110) compares this model with a model developed in Virginia (Kosidlak, 1999). The Virginia model also

relied on interviews with practicing public health nurses.

A sample of a population-based nursing intervention plan is presented in Figure 5-4 (page 111). The plan includes elements of the Minnesota Department of Health, Public Health Interventions II Wheel, identified earlier in Figure 5-3.

Evaluation

Outcomes of population-based nursing practice focus on health status, functional abilities, and quality of life of at-risk population groups. Data are collected that reflect the aggregated response of the total at-risk group for each specified outcome. Descriptive statistics, such as mean, range, and percentages as well as biometric measures such as rates are used in the analysis of group data. Case studies

(continues on page 114)

TABLE 5-3	Population-Based Health Determinants Assessment Template — Excerpt

Community Level

Physical Environment

- Housing and geographic location, safety of neighborhoods, community, and school quality
- Environmental quality: air, water, ground, chemical, physical, and biological hazards
- Availability of transportation, communication systems, parks, and recreation facilities

Social Environment

- Community norms, values, and patterns of behavior; political structures within community
- Incidence of crime and violence within the population group and the larger community
- Employment opportunities within community, economic viability of community

Policies and Interventions

- National, state, county, and city health and social policies
- Policies of public, private, and voluntary organizations that provide health and social services
- Policies of health insurance companies, health maintenance organizations, health systems, and health care provider groups

Health Systems Level

Access to Quality Health Care

- Appropriate primary, secondary, and tertiary health services and providers
- Health and social services workforce (numbers, diversity, interdisciplinary mix, deployment, sustainability); educational institutions offering health care provider education and training
- Availability of health and social services resources 24 hours a day, 7 days per week

Population Level

Biological

- Demographic data (age, gender, racial/ethnic patterns)
- Biological and genetic factors, patterns of health and disease (morbidity and mortality data)

Behavioral

- Education patterns and levels, cultural patterns (lifestyle, languages, religion)
- Socioeconomic status (employment patterns, housing, health and dental insurance)
- Cultural health patterns (health beliefs and self-care practices, nutrition, fitness, previous experiences with health care system, current health providers, family and intergenerational health patterns)

Data Analysis

- Prioritize the health needs of the community and prioritize the vulnerable and at-risk population groups based on need and health status.
- Identify the modifiable and nonmodifiable health risks of the at-risk population.
- Identify the biological, psychosocial, environmental, cultural, political, financial, and iatrogenic causes of the identified health risks.

TABLE 5-4	*Data Sources for Population-Based Assessment*

Data utilized may be primary (collected by group conducting assessment) or secondary (collected from other sources).

Common sources of primary data

- Key informant interviews and surveys of health and social services providers, community leaders, media, governmental agency officials and personnel
- Key informant interviews, surveys, and observations (participant and nonparticipant) of members of at-risk or vulnerable population groups (may require formal approval process if research done on human subjects)
- Windshield and walk-through surveys of the community and organizations involved

Common sources of secondary data

- Health data, vital statistics, and census data obtained from governmental sources
- Community planning documents
- Health reports on subpopulations from governmental, voluntary, private organizations, and consumer groups
- Scientific and professional literature and databases
- Proprietary client/member population data from health care insurers and providers—may be available only to employees of the organization
- The news and communications media, including newspapers, journals, television, radio, and the Internet

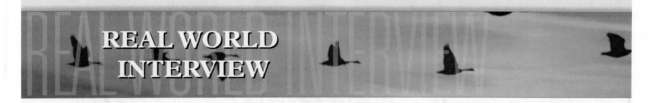

REAL WORLD INTERVIEW

Several years ago, I spent a month in Peru as a volunteer with a group of surgeons. This experience gave me insight into the health status of other countries. Before patients came into the hospital, they were given a "shopping list" of items they had to buy. The list included intravenous bags and tubing, dressings and tape, and needles for injections and IV lines. The families provided the sheets and blankets for the beds. Food was served a couple of times a day, but it was mostly soup. If the patients wanted more substantial food, their families had to cook it and bring it in. Some of the families came from rural areas, several days' walk from the town. Since they could not return home, they would sleep in the patient's bed, on the floor near them, or in the courtyard of the hospital. Having a family member in the hospital was a very expensive experience for these families. It took a large portion of their savings to provide basic needs for their family members. Since that trip, I try to be aware of the nurses and doctors who volunteer in Third World countries so we can save supplies for them.

Catherine Miller, RN
Degree Completion Nursing Student

TABLE 5-5	Comparison of Population-Based Nursing Practice Intervention Models	
	Minnesota Model (MDH, 2001)	**Virginia Model (Kosidlak, 1999)**
Surveillance	x	
Disease/health threat investigation	x	
Outreach	x	Community outreach
Screening	x	x
Case finding	x	
Referral and follow-up	x	
Advocacy	x	
Coalition building	x	x
Community organizing	x	
Consultation	x	
Policy development and enforcement	x	
Social marketing	x	Public awareness
Case management	x	
Counseling	x	
Delegated functions	x	
Health teaching	x	Public education
Provider education	x	x

Compiled with information from "Assessment, Program Planning, and Evaluation in Population-Based Public Health Practice," by L. O. Keller, M. Schaffer, B. Lia-Hoagberg, and S. Strohschein, 2002, *Journal of Public Health Management and Practice* and from "The Development and Implementation of a Population-Based Intervention Model for Public Health Nursing Practice," by J. G. Kosidlak, 1999, *Public Health Nursing, 16*(5), 311–320.

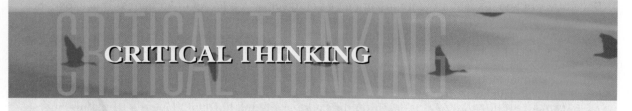

CRITICAL THINKING

Consider the implications of the following situation. Your community is experiencing a measles epidemic. You are asked to forgo your home visits to your hospice clients for 1 day so that you can staff a measles immunization clinic. You have three hospice visits scheduled, one to a family with a child near death. By staffing the immunization clinic, you would be able to vaccinate and protect 150 children.

What decision would you make? What alternative choices might you have in resolving this dilemma?

NURSING DIAGNOSIS: Female students, ages 13 to 15, in Data Middle School at risk for altered nutrition: less than body requirements related to nutritional habits, body image disturbance, sense of powerlessness, and lack of screening and outreach services as evidenced by:

- 10% of the female students are below the 5th percentile in weight but above the 25th percentile in height on standardized growth and development charts.

- 75% of the female students report that they routinely skip breakfast on 3 or more school days per week, and 50% routinely eat snacks from the vending machines for lunch.

- 90% of the female students agree with the statement, "I do not like my body the way it is."

- 80% of the female students agree with the statement, "It is very important to me and my friends to be thin."

- 20% of the female students report that their lives are out of control and one of the only things they have control over is their eating behaviors.

- The school staff has not been trained to refer girls who appear extremely thin or are not eating meals to the school nurse.

GOAL: Reduce the risk for altered nutrition among 13-to-15-year-old female students at Data Middle School.

MODIFIABLE RISK FACTORS: Nutrition habits, body image disturbance, powerlessness, lack of screening and outreach services

PROTECTIVE FACTORS: Friendship and peer network, school nurse, social worker, and counseling staff, school breakfast and lunch program, primary care clinic open at school

STRENGTHS, ASSETS, RESILIENCE: Most of the girls have parents they are willing to talk to about nutrition, students like health and fitness class and instructor at school, school district has small amount of money to start intervention program, most at-risk females visit health office often and appear motivated to improve their health and fitness.

OUTCOMES	INTERVENTIONS	PROVIDERS	EVALUATION
1. 75% of the students will obtain lunch from cafeteria rather than vending machines by 1/1/02. (P)	1.1 Health teaching: nutrition 1.2 Collaboration: redesigning how and where students eat lunch 1.3 Policy development: change school policies about use of vending machines during lunch hour	School nurse, health teachers Administration, food services, student council, school nurse School board	Student survey Cafeteria register count
2. 50% of students at risk will agree with the statement, "I like my body the way it is" by 5/01/02. (P)	2.1 Counseling: support group for at-risk students, peer counseling	Social workers, psychologist, school nurse, peer helpers and peer helper instructor	Survey or interview
3. 100% of the students at risk will agree with the statement, "I am more in charge of my life than I was 6 months ago" by 5/01/02. (P)	3.1 Counseling: support group for at-risk students, peer counseling	Social workers, psychologist, school nurse, peer helpers and peer helper instructor	Survey or interview

C: community-focused outcome; P: population-focused outcome related to individuals, families, small groups; S: system-focused outcome.

Figure 5-4 Sample Population-Based Nursing Intervention Plan

(continues)

OUTCOMES	INTERVENTIONS	PROVIDERS	EVALUATION
4. A screening and outreach program to identify and refer students at risk for eating disorders will be implemented by 1/30/02. (S)	4.1 Outreach and referral: program implemented school-wide for outreach and referral	Administration, school staff, peer counselors	Provider survey
	4.2 Screening: process for screening at-risk students will be developed and implemented	Administration, school nurse, social workers, psychologist	Log of students referred analyzed
	4.3 Provider education: workshop and information sheets will be provided to school staff	Administration, school staff, health education teacher, school nurse	
	4.4 Social marketing: parents association and school board will be targeted for informational meetings	Administration, PTA, school nurse, health education teacher, school board	Evaluation at end of meeting of school board
5. 25% of students with weight below the 5th percentile and height above the 25th percentile on a standardized growth grid will weigh above the 5th percentile by 6/1/02. (P)	5.1 Surveillance: a monitoring program for at-risk students will be developed and implemented	School nurse, administration	Review of student progress records
6. 75% of participants on community health education will agree at end of session that adolescents with eating disorders are an important health priority in their community. (C)	6.1 Social marketing and health teaching: Community education department will hold a communitymeeting on eating disorders and adolescencein June 2002	Panel: health educator, school psychologist, social worker, school nurse, nutritionist, physician	Exit survey

C: community-focused outcome; P: population-focused outcome related to individuals, families, small groups; S: system-focused outcome.

Figure 5-4 *(continued)*

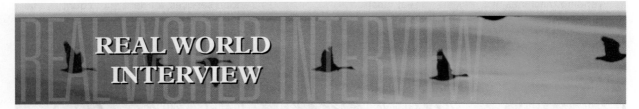

REAL WORLD INTERVIEW

The current philosophy within the state of Minnesota is to provide long-term care services where the elderly want those services delivered. Most frail elderly desire to have their needs for assistance met in their own homes. Care in the home setting puts these frail elderly at particular risk for abuse and neglect, as licensed professional nurses do not directly supervise care on a daily basis. Monthly supervision by a licensed professional is all that is currently required to maintain home care services. However, remaining in the home setting allows the elderly the independence they crave within the community where they reside. Until the needs of the frail elderly become a priority with lawmakers, home care services will not meet their needs. The ideal solution is to provide long-term care services where, when, and how the elderly desire the delivery of those services and to provide the level of supervision and case management services that guarantee safe care and decrease the risk of abuse and neglect. The practical solution, based on available resources, is to provide limited supervision and case management services in the home setting and to encourage frail elderly to enter institutional care when community-based care is not available at a safe level.

Holly Cain, BSN
Former Medicare Quality Improvement Coordinator

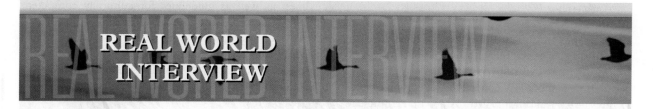

REAL WORLD INTERVIEW

I work with pregnant and parenting teens at an alternative high school program that provides educational options for teens whose lives don't fit the traditional school day. Our program includes teens from a variety of cultures and backgrounds. The program currently has eight young women who will deliver their babies during the school year. This year, we also have four young fathers enrolled. The program has an on-site child care center, so these students bring their children to school with them and are able to visit their child during the school day.

Another public health nurse and I share this assignment. We teach weekly prenatal classes in conjunction with the life skills class that all our students are required to take for graduation. Each student spends time working in the child care rooms, both in their own child's room as well as the next age group's room. This provides us with the opportunity to discuss growth and development, health care, and to role model parent-child interactions.

We also work with each student to look at family planning options for him or her and are very proud of a program we started called The Pregnancy Free Club. This is a voluntary "club" that allows each student to have private time with a public health nurse to talk about how to use birth control correctly and look at barriers that prevent the student from effectively using birth control.

Peer support has also become an unexpected part of this program, making it easier and more acceptable for the students to talk about their birth control choice or their choice of abstinence. Our program currently has a repeat pregnancy rate significantly lower than the national average.

Barbara Reilly, PHN
City of Bloomington Health Department

From Reilly, B. (2001). "Health Teaching" in Getting Behind the Wheel, *Public Health Nursing Online Newsletter, 13.* Section of Public Health Nursing, Minnesota Department of Health. Retrieved from http://www.health.state.mn.us/divs/chs/phn/phnnews13.html on 7/13/01.

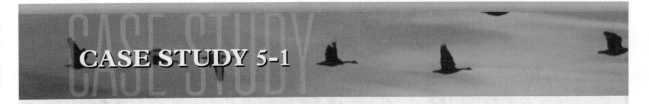

CASE STUDY 5-1

You are caring for a 72-year-old client, Mrs. Ramone, in her home. She lives mainly off her Social Security pension. She is getting weaker each time you visit her, yet she wants to stay in her home as long as she can.

What nursing advocacy initiatives might you undertake to ensure the provision of safe home care services to Mrs. Ramone? How might you justify the distribution of resources to assist Mrs. Ramone to stay in her home longer?

(continued from page 107)
illustrating how services are provided to clients are also very effective. The evaluation process involves the multidisciplinary team, health consumers, and community partnerships. After the evaluation of population outcomes is completed, the unmet needs of the at-risk population groups are determined to identify whether further interventions are necessary.

PROGRAM EVALUATION

Program evaluation is an integral part of the evaluation process when providing population-based care. Justification of resources and budget is necessary. A cost-benefit analysis, comparing improvements in health status, functional abilities, and quality of life of the targeted at-risk population with expenditures of human and material resources, is appropriate. Ethical guide-

lines, as well as guidelines for culturally competent care, should be used to evaluate the efficacy of health provider interactions with vulnerable or marginalized population groups. A set of questions that may be used to focus program evaluation is found in Figure 5-5.

KEY CONCEPTS

- The focus of population-based health care is to reduce health disparities that exist among diverse population groups.
- The goals of population-based health care and population-based nursing care are access, quality, cost containment, and equity.
- Population-based nursing practice focuses on at-risk, vulnerable, and underserved population groups.

	Program Evaluation of Population Based Nursing Practice
Access	Did we find the high-risk, underserved, vulnerable population groups in the community/service area and provide timely and accessible services?
	Did we offer service regardless of age, gender, race, ethnicity, health care status, or location?
Quality	Did our services meet the greatest unmet health needs of the community or the at-risk, vulnerable, underserved population groups?
	Did their health status improve?
	Were their health risks reduced?
	Were they satisfied with the services they received?
Cost	Were patients able to afford what we had to offer?
	Did we manage to stay within our budget?
	Are we reducing the cost of care over time?
Equity	Did we use our resources in a way that met the priority health needs of all of our high-risk patient groups?
	Did we target our services and use our resources to improve the health status of those who were the most underserved?
	Did we have enough resources left over to meet the essential health needs of lower-risk population groups?

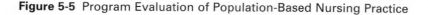

Figure 5-5 Program Evaluation of Population-Based Nursing Practice

- Traditional population-based nursing practice usually starts with a community health needs assessment that identifies health priorities and at-risk vulnerable population groups.
- Nontraditional population-based nursing practice starts with an identified at-risk group and is followed by a health assessment related to the at-risk group.
- Population-based health care involves multidisciplinary, health consumer, and community partnerships.
- Population-based intervention strategies focused at the population, health systems, and community levels are necessary to improve the health of the population as a whole.
- Outcomes of population-based health care are measured at the population level. Three domains of population outcomes are health status, functional abilities, and quality of life.
- Nurses play key roles in the successful development and implementation of population-based health care services.

KEY TERMS

activities of daily living
functional health status
health determinants
health-related quality
   of life
health risk factors
health status
instrumental activities
   of daily living

population-based
   health care practice
population-based
   nursing practice
protective factors
quality of life
resiliency
vulnerable population
   groups

REVIEW QUESTIONS

1. The four goals of population-based nursing practice are
   A. access, cost, empowerment, equity.
   B. access, cost, equity, resilience.
   C. access, cost, equity, quality.
   D. cost, equity, resilience, quality.
2. Population-based nursing interventions are directed at
   A. all individuals who need health services.

B. people without health care insurance.
C. the health needs of the total community.
D. only vulnerable groups within the community.

3. Major causes of international and U.S. health disparities include
   A. gender, race, ethnicity, and poverty.
   B. lack of sustainable health care systems.
   C. poverty and national economic conditions.
   D. TB, diarrhea, malaria, and AIDS.

4. Priority population-based nursing interventions for indigent families with limited access to health care and many unmet health needs should include
   A. advocacy, community organizing, social marketing, coalition building.
   B. disease and health event investigation, screening, referral, consultation.
   C. outreach, screening, referral and follow-up, health teaching and counseling.
   D. screening, referral and follow-up, case management, surveillance.

REVIEW ACTIVITIES

1. Compare and contrast individual-focused nursing practice with population-based nursing practice. What nursing knowledge and skills do you need to practice population-based nursing care?

2. Hilfinger (2001) believes that nurses should adopt a global framework for the empowerment of women to reduce health disparities. Discuss what you think this framework should include. How could you become a nursing advocate for this at the local, national, and international levels?

3. Survey your classmates using the health determinants assessment framework excerpt. Analyze your data and identify common health risk factors within the group.

EXPLORING THE WEB

- Where could you find information to help serve the health care needs of immigrants? National Institutes of Health: *http://www.nih.gov* Office of U.S. Surgeon General: *http://www. surgeongeneral.gov*

U.S. Department of Health and Human Services: *http://ww.os.dhhs.gov*
Center for Cross-Cultural Health: *http://www.crosshealth.com*
Race and health: *http://www.os.dhhs.gov/topics/minority.html*
Immigration and Refugee Services of America (IRSA): *http://www.refugeesusa.org*
United Nations: *http://www.un.org*
World Health Organization: *http://www.who.int*

- What sites could you review for data about your community and the nation?
  Statistics on any U.S. community: *http://www.scorecard.org*
  U.S. national statistics: *http://www.fedstats.gov*

REFERENCES

American Nurses Association. (1995). *Position statements—promotion and disease prevention.* Retrieved March 30, 2002, from http://nursingworld.org/readroom/position/social/scprmo.htm.

American Public Health Association. (2001). *The fourteen points for the campaign for universal health care—the nation's health.* Retrieved July 9, 2001, from http://www.apha.org/legislative/issues/reform.htm

Baldwin, J. H., Conger, C. O., Abegglen, J. C., & Hill, E. M. (1998). Population-focused and community-based nursing—moving toward clarification of concepts. *Public Health Nursing, 15*(1), 12–18.

Bastian, H. (1989). A guide to WHO and "WHO speak." *Consumer Health Forum, 9,* 15.

Bauer, H. M., Rodriguez, M. A., Quiroga, S. S., & Flores-Ortiz, Y. G. (2000). Barriers to health care for abused Latina and Asian immigrant women. *Journal of Health Care for the Poor and Underserved, 11*(1), 33–44.

Bellack, J. P., & O'Neil, E. H. (2000). Recreating nursing practice for a new century. Recommendations and implications of the Pew Health Professions Commission's final report. *Nursing and Health Care Perspectives, 21*(1), 14–21.

Centers for Disease Control. (2001). Tobacco use among adults—Arizona, 1996 and 1999. *Morbidity and Mortality Weekly Report May 25, 2001, 50:20; 402–406.* Retrieved from http://www.cdc.gov/mmwr/preview/mmwrhtml/mm5020a2.htm on March 27, 2002.

Crow, K., Matheson, L., & Steed, A. (2000). Informed consent and truth-telling: Cultural directions for healthcare providers. *Journal of Nursing Administration, 30*(3), 148–152.

Duncan, S. M. (1996). Empowerment strategies in nursing education: A foundation for population-focused clinical studies. *Public Health Nursing, 13*(5), 311–317.

Freeman, R. B. (1957). *Public health nursing practice* (2nd ed.). Philadelphia: Saunders.

Harris, P. A., Kerr, J., & Steffen, D. (1997). A state-based immunization campaign: the New Mexico experience. *Journal of School Health, 67*(7), 273–276.

Hartwig, M. S., & Landis, B. J. (1999). The Arkansas AHEC model of community-oriented primary care. *Holistic Nurse Practitioner, 13*(4), 28–37.

Hastings, D. P. (2001). The New Hampshire health initiative on domestic violence. *Nursing Forum, 36*(1), 31–35.

Healthy People. (n. d.). *What are the leading health indicators?* Retrieved January 20, 2002, from http://www.health.gov/healthypeople/document/pdf/uih/2010uih.pdf

Heller, B. R., Oros, M. T., & Durney-Crowley, J. (2000). The future of nursing education. Ten trends to watch. *Nursing and Health Care Perspectives, 21*(1), 9–13.

Her, M. (2001). "Outreach": Getting Behind the Wheel. *Public Health Nursing Newsletter, 15.* Retrieved July 13, 2001, from http://www.health.state.mn.us/divs/chs/phn/phnnews15.html

Hilfinger, D. K. (2001). Globalization, nursing, and health for all. *Journal of Nursing Scholarship, 33*(1), 9–11.

Holland, L., & Courtney, R. (1998). Increasing cultural competence with the Latino community. *Journal of Community Health Nursing, 15*(1), 45–53.

Keller, L. O., Schaffer, M., Lia-Hoagberg, B., & Strohschein S. (in press). Assessment, program planning, and evaluation in population-based public health practice. *Journal of Public Health Management and Practice.*

Keller L. O., Strohschein S., Lia-Hoagberg, B., & Schaffer, M. (1998). Population-based public health nursing interventions: A model from practice. *Public Health Nursing, 15*(3), 207–215.

Kindig, D. A. (1999). Purchasing population health: Aligning financial incentives to improve health outcomes. *Nursing Outlook, 47,* 15–22.

Lyons, W., & Scheb, J. M., II. (1998). Managed care and Medicaid reform in Tennessee: The impact of Tenncare on access and health-seeking behavior. *Journal of Health Care for the Poor and Underserved, 10*(3), 328–337.

McBride, A. B. (1999). Breakthroughs in nursing education: Looking back, looking forward. *Nursing Outlook, 47*(30), 114–119.

Minnesota Department of Health, Section of Public Health Nursing. (2001). *Public health interventions—applications for public health nursing practice.* St. Paul, MN: Minnesota Department of Health. Retrieved April 20, 2002, from http://www.health.state.mn.us/divs/chs/phn/manfrm.html

Mitchell, P. (1999). UK government aims to prevent 300,000 deaths over ten years. *Lancet, 354,* 139.

Mundt, M. H. (1998). Exploring the meaning of "underserved:" A call to action. *Nursing Forum, 33,* 5–6.

Nelson, M., Proctor, S., Regev, H., Barnes, D., Sawyer, L., Messias, D., Yoder, L., & Meleis, A. I. (1996). International population and development: The United Nations' Cairo action plan for women's health. *Image: Journal of Nursing Scholarship, 28*(1), 75–80.

Peters, R. M. (1995). Teaching population-focused practice to baccalaureate nursing students: a clinical model. *Journal of Nursing Education, 34*(8), 378–383.

Reilly, B. (2001). "Health Teaching" in *Getting Behind the Wheel, Public Health Nursing Online Newsletter, 13.* Section of Public Health Nursing, Minnesota Department of Health. Retrieved from http://www. health. state.mn.us/divs/chs/phn/phnnews13.html on July 13, 2001.

Rew, L., Taylor-Seehafer, M., Thomas, N. Y., & Yockey, R. D. (2001). Correlates of resilience in homeless adolescents. *Journal of Nursing Scholarship, 33*(1), 33–40.

U.S. Department of Health and Human Services. (2000). *Healthy people 2010: Understanding and improving health,* (2nd, ed.). Washington, DC: U.S. Government Printing Office.

Wald, L. D. (1915). *The house on Henry Street.* New York: Dover Publications.

Wells, M. I. (2000). Beyond cultural competence: A model for individual and institutional cultural development. *Journal of Community Health Nursing, 17*(4), 189–199.

Williams, C. A. (2000). Community-oriented population-focused practice: The foundation of specialization in public health nursing. In M. Stanhope & J. Lancaster (Eds.), *Community and public health nursing* (5th ed., pp. 2–19). St. Louis, MO: Mosby.

SUGGESTED READINGS

Abbasi, K. (1999). Healthcare strategy—the role of the World Bank in international health. *British Medical Journal, 318,* 933–936.

Beauchesne, M. F. (2001). When urban U.S. means urban underserved. *Reflections on Nursing Leadership, 27*(2), 24–27.

Brundtland, G. H. (2001). *Meeting of interested parties—opening remarks.* Retrieved January 20, 2002, from the World Health Organization web site: http://www. who.int/director-general/speeches/2001 /english/20010618_mipgeneva2001.en.html

Burkhardt, M. A., & Nathaniel, A. K. (2002). *Ethics & issues in contemporary nursing.* Clifton Park, NY: Delmar Learning.

Clark, M. J. (1996). The community context. In M. J. Clark (ed.), *Nursing in the community* (2nd ed., pp. 3–16). Stamford, CT: Appleton & Lange.

Coler, M. S., Filha, M. de O. F., Ozalting, G., Gorman, D., Rigol, A., & Oud, N. Violence: A NANDA nursing diagnosis targeted at a universal problem: One proposal for prevention and intervention. In M. J. Rantz & P. Lemone (Eds.), *Classification of nursing diagnoses. Proceedings of the thirteenth conference* (pp. 377–389). Glendale, CA: CINAHL.

Diekemper, M., Smith Battle, L., & Drake, M. A. (1999). Part I. Bringing the population into focus. *Public Health Nursing, 16*(1), 3–10.

Diekemper, M., Smith Battle, L., & Drake, M. A. (1999). Sharpening the focus on populations: An intentional community health nursing approach. Part II. *Public Health Nursing, 16*(1), 11–16.

Evans, R., & Stoddart, G. (1990). Consuming health care, producing health. *Social Science Medicine, 31,* 1347–1363.

Gordon, M. (2000). *Manual of Nursing Diagnosis* (9th ed). St. Louis, MO: Mosby.

Green, P. M., & Slade, D. S. (2000). Environmental nursing diagnoses for aggregates and community. *Nursing Diagnosis, 12*(1), 5–13.

Helvie, C. O., & Nichols, B. S. (1998). Reconceptualization of community health nursing clinicals for the undergraduate students. *Public Health Nursing, 15*(1), 60–64.

Her, M. (2001, April). St. Paul-Ramsey County Department of Public Health, St. Paul, Minnesota, case study: Target population, Hmong elderly at risk for depression—intervention, outreach behind the wheel. *Public Health Nursing Newsletter.* Retrieved July 13, 2001, from http://www.health.state.mn.us/ divs/chs/phn/phnnews15.html

Institute of Medicine. (1988). *The future of public health.* Washington, DC: National Academy Press.

Kosidlak, J. G. (1999). The development and implementation of a population-based intervention model for public health nursing practice. *Public Health Nursing, 16*(5), 311–320.

Kurland, J. (2000). Public health in the new millennium II: Social exclusion. *Public Health Reports, 115*(4), 298.

Lindeman, C. A. (2000). The future of nursing education. *Journal of Nursing Education, 39*(1), 5–12.

Minnesota Department of Health, Section of Public Health Nursing. (2001). Getting behind the wheel. *Public Health Nursing Newsletter.* Retrieved January 30, 2002, from http://www.health.state.mn.us/divs/ chs/phn/index.html

O'Neil, E. H. & the Pew Health Professions Commission. (1998). *Recreating health professional practice for a new century.* San Francisco: Pew Health Professions Commission.

Public Health Reports. (1998). Eliminating racial and ethnic disparities in health: Response to the president's Initiative on Race. *Author,* 113(4), 372–374.

Registered Nurses Association of British Columbia. (1992). *Determinants of health: Empowering strategies for nursing practice.* Vancouver, British Columbia, Canada: Author.

Schaal, M. G., Rose, M. A., Doherty, A., & Vilan, A. (2000). Global connections in a changing world: Romanian and U.S. nurses unite. *Journal of Community Health Nursing,* 17(4), 201–209.

Small, H. (1998, March). Paper presented at the States and Lamps Research Conference.

Uys, L. R. (2001). Universal access to health care: If not now, when? *Reflections on Nursing Leadership,* 27(2), 21–23.

Williams, C. A. (1996). Community-based population-focused practice: The foundation of specialization in public health nursing. In M. Stanhope & J. Lancaster (Eds.), *Community health nursing: Process and practice for promoting health* (4th ed., pp. 21–32). St. Louis, MO: Mosby-Year Book.

Willis, E. M., Biggins, A. L., & Donovan, J. E. (1999). Population-focused practice. In J. E. Hitchcock, P. E. Schubert, & S. A. Thomas, *Community health nursing* (pp. 209–223). Clifton Park, NY: Delmar Learning.

World Health Organization. (2000). *A massive effort for better health among the poor.* Retrieved July 7, 2001, from http://www.who.int/inf-new/conclu.htm

CHAPTER 6

Fundamentally who we are and how we work together is what our patients receive.
(Nancy Moore, 2000)

Personal and Interdisciplinary Communication

Jacklyn L. Ruthman, PhD, RN

OBJECTIVES

Upon completion of this chapter, the reader should be able to:

1. Detail current trends in society that affect communication.
2. Describe the communication process.
3. Relate characteristics of verbal and nonverbal communication.
4. Increase effectiveness of communication by using basic communication skills.
5. List barriers to communication.
6. Describe typical nursing communication activities in the workplace.

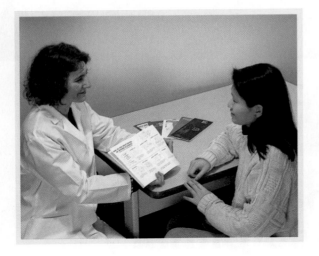

As a newly licensed RN working on a medical unit in your community hospital, you begin your shift by making rounds on your patients to perform initial assessments. You enter the room of Mr. Mason, who has a long history of chronic obstructive pulmonary disease. He was admitted yesterday with pneumonia. He is well known to the experienced staff. As you assess his breath sounds, he tells you, "I don't think I'm going to make it this time." His wife, who is at his bedside, replies, "Don't talk like that."

What are your thoughts about this situation?

What nonverbal cues might be used to help you interpret this message?

What communication skills will you use to respond appropriately?

Today's nurses use basic principles of communication to facilitate interactions with patients, family members, peers, and other disciplines. These principles allow nurses to adapt to trends that affect the profession of nursing and its practice. The dictionary defines communication as a process by which information is exchanged. Nurses follow a process of communication that is more universal than unique to nursing. They rely on communication skills to effectively promote patient care and professionalism in a variety of settings for an increasingly diverse society. These skills enable nurses to engage in the complex, interactive process of communication that uses both verbal and nonverbal modes. Nurses are aware of the context in which communication occurs. Nurses must be aware of potential barriers to communication to be able to overcome them. Awareness of principles and skills of communication empowers nurses to manage a variety of communication demands in the workplace.

TRENDS IN SOCIETY THAT AFFECT COMMUNICATION

Good communication will grow in importance because of trends in our culture. Among the trends affecting nursing practice is the increasing diversity in society. The United States has been called the melting pot, and that has never been more true than now when we see the influence of many different ethnic, racial, cultural, and socioeconomic backgrounds. Increased diversity causes once-dominant values and beliefs to be replaced or diluted with different values and beliefs. These differences become a source of possible misunderstanding that can be bridged by effective communication.

Another trend is our aging population. It is estimated that 20% of the population will be 65 years of age or older by 2020. Our aging society will challenge nurses to maintain effective communication to compensate for the diminished sensory abilities that typically accompany aging. Multiple sensory deficits can occur simultaneously so that patients may experience losses in a variety of combinations that include hearing, seeing, smelling, tasting, and touching. The potential diminished input challenges nurse and patient alike to creatively compensate for these deficits. At the same time that the population is aging, it is also shifting to an electronic mode, with computer technology playing an increasingly dominant role. As electronic communication assumes a greater role, nurses' ability to effectively communicate in writing will grow in importance. Reliance on written communication using electronic input shifts the source of input away from traditional visual, auditory, and kinesthetic modes to the written word. Therefore, tomorrow's nurses will require keen writing skills. These trends have influenced recommendations for current nursing competencies. Communication is so central to nursing that the majority of competencies identified in the Pew Health Professions Commission's report discussed in Chapter 1 contain a communication component (Bellack & O'Neil, 2000).

ELEMENTS OF THE COMMUNICATION PROCESS

Communication is the exchange of information or opinions. Communication is most often an interactive process that is a means to an end and is influenced by the context in which it occurs. Communication typically involves a sender, a message, a receiver, and feedback. Face-to-face communication allows the process to proceed almost immediately, that is, be synchronous. Electronic media can be either synchronous or asynchronous. Figure 6-1 illustrates the communication process.

Sender

A message originates with the sender. Laswell's classic model of communication (1948) describes the sender as the "who" in communication. If nurses initiate communication, they are the senders.

Message

The **message** originates with the sender. It consists of verbal and/or nonverbal stimuli that are taken in by the receiver. The message is the "what" in communication.

Receiver

The **receiver** takes in the message and analyzes it. When nurses listen to patient-initiated conversations, they are the receivers. When the receiver reacts by returning a new message, the receiver and sender reverse roles.

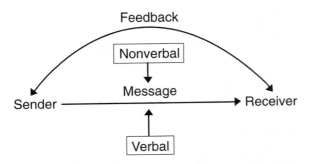

Figure 6-1 Basic Communication Model

Feedback

The new message that is generated by the receiver in response to the original message from the sender is the **feedback**. Bradley & Edinberg (1986) describe feedback as the "with what effect" and note that feedback is effective when the two communicators are sensitive to each other's messages and they change behaviors based on the message exchanges.

CHANNELS OF COMMUNICATION

In almost every nursing interaction, there is **visual** (seeing), **auditory** (hearing), and **kinesthetic** (touching) input. According to Bradley & Edinberg (1986), authors who are responsible for one of the earliest nursing communication texts, these sensory stimuli may be processed at different levels, with the simplest level being to report what is actually seen, heard, or touched. The next level of sensory processing orders and structures information from the usual auditory or kinesthetic input and integrates the stimulus so that one reports observing, listening, or feeling. The highest level of processing interprets and integrates information from all the inputs leading to perception and interpretation. The processing occurs in each person who is communicating and may occur at different levels depending on each person's cognitive abilities. For example, a toddler who is just beginning to communicate effectively using words delights in sharing labels such as "snow." This is the simplest level of communication. Upon touching the snow, the toddler might demonstrate his ability to integrate his experience with touching snow by exclaiming, "Snow cold." His mother delights in the child's sophistication and interprets the first encounter at the higher level of processing by responding to the child at the highest level and telling the child he's right and offering that snow is cold and white and beautiful and fun to play in.

The Visual Channel

All seeing people take in information from the surrounding environments through sight. The amount of detail available is limited primarily by how much one looks. For nurses, visual data offers a wealth of information that can lead to rapid interpretation. For example, a nurse who is caring for a fresh postoperative patient looks at the dressing to validate that it is dry, intact, and free of discharge. The nurse interprets these negative findings as being a stable situation.

The Auditory Channel

Hearing is another sensory channel that is focused on words that are spoken, as well as the volume, pitch, tone, rhythm, and speed with which they are delivered. Hearing involves identifying not only the words spoken but also how a message is delivered. Babies are typically born with the ability to hear, but they must learn to listen. Listening involves making sense out of what was said. To listen effectively, the nurse must put together accurately what is said and how it is said. The nurse who is assessing the fresh postoperative patient asks him, "How would you rate your pain on a scale of 0–10 with 0 being no pain and 10 being the worst pain you can imagine?" The patient replies, "Oh, I don't know, maybe a 4." The nurse begins the feedback by inquiring whether a pain rating of 4 is acceptable to him. The words she speaks to him are also filled with cues based on her volume, rhythm, tone, pitch, and speed. The patient tells her that his pain is acceptable, but for the nurse to truly listen, she must also process cues based on his volume, rhythm, tone, pitch, and speed.

The Kinesthetic Channel

All aspects of communication that relate to feelings are considered kinesthetic. At the most basic level, this involves touch and physiological responses. Kinesthetic stimuli have cognitive and emotional components that are integrated to become feelings, or the quality of things as imparted through touch. For example, as the nurse repositions the patient, she touches his skin and notes it is warm and dry. She interprets these stimuli favorably. However, she also notices that the patient grimaces as he moves. His body actions or body language communicate additional kinesthetic information. Body language is important because it may accompany, substitute, or modify input from other channels. Integrating information from all channels, the nurse perceives that the patient may be in pain that is unacceptable. She offers verbal feedback that matches her perception, thereby continuing the communication process using all channels until the exchange is complete.

MODES OF COMMUNICATION

The two traditional modes of communication, verbal and nonverbal, are exemplified in the nurse–patient scenario that follows. Because face-to-face encounters usually allow for verbal and nonverbal exchange, they have been regarded as the most effective modes of communication and hence have been preferred. When face-to-face encounters are not possible or practical, other approaches are used. Historically, the next most effective approach is the telephone, followed by voice messages, e-mail messages, and written documents. These electronic methods comprise the third mode of communication, and it will grow in importance as nurses increasingly rely on technology, particularly computers, to communicate interpersonally. As was previously mentioned, using e-mail requires that nurses have keen writing skills.

Verbal Communication

Verbal communication relies on speaking words to convey a message. It involves the use of the auditory channel previously discussed. The accuracy of the message is dependent on the sender's vocabulary and the receiver's ability to make sense of the words used to send the message. In addition, the verbal message is influenced by the sender's tone. According to Yogo, Hashi, Tsutsui, and Yamada (2000), the tone is more influential when conveying a message than the content. Another factor that influences verbal communication is the pacing or timing of a message. Verbal communication is a conscious process, so the sender has the ability to control what is said.

Nonverbal Communication

Nonverbal communication consists of aspects of communication that are outside what is spoken. The communicator's appearance, facial expressions, posture, gait, body movements, position, gestures, and touch all influence how the message is processed. And, while tone is more important than the words spoken, it has long been suggested that facial expression is even more important than either tone or the words used. Nonverbal communication tends to be unconscious and more difficult to control.

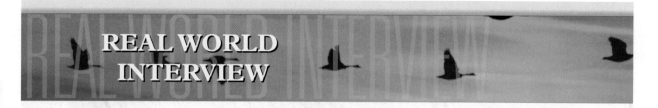

REAL WORLD INTERVIEW

I view my primary responsibility as a nurse to be that of patient advocate. As a team leader, I am responsible for coordinating patient care for a group of patients. I am responsible for setting patient care goals and then directing my team to achieve the goals. I make those patient care goals the focus of my team's efforts. Patient care is rendered with the assistance of subordinates, including certified nurse assistants (CNAs), nursing student externs, and occasional high school student volunteers. Communication is the key to a successful team. A recent patient typifies how I interact with my team.

An elderly nonverbal patient with a history of schizophrenia was admitted to our surgical unit for dehydration. She was in need of total care, especially with respect to hygiene, which had been neglected. She was dependent on staff to turn and position her. Her level of awareness suggested she was unable to use a call light for help.

This patient challenged staff for a variety of reasons. First, due to multiple other health problems, she was not a candidate for surgery. This placed her among the patients who don't really "fit" the surgical unit where she was admitted. Nonetheless, my goal was to advocate for comfort care with her physician while also encouraging subordinates to provide quality care even though the goal was not for cure with this particular patient. The patient's inability to communicate verbally added to the challenge. It was unclear how aware the patient was of the care she was receiving. Her nonverbal status blocked her ability to dialogue. This caused us to rely on nonverbal cues. Respect for patients with or without their verbal feedback is essential. The CNA and I tackled the needed bed bath together. Teamwork kept the focus on the goal for the patient, which was to optimize comfort and maintain skin integrity. It allowed me to complete a thorough assessment and to model desired communication with the patient, whom I addressed by name. I inquired whether she was in pain, to which she responded with twisting motions. I continued the one-way conversation, attempting to clarify what her nonverbal responses meant. She pointed to her shoulder, so we repositioned her and she settled down, resting quietly. As is often the case, the CNA willingly returned to reposition the patient with confidence the remainder of the shift. The patient's inability to verbalize needs was perceived as less of a barrier once we were successful in overcoming it together.

I find that CNAs will often volunteer to complete entire tasks they feel capable of performing independently. They also need to be assured that they will not be expected to handle clinical situations for which they do not feel qualified. This mutual respect for each other is essential to an ongoing working relationship. They honor my standard of care and will often complete tasks, going above and beyond what I ask. For example, later in the afternoon, the CNA returned to the patient and washed and braided her hair. Since this same patient would not likely use the call light, I also explained our goal to the high school student volunteer and I asked her to check the patient's position whenever she went by the room. I instructed her to let me know if the patient appeared uncomfortable, assuring her that I would reposition the patient as needed. The student expressed that she thought it was cool how nurses communicate with patients who can't talk. I believe through effective communication our team achieved the goal of optimizing this patient's comfort in spite of many potential barriers.

Lari Summa, RN, BSN
Team Leader

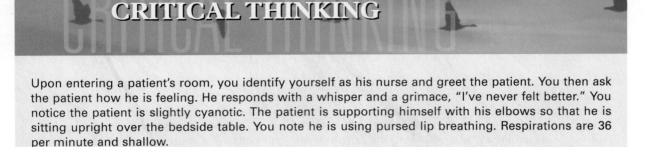

CRITICAL THINKING

Upon entering a patient's room, you identify yourself as his nurse and greet the patient. You then ask the patient how he is feeling. He responds with a whisper and a grimace, "I've never felt better." You notice the patient is slightly cyanotic. The patient is supporting himself with his elbows so that he is sitting upright over the bedside table. You note he is using pursed lip breathing. Respirations are 36 per minute and shallow.

What kinds of problems occur when verbal and nonverbal communications are incongruent? How will you handle the incongruent verbal and nonverbal communications? Which message, the verbal or nonverbal, is more difficult to control?

Electronic Communication

It was previously mentioned that communication is shifting to an electronic mode, with computer technology playing an increasingly dominant role. Patients are being monitored long distance and connecting to their health care providers using a variety of technologies, including telephones, voice mail, and e-mail. These methods, which may be asynchronous because caregiver and care receiver interact using technology rather than the traditional face-to-face or voice-to-voice encounter, require careful communication. For example, e-mail now allows almost instantaneous communication around the world, but it also accommodates individual preferences with respect to the timing of the response. This allows a patient to provide an update on a condition early in the day and affords the caregivers the opportunity to respond as their schedules permit. Using e-mail may save a patient and caregiver from travel or loss of work. However, using e-mail requires that nurses acting in such a caregiver role have keen writing skills. An explanation of all the considerations that are important to effective writing is beyond the scope of this text. However, a few tips are worth sharing. The speed with which exchanges can now be made using computers has reduced the acceptable response time. Therefore, the first tip when communicating using computers is to respond in a timely manner. Next, keep in mind that accurate spelling, correct grammar, and organization of thought assume greater impor-

tance in the absence of verbal and nonverbal cues that are given in face-to-face encounters. Finally, always proofread correspondences prior to sending them. Imagine yourself the recipient of the document. Look for complete sentences, logical development of thought and reasoning, accuracy, and appropriate use of grammar such as punctuation and capitalization.

LEVEL OF COMMUNICATION

The level of communication involves who the audience is when communicating. Consequently, communication can be thought of as having three levels: public, intrapersonal, and interpersonal.

Public Communication

Nurses rely primarily on interpersonal communication. However, they also use the other levels, so brief descriptions will be given for them. First, there is public communication. The nurse educator presenting a workshop on signs and symptoms of menopause to a room full of middle-aged women engages in public communication. Her audience is a group of people with a common interest. As presenter, she acts primarily as a sender of information. By design, feedback is typically limited in public speaking, though it does occur. Strategies abound to enhance public speaking skills, but it is beyond the scope of this text to discuss them.

Intrapersonal Communication

Another level is **intrapersonal communication**, which can be thought of as self-talk. As the name suggests, it is what individuals do within themselves and can present as doubts or affirmations. A new nurse may engage in intrapersonal communication as he simultaneously doubts and affirms his ability to complete a procedure. For example, the first time the newly licensed RN has to catheterize a patient, he may simultaneously doubt his ability to insert a Foley catheter with one message, "I haven't done this for months," while affirming his ability to insert a Foley catheter with an "I can do this" message to himself. He is engaging in intrapersonal communication. The so-called competing voices within himself act as sender and receiver in this intrapersonal conversation whose outcome will be influenced by the feedback that follows.

Simms, Price, and Ervin (2000) present communication with self or intrapersonal communication as the first important element in developing a sphere of communication. From self-awareness and understanding of oneself, a nurse can move confidently into one-to-one interactions with others, and then into interactions with smaller and larger groups. See Figure 6-2 for some spheres of communication and their related skills.

Interpersonal Communication

The last level, **interpersonal communication**, involves communication between individuals, person-to-person or in small groups. Not surprisingly, nurses engage in this level regularly. Interpersonal communication allows for a very effective level of communication to occur and incorporates all of the elements, channels, and modes previously discussed. The

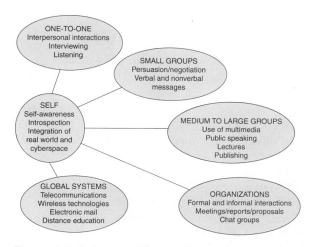

Figure 6-2 Spheres of Communication and Related Skills

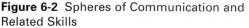

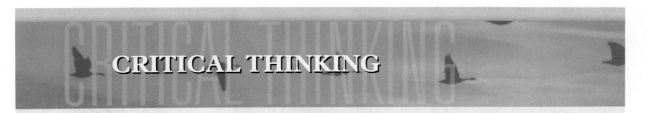

A diabetic patient who lives in the rural West is excited to have recently become "connected' to the World Wide Web with the acquisition of a computer and Internet services. His wife, who accompanies him to the office visit, wonders whether some of the monitoring that currently occurs during office visits might not be accomplished using e-mail. They reason that winters are hard and travel is difficult, the patient's circulation is poor, he fatigues easily, and it could save them the 6-hour round-trip. Furthermore, they're hoping to spend several weeks in the South this winter. They reason that using e-mail, they can maintain contact as needed without the drawbacks they identified.

What are the advantages of this suggestion for the patient? The caregiver? What are the drawbacks of this suggestion for the patient? The caregiver? What safeguards can you think of to facilitate communicating using e-mail and to ensure quality care?

nurse, who observes a patient grimace when he moves, interprets the nonverbal cue as indicating that the patient is experiencing pain. Using verbal communication, she clarifies her perception by asking the patient to describe and rate his pain. He describes it as tolerable and states he is expecting a visitor and he does not want to be drowsy. The communication goes back and forth until, ideally, both parties' understanding of the message match. This is the goal of communication.

ORGANIZATIONAL COMMUNICATION

Avenues of communication are often defined by an organization's formal structure. The formal structure establishes who is in charge and identifies how different levels of personnel and various departments relate within the organization. When the chief executive officer of an organization announces that the company will adopt a new policy that all employees will follow, that is downward communication. The message starts at the top and is usually disseminated by levels through the chain of communication. Upward communication is the opposite of downward communication. The idea originates at some level below the top of the structure and moves upward. For example, when a nurse recommends a more efficient approach to organizing care to his nurse manager, who takes the recommendation to her superior, who uses the recommendation to develop a new policy, that is upward communication. Lateral communication occurs among people with similar status. Two nurses discussing how to best change a patient's dressing are engaged in lateral communication. Diagonal communication occurs when members of the team who may be on different levels of the organizational chart discuss a patient care concern such as discharge planning. The organizational structure within nursing also determines who is responsible for representing nursing concerns in this type of interaction. For example, if the department practices within a primary nursing model, the primary nurse is responsible for representing nursing concerns. In team nursing, the team leader rather than the nurse delivering care is responsible. A final avenue worth mentioning, which is not a formal avenue, is the grapevine. The grapevine is an informal avenue in which rumors circulate. It ignores the formal chain of command. The major benefit of the grapevine is the speed with which information is spread, but its major drawback is that it often lacks accuracy. For example, nurses who inform an oncoming shift about a rumor that layoffs or mandatory overtime is imminent in the absence of any information from the hospital's administration are participating in grapevine communication.

COMMUNICATION SKILLS

Because nurses are often placed in positions of leadership and are responsible for representing nursing's concerns to others, including the patient, it is important they have the requisite skills to be effective communicators. There is no one correct way to ensure effective communication. Rather, effective communication requires that both parties engaged in communicating use skills that enhance that particular interaction. Baker, Beglinger, King, Salyards, and Thompson (2000) believe that the most important considerations for facilitating communication are to be open and to be willing to give and receive feedback. Some of the most important skills upon which nurses rely to do this are attending, responding, clarifying, and confronting skills. Additional skills are listed in Table 6-1.

Attending

Attending involves active listening, the most important skill used by nurses to gain an understanding of the patient's message. Active listening requires that the nurse pay close attention to what the patient is saying. In addition, the nurse uses the sensory and visual channels, looking for congruence between what is said and how it is said. Attending involves the nurse's nonverbal cues. Facing the patient and maintaining eye contact are two skills that facilitate attending. If possible, sitting down and leaning forward send a message that the nurse is willing to listen. Distracting behaviors, such as tapping, send a message that the nurse is not interested in the message; therefore, these types of behaviors should be avoided.

Responding

Responding entails verbal and nonverbal acknowledgment of the sender's message. When the nurse

TABLE 6-1	*Additional Communication Skills*
Skill	**Description**
Supporting	Siding with another person or backing up another person: "I can see that you would feel that way."
Focusing	Centers on the main point: "So your main concern is..."
Open-ended questioning	Allows for patient-directed responses: "How did that make you feel?"
Providing information	Supplies one with knowledge she did not previously have: "It's common for people with pneumonia to be tired."
Using silence	Allows for intrapersonal communication
Reassuring	Restores confidence or removes fear: "I can assure you that tomorrow..."
Expressing appreciation	Shows gratitude: "Thank you" or "You are so thoughtful."
Using humor	Provides relief and gains perspective; may also cause harm so use carefully
Conveying acceptance	Makes known that one is capable or worthy: "It's okay to cry."
Asking related questions	Expands listener's understanding: "How painful was it?"

nods affirmatively as she listens, she is responding nonverbally that the message has worth. A response can be as simple as an acknowledgment that the message was received, for example, "I hear you." Sometimes, however, responding involves more. Two verbal skills that elevate the level of responding are questioning and rephrasing. Questioning allows the nurse to clarify the message by asking related questions. Rephrasing involves restating what the nurse believes to be the important points. These techniques refine perceptions and enhance understanding.

Clarifying

Clarifying by using such skills as restating, questioning, and rephrasing, helps the message become clear. As with most communication, clarifying can be accomplished using a variety of approaches. For example, if the nurse does not follow a patient's account of his presenting complaint, the nurse can respond with "I lost you there." Perhaps the nurse tries to process information that is confusing or conflicting. She can restate what she heard in an effort to clarify the information. Clarifying involves com-

municating as specifically as possible. Questioning and rephrasing were described previously. They are used not only to respond but also to clarify.

Confronting

Confronting means to work jointly with others to resolve a problem or conflict. Given that definition, it is a very effective means of resolving conflict. It involves, first of all, identifying the conflict, which can arise from perceived or real differences. A nurse might identify a conflict with a simple "We have a problem here." Next, the problem is clearly delineated so that those involved understand what it is and what it is not. Then using knowledge and reason, attempts are made to resolve the problem. The goal is to achieve a win-win solution in which both parties' needs are met. This sounds easier to do than it sometimes is because emotions can get in the way and cloud reason. Cooling-off periods are sometimes needed between problem identification and conflict resolution. Acceptable motives for confronting are to resolve conflict, further growth, and improve relationships.

BARRIERS TO COMMUNICATION

Barriers are obstacles to effective communication. The nurse who can identify potential barriers to communication will be better equipped to avoid them or to compensate for them. Some of the most common barriers are gender, culture, anger, incongruent responses, and conflict.

Gender

Gender interferes with communication when men and women lack the understanding that they may process information differently. In general, some men are more interested in using reason while some women want to be heard and validated through communication (Gray, 1992). Gender differences and patterns do not preclude working together. Rather, both sides must realize the other's preference and make accommodations so that effective communication results.

Gender differences have been attributed, in part, to gender socialization in which males are provided with more opportunities to develop confidence and assertiveness than females. Fortunately, the feminist movement and increased sexual equality in Western society, in general, have lessened traditional sociological patterns of competitiveness and decisiveness in men and passivity and nurturing in women. However, remnants of the traditional model persist, particularly in health care settings. Nurses who lack assertiveness and confidence are encouraged to acquire the requisite skills to be assertive and confident to be an effective patient advocate and also to communicate in a confident manner.

Culture

As was stated previously, our culture grows increasingly diverse. This diversity reduces the likelihood that patients and nurses will share a common cultural background. In turn, the number of safe assumptions about beliefs and practices decreases and the probability for misunderstanding increases. For example, shortly after delivering a baby, women are often hungry and thirsty. Some cultures believe that for women to restore their energies appropriately, women are to eat hot foods and beverages while others believe cold foods and beverages are appropriate. A well-intentioned nurse who does not consult with the

patient about her preferences may arrange culturally inappropriate nourishment. Broadly defined, culture encompasses different groups' beliefs and practices by gender, race, age, economic status, health, and disability. Poole, Davidhizar, and Giger (1995) outline six phenomena that must be considered when delegating to staff with a culturally diverse background. They emphasize that culture and communication are intrinsically intertwined; see the literature application that follows. Nurses are responsible for bridging gaps between themselves and their patients through first being accepting of differences. They can also overcome cultural differences by learning about other cultures. Finally, nurses bridge cultural differences by vigilantly using the skills previously described to facilitate communication.

Anger

Anger is a universal, strong feeling of displeasure that is often precipitated by a situation that frustrates or prevents a person from attaining a goal or getting what is wanted from life. Anger is influenced by one's beliefs. Ellis (1997) describes anger as an irrational response that arises from one of four irrational ideas: (1) that the treatment one received was awful (awfulizing), (2) feeling that one can't stand having been treated so irresponsibly and unfairly (can't-stand-it-itis), (3) believing that one should not, must not behave as he did (shoulding and musting), and (4) because one acted in a terrible manner, he is a terrible person (undeservingness and damnation). He maintains that beliefs remain rational as long as the evaluation of the action does not involve an evaluation of the person. Rational and appropriate responses are feelings of disappointment. Anger, on the other hand, can be unmanageable and self-defeating. He believes that we all have the ability to choose our response to anger.

Anger can be dealt with in one of several ways. Three methods that may work from time to time but that may have serious and potentially destructive drawbacks are denying and repressing anger, which may lead to resentment; expressing anger, which may lead to defensiveness on the part of the respondent; and turning the other cheek, which may lead to continued mistreatment and lack of trust. Because anger stems from carrying things further and viewing the situation as awful, terrible, or horrible, Ellis (1997) advocates disputing irrational beliefs. Anger can stem

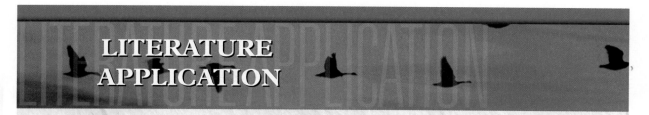

LITERATURE APPLICATION

Citation: Poole, V. L., Davidhizar, R. E., and Giger, J. N. (1995). Delegating to a transcultural team. *Nursing Management, 26*(8), 33–34.

Discussion: All cultural groups show evidence of six phenomena: communication, space, social organization, time, environmental control, and biological variations. However, the application and use of these phenomena vary within and among cultures. Nurses' cultural assessment is essential when delegating to a transcultural team. Suggestions for bridging variations are category specific. Regarding communication, the authors recommend assessing dialect, style, volume, the use of touch, context of speech, and kinesics. They identify that the 2 to 3 feet of socially acceptable space that some white American middle-class people find comfortable when talking is considered distant among other cultural groups, specifically African-Americans and the French. While family may dominate as the primary social organization among many individuals and groups, others may hold an individualistic view. Cultural groups may be past, present, or future focused with respect to time. Environmental control is concerned with locus of control, which can be internal or external. And finally, biological variations exist between racial and ethnic groups that cause varying susceptibility to disease. All staff are encouraged to maintain an optimal level of wellness to maintain their ability to deal with patient problems.

Implications for Practice: When delegating, all the previously mentioned phenomena must be considered for both individual and group interactions.

from deep-seated feelings of unassertiveness. Assertion involves taking a stand, while aggression involves putting another down. If unassertiveness is the source of anger, then a solution is to learn to act assertively.

Incongruent Responses

When words and actions in a communication do not match the inner experience of self or are inappropriate to the context, the response is incongruent. Some common incongruent responses are blaming, placating, being superreasonable, and using irrelevant information to make decisions. Blaming is finding fault or error and occurs when a response lacks respect for others' feelings. For example, a nurse who attributes a medication error to her overloaded assignment might blame the nurse who made the assignment, saying that "It's all her fault." This can be avoided by standing up for one's rights while respecting the rights of others. Placating is soothing by concession and occurs when one lacks self-respect. For example, a nurse who consents to a patient assignment that she

believes is unfair or unsafe just to keep the peace is placating. Placating can be overcome by paying attention to one's own needs and by negotiating what one believes to be a fair and safe assignment. Being superreasonable is to go beyond reason and lack respect for others' and one's own feelings. The nurse described previously, who when approached by the house supervisor agrees to whatever solution is offered, has become superreasonable when she says, "You're always right; I'll do whatever you need." This ineffective approach can be sidestepped by considering each other's feelings when arriving at a solution. Finally, using irrelevant information for decision making shows lack of respect for others' and one's own feelings. A nurse who challenges a colleague's abilities based solely on their out-of-work activities or political preference is using irrelevant information. Likewise, arguing against a colleague's ability to function as a charge nurse because of an incident that occurred a year prior during the nurse's orientation is often irrelevant. Respecting feelings and context can avert irrelevance.

Conflict

Conflict arises when ideas or beliefs are opposed. Not surprisingly, it occurs at different levels: interpersonal and organizational. As was previously stated, conflict resolution is one way to resolve conflict. To resolve conflict, the nature of the differences and the reasons for the differences must be considered. These differences arise for an array of reasons. Some of these reasons include variations in facts, goals, and methods to achieve goals, values, or standards (Kinney & Hurst, 1979). Conflict resolution typically occurs using one of five distinct approaches: avoiding, accommodating, competing, compromising, and collaborating (Yoder-Wise, 1999).

Avoiding or retreating disregards the needs of self and others but sometimes offers the benefit of allowing tempers to cool. An example of avoidance is the nurse who walks away from a heated discussion with a peer following a change of shift report. Accommodating satisfies the needs of others at the expense of self. The nurse who forfeits after-work plans to staff the unit by working overtime is accommodating. Accommodating sometimes leads to disappointment. Competing can lead to personal victory at the expense of others, which can lead to ill will. For example, two nurses who want the same weekend off may plead their cases to the nurse manager, each in hopes of getting her own way.

Compromising leads to a middle ground solution in which neither party gets all they want. The charge nurse who gives each of the nurses above a day off on the weekend they requested has resolved the conflict by compromising. Finally, collaborating resolves conflict so that both parties are satisfied. It involves seeking creative, integrative solutions, while also working through emotions. It is the best strategy for successful conflict resolution, but it is more difficult than it may appear. The charge nurse who clarifies the above nurses' requests for the same weekend off discovers one is for a sister's wedding while the other is for a getaway that can be moved to another weekend. Each nurse can be satisfied through collaboration.

Additional barriers to communication are seen in Table 6-2.

WORKPLACE COMMUNICATION

It is probably clear by now that how individuals communicate depends, in part, on where communication occurs and in what relationship. Patterns of communication in the workplace are sensitive to organizational factors that define relationships. Nurses have diverse roles and relationships in the workplace that call for different communication patterns with superiors, coworkers, subordinates, physicians and other health care professionals, patients, families, and mentors.

Superiors

Communicating with a superior can be intimidating, especially for a new nurse. Observing professional

TABLE 6-2	Additional Barriers to Communication
Barrier	**Description**
Offering false reassurance	Promising something that cannot be delivered
Being defensive	Acting as though one has been attacked
Stereotyping	Unfairly categorizing someone based on his or her traits
Interrupting	Speaking before other has completed her message
Inattention	Not paying attention
Stress	A state of tension that gets in the way of reasoning
Unclear expectations	Ill-defined tasks or duties that make successful completion unlikely

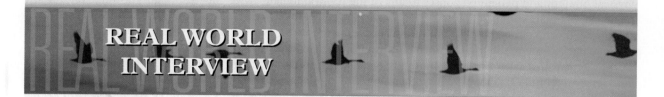

REAL WORLD INTERVIEW

My husband, Ted, was seriously ill from cancer last year. We went to a large university hospital for treatment, where we expected to receive the finest, state-of-the-art care. Most of the care we received was excellent. One day, however, Ted was scheduled to have two outpatient blood tests done prior to his dose of chemotherapy. One blood test had to be drawn from his port and the other test was to be drawn from his vein. The nursing staff usually did the tests at the same time, with Ted in a patient care room where he could rest after the tests and prior to his scheduled chemotherapy. This day, however, the nurse caring for him stated she could only perform the blood test from the port. She said she did not have the orders for both tests and that we had to go upstairs to another hospital unit to get the other blood test done. I said that I would go upstairs and get the other orders to avoid having my exhausted, sick husband go upstairs for the test and then have to come back down again to get his chemotherapy. I went upstairs and down a long hall to the nurse upstairs who said that the first nurse had the orders. I went back down the long hall and down the stairs to the first nurse. She still said she did not have the orders. I went back up the stairs where the nurse upstairs said again that the first nurse definitely had the orders. This process continued two to three times, with me going up and down several times, until finally, in frustration, I started to cry and asked the nurse downstairs to let me look at Ted's orders. The nurse said to me, you are just tired. I replied, I am not tired; I just care about doing the best thing for my husband. Finally, she admitted she had the orders and she drew the blood sample. It is hard for me to see how something like this could happen in a university hospital known for quality care. Where was the compassion? Where was the quality? Why didn't the staff communicate better both with each other and with me?

Florence Lebryk
Patient's Wife

courtesies is an important first step. For instance, begin by requesting an appointment to discuss a problem when it arises. This demonstrates respect and allows for the conversation to occur at an appropriate time and place. Dress professionally. Arrive for the appointment on time, and be prepared to state the concern clearly and accurately. Provide supporting evidence, and anticipate resistance to any requests. Separate out your need from your desires. State a willingness to cooperate in finding a solution and then match behaviors to words. Persist in the pursuit of a solution.

Coworkers

Nurses depend on their coworkers in many ways to collectively provide quality patient care. Nowhere is this more important than in the acute care setting where nursing services are nonstop around the clock.

Transfer of patient care from nurse to nurse is one of the most important and frequent communications between coworkers. It depends on fluid communication in end of shift reports to achieve quality nursing care. However, time constraints demand that the change of shift report be accurate, informative, and succinct. How the nursing care is organized influences who gets the report. For example, nurses who practice using a team model will require that, at a minimum, the team leaders get the report. The method of delivery of the report also varies from setting to setting and may include walking rounds, written communication, or tape recording. Regardless of the method used, information that is typically exchanged during a change of shift report either in writing or orally includes the patient's age, gender, admitting problem, needs, other health care concerns, activity, diet, intake and output, IV therapy, treatments, tests, and family concerns. Significant physical findings and patient responses to any of the items just listed are often elaborated. The organization of the information varies and may, for example, follow a head-to-toe model if assessment forms also use this organizing approach. The most important consideration for nurses as they organize their reports is to paint an accurate picture of the patient's condition and needs.

Subordinates

An excellent guide for directing communication with subordinates is the golden rule: "Do unto others as you would have them do unto you." As a nurse who will be responsible for overseeing others' work, a valuable perspective for you to maintain is that all members of the team are important to successfully realize quality patient care. Communication between nurses and subordinates will most likely involve delegating. This important topic is covered elsewhere in this book, and you are encouraged to review this material as it relates to subordinates. In addition to delegating, a few other communications skills are worth mentioning Offering positive feedback such as, "I appreciate the way you interacted with Mr. T. to get him to

ambulate twice this shift," goes a long way toward team building, and it improves subordinates' sense of worth. Nurses also have an opportunity to act as teachers to subordinates. Often in a hospital setting, nurses teach by example. Demonstrating the desired behavior allows the subordinate to copy the behavior. It is important to allow time for return demonstrations to evaluate that the subordinate has learned the intended skill. For example, as the nurse, you may demonstrate how to position a patient with special needs, encouraging the subordinate to assist and ask questions. The next time repositioning is indicated, accompany the subordinate and observe his or her ability to successfully complete the task. Offer constructive feedback. Be patient. Remember your own learning curves when mastering new skills and behaviors and allow those you supervise the opportunity to grow. Be open to the possibility that subordinates, particularly those with experience, may have a few pearls of wisdom to share with you as well. For example, this author is forever indebted to a nurse aide who shared how to really position patients comfortably. Likewise, a veteran LPN who knew the politics of the institution mentored a batch of new graduates as they learned to be charge nurses on the evening shift.

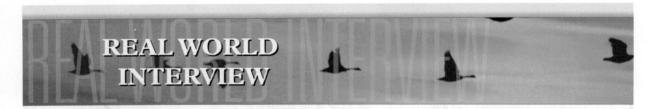

REAL WORLD INTERVIEW

A second shift occupational health nurse working in a factory setting was presented with a patient who entered the nursing office complaining that he didn't feel good. The nurse's initial assessment, including vital signs, revealed that the only abnormality was an elevated blood pressure. In this situation, like in any clinical situation, it is important to distinguish the urgent from the nonurgent. With hypertensive patients, it is important to realize that an urgent situation is suggested by evidence of acute end organ damage. Specifically, in this situation, it was important to know whether the patient was experiencing altered sensorium, headache, visual disturbance, chest pain, or dyspnea. The presence of any of these findings should be communicated to the physician and would dictate urgent transport to the hospital. In their absence, the patient can be referred for more elective blood pressure control.

In any clinical situation, such as the one above, the nurse can facilitate communications by being organized and objective. Be prepared to discuss the basics such as the patient's chief complaint, his vital signs, his medications, and any changes from baseline. Know why you are worried about observed changes and communicate this to the physician.

John C. Ruthman, MD

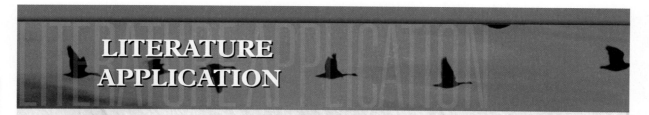

LITERATURE APPLICATION

Citation: Malone, G., and Morath, J. (2001). Pro-patient partnerships. *Nursing Management, 32,* 46–47.

Discussion: Effective nurse-physician partnership is a key factor influencing quality patient care. When nurses and doctors work well with each other, their patients' death and readmission rates improve. Individual nurses can successfully collaborate with physicians by using assertive communication. Be open, honest, and direct. Promote lifelong learning in both nursing and medicine. Ask questions about your coworker's profession. Foster support for nurses and doctors. Reach out. Make and seek commitments with physician colleagues. Ask them to serve on several of your committees. Have them review your unit's operational systems. Realign your goals and work together. Form and strengthen a proactive, shared vision with your facility's physicians. Finally, stay focused. Remember, it is not about personality and power; it is about the patients.

As a nurse-physician team, you can establish a shared vision. Form joint practice committees and standardize care orders. Make collective decisions and maintain shoulder-to-shoulder dialogue.

Implications for Practice: In forging an environment of nurse-physician partnerships, consider adopting a 20-60-20 leadership outlook. Realize that 20% of employees resist change, complain, and criticize; 20% remain committed and cooperative; and 60% fall in between. Develop a strategy that models success with the receptive 20% and engages the middle majority.

Physicians and Other Health Care Professionals

One of the most intimidating experiences for new nurses is to communicate with physicians. Despite gender and role challenges that have already been discussed, this need not be a stressful event. The nurse's goal is to strive for collaboration, keeping the patient goal central to the discussion. As was previously discussed, collaboration allows both parties to be satisfied. It involves seeking creative, integrative solutions while also working through emotions. To communicate effectively with the physician, the nurse presents information in a straightforward manner, clearly delineating the problem, supported by pertinent evidence. This is especially important when reporting changes in patient conditions. Nurses are responsible for knowing classic symptoms of conditions, orally apprising the physician of changes, and recording all observations in the chart (Sanchez-Sweatman, 1996). Dr. John Ruthman offers a recent real-life example from an occupational health care setting in the Real World Interview feature box. It is important that the nurse remain calm and objective even if the physician does not cooperate. Calfee (1998) offers suggestions for handling telephone miscommunications. For example, if a physician hangs up, document that the call was terminated and fill out an incident report. If the physician gives an inappropriate answer or gives no orders, for example, for a patient complaint of pain, document the call, the information relayed, and the fact that no orders were given. In addition, document any other steps that were taken to resolve the problem, for example, notifying the nursing supervisor. If a physician cannot be reached, first follow the institution's procedure for getting the patient treated and then document the actions taken.

Patients and Families

Communication with patients and families is optimized by the many skills previously described in this

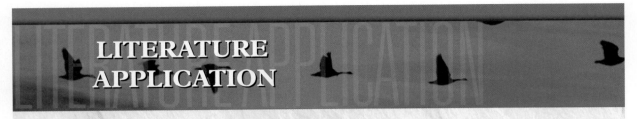

LITERATURE APPLICATION

Citation: DiBartola, L. (2001, June). Listening to patients and responding with care. *Joint Commission Journal on Quality Improvement, 27*(6), 315–323.

Discussion: Clinicians who want to improve their listening skills benefit from identifying the way in which patients are most comfortable interacting. A tool for assessing this is demonstrated. Once the patient's interaction style is identified, the clinician uses this information to move closer to where the patient is comfortable communicating. This article discusses a communication model for improving patient communication. Figure 6-3 describes behavioral characteristics of the four communication modes.

The framework for this model is the continuum of two intersecting axes. The horizontal axis poles are inquisitive and assertive. The vertical axis poles are objective and subjective. People who are most comfortable communicating in an inquisitive way and tend to be objective are called investigators. Those who are most comfortable communicating in an inquisitive way but are subjective in nature are called unifiers. People who are most comfortable communicating in an assertive way and favor subjectivity are called energizers. Those who are most comfortable communicating in an assertive way and tend to be objective are called enterprisers. Behavioral markers can be used to identify someone's preferred communication mode (Figure 6-4).

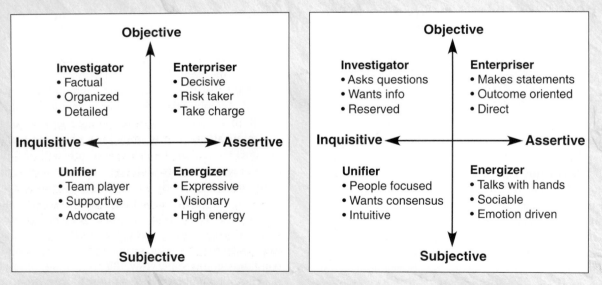

Figure 6-3 Behavioral Characteristics of the Four Communication Modes (From "Listening to Patients and Responding with Care," by L. DiBartola, 2001, *Joint Commission Journal on Quality Improvement, 27*(6), 319. Reprinted with permission.)

Figure 6-4 Behavioral Markers for the Four Communication Modes (From "Listening to Patients and Responding with Care," by L. DiBartola, 2001, *Joint Commission Journal on Quality Improvement, 27*(6), 322. Reprinted with permission.)

(continues)

Literature Application *(continued)*

Using your observation skills, determine where your patient is on the inquisitive-assertive scale. Typical markers that would identify someone who is close to the inquisitive side are asking questions, attending carefully to detail, listening carefully to what the other person is saying, showing caution in making a decision without having adequate time to think about it, and preferring facts over intuition. On the other side of the scale, markers for someone who prefers to communicate in an assertive way are showing concern about wasting time, being quick to make a decision, being more interested in outcomes than in process, being willing to take risks, and making strong statements rather than asking questions.

In addition, you will want to make observations about the patient's preference for objectivity or subjectivity. Whereas people with an objective preference are more interested in facts than intuition and in the project outcome than the process, people who are more subjective show more interest in the people who are working on the project than the project itself, are more willing to trust intuition than the facts, and show greater interest in being satisfied than in being right.

Nonverbal cues include the use of gestures or hands while talking for those on the assertive side, reserve and control for those on the inquisitive side, and high energy and expressiveness for those on the subjective side. To apply this model, think of an interaction that did not go well. Notice where both parties fit on the scale. The closer both parties are on the scale, the easier it will be for them to communicate.

Implications for Practice: Once you understand the way in which both you and your patient are most comfortable communicating, you can decide to communicate in a way that may be more comfortable for your patient. You are not expected to change who you are; the goal of this approach is to know yourself, understand the patient, and then move closer to the patient. This will build trust and respect, and result in the patient feeling satisfied in the interaction.

chapter. There are a few additional skills that have not yet been mentioned. The first is touch. Nurses routinely use touch as a way to communicate caring and concern. Occasionally, language barriers will limit communication to the nonverbal mode. For instance, a stroke patient who cannot process words can still interpret a gentle hand on his shoulder.

Communication requires an openness and honesty with concurrent respect for patients and families. In addition, it is important to honor and protect patients' privacy with the nurse's actions and words. Information that patients share with nurses and other health care providers is to be held in confidence. Verbal exchanges regarding patient conditions are private matters that should not occur in the hallway or just outside a patient's room where others will hear them. Nurses are obligated to not discuss patient conditions with others, even family members, without patient permission.

Mentor and Prodigy

The final pattern of communication that occurs in the workplace that will be discussed is between mentor and prodigy. Mentoring is typically an informal process that occurs between an expert nurse and a novice nurse, but it may also be an assigned role. This one-on-one relationship focuses on professional aspects and is mutually beneficial. The optimal novice is hardworking, willing to learn, and anxious to succeed (Shaffer, Tallarica, & Walsh, 2000). Communication entails using the skills previously described in this chapter to help the novice develop expert status and career direction. The novice accomplishes this by gleaning the mentor's wisdom. This wisdom is typically shared through listening, affirming, counseling, encouraging, and seeking input from the novice (Creasia & Parker, 1996). A couple of strategies that facilitate mentoring are to share the same work schedule so that the novice is exposed to

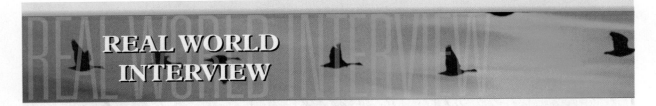

REAL WORLD INTERVIEW

A 16-year-old, first-time expectant mother presented to the labor and delivery department in labor anticipating an uncomplicated delivery. The admitting nurse completed normal admissions information and because of the patient's age, assessed whether a social service consult was indicated immediately. She established who the patient's social support network was, for example, mother, grandmother, or significant other. The delivery commenced uneventfully, and a healthy baby girl was born. Since the mother indicated on admission that she wanted to try to breastfeed, the nurse assisted the mother to breastfeed during the immediate postpartum period prior to the baby being taken to the nursery.

In this clinical situation where hospital stays are short, communication is critical for comprehensive care to occur. Several health care providers are responsible for ensuring quality care in this setting. Nurses play a central role in coordinating communication between the patient and her family/significant other, other nurses, physician or nurse midwife, and other health care providers such as the lactation consultant or a social worker. For example, a social worker could be contacted for challenging social situations identified during the admitting assessment, such as a report of physical abuse, incest, or active drug or alcohol use. The nurse also identifies potential teaching needs during the antepartum period, such as breastfeeding. These teaching needs will be addressed at a later time. These needs are communicated to the appropriate caregiver as responsibility for care is transferred between members of the health care team. The admitting nurse focuses on the patient's immediate needs during labor. This patient's age required specific attention to adolescent developmental needs. As with all patients, the nurse assesses readiness to learn. Whenever possible, she communicates using the patient's preferred communication style, for example, video, reading material, or demonstration.

During labor, the nurse explained what to expect, supported the patient and support person through the stages of labor, and constantly reassured the patient and support person using verbal and nonverbal modes. She used multiple communication skills, that is, attending, responding, and clarifying. A team of health care workers was involved in this delivery. The nurse often functions as informer, recorder, and coach. She communicates labor progress to the physician or midwife and documents the progress while simultaneously supporting the patient. Following delivery, communication with the patient and family continues. The nurse's responsibilities include ongoing assessment of the patient's postpartum status and the initial assessment of the baby's status. The nurse is responsible to communicate to the nursery nurse details of the pregnancy and delivery and the baby's initial status. She may also prepare the mother for transfer to a postpartum unit where other nurses will assume responsibility for care. Once again, communication regarding the multifaceted concerns of the new family unit is necessary in order to ensure quality care. Nurses' attention to accurate verbal reports and written records facilitates communication between patient, family, coworkers, and physicians while maintaining confidentiality.

Kay Kember, RN

the mentor. This allows for sharing and shadowing opportunities. The mentor can also anticipate added challenges that will likely occur with increasing responsibility. Outlining these challenges with suggestions for how to manage them prepares the novice for his expanding responsibilities. Role-playing, in which the expert preceptor nurse describes a theoretical situation and allows the novice to practice his response to new and sometimes challenging situations, is another strategy that can be used.

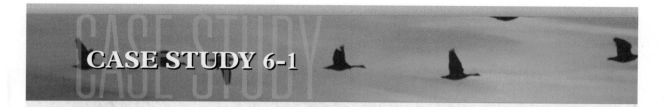

CASE STUDY 6-1

As a new graduate, you have finished orientation and received notice that you have passed your NCLEX exam. The nursing care manager is relieved because two of the other regular nurses are pregnant and will soon be off on maternity leave. One of them is your preceptor. These absences will create a staffing crunch. Therefore, the nursing care manager is anxious to acclimate you to the role of team leader because you will soon be expected to assume those responsibilities.

How can your preceptor help you to take on this additional responsibility? What techniques will you use to enhance your communication with subordinates?

KEY CONCEPTS

- Nurses rely on basic principles of communication to facilitate interactions with patients, peers, and other disciplines.
- Principles of communication allow nurses to adapt to trends, such as increasing diversity, an aging population, and computer technology, that affect the profession of nursing and its practice.
- Nurses follow a process of communication that is more universal than unique to nursing. At the most basic level, this process involves a sender, a message, a receiver, and feedback. The input comes from visual, auditory, and kinesthetic stimuli, which are delivered using verbal and nonverbal modes. Nurses engage in three levels of communication: intrapersonal, interpersonal, and public.
- Nurses participate in upward, downward, lateral, and diagonal communications that are typically defined by their organization. Additionally, nurses may take part in informal exchanges using the grapevine.
- Nurses rely on communication skills such as attending, responding, clarifying, and collaborating to effectively promote patient care and professionalism in a variety of settings.
- Barriers of gender, culture, conflict, and incongruent responses exist.
- Communication in the workplace involves many different relationships that shift the focus of effective communication. These include communicating with superiors, coworkers, subordinates, physicians and other health care workers, and mentors.

KEY TERMS

accommodating	grapevine
attending	interpersonal communication
auditory	intrapersonal communication
avoiding	kinesthetic
clarifying	message
collaborating	nonverbal communication
competing	receiver
compromising	responding
confronting	verbal communication
feedback	visual channel

REVIEW QUESTIONS

1. Which of the following is a trend in society that affects communication?
   A. Decreasing interest in technology
   B. Increasing diversity among Americans
   C. Increasing proportion of younger Americans
   D. Decreasing need for writing skills

2. What part of the communication process returns input to the sender?
   A. Feedback
   B. Message
   C. Receiver
   D. Sender

3. Which of the following characteristics pertains to verbal communication?
   A. Eye contact
   B. Nodding
   C. Smiling
   D. Tone

4. Which of the following skills involves active listening and is a very important skill used by nurses to gain an understanding of the patient's message?
   A. Attending
   B. Clarifying
   C. Confronting
   D. Responding

5. Nurses must be concerned about barriers to communication
   A. because they enhance interactions.
   B. so that they can use them when communicating.
   C. so that they can compensate for them.
   D. Nurses do not need to be concerned.

REVIEW ACTIVITIES

1. Your nursing care manager has asked you to serve on a committee to explore how your unit might communicate more effectively. What current trends in our culture might affect the group's plan?

2. The charge nurse apologizes as she informs you that your assignment includes the "problem patient" on the unit. What communication skills will you use to enhance communication with this patient? How will you avoid barriers of communication with this patient?

3. You found out that you passed your licensure exam last month. When you report for your evening shift, you discover you are assigned to be the team leader. What considerations will be given as you communicate with subordinates?

EXPLORING THE WEB

- What sites would you consider to improve your communication skills? It depends on what aspect is of concern. By using the *http://www.Yahoo.com* search engine and searching for the phrase *communication + skills,* more than 250 sites were identified. Try it and look at the incredible possibilities on-line.

- Keep up with what is happening in the field of nursing and technology. Visit *http://www.ania.org/.* What did you find?

- Are you curious how effectively you communicate? Take an online communication test at *http://www.queendom.com/cgi-bin/tests/transfer.cgi.*

REFERENCES

Baker, C., Beglinger, J., King, S., Salyards, M., & Thompson, A. (2000). Transforming negative work cultures. *JONA, 30*(7/8), 357–363.

Bellack, J. P., & O'Neil, E. H. (2000). Recreating nursing practice for a new century. *Nursing and Health Care Perspectives 21*(1),15–21.

Bradley, J. C., & Edinberg, M. A. (1986). *Communication in the nursing context.* Norwalk, CT: Appleton-Century-Crofts.

Calfee, B. E. (1998). Making calls to the physician. *Nursing 98, 10,* 17.

Creasia, J., & Parker, B. (1996). *Conceptual foundations of professional practice* (2nd ed.). St Louis, MO: Mosby.

DiBartola, L. (2001, June). Listening to patients and responding with care. *Joint Commission Journal on Quality Improvement, 27*(6), 315–323.

Ellis, A. (1997). *Anger: How to live with it and without it.* New York: Citadel Press, Kensington.

Gray, J. (1992). *Men are from Mars, women are from Venus.* New York: HarperCollins.

Kinney, M., & Hurst, J. (1979). *Group process in education.* Lexington, MA: Ginn Customs.

Laswell, H. D. (1948). The structure and function of communication in society. In L. Bryson (Ed.), The *Communication of ideas.* Institute for Religious and Social Studies.

Malone, G., & Morath, J. (2001). Pro-patient partnerships. *Nursing Management, 32,* 46–47.

Moore, N. (2000). In Malloch, K., Sluyter, D., & Moore, N. (2000). Relationship-centered care: Achieving true value in healthcare (p. 384). *JONA, 30*(7/8), 379–385.

Poole, V. L., Davidhizar, R. E., & Giger, J. N. (1995, August). Delegating to a transcultural team. *Nursing Management, 26*(8), 33–34.

Sanchez-Sweatman, L. (1996, September). *The Canadian Nurse, 92*(8), 49–50.

Shaffer, B., Tallarica, B., & Walsh, J. (2000). Win-win mentoring. *Nursing Management 31*(1), 32–34.

Simms, L. M., Price, S. A., & Ervin, N. E. (2000). *The professional practice of nursing administration* (3rd ed.). Clifton Park, NY: Delmar Learning.

Yoder-Wise, P. S. (1999). *Leading and managing in nursing* (2nd ed.). St. Louis, MO: Mosby.

Yogo, Y., Hashi, A. M., Tsutsui, S., & Yamada, N. (2000). Judgments of emotion by nurses and students given double-blind information on a patient's tone of voice and message content. *Perceptual and Motor Skills, 90*, 855–863.

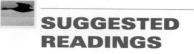

SUGGESTED READINGS

Anderson, K. (1998, October). 16 tips for reaching agreement. *Nursing Management, 29*(10), 89.

Heller, B. R., Oris, M. T., & Durney-Crowley, J. (2000, January/February). The future of nursing education. 10 trends to watch. *Nursing and Health Care Perspectives, 21*(10), 9–13.

Malloch, K., Sluyter, D., & Moore, N. (2000). Relationship-centered care: Achieving true value in healthcare. *JONA, 30*(7/8), 379–385.

CHAPTER 7

Politics and Consumer Partnerships

Terry W. Miller, PhD, RN

The days of building the health care experience around the desires and wishes of the professionals and administrators are over. Successful leaders in nursing and patient care will recognize that a major shift has occurred, and will build the experience of health care around the consumer's needs.

(Karleen Kerfoot, 2000, p. 98)

OBJECTIVES

Upon completion of this chapter, the reader should be able to:

1. Describe how politics defines health care services and affects nursing practice.
2. Recognize the need for nurses to be politically involved with the consumer movement in health care.
3. Describe the role of a nurse as a consumer advocate and political force.
4. Propose a political strategy for strengthening nurse-consumer relationships.
5. Articulate a service-oriented plan for providing nursing services to a selected consumer interest group.
6. Describe how demographic changes are affecting nurses and nursing services.

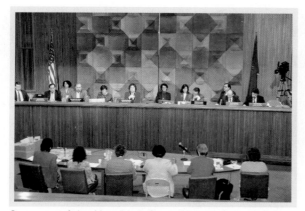

Courtesy of the New York State Nurses Association

The elderly man lying in a nursing home bed, pushing a call button and waiting for a nurse, is not thinking about Medicare, Medicaid, or any other payer for the service. All he knows is that he is not getting the service or care that he expected. And what service or care he is receiving is costing far more than his family anticipated. He probably does not know that Medicare cuts force nursing homes to make drastic changes. For example, Medicare cuts in 1997 were cited as the reason for 1 in 10 nursing homes filing for bankruptcy within a year. A report from the Health Care Financing Administration (HCFA) (2000) includes the claim that 54% of nursing homes do not have enough staff to meet a minimum standard of care. The Medicaid program has paid for almost 45% of the total cost of care for people using assisted living facilities or home health services in recent years. However, for those people who use more than 4 months of this long-term care, Medicaid pays for a much larger percentage. The data for 1998 show that Medicaid payments for nursing facility services and home health care totaled $41.3 billion for more than 3.3 million recipients of these services, an average 1998 expenditure of $12,375 per long-term care recipient. With the percentage of our population that is elderly or disabled increasing faster than that of the younger groups, the need for long-term care is expected to increase (HCFA, 2000).

Can we expect to improve the care of this elderly man given this scenario?

Does politics play a role in this elderly man's care?

Should nurses work with other consumer groups to improve care to elderly patients?

Politics is predominantly a process by which people use a variety of methods to achieve their goals. These methods inherently involve some level of competition, negotiation, and collaboration.

Nurses who can effectively compete, negotiate, and collaborate with others to get what they want or need have developed strong political skills. They have the greatest ability to build strong bases of support for themselves, patients, and the nursing profession.

Politics exist because resources are limited and some people control more resources than others. Resources include people, money, facilities, technology, and rights to properties, services, and technologies. Individuals, groups, or organizations that have the ability to provide or control the distribution of desirable resources are politically empowered. The consumer movement in health care is a political movement about health care resources. It reflects consumer perceptions and values about the largest industry in the United States and involves an assertion by consumers that they will have more direct control over their health care (Smith & Flarey, 1999).

The purpose of this chapter is to support the need for nurses to be politically active for the good of patients and the health care system. A major focus is how the consumer movement in health care creates new opportunities for nurses to advance nursing services by giving patients, including all people who receive health care, a stronger voice in their health care as consumers. Nurses are encouraged to develop a stronger political position by partnering with consumer groups instead of waiting for others to take the lead.

STAKEHOLDERS AND HEALTH CARE

Control of health care resources is spread among a number of vested interest groups called stakeholders. Everyone is a stakeholder in health care at some level, but some people are far more politically active about their stake in health care than others. See Table 7-1 for a list of Washington's most powerful lobbying groups. Many of these groups, as well as others such as insurance companies, consumer groups, professional organizations, health care providers, and educational groups, exert political pressure on health policy makers—local, state, and federal legislative bodies—in an effort to make the health care system work to their economic advantage.

Not all stakeholders in health care support the consumers' potentially dominant role in health care politics, for a variety of reasons. Some contend that consumers do not necessarily know what is best for

TABLE 7-1	Washington's Most Powerful Lobbying Groups

1. National Rifle Association
2. American Association of Retired Persons
3. National Federation of Independent Business
4. American Israel Public Affairs Committee
5. Association of Trial Lawyers
6. AFL-CIO
7. Chamber of Commerce
8. National Beer Wholesalers Association
9. National Association of Realtors
10. National Association of Manufacturers
11. National Association of Home Builders
12. American Medical Association
13. American Hospital Association
14. National Education Association
15. American Farm Bureau Federation

From "Fat & Happy in D.C.," *Fortune*, May 28, 2001, p. 95.

LITERATURE APPLICATION

Citation: Gebbie, K. M., Wakefield, M., & Kerfoot, K. (2000). Nursing and health policy. *Image: Journal of Nursing Scholarship, 32*(3), 307–314.

Discussion: The purpose of this qualitative study was to define ways nurses were or were not effectively involved in the development of health policy in the United States. The findings provide illustrations of world views that can be learned through nursing education and emphasize the importance of career decisions in moving nurses into policy roles. Participants in the study offered valuable suggestions about actions to strengthen the nurses' policy roles. Policy involvement is described as speaking for patients in arenas where patients' voices have been limited or absent. The authors discuss the need to change the way health care resources are allocated. They also discuss caring as a characteristic that distinguishes nurses in their policy roles from other stakeholders. The most important finding was that policy makers responded to nurses in the policy arenas when nurses presented their experiences regarding the determinants of health and illness.

Implications for Practice: "A nurse's knowledge of health issues and unmet needs, coupled with an understanding of what motivates people to get involved, is a potent combination in health policy. For example, a nurse can help policymakers understand the difference between regulations for physicians' decisions about home care and nurses' decisions in patients' homes" (p. 314). Nurses in practice and the patients they care for are directly affected by health care policy decisions. No one can represent nurses in practice to policy makers better than nurses themselves. Nurses in practice gain political power and help patients by offering experience-based perspectives of health and illness to policy makers. Neophyte nurses should not discount their need for understanding health care organizations, financing, and policy making.

them. Instead, they support the idea that health care experts, such as physicians, are better able to direct health care policy. Others maintain that only those directly paying for the services should make policy decisions and that health care is not necessarily a right because services should be based on ability to pay.

The growing cost of health care has led to increasing political activism by third-party payers, as well as consumers. As Johnson and Maas noted, "Payers and consumers want to know what they are getting for their money" (Cohen and DeBack, 1999, p. 38). Third-party payers include the government, business, and health insurance companies. Exposure of Medicare/Medicaid fraud has led to the very nature and control of professional practice being questioned by government payers. Nurses have come to understand how the control and distribution of resources in health care can drastically affect their incomes, workloads, work environments, and patients. Nurses across the country have reported that the patient load per nurse provider has increased significantly. However, these nursing concerns without political influence do little to change health care at any level.

Nursing has a long history of pulling together the various stakeholders and coordinating health care services around patients to ensure that patients obtain the health services they need. "Unfortunately, many nurses have little knowledge about their history" (Ogren, 2001, p. 7). Nurses who recognize that they have a critical role in addressing the major issues in health care delivery at the bedside will ensure that nursing enters into a partnership with agency executives who have control in the wider health care system of which the agency is a part. As partners, they will be able to compete, negotiate, and collaborate with other stakeholders at the system level to be politically effective. These nurses also must be concerned with the price of health care at the system level and understand that resources are controlled and distributed through health policy decisions.

Many authors of nursing articles, some books, and a few research studies support nurses' involvement in public policy and health care politics (Fagin, 1998; Williams, 1998; Mason & Leavitt, 1999; Milstead, 1999). Several other authors promote greater inclusion of policy content and political process in nursing curricula (Brown, 1996; Gebbie, Wakefield, & Kerfoot, 2000; Jones, Jennings, Moritz, & Moss, 1997). Nurses' involvement in policy arenas, such as policy-making committees and institutional boards, includes advocating for recipients of health care when those in need have little or no voice and advocating for those who need a stronger voice. Any professional nurse should understand and be able to articulate the relevance of politics to nursing practice. Making a difference in health care arenas is an outcome of involvement in policy making. As Margaret Mead said, "Never doubt that a small group of thoughtful committed citizens can change the world, indeed it's the only thing that ever has."

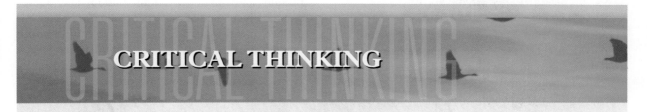

CRITICAL THINKING

Political conflict occurs because people may hold significantly different or conflicting opinions about any given topic. Consumers may disagree about what health care should be, who should provide it, how much it should cost, and who should pay for it. Nurses as providers have a professional responsibility to promote consumer dialogue and offer creative solutions to health care problems. Yet nurses, like consumers, disagree with each other in regard to the same issues consumers may have about health care.

What do you think your responsibility is as a consumer of health care? What is your responsibility as a health care provider? Do you think your responsibility as a consumer could conflict with your responsibility as a provider?

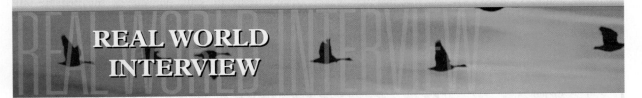

The nurse serves as an advocate and ally for consumers by helping consumers obtain what they perceive they need. Nurses have the opportunity to help consumers better understand what is available to them, as well as what they can legitimately expect to get from both the provider and system. Competent nurses understand how the system works because that is "where they live." The consumer moves in and out of the system so he is not as well acclimated to the limitations or pathways of the system. The consumer and the nurse become natural allies whether it is a patient care setting or a public policy setting. The reason is because the nurse seeks not only to make the patient successful in achieving wellness, the altruistic part, but also to improve her own work environment, the professional part. One of my biggest frustrations is when nurses fail to see themselves as connected to the patient and the whole health care system. They become myopic in their approach to problems in direct patient care because they do not see that they are a piece of something bigger. No nurse's practice occurs in isolation. We are all part of an interdependent, highly complex system with governing economic and political relationships. I found consumer partnerships to be most useful when working as a lobbyist for the Washington State Nurses Association because, as nurses, we were able to build politically powerful coalitions with consumer groups and subsequently define the direction of long-term health care policy, specifically, state policies governing the long-term care industry. Because we were successful in partnering with selected consumer interest groups, we were able to ensure passage and funding of seven significant legislative bills. These bills included the AIDS Omnibus legislation, a long-term care reform act, and an act enabling nurses to declare death for the purpose of preventing unnecessary stress, care, and cost to consumers.

Robert S. Ball, MSN, RN
Nursing Care Manager

THE POLITICS AND ECONOMICS OF HUMAN SERVICES

Many nurses want to avoid the political nature of their work because they believe that human service should not be politically motivated. They also may ignore the business aspects of health care until they find themselves responsible for a budget. Yet all health care is inextricably linked to politics and economics as well as to the availability and services of providers. As a human service, health care has yielded remarkable returns in terms of improving overall quality of life as well as in extending life spans. As a business, health care has afforded millions of people, including nurses, with economic opportunities and lifelong careers.

Health care in the United States depends heavily on a continuous supply of resources from both public and private sectors. These resources include people such as the providers of health care services and the money to educate and pay these providers. Buildings, technology, administration, and equipment are just some of the other resources needed for the health care system to be serviceable. With health care requiring so many resources on such a large economic scale, thousands of people are directly involved in the allocation of those resources, hence, the politics of health care. Most of those people have good intentions, but they often disagree about how the resources can best be used to support health care.

Many consumers are aware that the ongoing redistribution of health care resources may not meet their health care needs, especially as they age and become more dependent upon related services. They are frightened by media reports of increasing national health care expenditures. Although most consumers do not directly pay for the majority of their health care, their individual portions of expenses incurred are rapidly increasing.

Health policy is formulated, enacted, and enforced through political processes at the local, state, or federal levels. For example at the local level, policies would be established and implemented by an individual hospital board or by directors of a total health care system regarding whether or when flu injections would be available to high-risk populations being served by those institutions. At the state level, policies govern nurses within a state by defining nursing practice, nursing education, and nursing licensure. These policies are often governed by a state nurse practice act that designates a state nursing commission or health professions board as the authority for enforcing the policies. Federal policies are evident in the rules and regulations governing Medicare and Medicaid funding.

When bills affecting health care are being developed in state and federal legislative bodies, it is important that nurses be aware of those actions and obtain copies of those bills, thus adding to their political knowledge base.

Ultimately, health care will be defined and controlled by those wielding the most political influence. If nurses fail to exert political pressure on the health policy makers, they will lose ground to others who are more politically active. It is unrealistic to believe that other stakeholders will take care of nursing while the competition for health care resources increases. Historically, some stakeholders in health care have never supported nursing as a profession or acknowledged professional roles for nurses. Nurses, like other

health care providers, must compete, negotiate, and collaborate with others to ensure their future in health care.

Cultural Dimensions of Partnerships and Consumerism

The minority-group population in the United States includes approximately 80 million racially and ethnically diverse people (Leddy & Pepper, 1998). The authors recognized that "people's habits of promoting health, their ways of behaving when sick, theirs ways of recognizing and responding to illness, and their ways of defining health are strongly determined by their sociocultural background" (p. 35). Increasing racial and cultural diversity are indicated in the census data. Whereas whites in the United States are likely to remain a significant majority for some time at greater than 70% of the population, the percentage is rapidly declining. The proportions of Hispanic, African-American, Asian, Native American/Alaskan Native, and Pacific Islander people are increasing, with the largest increase occurring in the Hispanic group (U.S. Census Bureau, 2000).

If nurses intend to form partnerships with consumer groups distinguished by cultural heritage, racial makeup, or ethnic background, they must understand and value diversity. Strong partnerships will frame nursing services in ways that respect cultural differences.

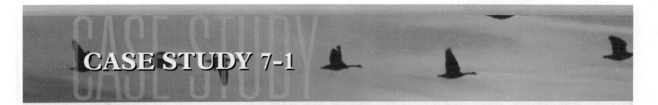

CASE STUDY 7-1

Maria is a maternity support nurse for First Steps, a specific state-funded program designed to provide care to underserved and underinsured pregnant women. Maria is in her third year of professional practice and has become highly resourceful as well as able to work in new situations with minimal supervision. Many of her case referrals come through a partnership with the local hospital's Teen Parent Resource Center, targeting girls under 20 who have dropped out of school during their pregnancy. Many of Maria's patients are from families at high risk for domestic violence and substance abuse. Recently, she was informed that the Teen Parent Resource Center will be discontinuing its partnership with First Steps because of funding issues.

What would you do if you were Maria?

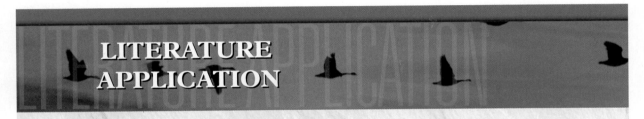

LITERATURE APPLICATION

Citation: Ferguson, S. L. (2001). An activist looks at nursing's role in health policy development. *Journal of Obstetric, Gynecologic, and Neonatal Nursing, 30*(5), 546–551.

Discussion: Nurses play a critical role in determining, developing, implementing, and evaluating health policies because of their knowledge of health care. A conceptual model (Longest, 1998) is useful to illustrate the public policy-making process. The model illustrated in this article depicts three phases: policy formulation, implementation, and modification.

Implications for Practice: Nurses will find the model illustrated in this article useful to influence public policy.

Politics and Demographic Changes

Certainly not all consumers agree about what health care should be, who should provide it, or how it should be paid for. The social, cultural, economic, psychological, and demographic characteristics of consumers largely determine their attitudes and inclination toward the health care system, its providers, and its services. Consumers also recognize some level of personal risk when changes are made in the system, especially involving payment for services and providers. If consumers, such as retired persons, perceive that their out-of-pocket cost for health care extends beyond their capacity to pay or will increase in the future, they are highly motivated to exert political pressure on their legislators to reverse the perceived trend.

The fastest growing consumer group for years to come is the elderly—people 65 years and older—because of the unprecedented reproductive growth rate in the United States between 1946 and 1964 (U.S. Census Bureau, 1996). The number of people aged 65 years and over is increasing almost three times as fast as the population as a whole. Between 1970 and 1994, while the overall U.S. population rose 28%, the number of people aged 50 and over climbed by 66%, and the number of people above age 85 years soared by 150%. It is estimated that 4.6 million people living in the United States are over 85. Seniors' share of the national wealth significantly

exceeds that of any other age group. People over 50 control fully one-half of the country's disposable income, as well as three-quarters of its financial assets and 80% of its savings. Yet most elderly Americans are not wealthy, with 20% projected as qualifying for Medicare benefits by the year 2020 (Shi & Singh, 2001).

Without a doubt, this aging of the U.S. population is profoundly affecting health care at every level. The dramatic increase in the number of elderly people in the Western world means that about one-half of all people who have ever reached age 65 are alive today (Roszak, 1998). Studies of voting behavior of U.S. citizens show that the elderly have no predictable political orientation on anything except obvious threats to perceived entitlements, the most widely recognized entitlement being Social Security benefits.

Many seniors are joining consumer groups to have a greater political voice, influence health policy decisions, and ensure that they receive the health care services they will need for years to come. A growing number are bridging the gap of social isolation, prominent in the past, through the Internet as well as through involvement in consumer groups. They are establishing closer contact with the outside world and are managing to successfully strengthen their relationships with other stakeholders in health care.

The American Association of Retired Persons (AARP), with more than 15 million members, constitutes a growing political powerhouse and an ideal

CRITICAL THINKING

Demographic changes present multiple challenges to health care. For example, as early as 1987, 1,600 health care experts identified the aging of America as the "number one public policy issue and the most critical issue affecting the future of our health care system" (Wesbury, 1988, p. 60). Buerhaus, Staiger, and Auerbach (2000) and others indicated the crisis would become especially evident in regard to the age mix of the health care workforce by 2010. Most, if not all, data indicate escalating age-related nursing and teacher shortages as well as a rapidly increasing demand for elder care services.

How do you see this affecting health care and your nursing practice? What are the political implications for health care providers with proportionally fewer people in the workforce and more people requiring health care services related to aging?

consumer partner for nursing in many ways. A large percentage of nurses are 45 years of age or older and within 5 years of qualifying for membership in the AARP. Few other consumer groups appear to have the potential that the AARP has for defining the health care system of the future.

NURSE AS POLITICAL ACTIVIST

Nurses who are politically active have a definitive voice in their work environments for patient welfare as well as for themselves. In addition to studying issues and voting, nurses will directly contact policy makers such as the chairperson of the hospital board or legislators through phone calls, letters, and e-mail messages. Nurses join professional organizations and actively participate to ensure a more collective, unified voice supporting health care issues and policies that have value for consumers and nursing. Nurses who are most involved will be seen supporting political activities and candidates, assisting during campaigns, helping to draft legislation, and running for political office.

As nurses develop politically, they come to understand the need for political strategy. The purpose of developing political strategies is to understand different ways to achieve one's goals, or the goals one is advocating for, while identifying the other stakeholders and their goals. Political strategy attempts to persuade those people supporting an issue, formulating a policy, or taking an action to take the position in support of those using the political strategy. To be feasible, a political strategy requires commitment by those using it, as well as their awareness of the other stakeholders. Effective political strategy implies considerable forethought and clarity of purpose in even the most ambiguous situations. Nurses who are most likely to wield political influence operate with strategy in mind before taking political action, voicing concerns, making demands, or even advocating for others. Unfortunately, some nurses may become involved in political issues or take overt political stands before adequately studying the political issue or the major stakeholders' positions regarding the issue.

Every nurse should be cognizant of what other involved groups think regarding any relevant political health issue. It is critical that nurses listen to other policy perspectives and understand as many facets of the issue as possible when making health policy proposals. Proposals need to include a rationale to neutralize opposing views. This ensures that unnecessary political fights can be avoided and that more collaboration will occur prior to any policy proposal being made to policy-making bodies such as hospital boards or state legislatures. The more support obtained from the various stakeholders in any policy arena, the better chance of a workable policy being developed and implemented.

To be most politically effective, nurses must be able to clearly articulate at least four dimensions of nursing to any audience or stakeholder: what nursing is, what distinctive services nurses provide to consumers, how nursing benefits consumers, and what nursing services cost in relation to other health care services. Although anecdotal stories and emotional appeals may be effective with certain audiences, it is far more powerful to present research-based evidence to support the political position of the nursing profession. Table 7-2 details responses to the four essential dimensions of nursing.

Politics and Advocacy

The nursing profession has embraced patient advocacy for several decades, even though nurses may compromise their employment positions as they advocate for patients. However, some concern has been voiced that the restructuring of health care is eroding the advocacy role of nurses (O'Connell, 2000). Part of that problem is that nurses doubt that they have the ability to advocate for their patients. They are not comfortable with the level of risk they associate with being a patient advocate. The greatest nurses throughout the profession's history have been strong advocates for patients and have taken far greater risks than a potential loss of a particular job.

Interestingly, some patients have begun advocating for nurses, a role reversal. Those patients perceived nurses as overextended by the nature of the work environment and contended that something had be done to improve the working conditions of

nursing. Nurses in California used consumer support to build their case for counteracting significant staffing cuts affecting nursing practice in their state. With strong consumer support, California nurses developed a legislative proposal in 1999 that has been enacted into state law. This law mandates a minimal staffing level of registered nurses for patient care. The intent is to protect patients from unqualified or dangerous staffing levels while receiving nursing services.

Advocacy and Consumer Partnerships

Nurses must understand the political forces that define their relationships with consumers. Consumers expect the best people to be health care providers, but they are confused about what the roles and responsibilities of professional nurses are. Informed consumers understand how health policy directly affects them but are less likely to recognize how health policy affects nurses. Consumers may expect nurses to be their advocates only in the context of providing direct patient care.

Working through their professional organizations, nurses can collaborate with consumer groups by creating formal partnerships, which serve to promote the role of nurses as consumer advocates in health policy arenas and strengthen the political position of both partners. These partnerships have a stronger political voice than either group has alone.

TABLE 7-2	*Four Essential Dimensions of Nursing*

1. *Nursing is* "attention to the full range of human experiences and responses to health and illness without restriction to a problem-focused orientation" (American Nurses Association, 1995, p. 6).

2. *Distinctive services nurses provide* include, but are not limited to, coordinating total patient care, completing ongoing health assessment, and advocating for quality care for patients. Nursing is perhaps the only profession whose focus is the patient's total health care.

3. *Benefits to consumers* include changes in policies such as reversing the short-stay maternity practice of the 1990s; better coordination of care; and greater access to health care services, especially in rural settings.

4. *Costs of nursing services* vary according to the care setting and role of the nurse. Primary care delivered by nurse practitioners and services provided by certified nurse midwives cost less than the same care delivered by physicians (Shi & Singh, 2001, pp. 138–139).

The partners gain power when interacting with any policy-making body because they represent (1) a larger **voting block**—a group that represents the same political position or perspective; (2) a broader funding base—a source of financial support, and (3) a stronger **political voice**—an increase in the number of voices supporting or opposing an issue—to any policy-making body. Increasingly, professional organizations in nursing recognize the value of partnering with consumers to build a better health care system.

See Table 7-3 for steps in establishing a partnership with a consumer group.

CONSUMER DEMANDS

As recipients of health care are required to pay a larger portion of the cost for health care services, consumers are demanding to be treated as something more than passive recipients of health care. They are

TABLE 7-3	Steps in Establishing a Partnership with a Consumer Group
1. Listen	Become sensitized to the health care needs and political nature of the potential consumer partner.
2. Study	Seek both representative and opposing perspectives from consumer group meetings, focus groups, relevant literature, and interviews.
3. Assess	Determine the need, value, context, and boundaries for establishing the partnership.
4. Focus	Mutually identify the purpose and articulate the goals and specific, realistic objectives for the partnership.
5. Compromise	Work through nonessential and noncritical points and issues.
6. Negotiate	Agree on one's position and responsibilities in the partnership.
7. Plan	Develop a political strategy for achieving the goals and fulfilling the objectives.
8. Test	Test the political waters. Gather feedback on the plan from key people before taking action.
9. Model	Model the political work. Define the structure for working the political strategy with partners.
10. Direct the political action	Understand the bigger picture and concentrate on what can be changed.
11. Implement	Line up political support and take action.
12. Network	Be committed to the mutually recognized goal and consistently work to have an adequate base of support in terms of people, money, and time.
13. Build political credibility	Participate in local, state, and national policy-making efforts that support the partnership and its political agenda.
14. Soothe and bargain	Downplay rivalry and address conflict in a timely, constructive manner.
15. Report, publicize, and lobby	Report, publicize, and lobby the group's political cause. Draw public attention to the needs of the consumer group.
16. Reaffirm, redefine, or discontinue	Regularly evaluate work with consumer group.

CRITICAL THINKING

The American public has become increasingly aware of and interested in health promotion (Leddy & Pepper, 1998). The relationship between personal lifestyle and the incidence of several diseases has been demonstrated through the mainstream media with public education campaigns. Many health promotion programs include the expectation that people invest in themselves, but people who live in poverty lead precarious lives. How do you think people in the lowest socioeconomic class perceive their health care? Do you assume most people will invest in themselves by living a lifestyle that promotes higher education, planned savings, healthy eating, regular exercise, deferred gratification, avoidance of smoking and excessive alcohol consumption, planned birth control, and regular physical checkups? Do you know people who seem to live only from one day to the next because their perspective of time is in the immediate and they do not seem to recognize the benefits of long-term planning?

very vocal in their requests to providers, payers, and agencies that they be more consumer friendly and service oriented, and they are seriously requesting a voice in how health care is regulated.

Nurses, working through professional organizations such as the American Nurses Association (ANA), have been strong, early supporters for patients' rights, regardless of the patient's ability to pay. Other professional groups, such as the American Medical Association (AMA) and the American Hospital Association (AHA), have received far more media recognition for their support of patients' rights. This is an indication that the AMA and AHA are better funded and wield more political power and may do a better job of presenting their positions on consumer issues to the media than the ANA.

Any political vision to make health care more consumer friendly and service oriented must address cost, access, choice, and quality. Perhaps the vision starts with the formula: the highest quality of care for all people at the least cost. Yet defining—much less evaluating—quality is culturally bound and very complicated. Many people cannot afford minimal health care services. Other people are increasingly unwilling to subsidize the care of other patients by paying increased costs for their health care. A vision for high-quality, low-cost care will require multiple stakeholders collaborating with one another to develop a workable philosophy, to include a mechanism for checks and balances to minimize abuse and

misuse and encourage intelligent, ethical decisions by those wielding the most political power.

TURNING A CONSUMER-ORIENTED VISION INTO REALITY

Nurses have opportunities to be more than supporters of a consumer-oriented vision for health care; they can be cocreators. To make this vision real, nurses will need to be more educated and articulate about what value they add to the overall health care system. Getting other stakeholders and the policy makers to understand and promote the value of nursing to consumers will take considerable political work. This work will have to be more than anecdotal pleas, or arguments in support of some consumer cause, or reactions to some particular health care issue or workplace injustice. Believing in a vision and working hard are not enough. Nurses must have a clear image of the vision; develop a sound philosophy; demonstrate intelligent, strategic thinking; and wield more political influence.

Although nurses may think they are the ones primarily affected by the changes in health care, it is more powerful and therefore strategic to understand that everyone, especially consumers, is affected. Rehtmeyer (2000) stated that "nurses need to seize the opportunity to use the confusion in the health care

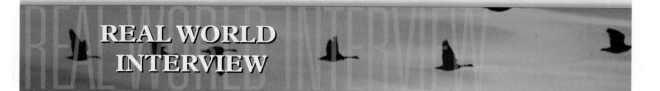

REAL WORLD INTERVIEW

Gary, age 46, and Laurie, age 42, have been married 7 years and have two daughters, ages 4 years and 6 years. Gary is a practicing commercial architect recently diagnosed with Ménière's disease. Laurie is a professional photographer working from home. She was recently diagnosed with sarcoidosis. Gary said the effectiveness of the U.S. health care system is "very restricted by the dictates of insurance companies and by what health care providers want. It's like doing the minimum for whatever reason. There's a reluctance to take a holistic approach." Laurie agreed, adding that "as it stands, service providers are needlessly competing with each other. As a consumer, I do not feel comfortable with how they collaborate with each other, much less the consumer. Nursing has been channeled into a corporate culture because so many nurses fail to think or practice as professionals." Gary said, "Nursing is taken for granted; we really do not see nurses as providers as much as technicians. There is a missed opportunity to meet the expanding needs of consumers. Create a system that is more accessible from a daily living or health maintenance standpoint." Consumers need their "concerns addressed openly and should be able to get answers or at least options without going through so many gatekeepers. I have come to believe that health care is a very inexact science. They are just guessing, or don't seem concerned enough to do more than what the provider wants or will get paid for." Laurie said, "Information is lost between service providers, hospitalizations, and clinic visits. You provide the same information several times and you wonder if anyone is really using or thinking about the information they are gathering. If nurses were better educated, they could be stronger advocates for the consumer." Gary adds, "Health care is becoming more inaccessible unless you are dying. Nurses certainly have the opportunity to do more and be first-level providers. We think that nurses did more to shape our hospital experiences to be a positive experience than anyone. They can be the worker bees of health care. They are vital, but they could do a better job of working with consumers of health care. We are willing to pay more if we trust the competence of the provider and can understand the need for the service. This includes nursing."

Gary and Laurie Maples, Consumers

arena as a source for trying or taking new directions" (p. 184). These new directions may include the strategies outlined in Table 7-4.

The Consumer Demand for Accountability

The vigilance of government, payers, and even attorneys is understandable when one looks at the behavior of some providers (Kavaler & Spiegel, 1997). Some providers focus on "What's good for the agency, my interest group, or me?" rather than "What is going to work for the consumers and all the other stakeholders over the long run?"

When stakeholders are motivated and directed solely by their own perceived needs, competitive polit-ical strategies replace more collaborative approaches to addressing the consumer's health care needs. Accountability becomes a serious issue because the goal of overtaking the competition supersedes the goal of offering the highest-quality services. People who will own the future of health care must address this growing problem of accountability. They will have to establish and sustain their credibility during a time when more people are distrustful of the health care system, its providers, third-party payers, and legislators.

Most people comprehend that being accountable requires being held responsible for one's behavior, decisions, and affiliations with others. Not withstanding, some nurses claim they are not culpable for their actions because they are merely doing what they must do as defined by their employer or some other larger entity. These nurses fail to understand that professional

TABLE 7-4 *Political Strategies for Mounting Consumer Campaigns*

1. Lobbying at state and federal levels for health care regulations and guidelines that serve a consumer group's interest
2. Consulting with representatives from a consumer group when health care regulations and guidelines are being debated or written
3. Monitoring the enforcement of health care regulations and exacting corrective or punitive action when noncompliance occurs
4. Encouraging providers and payers to make changes in delivery of services voluntarily to meet changing consumer demands
5. Changing consumer perceptions and behaviors through the distribution of educational materials or other media

CASE STUDY 7-2

Juan and Casey are study partners in the final semester of a nursing program. Juan served as a medical corpsman and worked as an emergency medical technician for several years whereas Casey entered college right out of high school, starting as a business major. One of their class assignments was to develop a strategy for reducing malpractice risks in a hospital setting. Casey proposes redefining the patient as the customer of health care services because adopting a more customer-oriented approach to health care services in hospitals would improve patient satisfaction and subsequently reduce malpractice claims. Juan opposes that strategy because he thinks that too many health care providers are adopting the culture of corporate America when they define patients as customers. He views patients as something more than customers but also thinks that patients do not know what is best for them in most health care situations.

Do you think that patients should be defined as health care customers?

Would patients be less likely to sue health care providers if they were approached as customers instead of patients?

accountability goes beyond responsibility in a particular employment situation. "The authority for the practice of nursing is based on a social contract that acknowledges professional rights and responsibilities as well as mechanisms for public accountability" (American Nurses Association, 1995, p. 3). In addition, the individual nurse practice acts of each state in the United States address those same concepts.

Increasingly, consumers are demanding positive results and are holding those in the health care system accountable for better health care outcomes. If the trend in increased litigation related to professional negligence and medical malpractice is any indication, just having an ethical process for providing care will not satisfy the consumer who experiences negative health outcomes (Cohen & DeBack,

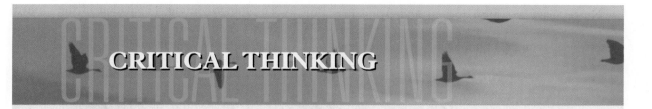

CRITICAL THINKING

Access, quality, and timing of information available to the public have greatly enhanced the consumer health care movement. Using the Internet, people can do customized searches on practically any health care concern; garner input from a wide audience; and do comparative shopping for services, providers, and products. Several uniform sources of information have been developed for the U.S. health care delivery system. These data sets offer information requested by the decision makers about some predetermined dimension of health care. They also establish standard definitions, classifications, and measurements for making evidence-based decisions. Nursing has been relatively absent from the data sought, collected, and disseminated to the decision makers.

Is there a need for nursing-sensitive consumer outcome measures that can be used by decision makers? What steps could be taken to make such information available to the public?

1999). The strongest potential for litigation in health care comes from too few health care professionals accepting personal responsibility for ensuring that health care services are provided in a safe, competent manner at a system level as well as at a personal level. Health care professionals, including nurses, depend upon each other to ensure the quality, consistency, and overall effectiveness of health care within their work environments.

CREDIBILITY AND POLITICS

To have credibility, nurses must demonstrate professional competence and a degree of professional accountability that exceeds consumer expectations. Nurses who are most able to successfully overcome these challenges assert their professional credibility in several ways. They are lifelong learners and demonstrate professional growth throughout their careers in nursing. They approach their vocation as a service to the public and to the nursing profession and an honorable way to make a living. They take ownership of the situations in which they find themselves and work to resolve problems and overcome obstacles to providing the best care possible. Nurses strengthen their political position by taking ownership of their problems in serving consumers. Leddy and Pepper (1998) stated, "When nurses blame others such as

physicians, administrators, or politicians for the state of the health care delivery system, or constantly look to others for improvement of this system, they weaken their position and power base [p. 331]. . . . Nursing is striving for a voice in setting policy for health care delivery at every level" (p. 342).

Nursing ownership, however, is not enough to guarantee the political credibility of nursing in the future. This is because others see the political gains to be made from identifying themselves as consumer advocates. An article titled "In Health Politics, It's Hip to Be Pro-Consumer" appeared in *The Business Journal of Milwaukee* (April 24, 1998). As other service providers board the consumer bandwagon, nurses will need to continuously demonstrate that they are more valuable to the consumer than providers of alternative services that cost less. Consumers increasingly will demand tangible evidence from nurses that their services are worth it.

KEY CONCEPTS

- Individuals or groups take political action to get what they want or prevent others from getting something they do not want them to have.
- Politics are inherent in any system in which resources are absolutely or relatively scarce and in which there are competing interests for those resources.

- Nurses have a critical role in addressing the major system-level issues in health care delivery.
- Political, economic, and social changes in the United States are transforming the health care system.
- Nurses must articulate what nursing is, what distinctive services they provide, how these services benefit consumers, and how much these services cost in relation to other health care services.
- If nursing is defined through politics to be less than critical or professional, nurses will be less empowered and paid less.
- The aging of the U.S. population constitutes a growing political force and affords nursing a wonderful opportunity to become stronger in health policy arenas.
- Consumer partnerships will become more critical for all stakeholders in health care to be politically effective.
- When a consumer group forms a political coalition with other groups such as nurses in a given community, the political influence of both is strengthened.

KEY TERMS

political voice   stakeholders
politics   voting block
resources

REVIEW QUESTIONS

1. Politics exists because
   A. it is required by law.
   B. resources cannot be limited by political process.
   C. some people control more resources than others.
   D. resources must be equally distributed among stakeholders.

2. The consumer movement in health care is
   A. a socialist movement about health care resources.
   B. growing because of the Internet and organizations such as the AARP.
   C. supported by all stakeholders in the health care system.
   D. losing its momentum because of managed care.

3. The minority-group population in the United States
   A. includes 80 million racially and ethnically diverse people.
   B. will surpass the white majority in another 10 years.
   C. has resisted the consumer movement.
   D. is a well-organized, cohesive group of consumers.

REVIEW ACTIVITIES

1. Find out who your congresspeople are. Write or e-mail them and find out what health care legislation they are supporting.

2. Notice who is supporting current health care legislation. Are consumer protections being emphasized in any proposed legislation?

3. Identify a consumer group in which you are interested. Use the steps identified in Table 7-2 to establish a partnership with the group. What did you learn?

EXPLORING THE WEB

- Identify some web sites for consumer groups. American Association of Retired Persons (AARP): *http://www.aarp.org/indexes* Citizens' Council on Health Care: *http://www.cchc-mn.org/* and *http://www.cchc-mn.org/directory.html*

- Note consumer tips at this site: *http://www.consumertips.com/politics.htm*

- Note this Consumers for Quality Care (CQC) site: *http://www.consumerwatchdog.org/healthcare*

- Note this site for consumer reports: *http://www.consumerunion.org/aboutcu/about.htm*

- Identify some sites for government bodies and health care agencies. U.S. Congress: *http://congress.org/* U.S. Department of Health and Human Services: *http://www.hhs.gov/about/profile.html*

- Note this site for collaboration between the Reforming States Group (RSG) and the Milbank Memorial Fund: *http://www.milbank.org/mringopolicy.html*

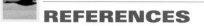

REFERENCES

American Nurses Association. (1995). *Nursing's social policy statement.* Washington, DC: American Nurses Publishing.

Brown, L. D. (1996). *Health policy in the United States: Issues and options.* New York: The Ford Foundation.

Buerhaus, P. I., Staiger, D. O., & Auerbach, D. I. (2000). Implications of an aging registered nurse workforce. *Journal of the American Medical Association, 283,* 2948–2954.

Cohen, E., & DeBack, V. (1999). *The outcomes mandate: Case management in health care today.* St. Louis, MO: Mosby.

Fagin, C. (1998). Nursing research and the erosion of care. *Nursing Outlook, 46*(6), 259–261.

Fat & happy in D.C. (2001, May). *Fortune,* p. 95.

Ferguson, S. L. (2001). An activist looks at nursing's role in health policy development. *Journal of Obstetric, Gynoecologic, and Neonatal Nursing, 30*(5), 546–551.

Gebbie, K. M., Wakefield, M., & Kerfoot, K. (2000). Nursing and health policy. *Image: Journal of Nursing Scholarship, 32*(3), 307–314.

Health Care Financing Administration. (2000, January). National health expenditure projections 1998–2008 [On-line]. Available: http://www.hcfa.gov/stats/NHE-Proj/

Kavaler, F., & Spiegel, A. D. (1997). *Risk management in health care institutions: A strategic approach.* Sudbury, MA: Jones and Bartlett.

Kerfoot, K. (2000). On leadership—"Customerizing" in the new millennium. *MedSurg Nursing: The Journal of Adult Health, 9*(2), 97–99.

Leddy, S., & Pepper, J. M. (1998). *Conceptual bases of professional nursing* (4th ed.). Philadelphia: Lippincott.

Mason, D., & Leavitt, J. K. (1999). *Policy and politics in nursing and health care* (3rd ed.). Philadelphia: Saunders.

Milstead, J. A. (1999). *Health policy & politics: A nurse's guide.* Gaithersburg, MD: Aspen.

O'Connell, B. (2000). Research shows erosion to advocacy role. *Reflections on Nursing Leadership, 26*(2), 26–28.

Ogren, K. E. (2001). The risk of not understanding nursing history. In E. C. Hein (Ed.), *Nursing issues in the 21st century: Perspectives from the literature* (pp. 3–9). Philadelphia: Lippincott.

Rehtmeyer, C. M. (2000). Seeing change as an opportunity. In F. L. Bower (Ed.), *Nurses taking the lead: Personal qualities of effective leadership* (pp. 173–198). Philadelphia: Saunders.

Roszak, T. (1998). *The longevity revolution and the true wealth of nations.* Boston: Houghton Mifflin.

Shi, L., & Singh, D. A. (2001). *Delivering health care in America* (2nd ed.). Gaithersburg, MD: Aspen.

Smith, S. P., & Flarey, D. L. (1999). *Process-centered health care organizations.* Gaithersburg, MD: Aspen.

U.S. Census Bureau. (1996, 2000). [On-line]. Available: http://www.census.gov/mp/www/censtore.html

Wesbury, S. A. (1988). The future of health care: Changes and choices. *Nursing Economic$, 6*(2), 59–62.

Williams, R. P. (1998). Nursing leaders' perceptions of quality nursing: An analysis from academe. *Nursing Outlook, 46*(6), 262–267.

SUGGESTED READINGS

Abeln, S. H. (1994). Quality as a risk management tool. *Rehab Management, 7*(2), 105–106.

American Nurses Association. (1991). *Standards of clinical nursing practice.* Washington, DC: American Nurses Publishing.

Anderson, E. T., & McFarlane, J. M. (2000). *Community as partner: Theory and practice in nursing.* Philadelphia: Lippincott, Williams & Wilkins.

Baird, K. (2000). *Customer service in health care: A grassroots approach to creating a culture of service excellence.* San Francisco: Jossey-Bass.

Edwards, T. (2000). *Contradictions of consumption: Concepts, practices, and politics in consumer society.* Buckingham, UK: Open University Press.

Glickman, L. B. (1999). *Consumer society in American history: A reader.* Ithaca, NY: Cornell University Press.

Jennings, C. P. (Ed.). (2000 to present). *Policy, Politics and Nursing Practice.* (Quarterly journal available through Sage Publications, Thousand Oaks, CA).

Jones, K., Jennings, B., Moritz, P., & Moss, M. (1997). Policy issues associated with analyzing outcomes of care. *Image: Journal of Nursing Scholarship, 29,* 261–268.

Maney, A., & Bykerk, L. (1994). *Consumer politics: Protecting public interests on Capitol Hill.* Westport, CT: Greenwood Press.

Mason, D., & Leavitt, J. K. (1998). *Policy and politics in nursing and health care.* Philadelphia: Saunders.

Miller, T. W. (1996). Health policy, politics, and community health advocacy. In B. W. Spradley & J. A. Allender (Eds.), *Community health nursing: Concepts and practices* (pp. 635–657). Philadelphia: Lippincott.

O'Reilly, P. (2000). *Health care practitioners: An Ontario case study in policy making.* Toronto: University of Toronto Press.

Pope, T. (2000). The rising tide of consumerism: How will it affect long-term care decision making? *Long-Term Care Interface, 1*(1), pp. 36–40.

Sherman, S. G., & Sherman, V. C. (1998). *Total customer satisfaction: A comprehensive approach for health care providers.* San Francisco: Jossey-Bass.

Smith, S., Heffler, S., & Freeland, M. (1999). The next decade of health spending: A new outlook. *Health Affairs, 18*(4), 86–95.

Spradley, B. W., & Allender, J. A. (1996). *Community health nursing: Concepts and practice.* Philadelphia: Lippincott.

Strasen, L. (1987). *Key business skills for nurse managers.* Philadelphia: Lippincott.

Wojner, A. W. (2001). *Outcomes management: Applications to clinical practice.* St. Louis, MO: Mosby.

World Health Organization. (1978). *Declaration of Alma Ata: Report of the International Conference on Primary Health Care.* Geneva, Switzerland: Author.

CHAPTER 8

Leadership is the essence of professionalism and should be considered an essential component of all nurse and other professional roles. (Joyce Clifford, PhD, RN, FAAN)

Leadership and Management

Linda Searle Leach, PhD, RN, CNAA

OBJECTIVES

Upon completion of this chapter, the reader should be able to:

1. Define management.
2. Describe the management process.
3. List 10 roles that managers fulfill in an organization.
4. Explain management theories.
5. Discuss motivation theories.
6. Define leadership and explain its importance for organizations.
7. Differentiate between leadership and management.
8. Describe characteristics of effective leaders.
9. Identify leadership styles.
10. Explain Hersey and Blanchard's situational theory of leadership.
11. Discuss transformational leadership theory.

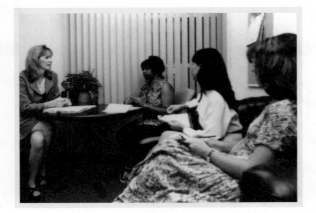

Ed was admitted to the cardiac observation unit earlier in the day. He had been diagnosed previously with heart disease and had experienced episodes of ventricular arrhythmias. His cardiologist had determined the need to change his antiarrhythmic medication to reduce the side effects Ed was experiencing. That evening, while Ed was talking to his wife on the phone and as his nurse was walking to his bedside, he suddenly stopped talking and went into ventricular tachycardia and cardiac arrest. His nurse reacted immediately and started cardiopulmonary resuscitation (CPR). Unable to use the phone to call for help, she gave a precordial thump to his chest. Normal sinus rhythm appeared on the monitor before anyone else could respond to the code. Ed was then transferred to the coronary care unit (CCU).

This nurse had been a registered nurse (RN) less than 1 year at the time, and although she had participated in code arrests a few times, she had never witnessed one occur right before her eyes. Her knowledgeable action saved this patient's life. In nursing, CPR is a mandatory skill and considered part of a nurse's ordinary work. Yet it is quite extraordinary work.

Earlier that evening, this nurse had agreed to work an extra shift in the CCU. After Ed was transferred there, she was assigned to him for the 11 P.M. to 7 A.M. shift. Everything had happened so quickly that evening that she never had a chance to talk to the patient before he was transferred. When she began the night shift, Ed was already asleep. He was fine all through the night, as if nothing had ever gone wrong. She entered his room the next morning, as the sun was just rising. As he awoke, she spent that quiet time with him. While he embraced the start of a new day, his thoughts must have been intense. What he chose to share was this acknowledgment: "You saved my life. Thank you." This precious moment was a celebration of both of their lives.

What leadership characteristics did this nurse demonstrate?

Why is this nurse considered a leader, even though she is not in an executive or management position?

Why is leadership important at all levels throughout a health care organization?

Professionals use their expertise and specialized knowledge to perform leadership roles. Many people think leaders are corporate executives, political representatives, military generals, or those who head organizations. Alfred DeCrane Jr., chairman of the board and chief executive officer of Texaco and a trustee of the University of Notre Dame, reminds us that this occurs because these leaders are in highly visible and high-profile positions. He says that we need leadership not just at the top of our organizations but across and throughout all levels (DeCrane, 1996). The Pew Health Professions Commission (1995) recommends that leadership be considered a competency for health professions and calls for leadership development as part of the preparation of health care providers.

Nurses make a critical difference every day in the lives of their patients and patients' families, yet nurses believe those accomplishments are part of their ordinary work. Nurses are leaders, and by using their expert knowledge and leadership, they provide caring that is extraordinary. This chapter introduces the process of management and explains management theories and functions. Management will be defined, and current trends will be discussed. This chapter also discusses leadership and provides a framework to differentiate leadership and management. Leadership characteristics, styles of leadership, and leadership theories are described.

DEFINITION OF MANAGEMENT

Management can be defined as a process of coordinating actions and allocating resources to achieve organizational goals. Descriptive research (Mintzberg, 1973; McCall, Morrison, & Hanman, 1978; Hales, 1986) about what managers do has been a helpful way to expand our understanding of management. Managers often seem to work at a hectic pace and sustain that effort through long hours, frequently working

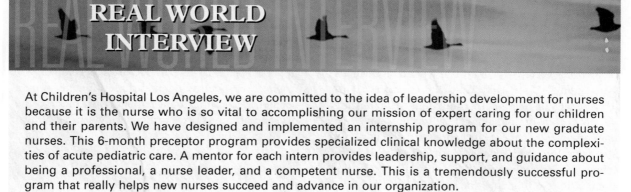

REAL WORLD INTERVIEW

At Children's Hospital Los Angeles, we are committed to the idea of leadership development for nurses because it is the nurse who is so vital to accomplishing our mission of expert caring for our children and their parents. We have designed and implemented an internship program for our new graduate nurses. This 6-month preceptor program provides specialized clinical knowledge about the complexities of acute pediatric care. A mentor for each intern provides leadership, support, and guidance about being a professional, a nurse leader, and a competent nurse. This is a tremendously successful program that really helps new nurses succeed and advance in our organization.

Mary Dee Hacker, RN, MBA
Vice President, Patient Care Services

without breaks. Yukl (1998) says that this reflects a preference by people in management positions who become adept at continuously seeking information and are constantly engaged in interactions with others who need information, help, guidance, or approval. The typical manager is on the go. Research by McCall, Morrison, and Hanman (1978) showed that the daily activities of managers are diverse and fast paced with regular interruptions. Priority activities are integrated among inconsequential ones. In the scope of one morning, a manager may engage in serious and far-reaching decisions about downsizing personnel, respond to a patient complaint, problem-solve a sick call, and participate in a celebration for an employee. Managerial work is driven by problems that emerge in random order, and that have a range of importance and urgency. These circumstances create an image of the manager as a "firefighter" involved in immediate and operational concerns. A significant proportion of a manager's time is spent in interaction with others, and more of the work is concerned with handling information than in making decisions (McCall, Morrison, & Hanman, 1978).

The Management Process

In the early 1900s, an emphasis on management as a discipline emerged with a focus on the science of management. In 1924, Mary Parker Follet wrote about management as an art of accomplishing things

through people. Henri Fayol, a manager, wrote a book in 1916 called *General and Industrial Management*. In it, he described the functions of planning, organizing, coordinating, and controlling as the management process (Fayol, 1916/1949). His work has become a classic in the way that we define the process of managing. Two other individuals, Gulick and Urwick, in some part as a result of their esteemed status as informal advisers to President Franklin D. Roosevelt, served to define the management process according to seven principles (Henry, 1992). Their principles form the acronym POSDCORB, which stands for planning, organizing, staffing, directing, coordinating (CO), reporting, and budgeting (Gulick & Urwick, 1937; Henry, 1992). Their work is also considered to be a classic description of management and is still a relevant description of how management is carried out today.

One of the most frequently referenced taxonomies of managerial roles is from an in-depth, monthlong study of five chief executives by Henry Mintzberg. A taxonomy is a system that groups or classifies principles. Mintzberg's observations led to the identification of three categories of managerial roles: (1) information processing roles, (2) interpersonal roles, and (3) decision-making roles (Mintzberg, 1973). A role includes behaviors, expectations, and recurrent activities within a pattern that is part of the organization's structure (Katz & Kahn, 1978). The information processing roles identified by Mintzberg (1973) are those of monitor, disseminator, and spokesperson and are used to manage people's information needs. The interpersonal roles consist of figurehead, leader, and liaison, and each of these is used to manage relationships with people. The decision roles are entrepreneur, disturbance handler, allocator of resources, and negotiator. Managers take on these roles when they make decisions.

More recently, Yukl (1998) and colleagues (Kim & Yukl, 1995; Yukl, Wall, & Lepsinger, 1990) described 13 managerial role functions for managing the work and for managing relationships. The role functions for managing the work are planning and organizing, problem solving, clarifying roles and objectives, informing, monitoring, consulting, and delegating. The role functions for managing relationships are networking, supporting, developing and mentoring, managing conflict and team building, motivating and inspiring, and recognizing and rewarding.

The amount of time a manager spends in particular roles varies by the level of the manager's position in an organization, ranging from the lowest level manager, to the middle level manager, to the highest or executive level manager. A low level managerial job is often the first-line manager, and in health care organizations that is the typical role of the nurse manager. The nurse manager spends the majority of her time supervising others as they deliver care as well as supervising the quality of care given. The next highest percentage of this manager's time is spent in planning with other responsibilities such as coordinating, evaluating, negotiating, and serving as a multispecialist and generalist taking less than 10% each of this nurse manager's time. In contrast, the middle-level manager, often called a director, such as the director of critical care nursing, spends less time supervising and more time in each of the other assignments, particularly planning and coordinating. At the highest level of the organization, usually described as the executive level, planning and being a generalist are greatly expanded role function, whereas monitoring is not the primary role function as it is in the other two levels. Nurses in executive-level roles in health care organizations usually have the title of chief nurse executive; in acute care hospitals, their title is often vice president of patient care services.

MANAGEMENT THEORIES

The current theories of management practice have evolved from earlier theories. Management practices

were actually a part of the governance in ancient Samaria and Egypt as far back as 3000 B.C. (Daft & Marcic, 2001). Most of our current understanding of management, however, is based on the classical perspective of management or the classical theories of management that were introduced in the 1800s during the industrial age as factories developed. The classical perspective includes three subfields of management: scientific management, bureaucratic theory, and administrative principles (Wren, 1979; Daft & Marcic, 2001).

Scientific Management

While practicing managers, such as Fayol, who was mentioned earlier, were describing the functions of managers, a man named Frederick Taylor was focusing his attention on the operations within an organization by exploring production at the worker level. Taylor is acknowledged as the father of scientific management for his use of the scientific method and as the author of *Principles of Scientific Management* (1911). Productivity was the area of focus in scientific management. Taylor, an engineer, introduced precise procedures based on systematic investigation of specific situations. The underlying point of view is that the organization is a machine to be run efficiently to increase production.

Working independently of Taylor, Frank and Lillian Gilbreth also contributed significantly to scientific management. They pioneered studies of time and motion that emphasized efficiency and culminated in "one best way" of carrying out work. Frank Gilbreth (1912) revolutionized surgical efficiency in the operating room, resulting in operations of shorter duration that substantially reduced risks from surgery for patients at that time.

Bureaucratic Theory

Max Weber is the German theorist recognized for the organizational theory of bureaucracy. Weber's beliefs were in stark contrast to the typical European organization that was based on a family-type structure in which employees were loyal to an individual, not to the organization—resources were used to benefit individuals rather than to advance the organization. Weber, however, believed efficiency is achieved through impersonal relations within a formal structure, competence should be the basis for hiring and promoting an employee, and decisions should be made in an

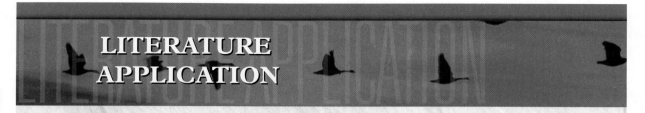

LITERATURE APPLICATION

Citation: Laborde, A. S., & Lee, J. A. (2000). Skills needed for promotion in the nursing profession. *Journal of Nursing Administration, 30*(9), 432–439.

Discussion: This research was designed to identify skills (interpersonal versus technical) needed for job promotion within the nursing field. As a nurse changes positions from primarily clinical practice to management, interpersonal skills seem to be more important than technical ones to move up the organizational ladder. Even though technical skills are necessary for those who supervise nurses, interpersonal skills become more important as tools to influence and lead others.

The hypotheses were as follows: more interpersonal skills would be important for promotion to upper-level management positions, whereas more technical skills would be important for promotion to lower-level management; a significant difference would exist between decision makers' perceptions of the importance of the skills and the skills' objective importance to promotion decisions. A stratified random sample of 219 nurse administrators was obtained from a large hospital in the southeastern United States. Sixty scenarios with hypothetical candidates were used to approximate the promotion situations. Hypothetical candidates were described in terms of their interpersonal and technical skills, and the participants were asked to decide how likely they would be to recommend this candidate for a promotion by using a Likert-type 5-point scale in which 1 was definitely not promote and 5 was definitely promote. No significant differences were found between the position and the number of interpersonal skills used. However, at the lower-level management position of clinical nurse 3 (CN3), a greater number of technical skills influenced promotion decisions more than for the middle management position.

Implications for Practice: The findings suggest that technical skills are more important for clinical nurse promotions than for nurse manager positions. The skills needed for success change as one moves from clinical practice to a managerial position. Several strategies were proposed to increase managerial effectiveness. A dual career ladder would provide a mechanism for retaining technical skills. It would give the employee a choice between developing technical skills and pursuing management. Succession planning may reduce the political influences and personal bias in the promotion process. Mentoring programs could provide valuable insights for new managers. Providing realistic job previews and complete job descriptions can clarify misunderstandings and reduce managerial burnout and turnover. Additional research is needed to improve management development programs for nurses and to evaluate designs for how managers are selected.

orderly and rational way based on rules and regulations. The bureaucratic organization was a hierarchy with clear superior-subordinate communication and relations, based on positional authority, in which orders from the top were transmitted down through the organization via a clear chain of command.

Administrative Principles

Administrative principles are general principles of management that are relevant to any organization. In addition to some of the principles described as the management process (e.g., planning, organizing, directing, coordinating, and controlling), principles such as unity of command and direction were identified. Unity of command and direction means that a worker would get orders from only one supervisor and related work would be grouped under one manager. These are examples of general principles generated during the early 1900s that were useful and relevant to all organizations (Fayol, 1916/1949).

Another key aspect of this perspective is attributed to Chester Barnard. Barnard (1938) is associated with the concept of the informal organization. The informal organization consists of naturally forming social groups that can become strong and powerful contributors to an organization. Barnard understood that these informal forces can be valuable in accomplishing the organization's goals and should be managed properly. He is also credited with the acceptance theory of authority. This theory identified people as having free will and that they actually choose to comply with orders they are given (Daft & Marcic, 2001). This view of people as making a difference in organizations was a precursor to the human relations movement that emerged from experiments at a Chicago electric company. See Table 8-1 for an overview of management theories.

Human Relations

The next focus in the development of management is the human relations movement. In contrast to the science of exact procedures, rules and regulations, and formal authority that characterized scientific management, the theories from the human relations school of thought espoused the individual worker as the source of control, motivation, and productivity in organizations. During the 1930s, labor unions became stronger and were instrumental in advocating for the human needs of employees. During this time, experiments were conducted at the Hawthorne plant of the Western Electric Company in Chicago that led to a greater understanding of the influence of human relations in organizations.

Electricity had become the preferred power source over gas; the Hawthorne plant experiments were run to show people that more light was necessary for greater productivity. This approach was designed to increase the use of electricity. Researchers Mayo (1933) and Roethlisberger and Dickson (1939) measured the effects on production of altering the intensity of lighting. They found that with more and brighter light production increased as expected. However, production also increased each time they reduced the light, even when the light was extremely dim. Their research findings led to the conclusion that something else besides the light was motivating these workers.

The notion of social facilitation or the idea that people increase their work output in the presence of others was a result of the Hawthorne experiments. They also concluded that the effect of being watched and receiving special attention could alter a person's behavior. The phenomena of being observed or studied, resulting in changes in behavior, is now called the **Hawthorne effect** (Hughes, Ginnet, & Curphy, 1999). Emerging from this study was the concept that people benefit and are more productive and satisfied when they participate in decisions about their work environment. This was the next phase in the evolution of management, called human relations management. In addition, social groupings, people's feelings, and their motivations became a focus of interest for future studies.

MOTIVATION THEORIES

The human relations perspective in management theory grew from the conclusion that worker output was greater when the worker was treated humanistically. This spawned a human resources point of view and a focus on the individual as a source of motivation. **Motivation** is not explicitly demonstrated by people but rather is interpreted from their behavior. Motivation is whatever influences our choices and creates direction, intensity, and persistence in our behavior (Hughes, Ginnett, & Curphy, 1999; Kanfer, 1990). Motivation is a process that occurs internally to influence and direct our behavior in order to satisfy needs (Lussier, 1999). Motivation theories are not management theories per se; however, they are frequently included along with management theories.

There are content motivation theories and process motivation theories (Lussier, 1999). The process motivation theories are expectancy theory and equity theory. The content motivation theories include Maslow's needs hierarchy, Aldefer's expectancy-relatedness-growth (ERG) theory, Herzberg's two-factor theory, and McClelland's manifest needs theory. Maslow's hierarchy of needs and Herzberg's two-factor theory are presented here along with Theory X and Y and Theory Z (Table 8-2).

Motivation theories are useful because they help explain why people act the way they do and how a manager can relate to individuals as human beings and workers. When you are interested in creating change, influencing others, and managing performance and outcomes, it is helpful to understand the motivation that is reflected in a person's behavior. Motivation is a critical part of leadership because we need to understand each other in order to be good leaders and good followers.

TABLE 8-1	*Management Theories*	

Management Theory	Main Contributors	Key Aspects
Scientific management	Frederick Taylor (1856–1915) Frank Gilbreth (1868–1924) Lillian Gilbreth (1878–1972)	Machinelike focus Analysis of elements of an operation Training of the worker Use of proper tools and equipment Use of incentives Use of time and motion studies to make the work easier
Bureaucratic theory	Max Weber (1864–1920): German sociologist	Division of labor, hierarchy of authority, and chain of command Rationality, impersonal management Use of merit and skill as basis for promotion/reward Use of rules and regulations, focus on exacting work processes Career service, salaried managers
Administrative principles	Mary Parker Follet (1868–1933): Trained in philosophy/political science at Radcliffe	The science of management Principles of organization applicable in any setting
	Henri Fayol (1841–1925): French mining engineer, head of major mining company	Fayol's principles: unity of command, division of work, unity of direction, scalar chain, and management functions—planning, organizing, coordinating, and controlling
	Chester Barnard (1886–1961): Harvard economics, president of New Jersey Bell Telephone	Concerned with the optimal approach for administrators to achieve economic efficiency
	Luther Gulick and Lyndal Urwick (1937): *Papers on the Science of Administration*	Planning, organizing, supervising, directing,controlling, organizing, reviewing, and budgeting = POSDCORB
	James Mooney (1939): *Principles of Organization*	Four principles: coordination, hierarchical structure (scalar), functional (division of labor), staff/line principle
Human relations (replaced later with the term *organizational behavior*)	Elton Mayo (1933) Fritz Roethlisberger (1939): Harvard University	Hawthorne studies led to the belief that human relations between workers and managers and among workers were main determinants of efficiency. The Hawthorne effect refers to change in behavior as a result of being watched.

TABLE 8-2	Motivation Theories	
Motivation Theory	**Main Contributors**	**Key Aspects**
Selected content of motivation theories	Abraham Maslow (1908–1970)	Hierarchy of satisfaction of physiological, safety, belonging, ego, and self-actualization needs
	Frederick Herzberg (1968) Two-factor theory	Hygiene-maintenance factors = prevent job dissatisfaction: provide adequate salary and supervision, safe and tolerable working conditions Motivators = job satisfaction: satisfying and meaningful work, development opportunities, responsibility, and recognition
	Douglas McGregor (1906–1964)	Theory X: leaders must direct and control as motivation results from reward and punishment Theory Y: leaders remove obstacles as workers have self-control, self-discipline; their reward is their involvement in work
	William Ouchi (1981)	Theory Z: Collective decision making, long-term employment, mentoring, holistic concern, and use of quality circles to manage service and quality; a humanistic style of motivation based on Japanese organizations

Maslow's Hierarchy of Needs

One of the most well-known theories of motivation is Maslow's hierarchy of needs. Maslow (1970) developed a hierarchy of needs that shows how an individual is motivated. Figure 8-1 applies Maslow's hierarchy of human needs to how organizations motivate employees. Motivation, according to Maslow, begins when a need is not met. For example, when a person has a physiological need, such as thirst, this unmet need has to be satisfied before a person is motivated to pursue higher-level needs. Certain needs have to be satisfied first, beginning with physiological needs, then safety and security needs, next belonging social needs, followed by esteem and ego needs before an individual is motivated by the needs at the next level. The need for self-actualization drives people to the pinnacle of performance and achievement.

Two-Factor Theory

Frederick Herzberg (1968) contributed to research on motivation and developed the two-factor theory of motivation. He analyzed the responses of accountants and engineers and concluded that there were two sets of factors associated with motivation. One set of motivation factors must be maintained to avoid job dissatisfaction. These factors are salary, job security, working conditions, status, quality of supervision, and relationships with others. These factors have been labeled maintenance or hygiene factors. Factors such as achievement, recognition, responsibility, advancement, and the opportunity for development also contribute to job satisfaction. These factors are intrinsic and serve to satisfy or motivate people. Herzberg proposed that when these motivation factors are present, people are very motivated and satisfied with their job. When these factors are absent from a work setting, people have a neutral attitude

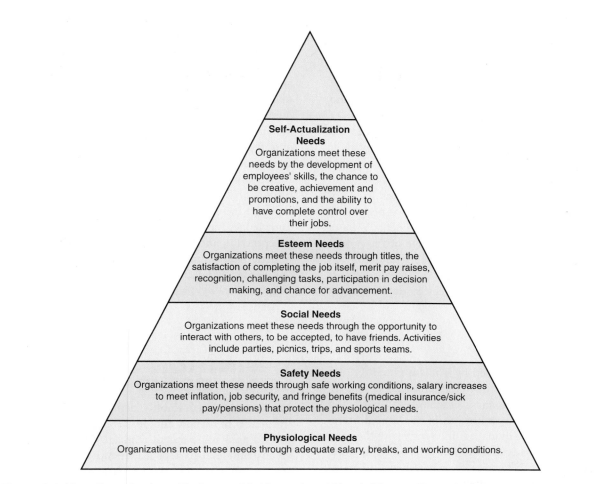

Self-Actualization Needs
Organizations meet these needs by the development of employees' skills, the chance to be creative, achievement and promotions, and the ability to have complete control over their jobs.

Esteem Needs
Organizations meet these needs through titles, the satisfaction of completing the job itself, merit pay raises, recognition, challenging tasks, participation in decision making, and chance for advancement.

Social Needs
Organizations meet these needs through the opportunity to interact with others, to be accepted, to have friends. Activities include parties, picnics, trips, and sports teams.

Safety Needs
Organizations meet these needs through safe working conditions, salary increases to meet inflation, job security, and fringe benefits (medical insurance/sick pay/pensions) that protect the physiological needs.

Physiological Needs
Organizations meet these needs through adequate salary, breaks, and working conditions.

Figure 8-1 How Organizations Motivate with Hierarchy of Needs Theory (From *Leadership: Theory, Application, Skill Building* [p. 81], by R. N. Lussier and C. F. Achua, 2001, Cincinnati, OH: South-Western College)

about their organization. In contrast, when the maintenance factors are absent, people are dissatisfied. Herzberg believed that by providing the maintenance factors, job dissatisfaction could be avoided, but that these factors will not motivate people.

New graduate nurses can use Herzberg's theory by evaluating the maintenance factors present in a health care organization when they apply for a job. The pay, working conditions, and the beginning relationship that has been established with the supervisor are aspects of the job that the nurse should consider. If these maintenance factors are not adequate to begin with, then the nurse may become easily dissatisfied with the job. The higher-level needs that Herzberg describes as motivation factors should also be evaluated by the nurse before joining an organization. Are there opportunities for the nurse to achieve professional growth, to take on new respon-

sibilities, to advance and be recognized for the contribution he has made?

Theory X and Theory Y

Continuing the emphasis on factors that stimulate job satisfaction and what motivates people to be involved and contribute productively at work, McGregor capitalized on his experience as a psychologist and university president to develop Theory X and Theory Y (McGregor, 1960). Theory X and Y are about two different ways to motivate or influence others based on underlying attitudes about human nature. Each view reflects different attitudes about the nature of humans. The Theory X view is that in bureaucratic organizations, employees prefer security, direction, and minimal responsibility. Coercion, threats, or punishment are necessary because people do not like the work to be done. These employees are not able to offer creative solutions to help the organizations advance. McGregor's beliefs about Theory X were related to the classical perspective of organizations that included scientific management, bureaucracy theory, and administrative principles.

The assumptions of **Theory Y** are that in the context of the right conditions, people enjoy their work; can show self-control and discipline; are able to contribute creatively; and are motivated by ties to the group, the organization, and the work itself. In essence, this view espouses the belief that people are intrinsically motivated by their work. Theory Y was a guide for managers to take advantage of the potential of each person, which McGregor thought was being only partially utilized, and to provide support and encouragement to employees to do good work (McGregor, 1960).

Theory Z

Theory Z was developed by William Ouchi (1981) based on his years of study of organizations in Japan. He identified that Japanese organizations had better productivity than organizations in the United States and that they were managed differently with their use of quality circles to pursue better productivity and quality. Theory Z focuses on a better way of motivating people through their involvement. Collective decision making is a hallmark of Theory Z as is a focus on long-term employment that involves slower promotions and less direct supervision. The organization and the worker are viewed more holistically. Through progressive development, the organization will be productive and quality goals will be achieved. The organization invests in its employees and addresses both home and work issues creating a path for career development. Democratic leaders, who are skilled in interpersonal relations, foster employee involvement (Ouchi, 1981).

The Changing Nature of Managerial Work

Current trends indicate that the numbers of managers in an organization, particularly at the middle level, are being reduced and that downsizing of staff has been a common phenomenon in most health care institutions. Those left in management positions after reorganizations are fewer in number and have

taken on more responsibility over more areas. As individual nurses become more involved in managing consumer relations and consumer care, managers will become managers of systems rather than managers of nurses per se. The systems they will manage include clinical systems, cost information systems, and data systems on consumer satisfaction and feedback. Leadership responsibilities will be integrated among all organizational participants who function as **knowledge workers** and provide their professional expertise. Knowledge workers are those involved in serving others through their specialized knowledge. Among nurses, specialized knowledge is the practice and science of nursing used to serve patients and families. So leadership responsibilities will be dispersed among all nurses, who are knowledge workers by virtue of their professional nursing expertise.

DEFINITION OF LEADERSHIP

Leadership is commonly defined as a process of influence in which the leader influences others toward goal achievement (Yukl, 1998). Influence is an instrumental part of leadership and means that leaders affect others, often by inspiring, enlivening, and engaging others to participate. The process of leadership involves the leader and the follower in interaction. This implies that leadership is a reciprocal relationship. Leadership can occur between the leader and another individual; between the leader and a group; or between a leader and an organization, a community, or a society. Defining leadership as a process helps us to understand more about leadership than the traditional view of a leader being in a position of authority, exerting command, control, and power over subordinates. What this means for nurses as professionals is that they function as leaders when they influence others toward goal achievement. Nurses are leaders. There are many more leaders in organizations than those who are in positions of authority. Each person has the potential to serve as a leader.

Leadership can be **formal leadership**, as when a person is in a position of authority or in a sanctioned, assigned role within an organization that connotes influence, such as a clinical nurse specialist (Northouse, 2001). An **informal leader** is an individual who demonstrates leadership outside the scope of a formal leadership role or as a member of a group rather than as the head or leader of the group. The informal leader is considered to have emerged as a leader when she is accepted by others and is perceived to have influence.

Not all leaders are managers. Another way to define leadership is through the differentiation of leadership and management (Zalenik, 1977). Bennis's work on differentiating the characteristics of managers versus leaders popularized the phrase "Managers are people who do things right and leaders are people who do the right thing" (Bennis & Nanus, 1985, p. 21).

Kotter (1990a) describes the differences between leadership and management in the following way: Leadership is about creating change and management is about controlling complexity in an effort to bring order and consistency. He says that leading change involves establishing a direction, aligning people through empowerment, and motivating and inspiring them toward producing useful change and achieving the vision, whereas management is defined as planning and budgeting, organizing and staffing, problem solving and controlling complexity to produce predictability and order (Kotter, 1990b).

Leadership Characteristics

According to Bennis and Nanus (1985), there are three fundamental qualities that effective leaders share. The first quality is a guiding vision. Leaders focus on a professional and purposeful vision that provides direction toward the preferred future. The second quality is passion. Passion expressed by the leader involves the ability to inspire and align people toward the promises of life. The third quality is integrity that is based on knowledge of self, honesty, and maturity that is developed through experience and growth. McCall (1998) describes how self-awareness—knowing our strengths and weaknesses—can allow us to use feedback and learn from our mistakes. Daring and curiosity are also basic ingredients of leadership from which leaders draw on to take risks, learning from what works as much as from what does not (Bennis & Nanus, 1985).

Certain characteristics are commonly attributed to leaders. These traits are considered desirable and seem to contribute to the perception of being a leader. They include intelligence, self-confidence,

determination, integrity, and sociability (Stodgill, 1948, 1974). Research among 46 hospitals designated as magnet hospitals for their success in attracting and retaining registered nurses emphasized the value of leaders who are visionary and enthusiastic, are supportive and knowledgeable, have high standards and expectations, value education and professional development, demonstrate power and status in the organization, are visible and responsive, communicate openly, and are active in professional associations (Scott, Sochalski, & Aiken, 1999; McClure, Poulin, Sovie, & Wandelt, 1983; Kramer & Schmalenberg, 1988). Research findings from studies on nurses revealed that caring, respectability, trustworthiness, and flexibility were the leader characteristics most valued. In one study, nurse leaders identified managing the dream, mastering change, designing organization structure, learning, and taking initiative as leadership characteristics (Murphy & DeBack, 1991). Research by Kirkpatrick and Locke (1991) concluded that leaders are different from nonleaders across six traits: drive, the desire to lead, honesty and integrity, self-confidence, cognitive ability, and knowledge of the business. While there is no set of traits that is definitive and reliable in determining who is a leader or who is effective as a leader, many people still rely on personality traits to describe and define leaders.

Leadership Theories

Many believe that the critical factor needed to maximize human resources is leadership (Bennis & Nanus, 1985). A more in-depth understanding of leadership can be gleaned from a review of leadership theories. The major leadership theories can be classified according to the following approaches: behavioral, contingency, and contemporary.

Behavioral Approach

Leadership studies from the 1930s by Kurt Lewin and colleagues at Iowa State University conveyed information about three leadership styles that are still widely recognized today. The three styles are autocratic, democratic, and laissez-faire leadership (Lewin, 1939; Lewin & Lippitt, 1938; Lewin, Lippitt, & White, 1939). **Autocratic leadership** involves centralized decision making, with the leader making decisions and using power to command and control others. **Democratic leadership** is participatory,

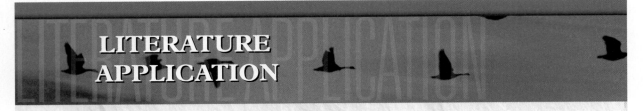

LITERATURE APPLICATION

Citation: Allen, D. W. (1998). How nurses become leaders: Perceptions and beliefs about leadership development. *Journal of Nursing Administration, 28*(9): 15–20.

Discussion: This article presents the factors that influence the development of leadership skills in nurses and the successful transition from a staff nurse role to a leadership role. Twelve registered nurses who had been in leadership positions for 9 to 29 years were interviewed. A set core of questions was used a guide, followed by additional questions that helped to clarify misunderstanding of the answers provided. Five dominant factors were identified that greatly influenced the nurses' leadership development. They are (1) self-confidence, (2) innate leader qualities/tendencies, (3) progression of experiences and success, (4) influence of significant others, and (5) personal life factors. For most of the nurses, there was at least one individual who fostered their sense of self-confidence through reinforcement and positive feedback. Education provided the participants with skills and knowledge that also contributed to their self-confidence. Innate leader qualities, going back as far as childhood, also contributed significantly to their leadership development. For example, most of the interviewed nurses, at some point in their life, were team captains or class officers. According to the author, a pattern of progressive successful experiences also emerged as a significant factor in leadership development. Education, especially that focused on leadership and management, provided the participants with new skills useful in their advancement. Mentors who recognized the strengths of the participants were able to improve their self-confidence and create opportunities for learning. Personal life factors, such as needing to work during the day shift or not being able to perform physically strenuous activities, led some of the participants to pursue nursing leadership and management. The factors that contributed to the development of these nurses were interconnected and promoted their gradual development as leaders.

Implications for Practice: While there are many individual and environmental factors that contribute to leadership development, each nurse can actively participate in designing and implementing a leadership development plan. An important avenue of growth is acquiring a mentor, who can help to create a progression of experiences that develop leadership skills and judgment in working with other people. Pursuing education to learn new skills that involve leadership behaviors and management practices is another excellent way to develop into a nurse leader. Sharing a desire to change and improve nursing practice with others through participation in professional nursing associations is another important vehicle for development as a leader and a professional.

with authority delegated to others. To be influential, the democratic leader uses expert power and the power base afforded by having close, personal relationships. The third style, laissez-faire leadership, is passive and permissive and the leader defers decision making. Lewin (1939) contrasted these styles and concluded that autocratic leaders were associated with high-performing groups but that close supervision was necessary and feelings of hostility were often present. Democratic leaders engendered positive feelings in their groups and performance was strong whether or not the leader was present. Low

productivity and feelings of frustration were associated with laissez-faire leaders.

Behavioral leadership studies from the University of Michigan and from Ohio State University led to the identification of two basic leader behaviors: job-centered and employee-centered behaviors. Effective leadership was described as having a focus on the human needs of subordinates and was called employee-centered leadership (Moorhead & Griffin, 2001). Job-centered leaders were seen as less effective because of their focus on schedules, costs, and efficiency, resulting in a lack of attention

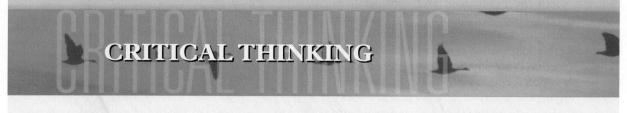

CRITICAL THINKING

Among the individuals commonly identified as leaders (Table 8-3), can you identify a set of traits that they all possess or traits that are associated with them? Are they perceived as leaders because they are characterized as intelligent, self-confident, and determined, have integrity, and are sociable? What other traits do (did) they have?

Table 8-3 Leaders Among Us: Past and Present

Mother Theresa	Martin Luther King
Princess Diana	John F. Kennedy
Oprah Winfrey	Mahatma Gandhi
Tiger Woods	Franklin Delano Roosevelt
Rosa Parks	Susan B. Anthony
H. Norman Schwarzkopf	Florence Nightingale
Colin Powell	Abraham Lincoln
Pope John Paul II	George Washington
Donna Shalala	Joan of Arc
Frances Hesselbein	Julius Caesar
Margaret Thatcher	Alexander the Great
Henry Kissinger	Cleopatra
Nelson Mandela	Jesus Christ

to developing work groups and high-performance goals (Moorhead & Griffin, 2001).

The researchers at Ohio State focused their efforts on two dimensions of leader behavior: initiating structure and consideration. **Initiating structure** involves an emphasis on the work to be done, a focus on the task and production. Leaders who focus on initiating structure are concerned with how work is organized and on the achievement of goals. Leader behavior includes planning, directing others, and establishing deadlines and details of how work is to be done. For example, a nurse demonstrating the leader behavior of initiating structure could be a charge nurse who, at the beginning of a shift, makes out a patient assignment.

The dimension of **consideration** involves activities that focus on the employee and emphasize relating and getting along with people. Leader behavior focuses on the well-being of others. The leader is involved in creating a relationship that fosters communication and trust as a basis for respecting other people and their potential contribution. A nurse demonstrating consideration behavior will take the time to talk with coworkers, be empathetic, and show an interest in them as people.

The leader behaviors of initiating structure and consideration define leadership style. The styles are as follows:

- Low initiating structure, low consideration
- High initiating structure, low consideration
- High initiating structure, high consideration
- Low initiating structure, high consideration

The Ohio State University studies associate the high initiating structure–high consideration leader behaviors with better performance and satisfaction outcomes than the other styles. This leadership style is considered effective, although it is not appropriate in every situation.

Another model based on these two dimensions is the managerial grid developed by Blake and Mouton (1985). Five styles identify the extent of structure, called concern for production, and consideration, called concern for people, demonstrated by the leader. The five leader styles are impoverished leader (1,1) for low production and people concern; authority compliance leader (9,1) for high production concern and low people concern; country club leader (1,9) for high people concern but low production concern; middle-of-the-road leader (5,5) for moderate concern in both dimensions; and team leader (9,9) for high production and people concern. Figure 8-2 shows the Leadership Grid with the dimensions of people and production from low to high on a scale from 1 to 9. Team management (9,9) is usually a more effective leadership approach than an overemphasis on either concern for people or concern for production.

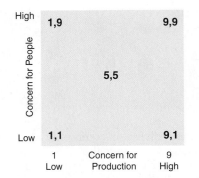

Figure 8-2 Blake, Mouton, and McCanse Leadership Grid (From *Leadership: Theory, Application, Skill Building* [p. 75], by R. N. Lussier and C. F. Achua, 2001, Cincinnati, OH: South-Western College)

Contingency Approaches

Another approach to leadership is **contingency theory**. Contingency theory acknowledges that other factors in the environment influence outcomes as much as leadership style and that leader effectiveness is contingent upon or depends upon something other than the leader's behavior. The premise is that different leader behavior patterns will be effective in different situations. Contingency approaches include Fielder's contingency theory, the situational theory of Hersey and Blanchard, path-goal theory, and the idea of substitutes for leadership.

Fielder's Contingency Theory. Fielder (1967) is credited with the development of the contingency model of leadership effectiveness. Fielder's theory of leadership effectiveness views the pattern of leader behavior as dependent upon the interaction of the personality of the leader and the needs of the situation. The needs of the situation or how favorable the situation is toward the leader involves leader-member relationships, the degree of task structure, and the leader's position of power (Fielder, 1967). **Leader-member relations** are the feelings and attitudes of followers regarding acceptance, trust, and credibility of the leader. Good leader-member relations exist when followers respect, trust, and have confidence in the leader. Poor leader-member relations reflect distrust, a lack of confidence and respect, and dissatisfaction with the leader by the followers.

Task structure refers to the degree to which work is defined, with specific procedures, explicit directions, and goals. High task structure involves rou-

tine, predictable, clearly defined work tasks. Low task structure involves work that is not routine, predictable, or clearly defined, such as creative, artistic, or qualitative research activities.

Position power is the degree of formal authority and influence associated with the leader. High position power is favorable for the leader and low position power is unfavorable. When all of these dimensions—leader-member relations, task structure, and position power—are high, the situation is favorable to the leader. When they are low, the situation is not favorable to the leader. In both of these circumstances, Fielder showed that a task-directed leader, concerned with task accomplishment, was effective. When the range of favorableness is intermediate or moderate, a human relations leader, concerned about people, was most effective. These situations need interpersonal and relationship skills to foster group achievement. Fielder's contingency theory is an approach that matches the organizational situation to the most favorable leadership style for that situation.

Hersey and Blanchard's Situational Theory. Situational leadership theory addresses follower characteristics in relation to effective leader behavior. Whereas Blake and Mouton focus on leader style and Fielder examines the situation, Hersey and Blanchard consider follower readiness as a factor in determining leadership style. Rather than using the words *initiating structure* and *contingency*, they use *task behavior* and *relationship behavior*.

High task behavior and low relationship behavior is called a telling leadership style. A high task, high relationship style is called a selling leadership style. A low task and high relationship style is called a participating leadership style. A low task and low relationship style is called a delegating leadership style.

Follower readiness, called maturity, is assessed in order to select one of the four leadership styles for a situation. For example, according to Hersey and Blanchard's situational leadership theory (2000), groups with low maturity, whose members are unable or unwilling to participate or are unsure, need a leader to use a telling leadership style to provide direction and close supervision. The selling leadership style is a match for groups with low to moderate maturity who are unable but willing and confident and need clear direction and supportive feedback to get the task done. Participating is the leadership style recommended for groups with moderate to high maturity who are able but unwilling or are unsure and who need support and encouragement. The leader should use a delegating style with groups of followers with high maturity who are able and ready to participate and can engage in the task without direction or support.

An additional aspect of this model is the idea that the leader not only changes leadership style according to followers' needs but also develops followers over time to increase their level of maturity (Lussier & Achua, 2001). Use of these four leadership styles helps a nurse manager assign work to others.

Path-Goal Theory.

In this leadership approach, the leader works to motivate followers and influence goal accomplishment. The seminal author on path-goal theory is Robert House (1971). By using the appropriate style of leadership for the situation (i.e., directive, supportive, participative, or achievement oriented), the leader makes the path toward the goal easier for the follower. The directive style of leadership provides structure through direction and authority, with the leader focusing on the task and getting the job done. The supportive style of leadership is relationship oriented, with the leader providing encouragement, interest, and attention. Participative leadership means that the leader focuses on involving followers in the decision-making process. The achievement-oriented style provides high structure and direction as well as high support through consideration behavior. The leadership style is matched to the situational characteristics of the followers, such as the desire for authority, the extent to which the control of goal achievement is internal or external, and the ability of the follower to be involved. The leadership style is also matched to the situational factors in the environment, including the routine nature or complexity of the task, the power associated with the leader's position, and the work group relationship. This alignment of leadership style with the needs of followers is motivating and believed to enhance performance and satisfaction. The path-goal theory is based on expectancy theory, which holds that people are motivated when they believe they are able to carry out the work and when they think their contribution will lead to the expected outcome and that the rewards for their efforts are valued and meaningful (Northouse, 2001).

Substitutes for Leadership.

Substitutes for leadership are variables that may influence followers to the same extent as the leader's behavior. Kerr and Jermier (1978) investigated situational variables and identified some aspects as substitutes that eliminate the need for leader behavior and other aspects as neutralizers that nullify the effects of the leader's behavior.

Some of these variables include follower characteristics, such as the presence of structured routine tasks, the amount of feedback provided by the task, and the presence of intrinsic satisfaction in the work; and organizational characteristics such as the presence of a cohesive group, a formal organization, a rigid adherence to rules, and low position power. For example, an individual's experience substitutes for task direction leader behavior (Kerr & Jermier, 1978). Nurses and other professionals with a great deal of experience already have knowledge and judgment and do not need direction and supervision to perform their work. Thus, their experience serves as a leadership substitute. Another substitute for leader behavior is intrinsic satisfaction that emerges from just doing the work. Intrinsic satisfaction occurs frequently among nurses when they provide care to patients and families. Intrinsic satisfaction substitutes for the support and encouragement of relationship-oriented leader behavior.

Contemporary Approaches

Contemporary approaches to leadership address the leadership functions necessary to develop learning organizations and lead the process of transforming change. These approaches include charismatic leadership and transformational leadership theory.

Charismatic Theory

A charismatic leader has an inspirational quality that promotes an emotional connection from followers. House (1977) developed a theory of charismatic leadership that described how charismatic leaders behave as well as distinguishing characteristics and situations in which such leaders would be effective. Charismatic leaders display self-confidence, strength in their convictions, and communicate high expectations and their confidence in others. They have been described as emerging during a crisis, communicating vision, and using personal power and unconventional strategies (Conger & Kanungo, 1987). One consequence of this type of leadership is a belief in the charismatic leader that is so strong it takes on an almost supernatural purpose and the leader is worshipped as if superhuman. Examples of charismatic leaders who have been worshipped by some include Adolf Hitler, Charles Manson, and Jim Jones.

Charismatic leaders can have a positive and powerful effect on people and organizations. Lee Iacocca, former chief executive officer (CEO) of Chrysler Corporation, and the current CEO of Southwest Airlines, Herb Kelleher, are described as effective charismatic leaders. This type of leader can contribute significantly to an organization, even though all the leaders in an organization are not charismatic leaders. There are effective leaders who do not exhibit all the qualities associated with charismatic leadership. Charisma seems to be a special and valuable quality that some people have and some people do not.

Transformational Leadership Theory

Burns defined transformational leadership as a process in which "leaders and followers raise one another to higher levels of motivation and morality" (Burns, 1978, p. 21). Transformational leadership theory is based on the idea of empowering others to engage in pursuing a collective purpose by working together to achieve a vision of a preferred future. This kind of leadership can influence both the leader and the follower to a higher level of conduct and achievement that transforms them both (Burns, 1978). Burns maintained that there are two types of leaders: the traditional manager concerned with day-to-day operations, called the **transactional leader**, and the leader who is committed to a vision that empowers others, called the **transformational leader**.

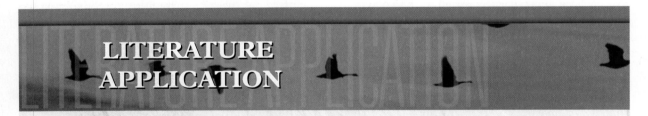

LITERATURE APPLICATION

Citation: Levi, P. (1999). Sustainability of healthcare environments. *Image: Journal of Nursing Scholarship, 31,* 4, 395–398.

Discussion: Will nursing play a significant role in advancing the future of health care? Using indicators such as access to care, infant mortality, children's health, and statistics on children living in poverty, the author questions whether nursing, as a profession with more than 2.6 million members, will be instrumental in influencing policies to address these issues. The author identifies transitions occurring in the health care industry, including a shift from hospital dominance to care delivery in the community, from acute care to community based and alternative care, from disease management to prevention, screening, and detection. These changes, along with advancing technologies from molecular and genetic research, are cornerstones in advancing our knowledge and changing health care practices.

Implications for Practice: The author calls for a strong culture of nursing in which nurses are socialized to succeed in a more complex environment. To have a significant role in the future of health care, nursing needs to provide transformational leaders who create ethical environments and nurses who involve themselves in forming and speaking out about health policy.

Transformational leaders motivate others by behaving in accordance with values, providing a vision that reflects mutual values, and empowering others to contribute. Bennis and Nanus (1985) describe this new leader as a leader who "commits people to action, who converts followers into leaders, and who converts leaders into agents of change" (p. 3). According to research by Tichy and Devanna (1986), effective transformational leaders identify themselves as change agents; are courageous; believe in people; are value driven; are lifelong learners; have the ability to deal with complexity, ambiguity, and uncertainty; and are visionaries. Yet transformational leadership may be demonstrated by anyone in an organization regardless of his position (Burns, 1978). The interaction that occurs between individuals can be transformational and motivate both to a higher level of performance (Bass, 1985).

Transformational leadership at the organizational level is about innovation and change. The transformational leader uses vision based on shared values to align people and inspire growth and advancement. It is both the inspiration and the empowerment aspects of transformational leadership that lead to commitment beyond self-interest, commitment to a vision, and commitment to action that creates change. Transformational leadership theory suggests that the relationship between the leader and the follower inspires and empowers an individual toward commitment to the organization.

Nurse researchers have described nurse executives according to transformational leadership theory and have used this theory to measure leadership behavior among nurse executives and nurse managers (Leach, 2000; McNeese-Smith, 1995; Dunham-Taylor, 1995, 2000; Trofino, 1995; Wolf, Boland, & Aukerman, 1994; McDaniel & Wolf, 1992; Young, 1992; Dunham & Klafehn, 1990). Additionally, transformational leadership theory has been the basis for nursing administration curriculum and for investigation of relationships such as between a nurse's commitment to an organization and productivity in a hospital setting (Leach, 2000; McNeese-Smith, 1997; Searle, 1996). Cassidy and Koroll (1998) explored the ethical aspects of transformational leadership, and Barker (1990) comprehensively discussed nursing in terms of transformational leadership theory. Of the contemporary theories of leadership, transformational leadership has been a popular approach in nursing.

FUTURE DIRECTIONS

The organizations that nurses are a part of are changing. They reflect the advance and the promise of the technology that enables us to perform our work. Peter Drucker (1994) identifies the organization of the future as a knowledge organization composed of knowledge workers. Knowledge workers are those who bring specialized, expert knowledge to an organization. They are valued for what they know. The knowledge organization will share, provide, and grow the information necessary

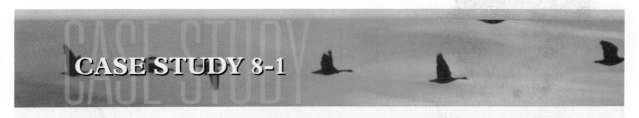

CASE STUDY 8-1

A nurse is making rounds on her new postoperative laryngectomy patient. As she enters the room, the patient begins to bleed from his neck incision. The nurse applies direct pressure with one hand and calls for assistance. Help arrives and the patient is taken to surgery with the nurse still maintaining pressure on the bleeding site. The patient lives and goes home a few days later.

What leadership characteristics does this nurse demonstrate?

Why is leadership important at all levels throughout a health care organization?

How can a nurse develop this type of leadership skill?

to work efficiently and effectively. Drucker says that knowledge organizations, in which the knowledge worker is at the front lines with the expertise and the information to act, will be the dominant organizational type (Drucker, 1994; Helgesen, 1995). In organizations such as these, the ideas of leadership at the top and leadership equated with the power of a position are obsolete notions. Workers with the expertise and information to act are the organization's leaders. They provide the service, interact with the customer, represent the organization, and accomplish its goals. Leadership will be needed at all levels within such an organization, not just at the top and not just with certain positions in the organization. Every worker will play a role in fulfilling the purpose of the organization and in so doing will be both a leader and a follower.

The New Leadership

Margaret Wheatley, in *Leadership and the New Science* (1992), says, "There is a simpler way to lead organizations, one that requires less effort and produces less stress than the current practices" (p. 3). She presents us with a new view of leadership, one encompassing connectedness and self-organizing systems that follow a natural order of both chaos and uncertainty, which is different from a linear order in a hierarchy. The leader's function is to guide an organization using vision, to make choices based on mutual values, and

to engage in the culture to provide meaning and coherence. This type of leadership fosters growth within each of us as individuals and as members of a group. The notion of connection within a self-organizing system optimizes autonomy at all levels because the relationships between the individual and the whole are strong (Wheatley, 1992). For nursing, such systems might be the infrastructure that will foster interdisciplinary decision making and strengthen the connection with nonprofessional workers. New possibilities may emerge that help nursing to move away from dependence on numbers of staff, numbers of patient care hours, cost and volume productivity measures, and the tools of an industrial age and Newton's physics toward the new science focused on naturally occurring events, wholeness, and interaction.

Generational Leadership Issues

Organizations have become more complex, and nursing's systems and ways of leadership must keep pace with the complexities and the advances of a highly technological, information-driven environment. Leadership will emerge from teams that self-organize and self-direct (Avolio, 1999). Organizational teams will become diverse, both racially and ethnically, but also in that different generations will participate in the workforce simultaneously. The generation known as

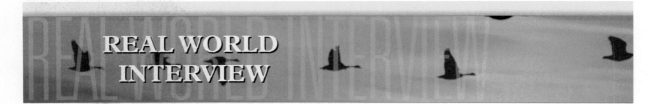

REAL WORLD INTERVIEW

Leadership in nursing is probably one of the more personal forms of leadership. Nursing is one of the most intimate leadership relationships because of the vulnerability the patient brings to the relationship. With patients who are dying or in terrible situations, the nurse provides them with two vital leadership characteristics: optimism and courage. With patients who have lost their courage, it is the nurse who shows courage and strength that supports a patient and their family. Optimism and courage are the trademarks of great leaders. Nurses lead the patient, their family, their nurse colleagues, and other health care providers. They have the courage to care in the face of fear and uncertainty, and in the face of disability or in death. Caring, hope, and support are a source of optimism that nurses provide. There are very few professions where you touch an individual's life so profoundly.

Jay Conger, PhD
Author, Learning to Lead

the baby boomers, born between 1946 and 1964, will work with different age-related groups such as the buster generation, born between 1965 and 1981 (Moats Kennedy, 1998). According to Moats Kennedy, the boomers and busters exhibit different values about work, motivation, lifestyle, and communication. For example, she points out that boomers tend to demonstrate loyalty to an employer whereas busters regularly change organizations to advance their development. Additionally, busters have a more individual approach to work and tend to value a work-family balanced lifestyle more highly than boomers, who tend to work hard with a strong emphasis on money and acquiring things. Such different styles reveal differences in how learning occurs and the methods best suited for busters, who are computer skilled and comfortable with high-tech tools versus boomers, who tend toward more personalized training methods.

Research among nurses has revealed that conflict and stress among these generations can occur regarding their feelings about work, job tenure, and work behaviors; for example, some boomers hold negative views about the degree of commitment and self-centered focus exhibited by busters (Santos & Cox, 2000). Leadership development must address embracing an understanding of generational differences and support the idea of maximizing the strengths of boomers, busters, and the most recent group, generation nexters, born between 1980 and 2000, within a team-based approach to organizational work.

KEY CONCEPTS

- Nurses are leaders and make a difference to health care organizations through their contributions of expert knowledge and leadership. Leadership development is a necessary component of preparation as a health care provider.
- Management is a process used to achieve organizational goals. It involves the management functions of planning, leading, organizing, and controlling.
- Motivation is an internal process that contributes to our behavior in an effort to satisfy our needs. Maslow's hierarchy of needs reflects the belief that the needs that motivate us have an order, and lower-level needs have to be satisfied first or we will not be motivated to address higher-level needs. Herzberg's two-factor theory

of motivation identifies maintenance factors, such as security and salary, that are needed to prevent job dissatisfaction, while motivators, such as development and opportunities to advance, contribute to job satisfaction.
- Leadership is a process of influence that involves the leader, the follower, and their interaction. Followers can be individuals, groups of people, communities, and members of society in general. Leadership can be formal and informal, occurring by being in a position of authority in an organization, such as manager, or outside the scope of a formal role, such as member of a group.
- Leadership and management are different. Management is viewed as actions employed to cope with changes, while leadership is the effort to envision and inspire change.
- Future directions for nurses in organizations will be influenced by technology. Nursing leadership in the future will be needed at all levels within an organization, not just at the top or from managers. Every knowledge worker, with specialized knowledge and expertise, will be both a leader and a follower in knowledge organizations.
- Organizations are being viewed as self-organizing systems in which, initially, what looks like chaos and uncertainty is indeed part of a larger coherence and a natural order. Such a living system, when understood better by participants, will be a less stressful and more holistic environment in which to carry out work.
- Work teams are becoming generationally diverse as more boomers are working alongside younger generations, called busters. Busters are less concerned with loyalty to an organization but value balance in personal and work life. Boomers show commitment to their employer, work hard, and are motivated by financial rewards. These differences can be a source of stress among nurses.

KEY TERMS

administrative principles
autocratic leadership
bureaucratic organization
consideration
contingency theory
democratic leadership
job-centered leaders

employee-centered leadership
formal leadership
Hawthorne effect
informal leader
initiating structure
motivation factors

knowledge workers
laissez-faire leadership
leader-member relations
leadership
maintenance or
  hygiene factors
management
management process
motivation

position power
substitutes for
  leadership
task structure
Theory X
Theory Y
Theory Z
transactional leader
transformational leader

5. According to Hersey and Blanchard and House, a participative leadership style is appropriate for employees who
A. are not able to get the task done and are less mature.
B. are able to contribute to decisions about getting the work done.
C. are unable and unwilling to participate.
D. need direction, structure, and authority.

REVIEW QUESTIONS

1. Why is leadership development important for nurses if they are not in a management position?
A. It is not really important for nurses.
B. Leadership is important at all levels in an organization because nurses have expert knowledge and are interacting with and influencing the customer.
C. Nurse leaders leave their jobs sooner for other positions.
D. Nurses who lead are less satisfied in their jobs.

2. Management as a process that is used today by nurses or nurse managers in health care organizations is best described as
A. scientific management.
B. decision making.
C. commanding and controlling others using hierarchical authority.
D. planning, organizing, coordinating, and controlling.

3. Motivation is whatever influences our choices. What factors did Herzberg say would motivate workers and lead to job satisfaction?
A. Being offered a substantial bonus when being hired
B. Realizing that no one ever gets fired from the organization and that job security is high
C. Having good relationships with colleagues and supervisors
D. Being offered opportunities for development and advancement

4. Leadership is defined as
A. being in a leadership position with authority to exert control and power over subordinates.
B. a process of interaction in which the leader influences others toward goal achievement.
C. managing complexity.
D. being self-confident and democratic.

REVIEW ACTIVITIES

1. Take the opportunity to learn about yourself by reflecting on the five predominant factors identified as being influential in a nurse's leadership development: self-confidence, innate leader qualities/tendencies, progression of experiences and success, influence of significant others, and personal life factors. Consider what reinforces your confidence in yourself. What innate qualities or tendencies do you have that contribute to your development as a leader? Consider what professional experiences, mentors, and personal experiences or events can help you influence and change nursing practice.

2. Describe the type of leader you want to be as a nurse in a health care organization. Identify specific behaviors you plan to use as a leader. In what way are the transformational leadership and the charismatic leadership theories useful to your development as a leader?

3. Rate each of these 12 job factors that contribute to job satisfaction by placing a number from 1 to 5 on the line before each factor.

Very important		Somewhat important		Not important
5	4	3	2	1

_____ 1. An interesting job I enjoy doing
_____ 2. A good manager who treats people fairly
_____ 3. Getting praise and other recognition and appreciation for the work I do
_____ 4. A satisfying personal life at the job
_____ 5. The opportunity for advancement
_____ 6. A prestigious or status job
_____ 7. Job responsibility that gives me freedom to do things my way

_____ 8. Good working conditions (safe environment, nice office, cafeteria)
_____ 9. The opportunity to learn new things
_____ 10. Sensible company rules, regulations, procedures, and policies
_____ 11. A job I can do well and succeed at
_____ 12. Job security and benefits

Write the number from 1 to 5 that you selected for each factor. Total each column for a score between 6 and 30 points. The closer to 30 your score is, the more important these factors (motivating or maintenance) are to you.

Motivating factors	Maintenance factors
1. _____	2. _____
3. _____	4. _____
5. _____	6. _____
7. _____	8. _____
9. _____	10. _____
11. _____	12. _____

Totals   _____   _____

From _Leadership: Theory, Application, Skill Development_ (pp. 15–16), by R. N. Lussier and C. F. Achua, 2001, Cincinnati, OH: South-Western College Publishing.

EXPLORING THE WEB

Search the Web, checking the following sites.

- Emerging Leader: _http://www.emergingleader.com_
- Leadership Directories: Who's who in the leadership of the United States: _http://www.leadershipdirectories.com_
- Health Leadership Associates: _http://www.healthleadership.com_
- Big Dog's Bowl of Biscuit's Leadership Page: _http://www.nwlink.com/~donclark_
- Population Leadership Program: _http://www.popldr.org_
- Leadership Knowledge Base: Information to Improve Your Leadership Skills: _http://www.sonic.net/~mfreeman_

REFERENCES

Allen, D. W. (1998). How nurses become leaders. Perceptions and beliefs about leadership development. _Journal of Nursing Administration, 28_(9), 15–20.

Avolio, B. (1999). _Full leadership development: Building the vital forces in organizations._ Thousand Oaks, CA: Sage.

Barker, A. (1990). _Transformational nursing leadership: A vision for the future._ Baltimore: Williams & Wilkins.

Barnard, C. (1938). _The functions of the executive._ Boston: Harvard University Press.

Bass, B. (1985). _Leadership and performance beyond expectations._ New York: Free Press.

Bass, B. (1990). _Bass and Stodgill's handbook of leadership._ New York: Free Press.

Bennis, W., & Nanus, B. (1985). _Leaders: The strategies for taking charge._ New York: Harper & Row.

Blake, R. R., & Mouton, J. S. (1985). _The managerial grid III._ Houston, TX: Gulf.

Burns, J. M. (1978). _Leadership._ New York: Harper & Row.

Cassidy, V., & Koroll, C. (1998). Ethical aspects of transformational leadership. In E. Hein (Ed.), _Contemporary leadership behavior: Selected readings_ (5th ed., pp. 79–82). Philadelphia: Lippincott.

Clifford, J. (1991). The practicing nurse leader. _MCN: American Journal of Maternal Child Nursing, 16_(1), 18–20.

Conger, J., & Kanungo, R. (1987). Toward a behavioral theory of charismatic leadership in organizational settings. _Academy of Management Review, 12,_ 637–647.

Daft, R. L., & Marcic, D. (2001). _Understanding management_ (3rd ed.). Philadelphia: Harcourt College.

DeCrane, A., Jr. (1996). A constitutional model of leadership. In F. Hesselbein, M. Goldsmith, & R. Beckhard (Eds.), _The leader of the future: New visions, strategies, and practices for the next era_ (pp. 249–256). San Francisco: Jossey-Bass.

Drucker, P. F. (1994). _The post-capitalist society._ New York: Harper & Row.

Dunham, J., & Klafehn, K. A. (1990). Transformational leadership and the nurse executive. _Journal of Nursing Administration, 20_(4), 28–34.

Dunham-Taylor, J. (1995). Identifying the best in nurse executive leadership: Part 2, interview results. _Journal of Nursing Administration, 25_(7/8), 24–31.

Dunham-Taylor, J. (2000). Nurse executive transformational leadership found in participative organizations. _Journal of Nursing Administration, 30_(5), 241–250.

Fayol, H. (1916/1949). (C. Storrs, Trans.). _General and industrial management._ London: Pitman.

Fielder, F. (1967). _A theory of leadership effectiveness._ New York: McGraw-Hill.

Gilbreth, F. (1912). _Primer of scientific management._ New York: Van Nostrand.

Gulick, L., & Urwick, L. (Eds.). (1937). _Papers on the science of administration._ New York: Institute of Public Administration.

Hales, C. P. (1986). What managers do: A critical review of the evidence. *Journal of Management Studies, 23,* 88–115.

Helgesen, S. (1995). *The web of inclusion: A new architecture for building organizations.* New York: Doubleday Currency.

Henry, N. (1992). *Public administration and public affairs* (5th ed.). Englewood Cliffs, NJ: Prentice Hall.

Hersey, P., & Blanchard, K. (2000). *Management of organizational behavior* (8th ed.). Englewood Cliffs, NJ: Prentice Hall.

Herzberg, F. (1968, January/February). One more time: How do you motivate employees? *Harvard Business Review,* 53–62.

House, R. H. (1971). A path-goal theory of leader effectiveness. *Administrative Science Quarterly, 16,* 321–338.

House, R. H. (1977). A 1976 theory of charismatic leadership. In J. Hunt & L. Larson (Eds.), *Leadership: The cutting edge* (pp. 21–26). Carbondale, IL: Southern Illinois University Press.

Hughes, R. L., Ginnett, R. C., & Curphy, G. J. (1999). *Leadership: Enhancing the lessons of experience* (3rd ed.). San Francisco: Irwin McGraw-Hill.

Kanfer, R. (1990). Motivation theory in industrial and organizational psychology. In M. D. Dunnette & L. M. Hough (Eds.), *Handbook of industrial and organizational psychology: Vol. 1* (pp. 53–68). Palo Alto, CA: Consulting Psychologists Press.

Katz, D., & Kahn, R. L. (1978). *The social psychology of organizations* (2d ed.). New York: John Wiley.

Kerr, S., & Jermier, J. (1978). Substitutes for leadership: Their meaning and measurement. *Organizational Behavior and Human Performance, 22,* 374–403.

Kim, H., & Yukl, G. (1995). Relationships of self-reported and subordinate-reported leadership behaviors to managerial effectiveness and advancement. *Leadership Quarterly, 6,* 361–377.

Kirkpatrick, S. A., & Locke, E. A. (1991). Leadership: Do traits matter? *The Executive, 5,* 48–60.

Kotter, J. (1990a). *A force for change: How leadership differs from management.* Glencoe, IL: Free Press.

Kotter, J. (1990b). What leaders really do. *Harvard Business Review, 68,* 104.

Kramer, M., & Schmalenberg, C. (1988). Magnet hospitals: Part II institutions of excellence. *Journal of Nursing Administration, 18*(2), (pp. 11–19).

Laborde, A. S., & Lee, J. A. (2000). Skills needed for promotion in the nursing profession. *Journal of Nursing Administration, 30*(9), 432–439.

Leach, L. S. (2000). *Nurse executive leadership and the relationship to organizational commitment among nurses.* Unpublished doctoral dissertation, University of Southern California, Los Angeles.

Levi, P. (1999), Sustainability of healthcare environments. *Image: Journal of Nursing Scholarship, 31*(4), 395–398.

Lewin, K. (1939). Field theory and experiment in social psychology: Concepts and methods. *Journal of Sociology, 44,* 868–896.

Lewin, K., & Lippitt, R. (1938). An experimental approach to the study of autocracy and democracy: A preliminary note. *Sociometry, 1,* 292–300.

Lewin, K., Lippitt, R., & White, R. (1939). Patterns of aggressive behavior in experimentally created social climates. *Journal of Social Psychology, 10,* 271–299.

Lussier, R. N. (1999). *Human relations in organizations: Applications and skill building* (4th ed.). San Francisco: Irwin McGraw-Hill.

Lussier, R. N., & Achua, C. F. (2001). *Leadership: Theory, application, skill development.* Cincinnati, OH: South-Western College.

Mahoney, T. A., Jerdee, T. H., & Carroll, S. I., Jr. (1965). The job(s) of management. *Industrial Relations, 4,* 97–110.

Maslow, A. (1970). *Motivation and personality* (2nd ed.). New York: Harper & Row.

Mayo, E. (1933). *The Human problems of an industrial civilization.* New York: Macmillan.

McCall, M. W., Jr. (1998). *High flyers: Developing the next generation of leaders.* Boston: Harvard Business School Press.

McCall, M. W., Jr., Morrison, A. M., & Hanman, R. L. (1978). *Studies of managerial work: Results and methods* (Tech. Rep.). Greensboro, NC: Center for Creative Leadership.

McClure, M., Poulin, M., Sovie, M., & Wandelt, M. (1983). *Magnet hospitals: Attraction and retention of professional nurses.* Kansas City, MO: American Nurses Association.

McDaniel, C., & Wolf, G. (1992). Transformational leadership in nursing service. *Journal of Nursing Administration, 12*(4), 204–207.

McGregor, D. (1960). *The human side of enterprise.* New York: McGraw-Hill.

McNeese-Smith, D. (1995). Job satisfaction, productivity, and organizational commitment: The result of leadership. *Journal of Nursing Administration, 25*(9), 17–26.

McNeese-Smith, D. (1997). The influences of manager behavior on nurses' job satisfaction, productivity, and commitment. *Journal of Nursing Administration, 27*(9), 47–55.

Mintzberg, H. (1973). *The nature of managerial work.* New York: Harper & Row.

Moats Kennedy, M. (1998). Boomers versus busters: Addressing the generation gap in healthcare management. *Healthcare Executive, 13*(6), 6–10.

Mooney, J. (1939). *Principles of Organization*. New York: Harper.

Moorhead, G., & Griffin, R. W. (2001). *Organizational behavior: Managing people in organizations* (6th ed.). Boston: Houghton Mifflin.

Murphy, M., & DeBack, V. (1991). Today's nursing leaders: Creating the vision. *Nursing Administration Quarterly, 16*(1), 71–80.

Northouse, P. (2001). *Leadership: Theory and practice* (2nd ed.). Thousand Oaks, CA: Sage.

Ouchi, W. (1981). *Theory Z: How American business can meet the Japanese challenge*. Reading, MA: Addison-Wesley.

Pew Health Professions Commission. (1995). *Critical challenges: Revitalizing the health professions for the 21st century*. San Francisco: UCSF Center for the Health Professions.

Roethlisberger, J. F., & Dickson, W. J. (1939). *Management and the worker*. Cambridge, MA: Harvard University Press.

Santos, S. R., & Cox, K. (2000). Workplace adjustment and intergenerational differences between matures, boomers, and Xers. *Nursing Economic$, 18*(1), 7–13.

Scott, J. G., Sochalski, J., & Aiken, L. (1999). Review of magnet hospital research: Findings and implications for professional nursing practice. *Journal of Nursing Administration 29*(1), 9–19.

Searle, L. (1996, January). 21st century leadership for nurse administrators. *Aspen's advisor for nurse executives, 11*(4), 1, 4–6.

Stodgill, R. M. (1948). Personal factors associated with leadership: A survey of the literature. *Journal of Psychology, 25*, 35–71.

Stodgill, R. M. (1974). *Handbook of leadership: A survey of theory and research*. New York: Free Press.

Taylor, F. (1911). *Principles of scientific management*. New York: Harper & Row.

Tichy, N., & Devanna, D. (1986). *Transformational leadership*. New York: Wiley.

Trofino, J. (1995). Transformational leadership in health care. *Nursing Management, 26*(8), 42–47.

Wheatley, M. J. (1992). *Leadership and the new science: Learning about organization from an orderly universe*. San Francisco: Berrett-Koehler.

Wolf, G., Boland, S., & Aukerman, M. (1994). A transformational model for the practice of professional nursing. Part 1. *Journal of Nursing Administration, 24*(4), 51–57.

Wren, D. (1979). *Evolution of management thought*. New York: Wiley.

Young, S. (1992). Educational experiences of transformational nurse leaders. *Nursing Administration Quarterly, 17*(1), 25–33.

Yukl, G. (1997). *Development of a new measure of managerial behavior: Preliminary report on validation of the MPS*. Paper presented at the Eastern Academy of Management, Boston.

Yukl, G. (1998). *Leadership in organizations* (4th ed.). Upper Saddle River, NJ: Prentice Hall.

Yukl, G., Wall, S., & Lepsinger, R. (1990). Preliminary report on validation of the managerial practices survey. In K. E. Clarke & M. B. Clark (Eds.), *Measures of leadership* (pp. 223–238). West Orange, NJ: Leadership Library of America.

Zalenik, K. A. (1977). Managers and leaders: Are they different? *Harvard Business Review, 55*(5), 67–80.

SUGGESTED READINGS

Bass, B. (1998). *Transformational leadership: Industrial, military, and educational impact*. Mahwah, NJ: Erlbaum.

Bower, F. L. (2000). Nurses taking the lead: Personal qualities of effective leadership. Philadelphia: Saunders.

Buerhaus, P. I. (2000). Implications of an aging registered nurse workforce. *Journal of the American Medical Association, 283*, 2948–2954.

Conger, J., & Spreitzer, G. Editors (1992). *Learning to Lead*. San Francisco: Jossey Bass.

Cronin, S. N., & Bechere, D. (1999). Recognition of staff nurse job performance and achievements: Staff and manager perceptions. *Journal of Nursing Administration, 29*(1), 26–31.

Evans, M. G. (1996). R. J. House's "A path-goal theory of leader effectiveness." *Leadership Quarterly, 7*(3), 305–309.

Gordon, S. (1997). *Life support: Three nurses on the front lines*. New York: Little, Brown.

Hesselbein, F., Goldsmith, M., & Beckhard, R. (Eds.). (1996). *The leader of the future: New visions, strategies, and practices for a new era*. San Francisco: Jossey-Bass.

Kanges, S., Kee, C. C., & McKee-Waddle, R. (1999). Organizational factors, nurses' job satisfaction and patient satisfaction with nursing care. *Journal of Nursing Administration, 29*(1), 32–42.

Kohles, M. K., Baker, W. G., Jr., & Donoho, B. (1995). Transformational leadership: Reviewing fundamental values and achieving new relationships in health care. Chicago: American Hospital.

Kramer, M. (1990). The magnet hospitals: Excellence revisited. *Journal of Nursing Administration, 20*(9), 35–44.

Kramer, M., & Schmalenberg, C. (1990). Fundamental lessons in leadership. In E. Simendinger, T. Moore, & M. Kramer (Eds.), *The successful nurse executive: A guide for every nurse manager* (pp. 42–56). Ann Arbor, MI: Health Administration Press.

Likert, R. (1967). *The human organization: Its management and value.* New York: McGraw-Hill.

Luthans, S. F., Hodgetts, R., & Rosenkratz, S. (1988). *Real managers.* Cambridge, MA: Ballinger.

Mahoney, T. A., Jerdee, T. H., & Carroll, S. I., Jr. (1963). *Development of managerial performance: A research approach.* Cincinnati, OH: South-Western College.

O'Neil, E., & Coffman, J. (Eds.). (1998). *Strategies for the future of nursing: Changing roles, responsibilities, and employment patterns of registered nurses.* San Francisco: Jossey-Bass.

Parse, R. (1997). Leadership: The essentials. *Nursing Science Quarterly, 10*(3), 109.

Porter-O'Grady, T., & Wilson, C. K. (1995). *The leadership revolution in health care: Altering systems, changing behaviors.* Gaithersburg, MD: Aspen.

Rosenbach, W. E., & Taylor, R. L. (1998). *Contemporary issues in leadership* (4th ed.). Boulder, CO: Westview Press.

Senge, P. (1990, Fall). The leader's new work: Building learning organizations. *Sloan Management Review,* 7–22.

Urwick, L. (1944), *The elements of administration.* New York: Harper & Row.

Vroom, V. H. (1964). *Work and motivation.* New York: McGraw-Hill.

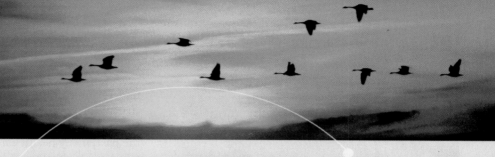

CHAPTER 9

The greater thing in this world is not so much where we stand as in what direction we are going.

(Oliver Wendell Holmes)

Strategic Planning and Organizing Patient Care

Amy Androwich O'Malley, RN, MSN
Ida M. Androwich, PhD, RNC, FAAN

OBJECTIVES

Upon completion of this chapter, the reader should be able to:

1. Describe the importance of an organization's mission and philosophy and the impact of these on the structure and behavior of the organization.

2. Define the purpose and identify the steps in the strategic planning process.

3. Be able to articulate the importance of aligning the organization's strategic vision both with the organization's own mission, philosophy, and values and also with the goals and values of the communities served by the organization.

4. Have a basic understanding of common organizational structures and a framework for examining the purposes and the advantages and the disadvantages of each.

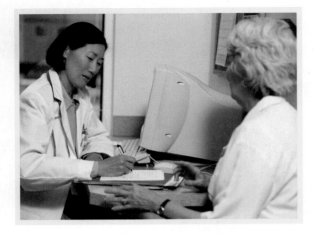

Your friend is discussing her plans to step down as the assistant unit coordinator on 3 West. You remember how pleased and excited she was to accept the position only a few months ago and wonder what has changed. She describes her frustration with either never having adequate information or not receiving the information in a timely manner. She feels this puts her in a poor position to be a staff and patient advocate for her unit. She states, "I feel like my manager has too many areas that are taking up all her time, and she really can't concentrate on our needs. It seems as if we are always putting out fires and never have a chance to step back and actually plan programs and processes that could make a big improvement on the unit. The organization's mission statement says that we value education, but I'm always having to turn down requests from staff for approval to go to educational programs because we are not recruiting and hiring nurses for all our budgeted positions. There are plenty of nurses routinely scheduled on days and not nearly enough on evenings. Most patients are now discharged in the early evening, and consequently we have our major needs for discharge planning and patient education then, but there is no plan for providing this necessary information. The result is dissatisfied patients, staff, and physicians."

What are your thoughts about this situation?
What advice do you have for your friend?
Is this situation unusual? How can it be improved?

There are increasing opportunities for nurses to become involved in strategic and tactical planning for the delivery of health care services in their organizations and communities. Yet, to be effective in leadership roles, nurses need a basic understanding of the way in which organizations are structured, how organizational systems function, and how to engage in the strategic planning process. In the past, many health care organizations were structured in a highly formal, top-down, militaristic manner. These bureaucratic organizations worked well in a relatively stable environment when communication channels could be hierarchical. They are not useful in a dynamic health care system in which information is rapidly changing. To be most effective, knowledge can and should be distributed throughout the organization (Hope & Hope, 1997). In addition, workers in today's health care systems are considered knowledge workers—professionals hired for their knowledge, skills, and expertise. They need a system that supports their ability to practice to the full extent of their professional accountability (Kanter, 1997).

Leadership in the health care organizations of the 21st century demands competent nurses with different skill sets than in the past. Functioning in a leadership role in today's highly complex health care environment requires an understanding of how systems function and how to improve health care delivery. Yet health care providers, including professional nurses, have been slow to integrate this information into their clinical practice. Planning for continuous improvement of quality, service, and cost-effectiveness is a critical competency of successful 21st century health care organizations and nurses.

The recent (1999) Institute of Medicine (IOM) report *To Err Is Human* states that preventable adverse events cause between 44,000 and 98,000 deaths each year at an annual cost of between $37.6 billion and $50 billion. The National Advisory Council on Nurse Education and Practice and the Council on Graduate Medical Education conclude that patient safety is dependent on the implementation of an interdisciplinary system that addresses the realities of practice and patient care and that education and service must stress interdisciplinary approaches ("National advisory councils in nursing and medicine collaborate," 2000). Other studies stress that the way a nurse's work is organized is a major determinant of patient welfare (Havens & Aiken, 1999). Consequently, nurses in leadership positions must be educationally prepared to be able to develop and implement sound models for the effective delivery of patient care. Although many health care organizations collect large sets of data and are beginning to use scientific methods to improve the services they render, these activities are typically fragmented, isolated from day-to-day nursing management, and lack alignment with organizational strategy. The American Nurses Association (ANA) concurs with the IOM that errors occur as a result of system failure rather than human failure (Meehan-Hurwitz, 1999). This chapter will discuss the strategic planning process and the importance of aligning the organization's strategic vision with the mission, philosophy, and values of the organization and the communities served by the organization.

ORGANIZATIONAL PURPOSE, MISSION, PHILOSOPHY, VALUES

Every organization has a purpose and a guiding philosophy. Most often, the purpose and philosophy are explicitly stated and detailed in a formal mission statement. Typically, this mission statement reflects the organization's values and provides the reader with an indication of the behavior and strategic actions that can be expected from that organization. Most health care organizations have mission statements that speak to providing high quality or excellence in patient care. Some mission statements focus exclusively on providing care, while others assume a broader view and consider the education of health care professionals and the promotion of research as contributing to their broader mission. The mission of other organizations may be community based, and these organizations consequently will focus on providing community outreach and population-based services to a specific community or population within a community.

Mission Statement

The **mission statement** is a formal expression of the purpose or reason for existence of the organization. It is the organization's declaration of its primary driving force or its vision of the manner in which it believes care should be delivered. (For examples of actual mission statements, refer to the Exploring the Web activity at the end of the chapter.)

Philosophy

The **philosophy of an organization** is typically embedded in the mission statement. It is, in essence, a value statement of the principles and beliefs that direct the organization's behavior. A careful reading of the mission statement will usually provide a good

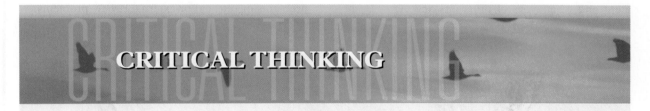

CRITICAL THINKING

Examine these two mission statements and then respond to the questions that follow.

Hospital A: "Our mission is to ensure the highest quality of care for the patients in our community. We believe that each patient has the right to the most innovative care that current science and technology can provide. To that end, we have assembled a world-renowned medical staff who will strive to ensure that the latest developments in medical science are used to combat disease."

Hospital B: "Our mission is to provide excellence in care to all. Our health care staff, nurses, physicians, and other professionals believe that care can best be provided in an atmosphere of collaboration and partnership with our patients and community. We believe in education—for our patients, for our staff, and for future health care providers. At all times we strive for optimal health promotion and the prevention of disease and disability."

Which of these institutions do you think would be more likely to have a patient lecture series on living with diabetes? Value the contributions of nursing? Provide experimental therapy for cancer? Be open to scheduling routine patient care visits for uninsured patients?

understanding of the institutional philosophy or value system. Mission statements with phrases such as "without consideration for ability to pay," "with respect for the dignity of each elderly resident," "a brighter future for all children," or "vigorous rehabilitation to maximize each individual's utmost potential" provide clues to the type of service that one could expect from an organization. In the best of worlds, there is congruence between the behaviors of the organization and the stated mission, philosophy, and values.

Sometimes an organization's values are formally stated and explicit, as in a mission statement. At other times, they are implicit and become part of the organizational culture. It is always important to assess an organization's values, as depicted in their mission statement, prior to considering employment because when important individual and organizational values collide, it is likely to be a constant source of frustration for the employee and employer.

STRATEGIC PLANNING

As Lewis Carroll observed in *Alice's Adventures in Wonderland*, "If you don't know where you are going, any road will do." A health care organization needs to have a good idea of where it fits into its environment and what types of programs and services are needed and demanded by its customers or stakeholders. This is true at a broad organizational level as well as at a unit level. It is important that a nurse manager in an ambulatory medicine clinic have an understanding of which programs and services are valued by the patient population the clinic serves and how the unit's ongoing activities fit in with the overall strategy of the larger organization. It is also important that staff consider patient needs when developing new services.

Strategic Planning Definition

The scenario described in the interview with Dr. Hernandez (below) is an example of factors that affect strategic planning. A strategic plan can be defined as the sum total or outcome of the processes by which an organization engages in environmental analysis, goal formulation, and strategy development with the purpose of organizational growth and renewal. Drucker (1973) defines strategic planning as "a continuous, systematic process of making risk-taking decisions today with the greatest possible knowledge of their effects on the future" (p. 125). Strategic planning is ongoing and is especially needed whenever the organization is experiencing problems or internal or external review problems.

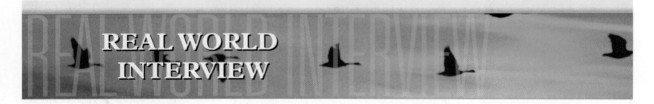

REAL WORLD INTERVIEW

Recent efforts to expand the range of dermatological services available at Loyola Chicago have centered on beginning a laser therapy center. Patients with a myriad of conditions such as port-wine stains, rosacea, and various pigmented lesions that are amenable to laser therapy would benefit from the addition of this type of health care service. Laser therapy could replace more antiquated methods of treating many types of cutaneous lesions, with a potential reduction in side effects and scarring. It would also result in a more cosmetically pleasing outcome. Currently, many individuals who require such procedures are referred out of our health care system. Several patients have complained that this results in additional time off from work to see another physician, increased travel times, and referral difficulties due to the constraints placed on many by their health insurance program. The expansion of available therapeutic options and improving ease of access to such procedures would benefit both patients and physicians.

Claudia Hernandez, MD
Dermatology

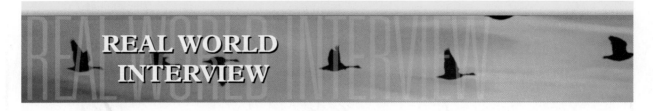

REAL WORLD INTERVIEW

The pivotal value of strategic planning is that it requires an organization to focus on its raison d'être, its mission, and to test how its operations are leading to accomplishment of that mission. Determined by the degree of dynamic change present in both its internal and external environments, an organization's strategic planning may extend years, or only months, into the future. However, at least annually, the strategic plan must be examined, reasserted as appropriate, and used as the standard against which short-term initiatives are measured for congruency with mission accomplishment.

Laura J. Nosek, PhD, RN
Health Care Consultant

Purpose of Strategic Planning

The purpose of strategic planning is twofold. First, it is important that everyone has the same idea or vision for where the organization is headed, and second, a good plan can help to ensure that the needed resources are available to carry out the initiatives that have been identified as important to the unit or agency. In addition, a clear plan allows the manager to select among seemingly equal alternatives based on the alternatives' potential to move the organization toward the desired end goal. Pesut (1998) states that nurses need to be involved with reengineering organizational processes to achieve higher productivity and quality. **Reengineering** is the fundamental rethinking and redesign of the process under review to bring about radical and dramatic improvements and increases in value. Often called business process reengineering, it implies an approach that will allow dramatic changes and yield dramatic improvements in the manner in which the business processes are carried out. Strategic planning is a major component of business process reengineering.

Steps in Strategic Planning Process

In any strategic planning process, there are steps to be followed. This process is similar to the nursing process. One assesses and plans before implementing a treatment. It is equally important when developing an organizational, unit, or program plan to progress in a systematic manner. The first step consists of an environmental assessment.

Environmental Assessment

An environmental or a situational assessment requires a broad view of the organization's current environment. For example, an environmental analysis of the type of undergraduate nursing education that would be needed for the 21st century professional nurse led one school of nursing to begin planning a curriculum revision that would incorporate the increasing emphasis on community-focused care. In addition, this analysis of the environment led faculty to understand that new models for clinical education will be needed to promote improved and expanded linkages between education and practice. This analysis is in line with Donaldson and Fralic's (2000) belief that the health care system is evolving, and this evolution makes uniting the academic and clinical practice settings more critical than ever.

SWOT Analysis

A **SWOT analysis** is a tool that is frequently used to conduct these environmental assessments. SWOT stands for strengths, weaknesses, opportunities, and threats. A SWOT analysis identifies strengths and weaknesses in the internal environment and opportunities and threats in the external environment. The

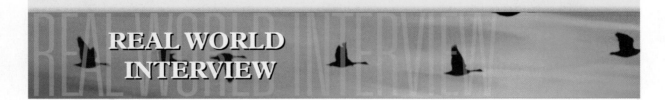

SWOT analysis is useful both for initial brainstorming and for a more formal planning document. Figure 9-1 is an example of a SWOT analysis that could be conducted by a university health care center (Jones & Beck, 1996).

Community and Stakeholder Assessment

A frequently overlooked but highly important area for analysis is the stakeholder assessment. A **stakeholder** is any person, group, or organization that has a vested interest in the program or project under review. A **stakeholder assessment** is a systematic consideration of all potential stakeholders to ensure that the needs of each of these stakeholders are incorporated in the planning phase.

For a program to be successful, the involvement of those who will be affected is essential. This is true whether the stakeholders are in the community or the stakeholders are the unit staff who will be affected by a proposed strategic plan. When stakeholders are not involved in the project planning, they do not gain a sense of ownership and may accept a program or strategic goals only with limited enthusiasm, or not at all.

Other Methods of Assessment

A number of methods can be used to support involvement in the strategic planning process. Thoughtful planning is required to determine the method and when to use the method.

Surveys and Questionnaires. Frequently, surveys or questionnaires are used when there are a large number of stakeholders and there is a general idea of the options available. For example, staff might be polled to see whether they would attend continuing education and which days and times would be most desirable.

Focus Groups and Interviews. Focus groups are small groups of individuals selected because of a common characteristic, such as a recent diagnosis of diabetes. The focus group is invited to meet in a group and respond to questions about a topic in which they are expected to have interest or expertise. An example of a focus group would be a group of patients who have recently had experiences with childbirth. They might be asked to come

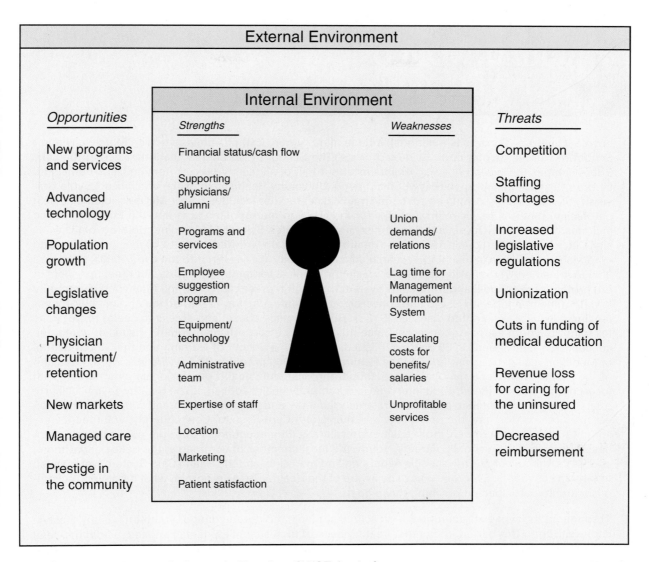

Figure 9-1 Key to Success in Strategic Planning: SWOT Analysis

together to discuss their obstetric experiences at the institution in the hope that the discussion will lead to insights or information that could be used for improving care or marketing services in the future. Focus groups are usually more time-consuming and expensive to conduct than questionnaires or surveys. They work best when the topic is broad and the options are not clear.

Advisory Board. Large projects often benefit from the formation of an advisory board, selected from various constituencies affected by a proposed program. The advisory board does not have formal authority over a program, but it is instrumental in reviewing the planned program and making recommendations and suggestions. Because the advisory board is deliberately selected to reflect representation from various stakeholders and areas of expertise, it is expected that the board will be able to identify potential concerns and provide sound guidance for the program.

Review of Literature Related to Identified Programs. A review of the literature should be completed prior to strategic planning or beginning any new project or program. This will allow the project team to identify similar programs, their structures and organization, potential problems and pitfalls, and

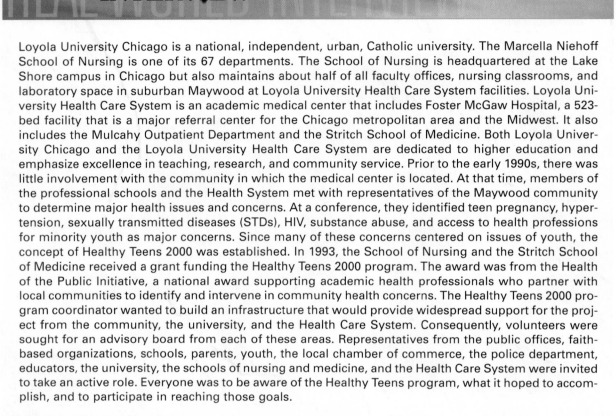

REAL WORLD INTERVIEW

Loyola University Chicago is a national, independent, urban, Catholic university. The Marcella Niehoff School of Nursing is one of its 67 departments. The School of Nursing is headquartered at the Lake Shore campus in Chicago but also maintains about half of all faculty offices, nursing classrooms, and laboratory space in suburban Maywood at Loyola University Health Care System facilities. Loyola University Health Care System is an academic medical center that includes Foster McGaw Hospital, a 523-bed facility that is a major referral center for the Chicago metropolitan area and the Midwest. It also includes the Mulcahy Outpatient Department and the Stritch School of Medicine. Both Loyola University Chicago and the Loyola University Health Care System are dedicated to higher education and emphasize excellence in teaching, research, and community service. Prior to the early 1990s, there was little involvement with the community in which the medical center is located. At that time, members of the professional schools and the Health System met with representatives of the Maywood community to determine major health issues and concerns. At a conference, they identified teen pregnancy, hypertension, sexually transmitted diseases (STDs), HIV, substance abuse, and access to health professions for minority youth as major concerns. Since many of these concerns centered on issues of youth, the concept of Healthy Teens 2000 was established. In 1993, the School of Nursing and the Stritch School of Medicine received a grant funding the Healthy Teens 2000 program. The award was from the Health of the Public Initiative, a national award supporting academic health professionals who partner with local communities to identify and intervene in community health concerns. The Healthy Teens 2000 program coordinator wanted to build an infrastructure that would provide widespread support for the project from the community, the university, and the Health Care System. Consequently, volunteers were sought for an advisory board from each of these areas. Representatives from the public offices, faith-based organizations, schools, parents, youth, the local chamber of commerce, the police department, educators, the university, the schools of nursing and medicine, and the Health Care System were invited to take an active role. Everyone was to be aware of the Healthy Teens program, what it hoped to accomplish, and to participate in reaching those goals.

Throughout its 8 years of operation, high school students mentored younger youth on healthy lifestyle choices. During this period, the unmet health needs of high school students surfaced, as did the need to establish a school-based health center at Proviso East High School, which is located in Maywood. In 1999, to begin the process of generating funding for the site, a survey was administered to a sample of Proviso East students to determine health needs and feelings toward the creation of a school-based health center. In November of 2000, the School of Nursing was awarded over $2 million in grants from the Health Resources Services Administration and the Illinois Department of Human Services to develop a school-based health care center at Proviso East High School. Members of the Healthy Teens advisory board were the first to envision such a project. The young people involved in the Healthy Teens program continue to meet twice a month, to prepare themselves as teen mentors and peer role models.

Carolyn Johnson, MSN
Program Coordinator — Healthy Teens 2000

successes. In the case described in the Johnson interview above, it was important, prior to designing the program, to have an understanding of the methods and strategies identified in the literature as effective in working with teens. This is an ongoing process. As programs are tentatively identified, the literature is searched for best practices and best evidence of how to conduct a program, and then the program ideas are refined.

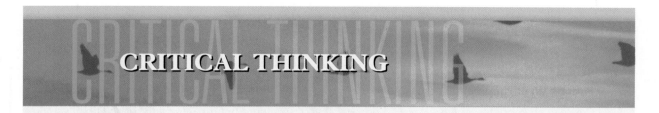

CRITICAL THINKING

You have just read about the Healthy Teens 2000 project. Use the description of that program to answer the following questions.

Do you think that community involvement was important in the success of this program? Why? Why weren't the health problems identified earlier by the Health Care System?

What do you think would have been the response of the community if Loyola attempted to tell the community members their problems instead of working collaboratively to identify major health issues? What kinds of strategies did the project use for building community support?

Are there any stakeholders who you think could have been included but were not? What do you see as key ingredients for making a community program such as this one successful?

Relationship of Strategic Planning to the Organization's Mission

All strategic planning and goals and objectives must be examined with an eye to the purpose or mission of the organization. Sometimes organizations get into trouble when they move too far afield of their core mission. Consequently, each new project needs to be evaluated in light of its congruence with the main mission that has been identified. It is fine for an organization to move to another project, but only if the new project is in line with the mission. Otherwise, there is a risk that the new programs will drain energy from the main mission.

Planning Goals and Objectives

Once all strategic goals and objectives have been identified, they need to be prioritized according to strategic importance, resources required, and time and effort involved. A timeline should be set. This will allow a thoughtful evaluation of each goal and objective and the degree to which each can be implemented in the specified time frame and with the available resources. This should be communicated to

all stakeholders. This will help to avoid misunderstandings and unmet expectations.

Developing a Marketing Plan

If a part of the strategic planning involves new programming for external audiences or if only internal redesign or restructuring is involved, the strategic plan and the goals and objectives will need to be communicated to all involved constituencies. Such communication will be needed, for example, when an institution is planning to implement a new information system to ensure that it remains competitive in the market. Designing, implementing, training, and evaluating this new system will require substantive changes in work flow and in the way that employees carry out their day-to-day work processes. If there has not been adequate thought to communication across the organization about the project, there is less chance of success and a greater risk of poor cooperation. See Table 9-1 for a summary of the steps involved in strategic planning.

ORGANIZATIONAL STRUCTURE

Organizations are structured or organized to facilitate the execution of their mission, strategic plans, report-

TABLE 9-1	*Summary of Steps in Strategic Planning*

1. Perform an environmental assessment.
2. Conduct stakeholder analysis.
3. Review literature for evidence and best practices.
4. Determine congruence with organizational mission.
5. Identify planning goals and objectives.
6. Estimate resources required for the plan.
7. Prioritize according to available resources.
8. Identify time lines and responsibilities.
9. Develop a marketing plan.
10. Write and communicate the business or strategic plan.
11. Evaluate.

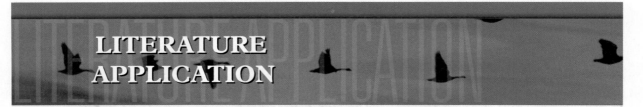

LITERATURE APPLICATION

Citation: Chezem, J., Friesen, C., Montgomery, P., Fortman, T., & Clark, H. (1998). Lactation duration: Influences of human milk replacements and formula samples on women planning postpartum employment. *Journal of Gynecological and Neonatal Nursing, 27*(6), 646–651.

Discussion: An institution, aware of the impending nursing shortage, identified a strategic planning goal of increasing nurse employee satisfaction in the organization. They determined that one method of supporting the large number of staff currently breastfeeding was to improve the work environment in this area. The positive benefits of breastfeeding are well documented in the literature, yet there are many barriers associated with successful breastfeeding in the workplace. Because the institution was interested in increasing nurse satisfaction and improving retention, it developed the following protocol.

The protocol was based on the two areas focused on in most of the literature: available support in the work environment and education for the mother. Staff members requesting a maternity leave would receive informational materials outlining the types of physical and emotional support available in the workplace as well as the educational resources. This is consistent with evidence suggesting that early education, motivation, support, and planning promote successful breastfeeding. Support was demonstrated in the work environment through the provision of a comfortable, appealing, private room for pumping milk. Refrigeration and needed supplies were made available. Unit managers were expected to provide break coverage for nurses to pump milk in the same manner as for work breaks and lunch hours. A business case can be made for the cost-effectiveness of the program in that the costs of the break coverage and environmental adaptations would be expected to be balanced positively by lower absenteeism and turnover. In addition, the literature supports that breastfed infants have fewer illnesses, which is associated with less maternal absenteeism.

Implications for Practice: When planning a program that involves workplace redesign, it is important to assess the evidence in the literature to determine what methods and strategies have worked well in the past.

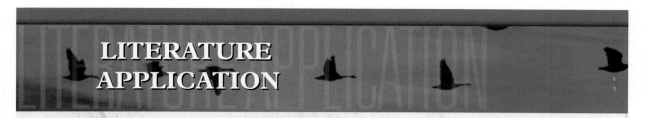

LITERATURE APPLICATION

Citation: Tonges, M., Rothstein, H., & Carter, H. (1998). Sources of satisfaction in hospital nursing practice: A guide to effective job design. *Journal of Nursing Administration, 28*(5), 47–61.

Discussion: A dilemma facing nursing and the health care field is the nursing shortage. There are many different reasons for this nursing shortage, including the aging of the nursing workforce and an increased number of opportunities for nurses in areas outside traditional practice areas. The peak of the nursing shortage is anticipated in the years from 2002 to 2007. As a result of this shortage, it is essential for hospitals to evaluate current retention strategies to keep valued employees because there will be a greater demand for nurses. The primary reason for the aging of the RN workforce is the decline in younger women choosing nursing. Unless this trend is reversed, long-term workforce needs will not be met. Extensive research has been done on nursing turnover in organizations and its costs. Job satisfaction is closely linked with retaining nurses. It is essential in the future that hospitals find new and different ways to retain nurses, or the turnover cycle will continue. If an institution is not successful in retaining nurses, nurses will leave institutions for a new hospital with such attractions as sign-on bonuses.

There are many different reasons for retaining nursing staff, including the fact that increased nursing satisfaction leads to increased patient satisfaction. The latest research shows that not only is the cost of orientation lost when a nurse leaves a position prematurely, but there is also a loss to the hospital in terms of lost productivity. Innovative ways to retain nurses must be developed. The role of nurse recruiter must be changed to focus on retaining current employees. This new role of nurse recruiter/nurse retainer (NR) will focus on the human capital of nursing and help keep it within an institution.

One of the main focuses of the NR will be to track turnover data and conduct exit interviews. In the past, there has not been enough review of the causes of nurse turnover and ways to prevent turnover. The NR can be expected to work with nurse managers to address unit-based issues, including promoting early employee interventions and facilitating potential transfers in and out of the unit. The NR can help to facilitate this transfer process, including using "the right fit" interview to ensure an employee transfers to the best area. The NR can provide in-services on the clinical ladder, the method for staff recognition and for promotion to higher nursing positions. In the past, clinical ladders have proven to be effective ways to retain staff and provide greater nursing satisfaction. The NR can work to help decrease the total number of nursing vacancies. In the recruitment role, the NR can continue to attract external candidates. In the retaining role, the NR can focus on increasing the satisfaction of current nursing staff. This reduces the number of external positions being recruited for. As the latest nursing shortage emerges, it is essential that recruitment and retention efforts be focused on decreasing nursing vacancies. Because all hospitals are facing the same shortage, new and different techniques must be applied to retain staff.

Implications for Practice: The dual role of nurse recruiter/nurse retainer has the potential to pave the way not only for an increase in nursing staff satisfaction but also for significant savings in orientation costs.

ing lines, and communication within the organization. This is true of entire organizations as well as individual nursing units. There are a number of ways to describe organizational structures that involve classifying them by identifying selected characteristics. Each of these characteristics tends to exist on a continuum.

For example, under the category of type or level of authority in an organizational structure, a highly bureaucratic, highly authoritarian structure is at one end of the continuum and a highly democratic, participative structure is at the other end. The highly authoritarian model is seen in the military and is well suited for the purpose of the military. When decisions need to be made quickly, with clarity and not with challenges or discussion, as in a battle situation, a highly authoritarian organizational structure works well.

An example at the other end of the continuum would be a multidisciplinary group of professionals meeting to determine the care management of a patient or patient population. An example of this group might be a hospice team task force made up of nurses, social workers, physicians, home care aides, bereavement specialists, and chaplains, all meeting to discuss the care planning for a dying patient. In this situation, it will be important for team members of each discipline to freely contribute according to their particular area of knowledge and expertise. An organizational structure such as this can function successfully only in a participative, democratic manner.

Types of Organizational Structures

Most often, the existing organizational structures are communicated by means of an organizational chart. Figure 9-2 is an example of an organizational chart for a typical acute care general hospital (Shortell & Kaluzny, 2000). This organization has a tall bureaucratic structure with many layers in the hierarchy or chain of command and a centralized formal authority in the board of trustees. It represents a formal, top-down reporting structure.

Matrix Structure

Today, given the greater complexity of the health care system, more organizations are using matrix structures. Figure 9-3 shows a matrix design (Shortell & Kaluzny, 2000).

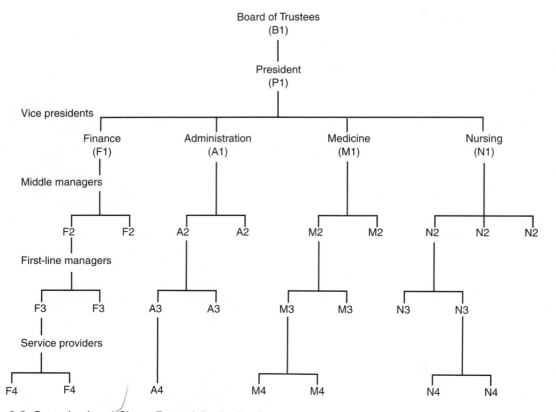

Figure 9-2 Organizational Chart, Formal Authority Structure: Acute Care General Hospital

Flat versus Tall Structure

Organizations are considered flat when there are few layers in the reporting structure. A tall organization would have many layers in the chain of command. An example of a flat organizational structure is a school of nursing that has no departments and many faculty members reporting to one dean of nursing.

Decentralized versus Centralized Structure

The terms *centralized* and *decentralized* refer to the degree to which an organization has spread its lines of authority, power, and communication. A tall, bureaucratic design like that in Figure 9-2 would be considered highly centralized. A matrix design like

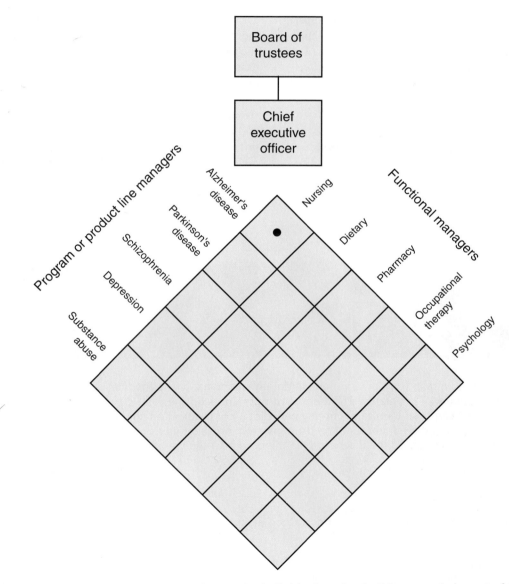

Figure 9-3 Matrix Design: A Psychiatric Center. An individual worker in this example is part of the Alzheimer program as well as a member of the nursing department.

that in Figure 9-3 would be on the decentralized end of the continuum. As can be seen in Figure 9-3, the nursing manager can interface with the Alzheimer's disease program manager without going through a central, hierarchical core, as would happen in a bureaucratic structure like that in Figure 9-2.

Other characteristics or attributes can be used to assess organizations. Many typologies exist that may be used for this purpose. For example, Shortell and Kaluzny (2000) suggest using external environment, mission/goals, work groups/work design, organizational design, interorganizational relationships, change/innovation, and strategic issues. Refer to Table 9-2 for an example of how these attributes can be assessed in four different health service organizations (Shortell & Kaluzny, 2000).

Division of Labor

The way the labor force is divided or organized has an effect on how the mission is accomplished. The functional organizational chart in Figure 9-4 graphically depicts how the formal authority in this organization is structured (Shortell & Kaluzny, 2000). At the highest level, the board of trustees delegates authority to the chief executive officer, who delegates to the vice presidents and so on. At the vice presidential level, there are five department directors for each branch. The department directors each report to their respective vice president. The nurse managers report to their department director of nursing. The charge nurse reports to the nurse manager of her unit. The treatment nurse and the medication nurse report to the charge nurse. In this functional design, the division of labor is quite efficient and specialized. A danger with functional division of labor is that each individual may be so focused on her specific area that she has little perspective about the overall picture. For example, a treatment nurse may focus on treatments and have little information about the total patient.

In the matrix structure shown in Figure 9-3, the structure was less important and the workforce roles and reporting relationships are based on the project or task to be accomplished, rather than on a rigid hierarchy. An example of this is the planning involved in the preparation for a Joint Commission on Accreditation of Healthcare Organizations (JCAHO) review. The JCAHO team could be composed of various

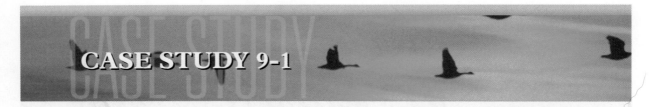

CASE STUDY 9-1

A patient developed a rash from a new medication, unbeknownst to the medication nurse, who never asked about any signs of problems. The treatment nurse noticed the rash during a routine dressing change but never thought to inquire about any new dietary or medication changes. It was not until the time of discharge when the patient read the drug information sheet advising that any skin changes be reported that the patient asked the discharge planning nurse if the week-old rash was significant.

What could have been done differently?

Was anyone at fault? Who?

Why is good communication especially important in a situation in which there is a functional division of labor?

What types of problems could you expect if staff members focused on their own tasks and failed to communicate with each other about the patient's emotional, psychosocial, educational, and discharge needs?

individuals at varying levels of responsibility and from programs across the organization, but they could interact with staff at all levels and report as a task force at a high level in the organization.

Roles and Responsibilities

Note that exact roles and responsibilities within each level and division are not defined on the organiza-

TABLE 9-2	Typology of Four Health Services Organizations			
Attribute	Health Maintenance Organizations (HMOs)	Home Health Care Agencies	Hospitals	Pharmaceutical Companies
External environment	Moderate complexity Moderate change Highly competitive	Relatively simple Moderate change Increasingly competitive	Complex High change Highly competitive	Moderate complexity Moderate change Highly competitive
Mission/goals	Primary care emphasis; keep people well	Quality of life Maintaining functional status	Acute care emphasis; curing illness	Research and development (R&D) emphasis; new product development
Work group/ work design	Primary care team; coordinate referrals	Simple design; primarily one-on-one patient contact	Departmental and cross departmental teams; high need for coordination	Separation of functions possible; R&D versus sales; relatively low need for coordination
Organization design	Functional and divisional integrating; primary care physicians and specialists	Functional	Divisional and matrix	Divisional and strategic business units
Interorganizational relationships	Link to expand primary care patient base	Expand patient base and gain economies of scale	Key to becoming part of vertically integrated health systems	Important for global expansion
Change/ innovation	Respond to and create new patient care management approaches	Respond to demographic and social changes	Respond to the new paradigm; implement new role within vertically integrated systems	Respond to new product development demands
Strategic issues	Expand the concept of managed care	Demonstrate continuing value, and therefore, reimbursement for services	Fit into an expanded and changing delivery system	Decrease time to develop new drugs

tional charts beyond specifying the given division, for example, nursing. Scope of responsibilities, specific duties, and specific job requirements are found in documents such as individual job or position descriptions.

Reporting Relationships

An organizational chart, such as the one that appears in Figure 9-4, allows one to determine the formal reporting relationships. These are shown with a solid line. Sometimes dotted lines are used in an organizational chart to depict dual or secondary reporting relationships. An example of this might be the role of the director of performance improvement. This individual might directly report to the chief executive officer but also have position accountabilities to the board of trustees. The formal reporting relationships may or may not reflect the

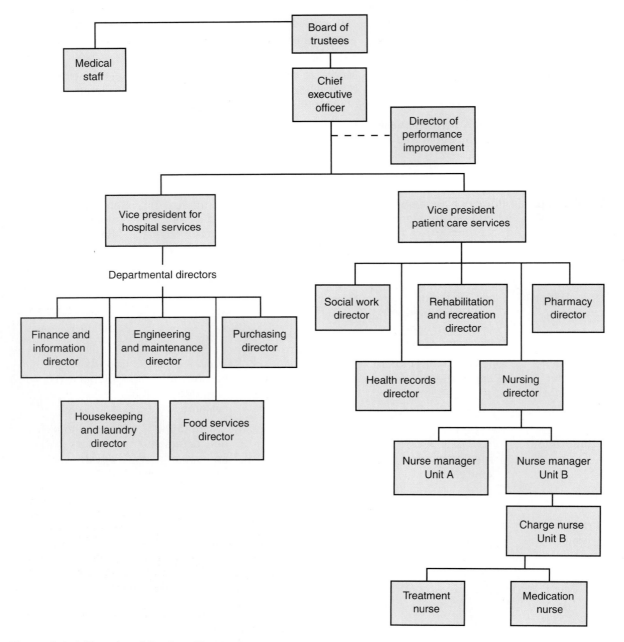

Figure 9-4 A Functional Design: Nursing Home

actual communications that occur within the institution.

Division of Labor by Geographic Area.

Care delivery divided according to geography or location can be efficient. It might consist of the hospital and ambulatory care, or at smaller unit levels, the North Team and the West Team. Frequently, care provided by home health agencies is divided by geographic district for efficiency in travel. At the health care system level, geographical division could mean that each major area, such as the hospital or the clinics, would have separate supporting services, such as two pharmacies, one in the outpatient clinic and one in the hospital. Both clinic and inpatient areas could, and often do, have separate medical records departments. An obvious concern in such arrangements is lack of coordination and duplication of services.

Division of Labor by Product or Service.

Sometimes, care delivery is organized around product lines or service lines. This is a type of functional division of work, but it is based on a patient's diagnosis or the specialty care required by a patient. For example, there might be a cardiology service line, a woman's health service line, and an oncology service line. This can lead to improved quality of care and decreased confusion for the patient because the information and protocols used in the outpatient side would be consistent with the information and protocols used in the hospital and across the entire health care system. Figure 9-5 demonstrates a product line design (Shortell & Kaluzny, 2000).

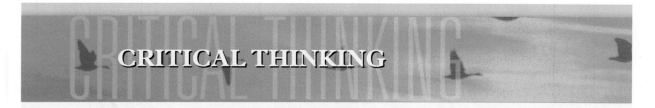

CRITICAL THINKING

There have been a number of studies that have demonstrated that primary nursing leads to improved patient and nurse satisfaction.

Why do you think this might be? Can you think of any disadvantages to a primary nursing care model for organizing care?

CRITICAL THINKING

You, as a nurse, have been asked to take a leadership role in identifying potential depression management programs that could be implemented in the community-based psychiatric center where you work. Suppose that you would normally report to the depression product line manager, but for this project you are designated as the coordinator of depression management programs. As you begin your assessment of potential programs, you will need to interact with a number of functional departments across the organization, such as dietary, pharmacy, occupational therapy, and psychology. In addition, you will have to examine the other product lines to be sure that you are not duplicating services.

Given this situation, what would be some advantages of working in an institution that had a matrix design such as that depicted in Figure 9-3? What might be disadvantages?

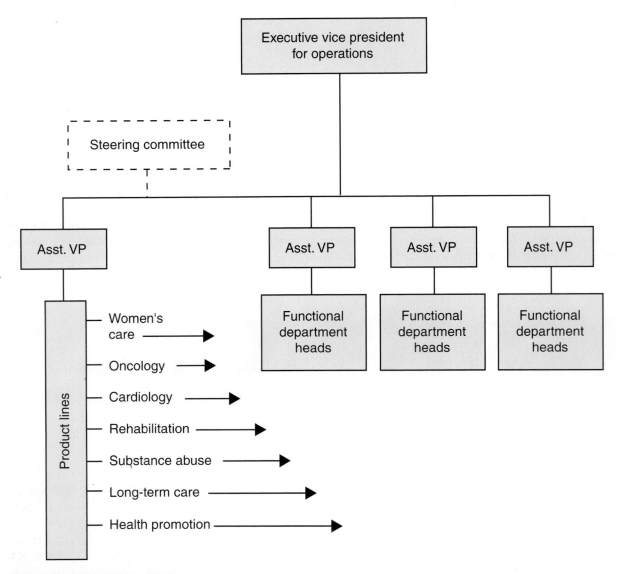

Figure 9-5 Product Line Design

Primary Nursing. Primary nursing care describes a model of care in which one nurse is primarily responsible for all aspects of patient care for a given patient or patients. The patient is assigned a primary nurse upon admission, and, when possible, that nurse will be the patient's primary caregiver throughout the hospitalization. In this model, there is usually an associate nurse to assume care responsibilities if the primary nurse is not available.

Many factors affect strategic planning, as the SWOT analysis discussed in this chapter highlighted. Nurses need to prepare to address these many factors.

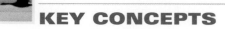

KEY CONCEPTS

- There are increasing opportunities for nurses to become involved in strategic planning for the delivery of health care services in their organizations and communities. To do so effectively, however, they will need a basic understanding of the way in which organizations are structured, how organizational systems function, and how to engage in the strategic planning process.
- Every organization has a purpose and a guiding

philosophy, which are typically explicitly stated and detailed in a formal mission statement.

- The mission statement reflects the organization's values and provides the reader with an indication of the behavior and strategic actions that can be expected from that organization.

- A health care organization needs to have a good idea of where it fits into its environment and what types of programs and services are needed and demanded by its customers or stakeholders.

- The pivotal value of strategic planning is that it requires an organization to focus on its raison d'être and its mission and to test how its operations are leading to accomplishment of that mission.

- The purpose of strategic planning is twofold. First, it is important that everyone has the same idea or vision of where the organization is headed; second, a good plan can help to ensure that the needed resources are available to carry out the initiatives that have been identified as important to the unit or agency.

- A stakeholder assessment is a systematic consideration of all potential stakeholders to ensure that the needs of each of these stakeholders are incorporated in the planning phase. For a program to be successful, the involvement of those who will be affected is essential.

- Organizations are structured or organized in a manner that is designed to facilitate the execution of their mission and their strategic plans.

- There are a number of ways to describe organizational structures that involve classifying them by identifying selected characteristics.

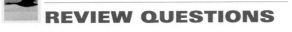

KEY TERMS

focus groups
mission statement
philosophy of an
  organization
reengineering

stakeholder assessment
stakeholder
strategic plan
SWOT analysis

REVIEW QUESTIONS

1. A document that describes the institution's purpose and philosophy is
   A. the organizational chain of command.
   B. the organizational chart.
   C. the mission statement.
   D. the strategic plan.

2. Which of the following is the outcome of the processes by which an organization engages in environmental analysis, goal formulation, and strategy development with the purpose of organizational growth and renewal?
   A. Stakeholder assessment
   B. SWOT analysis
   C. Strategic planning
   D. Mission development

3. The most formal and hierarchical organizational structure would be expected to have an organizational chart with
   A. a matrix design.
   B. many layers of command.
   C. a product line design.
   D. a number of dotted lines representing reporting relationships.

4. SWOT means
   A. strengths, weaknesses, opportunities, threats.
   B. strengths, worries, outcomes, threats.
   C. strengths, weaknesses, opportunities, treatment.
   D. structures, worries, outcomes, threats.

REVIEW ACTIVITIES

1. Having a strategic plan in place can help an organization to make a decision about one alternative over another. For example, an institution whose strategic plan calls for positioning itself as the leading cancer care provider in the area would be well served to advertise for nurses in the *Oncology Nursing Society Journal* rather than in a local newspaper, even if the costs of advertising in the journal were higher. Identify another situation in which a strategic plan could guide an organization in its choices among alternative actions.

2. Write a beginning mission statement and strategic plan for your professional nursing career. Do you plan to care for vulnerable populations in the community, become expert in critical care nursing, or seek advanced education to become a midwife? Once you have identified your mission, outline a strategic plan with objectives to attain your nursing goals. For example, you might want to conduct a SWOT analysis, looking at the external environment; your internal environment

(your skills, talents, and preferences); and the strengths, weaknesses, threats, and opportunities that exist in each. Once you have completed this exercise, you will have a better idea of which opportunities to pursue. For example, if you know that you want to work in pediatrics, you might ask for a pediatric journal subscription for your birthday. Additionally, you may be able to select or have input into the selection of your final clinical rotation in school, or you may be able to look for meetings, conferences, or educational sessions in your area of interest.

3. You are asked to help establish the advisory board for your institution's proposed hospice program. How would you recommend people to include on the advisory board? What groups of professionals and consumers would you want to see represented on a hospice advisory board? Identify at least 10 candidates and the stakeholder groups that they might represent. Remember to include both professionals and consumer/community representatives. It would be important to assess each individual's support for hospice concepts and his or her level of interest in becoming involved prior to inviting those individuals to join the advisory board. How might you go about doing this?

4. Examine the organizational structure of an organization or institution with which you are familiar. How would you characterize it using the types of structures that were discussed in this chapter? Look at organizational communication, reporting structure, and division of labor. Is the organization a hierarchy or a matrix? Does the way that the institution or organization is structured assist it in meeting its goals? Why or why not?

EXPLORING THE WEB

Upon completion of your nursing degree, you are planning to interview for a position at an area hospital. In preparation for your interview, you want to understand the mission as well as other information about that institution. Today that information is readily available on the web. For example, if you were planning to apply at Loyola University Chicago (*http://www.luc.edu*) you would go to *http://www.luhs.org/jobs.htm* (the exact address of the mission statement of the health system is *http://www.luhs.org/under/mission.htm*). Another

example is Children's Memorial Hospital in Chicago at *http://www.childrensmemorial.org* (the exact web address of the mission statement is *http://www. childrens memorial.org /hosp_info/mission.asp*).

Look at these web pages, paying particular attention to the descriptions they provide of the organizations' missions. What impressions do you form about these organizations and their missions? Does the stated mission seem to fit with the general "feel" that you get from the web site? Could you easily find information about positions available? About the institution? Try this exercise with your local hospital or medical center.

REFERENCES

Chezem, J., Friesen, C., Montgomery, P., Fortman, T., & Clark, H. (1998). Lactation duration: Influences of human milk replacements and formula samples on women planning postpartum employment. *Journal of Gynecological and Neonatal Nursing, 27*(6), 646–651.

Donaldson, S., & Fralic, M. (2000). Forging today's practice-academic link: A new era for nursing leadership. *Nursing Administration Quarterly, 25*(1), 95–101.

Drucker, P. (1973). *Management tasks, responsibilities, and practices.* New York: Harper & Row.

Havens, D. S. & Aiken, L. H. (1999). Shaping systems to promote desired outcomes: The magnet hospital model. *Journal of Nursing Administration, 29*(2), 14–20.

Hope, J., & Hope, T. (1997). Competing in the third wave. Boston: Harvard Business School Press.

Institute of Medicine. (1999). *To err is human.* Washington, DC: National Academy Press.

Jones, R., & Beck, S. (1996). *Decision making in nursing.* Clifton Park, NY: Delmar Learning.

Kanter, R. M. (1997). On the frontiers of management. Boston: Harvard Business School Press.

Meehan-Hurwitz, J. (1999). ANA applauds White House for steps to reduce medical errors. *SNA Insider, 12,* 1–2.

National advisory councils in nursing and medicine collaborate to develop new approaches for enhancing patient safety. (2000, Fall). *Health Workforce Newslink, 7*(1), 5.

Pesut, D. (1998). Twenty-first century learning. *Nursing Outlook, 46*(1), 37.

Shortell, S., & Kaluzny, A. (2000). *Health care management: Organization design and behavior,* (4th ed.). Clifton Park, NY: Delmar Learning.

Tonges, M., Rothstein, H., & Carter, H. (1998). Sources of satisfaction in hospital nursing practice: A guide to effective job design. *Journal of Nursing Administration, 28*(5), 47–61.

SUGGESTED READINGS

Aikman, P., Andress, I., Goodfellow, C., LaBelle, N., & Porter-O'Grady, T. (1998). System integration: A necessity. *Journal of Nursing Administration, 28*(2), 28–34.

Bates, D., & Gawande, A. (2000). Error in medicine: What have we learned? *Annals of Internal Medicine, 132,* 763–767.

Bennis, W. (1999, Summer): The end of leadership: Exemplary leadership is impossible without full inclusion, initiatives, and cooperation of followers. *Organizational Dynamics,* 71–80.

Blouin, A. S., & Tonges, M. C. (1996). The content/context imperative: Integration of emerging designs for the practice and management of nursing. *Journal of Nursing Administration, 26*(3), 38–46.

Bodenheimer, T. (1999). The movement for improved quality in health care. *New England Journal of Medicine, 340,* 488–492.

Buerhaus, P., Staiger, D., & Auerbach, D. (2000). Why are shortages of hospital RNs concentrated in specialty care units? *Nursing Economic$, 18*(3), 111–116.

Buerhaus, P., & Staiger, D. (1997). Future of the nurse labor market according to health executives in high managed-care areas of the United States. *Image: Journal of Nursing Scholarship, 29*(4), 313–318.

Chassin, M. R. (1996). Quality of health care part 3: Improving the quality of care. *New England Journal of Medicine, 335*(14), 1060–1063.

Chassin, M. R., Galvin, R. W., & the National Roundtable on Health Care Quality. (1998). The urgent need to improve health care quality. *Journal of the American Medical Association, 280,* 1000–1005.

Chezem, J., Montgomery, P., & Fortman, T. (1997). Maternal feelings after cessation of breastfeeding: Influence of factors related to employment and duration. *Journal of Perinatal and Neonatal Nursing, 11*(2), 61–70.

Clemmer, T. P., Spuhler, V. J., Berwick, D. M., & Nolan, T. W. (1998). Cooperation: The foundation of improvement. *Annals of Internal Medicine, 128,* 1004–1009.

Cormak, M., Brady, J., & Porter-O'Grady, T. (1997). Professional practice: A framework for transition to a new culture. *Journal of Nursing Administration, 27*(12), 32–41.

Duckett, L., Henly, S., Avery, M., Potter, S., Hills-Bonczyk, S., Hulden, R., & Savik, K. (1998). A theory of planned behavior-based structural model for breast-feeding. *Nursing Research, 47*(6), 325–336.

Gessner, T. L. (1998). Job design and work process in patient care. In J. A. Dienemann (Ed.), *Nursing administration: Managing patient care.* (2nd ed., pp. 359–378). Stamford, CT: Appleton & Lange.

Hawke, M. (1999, November 15). Nursing workforce 1999: A year of challenges and opportunities. *Spectrum,* 8.

Hornberger, J. & Wrone, E. (1997, October 15). When to base clinical policies on observational versus randomized trial data. *Annals of Internal Medicine, 127*(8 pt. 2), 697–703.

Jones, K. R., DeBaca, V., & Yarbrough, M. (1997). Organizational culture assessment before and after implementing patient-focused care. *Nursing Economic$, 15*(2), 73–80.

Kreitzer, M. J., Wright, D., Hamlin, C., Towey, S., Marko, M., & Disch, J. (1997). Creating a healthy work environment in the midst of organizational change and transition. *Journal of Nursing Administration, 27*(6), 35–41.

Leape, L., Woods, D., Hatlie, M., Kizer, K., Schroeder, S., & Lundberg, G. (1998). Promoting patient safety by preventing medical error. *Journal of the American Medical Association, 280*(16), 1444–1447.

Levi, P. (1999). Sustainability of healthcare environments. *Image: Journal of Nursing Scholarship, 31*(4), 395–398.

Mark, B. A. (1996). Organizational culture. *Annual Review of Nursing Research, 14,* 145–163.

Mills, A., & Blaesing, S. (2000). A lesson from the last nursing shortage: The influence of work values on career satisfaction with nursing. *Journal of Nursing Administration, 30*(6), 309–315.

Olson, L. L. (1998). Hospital nurses' perceptions of the ethical climate of their work setting. *Image: Journal of Nursing Scholarship, 30*(4), 345–349.

O'Neil, E. (1999, January/February). The opportunity that is nursing. *Nursing and Health Care Perspectives, 20*(1), 10–14.

Prescott, P. (2000). The enigmatic nursing workforce. *Journal of Nursing Administration, 30*(2), 59–65.

Rambur, B. (1999). Fostering evidence-based practice in nursing education. *Journal of Professional Nursing, 15*(5), 270–274.

Regenstein, M. (2000). *Medical errors and patient safety: Issue for public hospitals.* Washington, DC: National Public Health and Hospital Institute.

Schuster, M. A., McGlynn, E. A., & Brook, R. H. (1998). How good is the quality of health care in the United States? *Milbank Quarterly, 76*(4), 517–563.

Visness, C., & Kennedy, K. (1997). Maternal employment and breast-feeding: Findings from the 1998 National Maternal and Infant Health Survey. *American Journal of Public Health, 87*(6), 945–951.

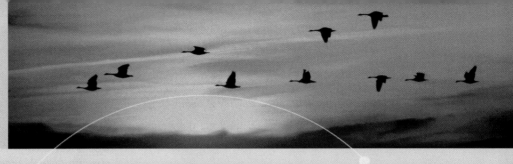

CHAPTER 10

Effective Team Building

Karin Polifko-Harris, PhD, RN, CNAA

OBJECTIVES

Upon completion of this chapter, the reader should be able to:

1. Identify the differences between teams and committees.
2. Discuss the stages of group process.
3. Review key concepts of effective teams.
4. Discuss ways in which a nurse manager can create an environment conducive to team building.

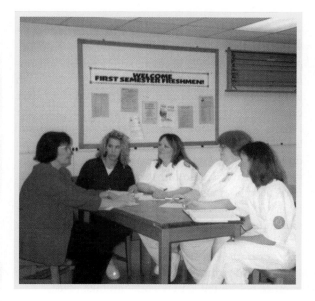

As a new nurse, you are making the day's assignments for a 34-bed medical-surgical unit. Working with you today will be another two registered nurses, two licensed practical nurses, and one nursing assistant. You graduated only months ago but were recently promoted to the role of charge nurse. Today, one of the licensed practical nurses and the nursing assistant are challenging your patient care assignments, saying you do not have enough experience to make a fair assignment, and they are trying to get the two registered nurses to side with them. It appears that the two registered nurses often work together, as do the two licensed practical nurses. You know you made the best assignment given the staff available, yet you are wondering if there is a better solution.

What are your thoughts on how to proceed?

What would be the best way to address their concerns?

How could you more actively involve them in the patient assignment responsibility?

Essential leadership and management skills in nursing always include some element of effective teamwork. Working together in a successful team requires more than good luck or chance. The health care delivery system continues to increase in complexity. Issues such as changing reimbursement schedules, more seriously ill hospitalized patients, and a move from acute health care to nonacute health care delivery may challenge nurse managers to alter how nursing care is provided to patients.

A critical trend in human resource development is team training. While American business culture has placed emphasis on the importance of the individual for success, the nursing profession has begun refocusing on teamwork and team building as a method for meeting the needs of a changing health care delivery model. Nurses generally do not work in isolation but provide care that is interdependent, providing a level of expertise to help the patient achieve optimal wellness. This chapter discusses the key factors that contribute to a successful nursing team, including team building. It also discusses characteristics and skills of an effective team leader.

DEFINING TEAMS AND COMMITTEES

Katzenbach and Smith (1993) define a **team** as "a small number of people with complementary skills who are committed to a common purpose, performance goals, and approach for which they hold themselves accountable (p. 45)." Senge, Roberts, Ross, Smith, and Kleiner (1994) further elaborate that a team is a group that has a purpose and needs each member's contributions to succeed. On some teams all members may have similar backgrounds and abilities, such as a nursing policy and procedure team. Other teams may be developed with members who have a variety of skills and talents, to provide different perspectives and ideas on how to solve problems.

An **interdisciplinary team** is composed of members with a variety of clinical expertise. An advantage to having an interdisciplinary team is the different strengths and viewpoints everyone can contribute. Everyone on the interdisciplinary team is trained in his or her specialty and looks at care delivery with a different focus: nurses, physicians, social workers, dieticians, case managers. Sometimes having so many viewpoints can be difficult, though, especially if a single decision is needed and everyone has varying opinions. The best way to work with an interdisciplinary team is to allow everyone to be heard, and to entertain various problem-solving methods and potential solutions. It is the role of the team leader to ensure that all members have the opportunity to participate to accomplish the work of the team.

To get the work of an organization completed, multiple committees may develop to assist in communication. A **committee** is a work group with a specific task or goal to accomplish. An ad hoc committee is generally temporary and formed for a specific purpose, for a specific time frame, or to accomplish a certain short-term goal. An example of an ad hoc committee may be the sick call policy committee that meets only until the new policy is adopted by the institution. Unlike ad hoc committees, standing committees may be an integral component of the organizational structure, with an example being the Quality Improvement Committee that meets on a monthly basis. Standing committees may be mandated through organizational bylaws, such as medical staff meetings. They may also be mandated by outside accrediting agencies, such as the Hospital Ethics Committee that the Joint Commission on Healthcare Organizations recommends. Other committees may exist because there is a need to have a formal process in place for decision making, as in the Critical Care Policy and Procedure Committee.

A committee may also be advisory, such as a committee that meets to discuss concerns of the professional nursing staff and then reports back to the chief nurse executive (CNE). Marquis and Huston (2000) point out that if a positive change in an organization is the desired result, then it is imperative to include as early as possible all those who would be affected by the change.

STAGES OF TEAM PROCESS

All teams go through predictable phases of development, much like a person, as they evolve from an immature stage to (one hopes!) a mature stage. It is critical to note that not all teams reach maturity, for a variety of reasons: perhaps there are ineffective leadership, problematic members, unclear goals and directives, or lack of focus or energy. Similar to individuals on the continuum of maturity, some teams may become fully functional and mature quickly, bypassing a stage or two along the way. It is usual for high-functioning teams whose members are familiar with one another to be able to make decisions quickly and accurately; it may take longer for other teams, whose members need to get to know and trust one another before the actual work can take place.

Tuckman and Jensen (1977) and Lacoursier (1980) identified five stages that a group normally progresses through as it reaches maturity. These stages are known as **group process** and consist of: forming, storming, norming, performing, and adjourning (Figure 10-1).

The first stage is the forming stage, in which several critical phases begin: the expectation phase, the interaction phase, and the boundary formation phase. The expectation phase starts when the first meeting begins. Everyone is curious what the group is all

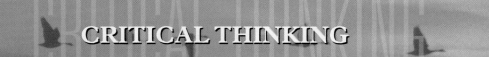

CRITICAL THINKING

You are the nurse who is working with Mr. Ward, a 76-year-old male who is admitted for congestive heart failure and chronic kidney disease. Mr. Ward is well known to the staff at Memorial Hospital for his multiple admissions. During this admission, his blood pressure is unusually high and he appears sluggish. His wife is visiting her relatives out of town, and he is by himself. When you attend the daily care management conference, you note most of the interdisciplinary team is present: the nurse case manager, the social worker, the nurse caring for him, the hospital chaplain, the dietician, the pharmacist, and his primary care physician.

What are some key issues that are concerning you? What perspective does each of the team members bring to the discussion on the care of Mr. Ward? How would you proceed to develop or alter Mr. Ward's plan of care? Are there any other team members who may be able to assist you with Mr. Ward's care?

Forming	Storming	Norming	Performing	Adjourning
• Expectations	• Tension	• Positioning	• Actual work	• Closure
• Interactions	• Conflict	• Goal setting	• Relationships	• Evaluation
• Boundary formation	• Confrontation	• Cohesiveness	• Group maturity	• Outcomes review

Figure 10-1 Stages of Group Process (Drawing on Tuckman & Jensen, 1977, and Lacoursier, 1980)

about—how will it meet their needs, what they will need to do to fit in, and what they can gain from group membership. During the interaction phase, opinions are beginning to be formed as the group takes shape, and expectations and boundaries are more clearly defined. The group is establishing its identity, with the help of the group leader. The group leader needs to provide the team with information on the purpose of the group meeting and the vision and boundaries of what the group is expected to accomplish.

The second stage of the group process is the storming phase. As everyone begins to feel more comfortable in the group setting, certain feelings and statements are made that may result in members finding a position within the group to which they can contribute. The storming phase is generally difficult because of conflict that may, at times, be quite apparent. Differences among group members—including even the group leader, perhaps—become obvious, with people often taking sides on certain concerns or issues. Although this phase is tension filled and confrontational, it is often necessary for a group to journey through the storming phase to encourage resolution of the emerging problems and to actively solve the issues at hand.

Stage three is the norming phase, which follows the conflict and confrontation of the storming stage. While the problems are not yet solved and decisions may not be made, there is a general understanding at least of what the issues are and who will be progressing toward solving them. Positions within the group are now established, with members having a sense of belonging and of setting goals to meet the expectations outlined in the forming stage. Conflict has converted into cohesiveness.

Performing is the fourth stage in the maturity of a group and is probably the most enjoyable phase. Agreement is a foremost activity—everyone knows what their role is and what they are supposed to do, and obvious progress is made toward the plan to achieve the overall group goal. The group is considered mature at this stage, and the individual members are now ready to focus on the actual work that will meet the group's objectives. Another strength of the performing stage is the emphasis placed on maintaining effective relationships with group members, as the individual members function as a whole (Tappen, 2001).

The final stage of group processing is adjourning. The group has met its stated and some unstated objectives, with closure activities the primary focus. Closure is the process by which the team members review the team's progress. Were the goals and objectives of the team met? Was there anything that would be done differently if the team were to start all over? During the final stage, the group should evaluate whether the stated purpose was accomplished. What were the outcomes of both the group process and the individuals' participation? So many times groups are disbanded without this closing review, leaving some members feeling empty and without a feeling of accomplishment.

Team Roles

As in any gathering, when people come together in a team, everyone takes on a different role. Some may want the role to be self-serving, as with the person who wants to be the center of attention and insists on being in the middle of any decision. Others play a

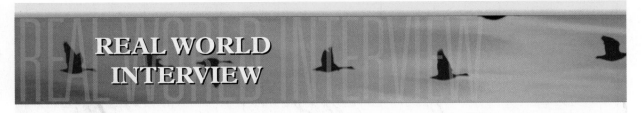

What makes a good team? Well, I believe, it happens when everyone works together. It's not looking the other way when someone needs help, its answering another nurse's patient call light. It's not putting your head down when you see family members approaching. It's taking responsibility for what you are expected to do as a professional.

Linea R. Murphy, RN
Team Leader

role that is clearly supportive: they are there to contribute in any way they can to the betterment of the whole but do not need or want any limelight thrown their way. There are numerous other roles that people may take on, though some roles not always clearly defined.

Functional versus Dysfunctional Members

In any team, there are bound to be both participants who are functional and those who are somewhat dysfunctional in their behaviors. Sometimes the behaviors are unconsciously acted out—perhaps in the form of a defense mechanism such as denial. At other times, a team member is quite clear and focused about the role she is playing, such as the antagonizer. In any case, it is imperative that the astute group leader be aware of everyone's roles to facilitate the most optimal team process possible.

So what role would a functional team member perform? Several roles are critical to the successful meeting of a team's goal (Bradford, 1978). When a project first begins, a group member is needed to fill the role of creator—someone who initiates the first move, someone who gets the ball rolling. A role complementary to the creator is that of coordinator—someone who is aware of the project flow and who keeps it moving in the right direction. Likewise, the team needs a mobilizer, whose job is to keep things energized and who provides the spark needed to keep team members interested in the project. Other functional roles include the questioner, who asks the questions that are on everyone's mind; the antago-

nist, who looks at the situation in an opposite manner to everyone else; and the recorder, who chronicles the details of the team meeting and process. It is not necessary to have all the roles filled at all times in a functional teams.

What are the dysfunctional roles that hinder the progress of a team? Unfortunately, there are numerous personality types that may be difficult, especially during the team's formative stages. Criticizers find fault with everything and everybody yet seldom contribute positively when asked. Everything is a strong "No!" and if it is not done their way, they believe it will not be done correctly. Passive ones will rarely take a stand on anything. It is their passivity and inability to make a decision that is often frustrating. They will not say a word for fear of rebuttal.

Detailers get so caught up with the facts that it is hard for them to see the big picture or to keep heading toward the goal. Likewise, controllers monopolize the group discussion—no one else can be heard. The only opinion that matters is theirs. They need constant refocusing by the leader to keep them on track. Finally, pleasers want to do just that—please. They will not make a comment or decision that may be unfavorable to anyone else. Refer to Table 10-1 for suggestions on how to cope with difficult personalities.

KEY CONCEPTS OF EFFECTIVE TEAMS

A familiar saying is that "the whole is greater than the sum of the parts." An effective team is one in which all members are equally important, everyone's voice and opinions are heard, and progress is made toward the stated goal on a steady basis. While in the past, American business valued the notion of individualism (Hofstede, 1997), in the past decade the focus has shifted to the concept of teamwork. How does one encourage the energy that comes from placing people of different backgrounds and specialties together to mutually solve problems and make decisions? What are the necessary skills to work with

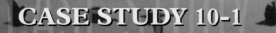

TABLE 10-1	Strategies for Coping with Difficult Personalities
Personality Type	**Coping Strategies**
Criticizer	Do not argue—it will add only fuel to the fire! Ask for input and practice active listening by reflecting on what you heard. Give criticizers a project to which they can directly contribute.
Passive one	Engage in communication, ask direct questions, ask for direct responses.
Detailer	Allow the detailer to give details at certain points in the meeting. Begin with the objective for the session, repeat information when necessary, summarize.
Controller	Keep focused on the task at hand; note any inconsistencies in the controller's conversation.
Pleaser	Let pleasers know that their comments are safe from attack and that their opinions are valued.

CASE STUDY 10-1

Your nurse executive has assigned you as the new team leader of the task force on patient falls. This task force has been meeting for almost a year without making much progress. In coming to your first meeting, you note that there are several challenging personalities on the team and wonder if maybe they will ever be able to work together effectively.

Jamie is a new graduate nurse and volunteers for everything so that he will be liked. Angela is the detailer, often asking everyone to repeat what they said so that she can get more information on the topic. Samantha is the passive one and just looks annoyed at having to be there. You noticed she was doing some of her patient charting while in the meeting. Anabelle attempts to keep the team on track, but with her soft-spoken voice, she is not well heard. Finally, no matter what anyone says, Beth is critical and comes up with a reason why something will not work.

Where do you begin?

How would you deal with the five team members?

What is your primary focus at the beginning of your time as team leader and why?

interdisciplinary team members in an increasingly complex health care delivery system?

Great Team Guidelines

Great teams don't just happen; there is behind-the-scenes planning, preparation, and forward thinking before anyone even meets. Theories of effective teams have been discussed in the literature for several decades by Lewin (1951), McGregor (1960), Argyris (1964), Burns (1978), Bennis (1989), and Senge (1990). What are the guidelines for encouraging great teams? A great team accomplishes what it sets out to do, with everyone on the team participating to achieve the desired outcomes. See Figure 10-2 for great team guidelines.

First and foremost, the team must have a clearly stated purpose: what are the goals, what are the objectives, and how long and how often will the team meet? What is the vision of the team? What does the leader see the team accomplishing? An effective team keeps the larger organization's mission in mind as it progresses; otherwise, its goals will be inconsistent with those of the parent organization. Second is an assessment of the team's composition: what are the team members' personal strengths and weaknesses? How do the team members see themselves—all as individuals? Do they see themselves as part of a cohesive team? Are any additional members needed? What are the roles of each team member?

Third is the communication link. Are effective communication patterns in place? Is there a need to improve communication, either in written format or verbal format? Does the team work well with e-mail and voice mail, or does it need the traditional paper trail to stay connected? Is communication open, with minimal hidden agendas by the members? Can the truth be told in order to reach a difficult decision, in a compassionate and sympathetic manner?

Active participation by all team members is a critical fourth item. Does everyone have a designated responsibility? Do people listen to one another, or is everyone trying to be heard at the same time? What are the relationships of the team members? Is there mutual trust and respect for members and their decisions, however unpopular? Are there turf issues that must be resolved before proceeding? *Turf*, according to Husting (1996), is the primary reason that early team-building efforts may not work. Therefore, it is important for the team leader to work on resolving turf-related problems first. The climate of the team should be relaxed but supportive, especially during brainstorming of new ideas or discussion of problems and problem solving.

Is there a clear plan as to how to proceed? This fifth element leads to an action plan that everyone

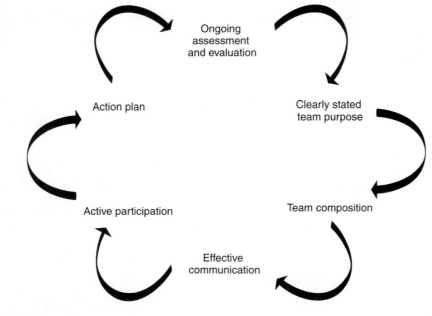

Figure 10-2 Great Team Guidelines

agrees with early on, and one that is revisited at certain designated times. Feedback by team members and others affected by the team's decisions is necessary to keep focus. The sixth guideline is actually ongoing, in that assessment and evaluation are continuous throughout the team's history. Outcomes have to be consistent and related to the expectations of the organization. Creativity is also encouraged at the team level; perhaps a member has an idea to solve a problem that no one has ever tried. In a supportive environment, pros and cons of all reasonable ideas should be freely discussed. A team needs to periodically assess its progress.

CREATING AN ENVIRONMENT CONDUCIVE TO TEAM BUILDING

Before any members can be effective in a team, whether the team is a committee or is part of the staff on a nursing unit, a team leader needs to ensure that the environment is conducive to team building. The attitudes, organizational culture, policies, and procedures all help determine how successful the team will be in accomplishing its directives. Developing an environment that is supportive and

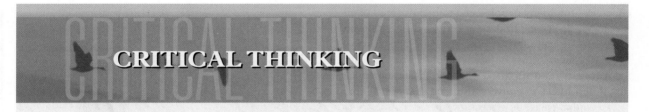

CRITICAL THINKING

The chief nurse executive has asked your nurse manager to initiate a new committee to review the issues of staffing in the hospital. She has asked you to join the committee. You are a nurse on a well-staffed oncology unit. You know that there are more challenging staffing issues elsewhere in the hospital. So far, no one else has volunteered to be on the committee, even though the nurse manager posted the request for members several weeks ago.

Who are you interested in having on the committee? Are they all registered nurses? Why or why not? How will you encourage people to join the committee? How will the nurse manager initiate the group process? Discuss several types of staff that you have worked with that were either functional or dysfunctional in a group and why.

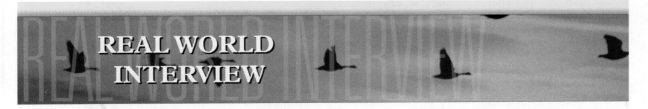

REAL WORLD INTERVIEW

One of the most important things to working with a team, especially a multidisciplinary team, is to really understand who everyone is: what do they represent, what is their knowledge base, what is important to them? You also have to become very good at not only listening to verbal cues, but to look for the nonverbal communications, which may actually describe the real situation.

Jan Wallace, RN
Quality Assurance Manager

exciting to work in is an ongoing process rather than a one-shot event.

Many hospitals employ authoritarian styles of management and leadership rather than true participatory or democratic styles. If the team members work in an authoritarian environment, they may be hesitant or uncomfortable in making decisions for themselves and may prefer the leader to make clear the parameters for decision making. Creativity and creative solutions to problems may be a challenge in this environment, but creativity is critical for progress to occur. Organizational hierarchy needs to be carefully looked at. Is it a formal or informal hierarchy? Who has the power to make decisions or to derail solutions? Having a top-heavy organizational structure and power base may discourage a team from being effective—too many people need to be informed of all the steps, decisions, and solutions of the team, and some may actually thwart progress from occurring.

Resources must be made available to the team for it to carry out its work. Is there a meeting space that is conducive to conversation and that is available on a regular basis? Is necessary secretarial support available to set up the meetings and take and distribute minutes? Is there adequate staffing to allow team members the time to meet? Are the communication systems reliable?

Are the administrators supportive of the team's efforts? For example, if there is a problem in having key members attend meetings, whether it is lack of commitment or other conflicting duties, will the administrator support efforts to change this situation? Often, a staff nurse is assigned to a team that is focused on solving an institutional problem, such as restraint usage, but may not have anyone assigned to take care of his patients during the committee meetings.

Team members also need to see that progress is made and that it is made on a consistent basis. Does the environment reward team members' contributions? Is team membership an expectation? Can the team's work be linked to the continuous improvement process so that members can see how they are making a difference in either the patient's care, the families or community they serve, system enhancement, or overall improvement of the quality of the organization? Continuous improvement is a process in which the status quo is never accepted and in which the care delivered is always being reviewed for better ways to improve satisfaction, decrease errors, or smooth care delivery processes.

Likewise, it is imperative to notify administration if the team's progress is not coming along as expected. It is better to share the unfavorable news as early as it is discovered, unless there is a good chance the direction may be changed with time or additional changes. Involving others early in the process may deflect more serious issues later on, because other people may be able to offer additional resources or information that team members may not have access to.

Table 10-2 offers a team evaluation checklist to evaluate whether your team environment is healthy and receptive. Any areas checked "no" may be opportunities for further improvement.

Teamwork on a Patient Care Unit

The role of the nurse is multifaceted. Depending on the scenario, a nurse may work directly or indirectly with a wide variety of staff on the health care team. A registered nurse (RN) is directly responsible for the care of the patient, but that care encompasses ensuring that the physician and nursing orders are carried out and that unlicensed assistive personnel document the intakes and outputs accurately for the shift. The RN ensures that the licensed practical nurse completes the ordered treatments; that discharge planning is coordinated with the social worker, the case manager, the pharmacist, and the administration; that the family understands how to dress the patient's wound; and finally, that the patient understands the discharge instructions. The role of the RN team leader incorporates the entire spectrum of care provided to the family by a wide variety of people. The effective nurse will possess excellent communication skills, both written and verbal; be sensitive of others' cultural and value differences; be aware of others' abilities; and show genuine interest in the team members. An open and objective communication style is needed, and communication should be done in an unbiased, constructive manner.

Effective Team Meetings

To run an effective team meeting, the team leader needs to plan and coordinate the work of the team. The leader needs to have a clear understanding of the purpose and goals of the team, facilitating members'

TABLE 10-2	Team Evaluation Checklist		
Question		**Yes**	**No**
1. Is the environment/climate conducive to successful team building?			
2. Do the team members have mutual respect and trust of one another? Are the team members honest with one another?			
3. Does everyone actively participate in the decision making and problem solving of the team?			
4. Are the purpose, goal, and objectives of the team obvious to all participants?			
5. Are creativity and mutual support of new ideas encouraged by all team members?			
6. Is the team productive and does it see actual progress toward goal attainment?			
7. Does the team begin and end its meetings on time?			
8. Does the team leader provide vision and energy to the team?			

REAL WORLD INTERVIEW

One thing that I always try to keep in mind is how important communication really is. As a team leader, you need to have strong communication skills and need to be able to communicate up the ladder to your boss, other administrators, and to physicians, as well as being able to communicate effectively with ancillary personnel. If you can say things in a positive way, you will be met with a lot less resistance and people are more likely to want to listen to you and what you have to say.

Jennifer Bialk, RN
Clinical Coordinator

full participation in the team. People are more apt to accomplish objectives when the vision is clearly stated and mapped. The leader should embrace and understand the change process and be able to teach staff members (Whittier, 1999). Another critical function of the leader is to prepare the team members ahead of time, perhaps meeting with them individually to get them fully engaged in the team. This time spent between the nurse leader and the team member is critical.

When the team meeting is in session, the leader will often be the (1) time keeper, to ensure that the meeting begins and ends when stated; (2) coordinator, making sure that necessary items and information are available to the team; (3) peacemaker, especially when opposite viewpoints are discussed in meeting sessions; (4) delegator, assigning tasks as needed, such as appointing someone to set up future meetings, and ensuring that the rooms, refreshments, and minutes are available; (6) feedback loop, providing information on the status of goals; and (7) role model, inspiring others on the team to continue their focus on the goals of the team, especially when performance does not show progress.

An effective team does not get results on its own. In addition to providing a supportive environment that nurtures success for its members, an effective team has a leader with vision. This leader has a clear idea of the team's strategic plan and will help others see the plan clearly, as well as its place in the institution. The leader readily inspires trust, and respects all members of the team, regardless of their status in the organization. Davis, Hellervik, Sheard, Skube, and Gebelein (1996) offer the following suggestions for building a successful team through effective leadership:

- Value the contributions of all team members: all members are critical to the success of the team regardless of their position on the team.
- Encourage interaction among group members: know when verbal and nonverbal behavior is appropriate and inappropriate and keep the flow of communication going.

- Discourage "we versus they" thinking: build teamwork that encourages inter-team participation and relationships.
- Involve others in shaping plans and decisions: involving the total team in the problem solving and decision making will strengthen any suggested changes made by the team because the entire team is able to support the decisions.
- Acknowledge and celebrate team accomplishments: publicly and frequently acknowledge positive contributions by team members, and keep the team members abreast of the positive changes they are actively involved in making.
- Evaluate your effectiveness as a team member: being an effective team leader includes being an effective team member. Are you carrying your weight, or are you expecting others to carry out your directives?

Developing Decision-Making and Problem-Solving Skills

Huber (2000) discusses a range of decision-making approaches that assist in accomplishing the stated goals and objectives during a nursing team's existence. Knowing when to have the entire team partic-

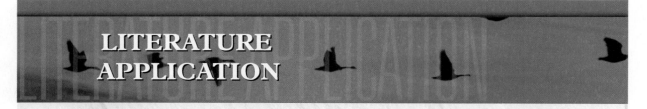

LITERATURE APPLICATION

Citation: Kerfoot, K. (1998). Micro-managing or leading: The clinician's challenge [On-line]. *MedSurg Nursing, 7*(5), 310. Available: InfoTrac/Expanded Academic.

Discussion: At times, there is a fine line between leading and managing. Kerfoot advises that many clinicians micromanage patient care due to low self-esteem with possibly the fear of failure: if you do it yourself, then you know it's done right, as the old saying goes. Leaders need to first recognize that while they may have the skills to complete the task, it is more prudent to work through others. Leaders should surround themselves with those who have special expertise and abilities, rather than relying on themselves to carry out the complete project.

Implications for Practice: Nurse leaders who learn to work through others will instill confidence and trust in their subordinates.

ipate in the decision-making process or when to have only the leader make the decision varies with the situation and desired outcome. The *autocratic* decision process is used by the leader in situations in which (1) the task or outcome is relatively simple (e.g., finding space to meet); (2) most team members would agree with the decision and provide consensus; and (3) a decision has to be made promptly.

In the *consultative* decision process, the leader will ask the opinions of the entire team, but the final decision lies with the leader. A fully developed team may use the *joint* decision process, in which there is mutual decision making by both team members and the leader, with everyone having an equal vote. This process encourages everyone to fully accept the team's conclusion. The joint decision process is also the most creative because all have the opportunity to provide input and differing perspectives into the decision. On the opposite end from the autocratic decision process is the *delegated* decision process, in which the leader is not involved with the final verdict. Instead, the team is truly self-governed and accountable for its decisions. An example of delegated decision process is setting up a unit orientation program for new graduate nurses. Once the leader provides the necessary parameters, the team would develop its own orientation program and merely report its decision to the nurse executive.

What are some common problems teams have when charged with decision making and problem solving? A primary issue is that of actually coming to a decision. An autocratic decision is made by one person, regardless of input from others. A joint decision is made together by everyone, with some members winning (e.g., their idea was chosen) and some losing (e.g., their idea was not chosen). Another common style of decision making is that of consensus: in this style, everyone has to agree with the final outcome, or else everyone must agree to work together until an acceptable decision is made.

Teams must also grapple with the issue of low productivity, or minimal results. People sometimes cannot focus in the right direction, and if a team meets infrequently, an entire year can go by without the team accomplishing anything significant. In contrast, there are some teams that believe that group members do not have any other commitments except to work on their team's goals and objectives. These high-powered teams expect team members to devote a fair amount of nonteam time to writing, research-

ing, and producing results for the next team meeting, regardless of other organizational obligations.

Successful Team Membership

Within any group, there are members who are productive, results-oriented team players, and there are members who are perfectly content to let others do the work. Some members may be destructive. Some of the destructive behaviors that group members may exhibit include being the aggressor or disapprover or blocker of others' suggestions; being a recognition seeker; being a self-confessor of personal, nongroup-oriented feelings or comments; being a playboy or playgirl; being a group dominator or help seeker; or using the group to meet personal needs or plead special interests (Northouse & Northouse, 1992).

If a team is to succeed, it is critical to get the right blend of personalities, experience, and temperaments to work toward a common goal. For example, if a new graduate nurse is placed on a critical committee responsible for developing a new sick call policy, it is important to include senior staff nurses for their experience. If an entire team is composed of aggressive, visionary members who are not detail oriented, many fine points may be missed. However, if a team is predominantly composed of people who get caught up with specific issues, the team members may miss the overall goal, because they are bogged down in details.

For a team to have positive outcomes, an astute team leader will keep in mind that some personality types complement others. One tool that some organizations use to assist them in devising effective work teams and team building is the Myers-Briggs Type Indicator, a psychological instrument that identifies different personality types. This tool is discussed in Chapter 15. Successful teams are those that use the right blend of personalities to achieve their goals.

KEY CONCEPTS

- Teams and committees are essential to the effective functioning of any health care organization.
- Teams may be formed for a variety of reasons, including the need for professional affiliation, the

need for socialization, and the need for psychological fulfillment.

- Teams and committees consist of people who come together for a common purpose and who need each other's contributions to achieve the overall goal.
- Each group goes through defined stages of increasing maturity.
- Team members can perform functional or dysfunctional roles, which may ultimately enhance or hinder the team's progress toward goal attainment.
- Great teams have clearly stated purposes, effective communication, an action plan, and continuously evaluate their progress.
- The team leader has certain designated responsibilities and tasks to ensure team productivity.
- An environment conducive to team building should be in place for maximum success.
- The team has various decision-making and problem-solving abilities and methods.

KEY TERMS

committee

group process

interdisciplinary team

team

REVIEW QUESTIONS

1. In forming a team, the leader should keep in mind that
   A. the team should decide the goals and objectives.
   B. the team is responsible for developing its vision.
   C. the team should be constructed of similar personality types.
   D. the team should encourage active participation by all members.

2. Which is the normal sequencing of group process?
   A. Forming, norming, storming, performing, adjourning
   B. Norming, forming, storming, performing, adjourning
   C. Forming, storming, norming, performing, adjourning
   D. Forming, storming, conforming, norming, adjourning

3. Which of the following team roles is considered functional?
   A. Creator
   B. Detailer
   C. Pleaser
   D. Controller

4. One of the primary duties of effective team leaders to their team is to
   A. ensure that all the details are taken care of all the time.
   B. enable the team to envision their goals and objectives.
   C. take effective minutes of the meetings.
   D. allow everyone a chance to participate, even if the meeting goes longer than expected

5. In maintaining an environment conducive to team building, it is important to
   A. have an autocratic management style by leaders.
   B. encourage creativity within the organization.
   C. reward employees who consistently revise the team's objectives.
   D. hold an evaluation session at the completion of the team's duration.

REVIEW ACTIVITIES

1. You are the manager of a 38-bed medical surgical unit. In light of several vacancies, you have hired three licensed practical nurses to fill positions in which you had only registered nurses working before.
   - How would you plan for them to become part of the team?
   - What are some important considerations for you, your established staff, and the new employees?
   - What are some things you can do to assist them in becoming members of your team?

2. Because of the increase in patient complaints about the quality of care, you have been asked to develop a team to address these patient care issues.
   - What are your expectations of the five stages of group process?

- How will you encourage the team members to progress though each stage?

3. On the unit on which you work as a registered nurse, the team is quite interdisciplinary in nature: you directly work with licensed practical nurses, unlicensed assistive personnel, a secretary, one housekeeper, one respiratory therapist, one case manager, and one clinical nurse specialist.
   - What are some of the advantages of working with interdisciplinary teams?
   - What are some of the challenges of working with interdisciplinary teams?
   - How does one best communicate with an interdisciplinary team?

EXPLORING THE WEB

- Where would you find additional information on effective team building on the Internet?
  http://www.accel-team.com

- What type of leadership style do you have in a team situation?
  http://www.onlinewbc.gov/Docs/manage/team.html

REFERENCES

Argyris, C. (1964). Integrating the individual and the organization. New York: Wiley.

Bennis, W. (1989). *Why leaders can't lead*. San Francisco: Jossey-Bass.

Bradford, L. P. (1978). *Group development*. La Jolla, CA: University Associates.

Burns, J. M. (1978). *Leadership*. New York: Harper & Row.

Davis, B. L., Hellervik, L. W., Sheard, J. L., Skube, C. J., & Gebelein, S. H. (1996). *Successful manager's handbook*. N. p.: Personnel Decisions International.

Hofstede, G. (1997). *Cultures and organizations*. New York: McGraw Hill.

Huber, D. (2000). *Leadership and nursing care management* (2nd ed.). N.p.: Saunders.

Husting, P. M. (1996). Leading teams and improving performance [Electronic version]. *Nursing Management, 27*(9), 35.

Katzenbach, J. R., & Smith, D. K. (1993). *The wisdom of teams: Creating the high-performance organization*. New York: Harper Business.

Kerfoot, K. (1998). Micro-managing or leading: The clinician's challenge [On-line]. *MedSurg Nursing, 7*(5), 310.

Lacoursier, R. B. (1980). *The life cycle of groups: Group development stage theory*. New York: Human Sciences Press.

Lewin, K. (1951). *Field theory in social sciences*. New York: Harper & Row.

Marquis, B. L., & Huston, C. J. (2000). *Leadership roles and management functions in nursing* (3rd ed.). Philadelphia: Lippincott.

McGregor, D. (1960). *The human side of enterprise*. New York: McGraw-Hill.

Northouse, P. G., & Northouse, L. L. (1992). *Health communication: Strategies for health professionals* (2nd ed.). Norwalk, CT: Appleton & Lange.

Senge, P. M. (1990). *The fifth discipline*. New York: Doubleday Books.

Senge, P. M., Roberts, C., Ross, R. B., Smith, B. J., & Kleiner, A. (1994). *The fifth discipline fieldbook: Strategies and tools for building a learning organization*. New York: Doubleday/Currency.

Tappen, R. M. (2001). *Nursing leadership and management: Concepts and practice* (4th ed.). Philadelphia: F. A. Davis.

Tuckman, B. W., & Jensen, M. A. C. (1977). Stages of small group development revisited. *Group and Organizational Studies, 2*(4), 419.

Whittier, S. (1999). Manager's corner: Effective team-building: More important than ever. *Home Care Nurse News, 6*(3), 1–3.

SUGGESTED READINGS

Bellack, J., & O'Neil, E. (1999). Recreating nursing practice for a new century: Recommendations and implications of the Pew Health Professions Commission's final report. *Nursing & Health Care Perspectives, 21*(1), 14–21.

Bennis, W. (1989). *On becoming a leader*. Reading, MA: Addison-Wesley.

Brown, B. (1998). 10 trends for the new year: Nurse managers predict the skills, technology and mind-set you'll need to prosper in 1999. *Nursing Management, 29*(2), 33–36. Carley, M. S. (1996). Teambuilding: Lessons from the theater [Electronic version]. *Training & Development, 50*(8), 41.

Farrell, M. P., Schmitt, M. H., & Heinemann, G. D. (2001). Informal roles and the stages of interdisciplinary team development. *Journal of Interprofessional Care, 15*(3), 281–295.

Grohar-Murray, M. E., & DiCroce, H. R. (1997). *Leadership and management in nursing.* Stamford, CT: Appleton & Lange.

Harwood, A. (1997). Spot the saboteurs. *Nursing Times, 93*(25), 72–75.

Jain, V. K., & Lall, R. (1996). Nurses' personality types based on the Myers-Briggs Type Indicator. *Psychology Reporter, 78*(3 pt. I), 938.

Keirsey, D., & Bates, M. (1978). *Please understand me: Character and temperament types.* Del Mar, CA: Prometheus Nemesis Books.

Kennedy, M. M. (2001). What do you owe your team? Survival tips for people who dread teamwork. *Physician Executive, 27*(4), 58–60.

Lengacher, C. A., Mabe, P. R., VanCott, M. L., Heinemann, D., & Kent, K. (1995). Team-building process in launching a practice model. *Nursing Connections, 8*(2), 51–59.

Leppa, C. J. (1996). Nurse relationships and work groups disruption. *Journal of Nursing Administration, 26*(10), 23–27.

Millward, L. J., & Jeffries, N. The team survey: A tool for health care team development. *Journal of Advanced Nursing, 35*(2): 276–287.

Monty, V. (1994). Effective team building and personality types [On-line]. *Special Libraries, 85*(1), 1.

Myers, I. B. (1995). *Introduction to type.* Palo Alto, CA: Consulting Psychologists Press.

Opt, S. K., & Loffredo, D. A. (2000). Rethinking communication apprehension: A Myers-Briggs perspective. *Journal of Psychology, 134*(5), 556–570.

Prager, H. (1999). Cooking up effective team building: *Training & Development, 53*(12), 14.

Shope, T. C., Frohna, J. G., & Frohna, A. Z. (2000). Using the Myers-Briggs Type Indicator (MBTI) in the teaching of leadership skills. *Medical Education, 34*(11), 956.

Sovie, M. (1992). Care and service teams: A new imperative. *Nursing Economic$, 10*(2), 94–100.

Wilson, R. D., Mateo, M. A., & Brumm, S. K. (1999). Revitalizing a departmental committee. *Journal of Nursing Administration, 29*(3), 45–48.

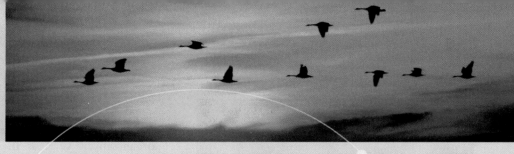

CHAPTER 11

There is nothing more difficult to take in hand, more perilous to conduct, or more uncertain in its success than to take the lead in the introduction of a new order of things. (Jean-Jacques Rousseau, 1712–78)

Budget Concepts for Patient Care

Corinne Haviley, RN, MS

OBJECTIVES

Upon completion of this chapter, the reader should be able to:

1. Describe the budget preparation process for health care organizations.
2. Define commonly used budgets for planning and management.
3. Describe key elements that influence budget preparation.
4. Identify services and products that generate revenue.
5. Identify expenses associated with the delivery of service.

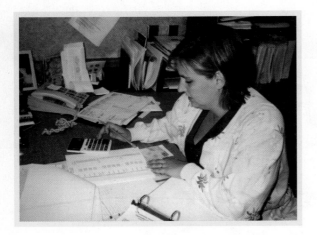

You are assigned to a patient care unit for your clinical experience. You are wondering what types of services are provided to patients on this unit. You talk with your instructor and, if appropriate, the nursing manager of the unit to review the unit's budget. You review the unit's scope of service and budget.

What kinds of patients are cared for on this unit?

What kinds of services are provided to patients on this unit?

How does the unit's budget help ensure provision of care for patients on this unit?

A key factor that influences patient care is the cost involved in the delivery of service. Resources—people, equipment, and time—are required to support the services delivered by nurses. These resources cost money. The economic success of a health care organization depends on those who are involved with service delivery. The decline in health care reimbursement as well as escalating costs, and increasing competition, have required hospitals to improve operational efficiency and to make economically sound decisions. The challenge in health care is to ensure that the quality of care and the caliber of the staff are not compromised in this ever-changing, cost-controlled environment.

Nurses need to understand how to manage the cost of patient care as it relates to their own clinical practice. Nurses are accountable for the distribution and consumption of resources, whether that equates to time, supplies, drugs, or staff. It is essential that appropriate decisions be made regarding cost-effective practices. Cost containment affects the patient's bill and the financial viability of a nursing department or unit. Hence, nurses need to be

informed and partner with the management team to generate revenue and control expenses in relation to patient care. According to regulatory and accrediting organizations such as the Joint Commission on Accreditation of Healthcare Organizations, departmental budgets need to be developed in collaboration with staff from respective services involved in care. (Joint Commission on Accreditation of Healthcare Organizations, 2001).

The purpose of this chapter is to provide an overview of the operational budget process, including budget development, implementation, performance, and evaluation. Common financial language and tools are discussed so nurses can understand the process involved in cost-effective care.

TYPES OF BUDGETS

Hospitals use several types of budgets to help with future planning and management. These include operational, capital, and construction budgets.

Operational Budget

An **operational budget** accounts for the income and expenses associated with day-to-day activity within a department or organization. Revenue generation is based upon billable services and expenses associated with equipment, supplies, staffing, and other indirect costs. Revenue may be based on the number of days that a patient stays on an inpatient unit or the number of hours spent in a procedure room. Revenue may be also based on the types of procedures delivered to a patient. Depending on reimbursement rates and requirements, expenses are sometimes bundled or included into a procedure or room charge, for example, an admission packet that includes a washbasin, cup, soap holder, and so on. In other situations, supply items may be billed separately, such as IV start kits, leukocyte removal filters, and so on.

Capital Budget

A **capital budget** accounts for the purchase of major new or replacement equipment. Equipment is purchased when new technology becomes available or when older equipment becomes too expensive to maintain because of age-related problems such as inefficiencies resulting from the speed of the equipment or downtime (amount of time it is out of service for repairs). Sometimes the expense and availability of replacement parts make it prohibitive to maintain equipment. Finally, equipment may become antiquated because of its inability to deliver service consistently, meet industry or regulatory standards, or provide high-quality outcomes.

Because there is a significant expense associated with equipment acquisition, organizations want to make the best and most economical and informed decisions. Staff members from a variety of areas, including materials management, clinical experts, legal counsel, biomedical engineering, information technology, finance, and management, often participate in planning for equipment purchases because they may have important input. Substantial analysis is required because equipment features, benefits, and limitations have to be understood as they relate to a department or institution's needs and goals. Often multiple vendors or companies sell similar or varying products with different terms, conditions, and warranty and maintenance agreements that can have short- and long-term effects.

Organizations differ regarding the dollar amount that is considered a capital purchase (Sullivan & Decker, 1997). Capital purchases are based upon the equipment cost and the life expectancy (also known as shelf life) or how long the equipment is expected to perform over time. Generally, capital purchases cost more than $500 and last 5 years or longer. For example, in one organization, a stent costing $2,000 is a supply item used during a surgical procedure. This supply is considered an operational expense because its life expectancy is 2 years, whereas a CT scanner costing more than $500 with a life expectancy of 7 years is considered a capital expense.

Construction Budget

A construction budget is developed when renovation or new structures are planned. The construction costs generally include labor, materials, building permits, inspections, equipment, and so on. If it is anticipated that a department will need to close during construction, then projected lost revenue is accounted for in the budget. Revenue and expenses may also be shifted to another department that absorbs the services on a temporary basis.

BUDGET OVERVIEW

An operational budget is a financial tool that outlines anticipated revenue and expenses over a specified period. A process called accounting, which is an activity that managers engage in to record and report financial transactions and data, assists with budget documentation. The budget translates operational plans into financial and statistical terms so that income can be projected with associated costs. Budgets serve as standards to plan, monitor, and evaluate the performance of a health care system. Details regarding a budget are specific to the area governed. Budgets account for the income generated as compared to the expenses needed to deliver the service. Profit is determined by the relationship of income to expenses. Profitability results when the income is higher than the expenses.

Budgets make the connection between operational planning and allocation of resources. This is especially important because health care organizations measure multiple key indicators of overall performance. For example, along with financial performance, organizations routinely evaluate quality patient outcomes and customer and staff satisfaction. All these indicators are intertwined and hold value in terms of patient care. Collectively, they reflect organizational success.

Figure 11-1 is a balanced scorecard or dashboard showing a variety of indicators that illustrate the connectivity between performance and quality outcomes. A dashboard is a documentation tool providing a snapshot image of pertinent information and activity at a particular point in time. A dashboard or balanced scorecard identifies any of four perspectives about an organization: finances, customer satisfaction and services, internal operating efficiency, and learning and growth (Norton & Kaplan, 2001). Figure 11-1 shows two separate units, the gastrointestinal laboratory (GI lab) and a medical nursing unit. These dashboards display measurable unit activity such as number of procedures delivered in the GI lab and the number of patient days accrued on the medical nursing unit. They illustrate the amount of revenue generated and the expenses incurred. Variance, or the difference between what was budgeted and the actual result, can be tracked (Grohar-Murray & DiCroce, 1997). A key activity that affects the number of patients that can be cared for, such as the room turnaround time, is also monitored. Finally,

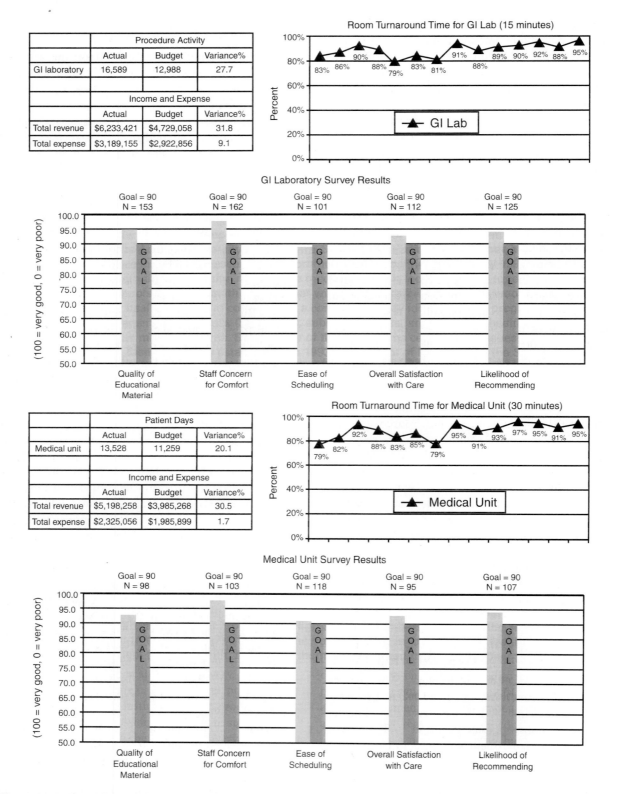

Figure 11-1 Patient Satisfaction, Turnaround Time, and Budget Activity Dashboard (Adapted with permission of Northwestern Memorial Hospital, Chicago, IL)

specific patient satisfaction indicators are visualized to determine whether the goals are met in high-priority areas.

Similar to controlling personal funds, such as managing one's checking or savings account, budgeting helps to define services by projecting how much cash is generated (revenue) and how much services will cost to operate (expenses). Budgeting requires forward thinking so that problems can be planned for and ways to work around any obstacles can be anticipated. Budgets also serve as a benchmark to measure whether the planning expectations are being met. Typically, budgets are monitored monthly, so that if deficiencies arise throughout the year, financial improvement plans can be instituted early. Corrective action is often initiated to prevent long-term effects in a particular area, such as wastage or loss of supply items. The budget functions as a tool to foster collaboration because individuals within departments must work together to achieve its goals.

BUDGET PREPARATION

Formulating a budget involves a systematic approach that begins with preparation (Grohar-Murray & DiCroce, 1997). Budgets are generally developed for a 12-month period. The yearly cycle can be based on a fiscal year as determined by the organization (e.g., September 1 through August 31) or a calendar year (e.g., January 1 through December 31). Shorter- or longer-term budgets may also be developed depending upon the organizational planning process.

Prior to the beginning of the budget year, most organizations devote approximately 6 months to preparing and developing the operational budget. To prepare a budget, organizations gather fundamental information about a variety of elements that influence the organization, including demographic information, competitive analysis, regulatory influences, and strategic plans. Additionally, it is helpful to review the department's scope of service, goals, and history.

Demographic Information

Pulling together demographic information relative to the population that the organization serves is most helpful because it identifies unique market characteristics, such as age, race, sex, income, and so on, that influence patient behavior. For example, an obstetrical practice would be expected to attract women of childbearing age rather than an older male population. Therefore, understanding the demographics and capture rate (the percent of the population that has been "captured" by the organization as a consumer) of the immediate or distant market region helps paint a clear picture regarding the patient population.

Competitive Analysis

A competitive analysis is important because it probes into how the competition is performing as compared to other health care organizations. A competitive analysis examines other hospitals or practices' strengths and weaknesses, in addition to other details such as location and new or existing services and technology. Having this knowledge can influence decisions regarding the implementation of new programs, hiring of specialty staff, and purchasing of equipment. Figure 11-2 presents a competitive analysis of three different hospitals.

Regulatory Influences

Regulatory requirements and reimbursement rates have an effect on financial performance. Regulatory changes are influenced by several governing bodies. A government agency that has high visibility in the area of reimbursement is the Centers for Medicare and Medicaid Services (CMS), whose mission is to ensure health care security for beneficiaries. CMS (www.cms.hhs.gov) administers federal control, quality assurance, and fraud and abuse prevention for Medicare, Medicaid, and the State Children's Health Insurance Program (SCHIP). Under the aegis of the Department of Health and Human Services, it is also responsible for coordinating health care policy, planning, and legislation.

Other regulatory bodies play a role in reimbursement by ensuring that federal and state laws are adhered to through approval and accreditation. For example, the Food and Drug Administration (www.fda.gov) regulates the use of drugs, food products, and medical devices in the United States. If equipment or drugs under its jurisdiction are not approved, then organizations cannot bill for their use, by law. The JCAHO (www.jcaho.org) accredits

Competitive Analysis: Hospital A

Location: Rural—100 miles from metropolitan area
Affiliation: Currently negotiating with three academic
    hospitals
General clinical description:
- Scattered bed approach to inpatient oncology
- Ambulatory chemotherapy clinic
- Many of the same physicians on staff at Hospital J
Radiation capability: None—refers to Hospital J
Support services: Cancer screenings offered sporadically
Miscellaneous:
- Tumor board
- Cancer committee

Competitive Analysis: Hospital B

Location: Suburb of large metropolitan city
Affiliation: University hospital
General clinical description:
- Dedicated oncology inpatient unit
- Ambulatory chemotherapy department
- Comprehensive breast center
- Head and neck oncology team
Radiation therapy:
- Linear accelerator—two units
- High dose rate
- Intraoperative radiation therapy
- Stereotactic radiosurgery
Support services:
- Home infusion and home care program
- Hospice care program
- Annual cancer awareness fair
- Support group—general cancer patients
Miscellaneous:
- Tumor registry
- Tumor board
- Committee on cancer
- Head and neck patient conferences
- Stereotactic radiosurgery conferences

Competitive Analysis: Hospital C

Location: Urban city with a population of 150,000
Affiliation: For-profit corporation
- Medical oncology affiliation with University K
- Radiation Therapy Department affiliation with
  University K Radiation Therapy Department
General clinical description:
- Dedicated inpatient medical oncology unit
- Dedicated inpatient surgical oncology unit
- Four-bed autologous and stem cell bone marrow
  transplant unit (Eastern Cooperative Oncology Group
  Referral Center for autologous bone marrow trans-
  plants)
- Coagulation laboratory
- Therapeutic pheresis
- Pain clinic
- Oncology clinic
- Oncology rehabilitation
- Breast cancer rehabilitation program
- Ambulatory care chemotherapy unit
- Medical oncologist on staff at two hospitals
Radiation therapy:
- Linear accelerator
- Stereotactic radiosurgery
- Hyperthermia
- Brachytherapy
Support services:
- Home health and hospice program
- Cancer registry
- Cancer committee
- Physician update—quarterly cancer newsletter
- Cancer information line
- Cancer advisory council
- Cancer Survivor's Day offered annually
- Cancer screenings offered routinely
- Cancer support group—general cancer patients

Figure 11-2 Competitive Analysis of Three Hospitals

hospitals and ambulatory care and home health agencies and departments to ensure that organizations meet specific standards. Medicare and Medicaid will not reimburse for services unless a hospital is accredited by JCAHO.

Regulatory requirements may change regarding who may deliver a specific service and in what type of setting; for example, a procedure may have to be done in the hospital rather than in a physician's office if it is to be reimbursed by the insurance company. Medicare and Medicaid change their reimbursement rates periodically. Total and partial coverage of spe-

cific procedures can change and may not be predictable from year to year. For example, as of the year 2001, Medicare reimburses physicians but not nurses to perform a flexible sigmoidoscopy for patients over the age of 55 years. However, insurance companies often reimburse for either a nurse or physician to provide the service regardless of age.

Managed care organizations and insurance companies typically negotiate rates on a yearly basis, which can affect hospital revenue. Consumers' willingness to pay out of pocket when not covered by insurance affects revenue as well.

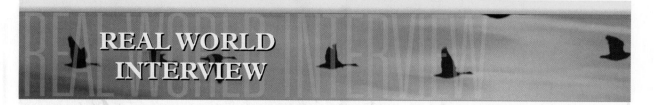

Staff nurses need to understand their own department's patient volume, what their case load is like, the effects of patient acuity, and how it may change. As patient acuity changes, so does patient care delivery. It may be that we can anticipate what services will be needed based upon patient acuity and how it affects the patient's stay. Communicating this information to management is most helpful. Remember that the budget process is fluid and not stagnant. Situations change and can alter the budget over time. A budget is not made in stone; it is only a guideline. Nurses can have an impact upon cost by understanding through cost accounting what supplies are being used with different types of admissions or procedures. Once calculated, this data can be shared with physicians. The use of standardized products can be compared when analyzing procedures or admissions by physicians and nurses. This process should assist in understanding both practice patterns and costs related to patient care. Physicians and nurses control major costs.

Nurses need to be stewards in recognizing expenses. For example, nurses are key to the patient length of stay and when and how resources are allocated during a patient stay. Nurses need to act on things before they become critical. Wastage is a good area to focus on because it adds to the cost of a patient stay. If a nurse wastes four gloves, the cost may only be $10 to cover the items. But think further about additional cost such as packaging, shipping, stocking, charging, and tracking, which may inflate the cost to $30. If this expense occurs during all 3 shifts times 30 beds, then the dollar amount adds up considerably. This cost in turn cuts into the profit or break-even point for one unit. Without elements of profit, the medical center cannot possibly meet payroll, fund programs that are critical to the community, purchase new equipment, or plan for construction. It all has a cycle and is important to performance.

Ron Andro, RN, MS, HSM
Program Administrator for Surgery

Strategic Plans

Generally, hospitals have strategic plans that map out the direction for the organization over several years. Strategic plans guide the staff at all levels so that the entire organization can have a shared mission and vision with clearly defined steps to meet the goals.

Each department develops unit-specific plans to help the organization follow its overall strategic plan. For example, a goal may be to become the most preferred GI lab or site for inpatient hospital care in the surrounding region. To meet the goal, one department may focus on patient satisfaction and room turnaround time to increase volume and decrease patient wait time for a procedure appointment. This goal is part of the organization's overall plan.

SCOPE OF SERVICE AND GOALS

During the budget preparation phase, it is important to examine the individual nursing or hospital department or section thoroughly. Hospital systems are frequently divided into sections, departments, or units to compartmentalize them for organizational purposes. These subsections or units, commonly called **cost centers**, are used to track financial data.

Each department or cost center defines its own scope of service (Figure 11-3 and Figure 11-4 provide examples of scope of service). The scope of service is helpful because it provides information related to the types of service and the sites at which services are offered, including the usual treatments and

The gastrointestinal laboratory (GI lab) may be defined as a specialized department that performs major procedures that are both diagnostic and therapeutic in nature such as upper endoscopies, colonoscopies, flexible sigmoidoscopies, and endoscopic retrograde cholangiopancreatography (ERCP). Conscious sedation is typically delivered to patients to provide comfort during the procedures. The gastrointestinal laboratory is operational Monday through Friday from 7 A.M. to 5 P.M., and provides after-hours service for emergent cases. Preprocedure, intraprocedure, and postprocedure care, including full recovery, is provided on site. Services are provided to critical in-house patients at the bedside via the staff assigned to travel to inpatient units. The department employs nurses, technicians, and receptionists, who work with gastroenterologists and surgeons to provide care. The unit is equipped with 10 procedure rooms, 25 recovery bays, and a gastrointestinal scope cleaning facility on site.

Figure 11-3 Gastrointestinal Laboratory Scope of Service

A medical nursing unit provides primarily inpatient care to patients with acute or chronic medical problems, such as congestive heart failure, diabetes, pulmonary disease, cancer, and so on. The unit, equipped with 30 private beds, a full kitchen, a lounge, and conference/consultation rooms, is operational 24 hours per day, 7 days per week. Patient education and support groups are held routinely in the library located directly on the unit. Team nursing is employed as the model of care. Nurses, patient care technicians, and unit secretaries are employed, with a social worker and diabetes educator providing additional patient support. Patients admitted to the unit for longer than 48 hours are discussed during daily multidisciplinary rounds. The rounds include case management personnel; psychosocial counselors; and nutrition, nursing, and medical staff. Staff discuss patient problems to facilitate future care, including discharge planning.

Figure 11-4 Medical Nursing Unit Scope of Care

procedures, hours of operation, and the types of patient/customer groups.

Departmental goals may include the introduction of new technology or treatments, patient education, and creation of a special patient care environment. Staff members are generally queried to determine whether they have any proposed quality initiatives that should be included in the plans for the upcoming year. Generally, new treatments, patient education materials, and documentation tools require different types or amounts of supplies. Technically trained staff members are often needed to implement new services. Both the staff and supplies can have varying costs during the early induction phase through full implementation. Creating a new environment or "best patient" experience may require additional funding that must be identified early in the planning stages. If new services are offered that are billable to the insurance company, then a method for charging patients has to be established to ensure that the hospital can receive appropriate payment. The manager is responsible for identifying the expenses associated with patient care up front so that they are covered by the charges. A charge is the dollar amount that the patient is responsible for paying as a result of service.

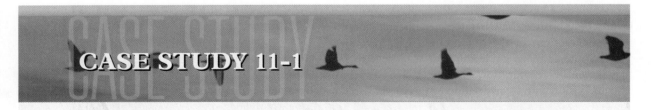

CASE STUDY 11-1

The manager from an inpatient unit asks for staff input into identifying ways to decrease use of medical supply and paper items. These items have been identified as in excess of the budget by 10% to 20% during the past 3 months. This is the first time that the staff members have been involved in helping with cost containment. Clinical nurses and assistants have been invited to participate.

When approaching an analysis of medical supply use, what might be the first step in the process? If you were to break the staff into work groups, which members should be chosen to analyze the use of clerical supplies? How would you proceed if you were trying to determine the supply costs associated with starting an IV with continuous infusion?

History

Organizations typically use history or past performance as a baseline of experience and data to better understand activity in a department or unit. These data are used to assist in interpreting associated expenses with staff productivity and unit performance. Most often, adjustments are made to planned budgets because of the ever-changing cost of products, supplies, and buying contracts. Buying contracts are negotiated so that predetermined reduced rates can be realized when organizations purchase large quantities of supplies. For example, if a hospital purchases a large quantity of one product, the vendor may reduce the price below the list price as an incentive. If a hospital can demonstrate that a particular product is used in a certain percentage, in 60% of all procedures or departments (called penetration rate), for example, then a reduced rate may be offered.

Additionally, knowledge about historical volume (e.g., procedures, admissions, or patient visits and average length of stay) provides a perspective as to how a department has grown or declined over time. This information may help with anticipating future demand and capacity. The story behind a unit and its heritage related to how the department developed is equally important because the financial numbers are tracked over time. Often the culture and complexity of a unit unfold by interviewing staff that may have been involved in the unit during the past, including physicians, nurses, technologists, assistants, housekeeping, dietary counselors, and so on. This information may provide further insight into why and how decisions were made in the past. Hence, multiple phases of data gathering are imperative to building a budget with a full knowledge base.

BUDGET DEVELOPMENT

Once background data have been gathered, the development of the budget can follow. This includes projecting revenue and expenses.

Revenue

Revenue is income generated through a variety of means, including billable patient services, investments, and donations to the organization. Specific unit-based revenue is generated through billing for services such as x-rays, invasive diagnostic or therapeutic procedures, drug therapy, surgical procedures, physical therapy, and so on. Revenue can also be generated through the delivery of multiple services over time, such as hourly rates for chemotherapy administration or blood transfusions. The specific number and types of services and procedures have to be projected for the budget. Each type of service may have varying volume associated with it. For example, projecting the volume and type of procedures to be conducted in a gastrointestinal laboratory is based upon feedback from referring physicians and technical staff, in addition to conclusions from historical data.

Similarly, the same types of projections occur for inpatient units, including the number of patients anticipated to be admitted, along with the average length of stay (e.g., 3 to 5 days) and the projected occupancy rate. The type and amount of services and patient days can be measured. The number of patient days or the services delivered are commonly called service units or primary statistics so that productivity and efficiency can be tracked.

It is important to note that the reimbursement rates of third-party payers affect revenue and can change from year to year. Uniform rates are often used, which transfers significant financial risk to the provider. Medicare, Medicaid, managed care companies, and insurance companies dictate or negotiate rates with health care organizations that may include discounts or allowances. Payers determine what costs are allowable for procedures, visits, or services. Payment schedules vary from state to state and among plans. Additionally, the rates can change monthly such as with the ambulatory payment classification (APC) system from Medicare, which applies to the outpatient setting. The reimbursement rates or payments received by hospitals often do not equal the actual hospital or unit charges for the services rendered. For example, there may be a fixed or flat reimbursement rate per case regardless of how long the patient stays in the hospital or how much the hospital pays for the service. If the costs exceed the reimbursement rate, then the provider absorbs the remaining costs.

Another payment classification system called diagnosis-related groups (DRGs) is used to group inpatients into categories based upon number of inpatient days, age, complications, and so on. Reimbursement covers room and board, tests, and therapy during a predetermined length of stay.

Some patients will not have health care insurance nor the ability to pay their bills. Therefore, the hospital may receive only a portion of the payment for services, if any.

Typically, organizations will review their payer mix to determine the percentage of patients carrying different types of health care coverage (Figure 11-5). The proportions help measure the anticipated dollars to be received for services delivered and projections for the coming year.

If charges for patient care are negotiated with a third-party payer such as insurance companies and managed care corporations, they are preestablished and are not negotiable once established. Third-party payers often impose a penalty fee, as a disincentive, if a health care organization changes a charge under contract. The penalty often exceeds the charge amount and will usually create a loss for the organization.

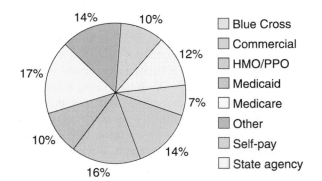

The reimbursement rates vary depending upon the payor. For example, Medicare may reimburse 40% of charges, Medicaid's rate may be 30%, and managed care may be at 60%. Factoring in reimbursement rates leads to profit and loss calculations for an organization.

Figure 11-5 Inpatient Payer Mix

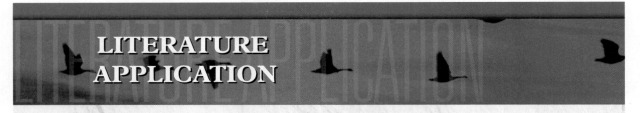

LITERATURE APPLICATION

Citation: Elser, R., & Nipp, D. (2001). Worker designed culture change. *Nursing Economic$, 19*(4), 161–163, 175.

Discussion: To effect operational efficiency and to improve employee performance, these authors proposed specific actions to change nursing culture. Work groups called resource utilization teams were organized to evaluate the unit values and the emotional components that affect relationships. Staff received educational support regarding communication and relationships so that differences and conflicts could be resolved. The staff was surveyed to determine their perceptions of their work environment based upon the cumulative responses. The team formulated a plan to staff the unit using the knowledge that they had gained and budgetary dollars that had been allocated. The team further identified role responsibilities and tasks that should be assigned to change the unit operations.

The strength of this article was in the creative proposal to capitalize on the knowledge and insight of staff to influence unit productivity. Every department or unit has its own unique characteristics and culture that influence the ability to produce and deliver quality care. Engaging staff in problem solving and role development is key to successful financial and operational management.

Implications for Practice: There are many creative ways to analyze expenses and productivity by using the workforce to improve operations and care. Imagine the potential if a work group were continually analyzing quality data points over time. The power of these work groups lies in their diverse members, who can see the department from different perspectives. When the work group is empowered, constructive measures can be identified to address problems that challenge departmental productivity, patient flow, and expenses.

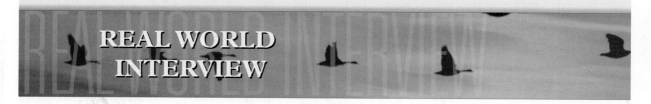

REAL WORLD INTERVIEW

Nurses need to have a good understanding of the financial aspects of the business, which includes the budget process. In addition, they also need to know how their everyday actions affect the bottom line. I also think that staff on a unit or outpatient clinic needs to "own" their budgets. It is not just the manager's budget; it is everyone's budget. I also think it is the role of nursing leaders to make the budget "real" for staff by education and implementing tools to aid in the process. For example, there are a number of staffing guideline tools that can be implemented to help staff calculate the cost of the shift, as well as the cost of the day. I have found these tools to be very beneficial in helping staff make better and more-cost-conscious staffing decisions.

The most important factor in developing an annual operating budget is to assess your current environment in light of the department's goals and objectives. Where am I now and where do I plan to be a year from now? Determining services and programs that are going to be added, as well as eliminated, is essential information needed to establish an annual budget. Analyzing historical data related to patient volume, patient days/visits, patient type and acuity are also important factors to consider. In addition, assessing equipment and supply needs based on current as well as projected future needs is also essential.

There are a number of ways that staff can assist in controlling costs. One way that I have found to be extremely useful is to have staff "own" certain line items. For example, I have had my staff responsible for ordering office supplies and forms and become responsible and accountable for the variances (positive and negative). I believe that using this approach has helped staff make more economical supply choices. In addition, it has also helped reduce supply usage because they become much more actively involved in monitoring the use of supplies.

Beth Kelly-Hayden, RN, BSN, MBA
Director of Nursing and Clinic Operations

Expenses

Expenses are determined by identifying the costs associated with the delivery of service. Expenditures are resources used by an organization to deliver services and may include supplies, labor, equipment, utilities, and miscellaneous items.

It is important to understand what it takes to deliver patient care services so that there are appropriate charges in place to pay for or cover the services. Expenses are commonly broken down into line items that represent specific categories that contribute to the cost of the procedure or activity such as paper supplies, medical supplies, drugs, and so on. This breakdown helps identify where the significant expenses lie related to a service. For example, a colonoscopy may have a high medical supply cost whereas chemotherapy administration may have a high drug cost associated with it.

Supplies

As new procedures are introduced, or when a manager wants to ascertain the actual supply expenses associated with a procedure or activity, zero-based budgeting may be instituted. Zero-based budgeting is a process used to drill down into expenses by detailing every supply item and the quantity of items typically used. A list of supplies is developed, including large and small items, along with the itemized expense. Often supplies are packaged in bulk and sold in quantity. Hence, the expense of the items has to be calculated and backed out of the bulk figure to accurately depict the expense.

Figure 11-6 illustrates the zero-based budgeting that may be necessary to understand all of the expenses associated with delivering a procedure. This example can be expanded further to calculate the total expense associated with the anticipated number of procedures. This calculation can be achieved by multiplying the number of anticipated procedures by the total expense per procedure, which leads to authentic projections.

Labor

Labor is another significant expense associated with medical and nursing care. Health care services are very labor intensive. It is estimated that salaries and benefits account for 50% to 60% of operational costs. Hence, it is very important to calculate the amount of time the staff members are involved with the service. This analysis includes professional, technical, and support staff. For example, the time that it takes to schedule an appointment, register a patient, and take a patient to a procedure room or unit needs to be calculated into the overall cost of care for the patient.

In the ambulatory area, staff time is calculated relative to the delivery of a specific procedure, including preparation for the procedure, intraprocedure care, and postprocedure care. Preprocedure preparation entails gathering of supplies, assembling equipment, and preparing the environment. Preparing the

General Supplies	Quantity	Price	Drugs	Quantity	Price
4 Chux	4	$ 3.00	Fentanyl	1	$ 0.25
Tri Pour Container	1	$ 0.20	Versed	1	$ 2.10
Sterile Water 1,000ml	1	$ 0.40		**Total**	**$ 2.35**
Normal Saline Vial	2	$ 0.10			
Cannister/Lid	2	$ 3.25			
Tubing	2	$ 0.50			
02 Cannula	1	$ 0.05	**Printed Forms**	**Quantity**	**Price**
Suction Catheter	1	$ 0.02			
Disposable Gowns	2	$ 3.80	Hospital Consent	1	$ 0.10
Gloves	6	$ 0.35	Procedure Consent	1	$ 0.75
4X4's	10	$ 0.25	Nursing Form	1	$ 0.75
Surgilube	2oz.	$ 0.15	Vital Sign Sheet	1	$ 0.05
Photos	2	$ 4.30	Doctors Orders	1	$ 0.15
Syringe 10cc	2	$ 0.15	History/Physical	1	$ 0.10
Syringe 60cc	1	$ 0.35	Discharge Instruction	1	$ 0.20
Emesis Basin	1	$ 0.10	Education Sheet	1	$ 0.80
Denture Cup	1	$ 0.15	Charge Voucher	1	$ 0.10
Recording Paper	1	$ 0.05	Procedure Education	1	$ 0.10
Alcohol Pads	2	$ 0.05		**Total**	**$ 3.10**
Slippers	1	$ 0.75			
Mask	2	$ 0.25			
Goggles/Face Shield	1	$ 1.20	**Clerical Supplies**	**Quantity**	**Price**
Cetacaine Spray	1	$ 0.10			
Bite Block	1	$ 2.00	Patient File	1	$ 0.80
Patient Bag	1	$ 0.20	Labels	2	$ 0.05
Cleaning Brush	1	$ 2.20	Xerox Paper	6	$ 0.05
	Totals	**$23.72**	Pen	1	$ 0.05
			Pencil	1	$ 0.05
			Marker	1	$ 0.05
IV Start	**Quantity**	**Price**	Highlighters	1	$ 0.05
				Total	**$ 1.10**
Tourniquet	1	$ 0.15			
Alcohol Wipes	2	$ 0.05			
Angiocath	1	$ 0.05			
IV Solution	1	$ 0.60			
IV Primary Set	1	$ 4.00			
Tegaderm	1	$ 0.15			
Tape	6 inches	$ 0.05	**Grand Total**		
Band-Aid	1	$ 0.05			
4X4	4	$ 0.10			
	Totals	**$ 5.20**			

Figure 11-6 Zero-Based Budgeting for GI Lab (Adapted with permission of Northwestern Memorial Hospital, Chicago, IL)

CRITICAL THINKING

Staff working day to day handling patient care activities are in an optimal position to identify the best practices that impact upon efficiency and cost-effectiveness. Managers can learn from staff and organize processes to assist with unit-based improvement. Think back on the steps taken by a nurse during the first hour of a shift. Reflect on communication and how information is received. Examine the amount of time spent in patient care versus other activities. Create a journal of activity from different time increments during a shift. Discuss your observations with your coworkers and manager. What problems in flow of activity and gaps in communication or efficiency did you find? How can you drill down further into understanding how the unit operates and ways to increase productivity? How could you improve your team's functioning?

patient may involve taking a history, completing a physical, administering medication or taking specimens, placing tubes or establishing an intravenous line, and positioning the patient. Intraprocedure care is the actual care delivered once the procedure has been initiated. Postprocedure care may require activity such as educating and discharging a patient, or extensive recovery activity requiring several hours of

direct nursing care and removal of equipment and supply items. Refer to Table 11-1 for a sample time analysis related to labor.

Staffing. The amount of staff and types of staff are often accounted for in a staffing model. The model outlines the number of staff required based upon the primary statistic such as procedures or patients. An

| TABLE 11-1 | Time Analysis per Procedure | | |

Preprocedure Care	Time (minutes)	Intraprocedure Care	Time (minutes)
Appointment schedule	5	Positioning	5
Registration	10	Initiation of conscious sedation	10
Escort to changing room	5	Procedure	10
Subtotal	20	Subtotal	25
Direct Patient Preparation		**Postprocedure Care**	
History	5	Recovery	120
Patient education and consent	10	Education	10
IV start	10	Changing and discharge	10
Subtotal	25	Subtotal	140

Grand total = 210 minutes per procedure

CRITICAL THINKING

"Staying in the loop" is key to becoming energized and feeling engaged as a part of the patient care team and as a vital part of the organization (Nelson, 1997). When you walk onto a unit, ask a staff member what the key quality initiatives are that the unit is working on that reflect process improvement. Ask what the goals are for the unit and how staff is participating in decisions so that the goals may be achieved. Think about how these initiatives may increase productivity, or staff or patient satisfaction or decrease expenses. Ask the staff what impact their efforts are having.

How are the staff involved in helping the organization to meet its goals?

outpatient model may focus on the number of procedure rooms that require staff. One nurse may be required to staff a gastrointestinal laboratory procedure room and one shared technician may staff two procedure rooms.

Models may help in analyzing productivity as illustrated in the following:

Scenario 1: One nurse is assigned to a procedure room during a 4-hour period in which 8 patients are treated.

Scenario 2: One nurse and a technical assistant are assigned to a procedure room for 4 hours, and 16 patients are treated.

The second scenario depicts greater productivity because the number of procedures delivered doubled by using two staff, recognizing that the assistant staff member will cost the organization less in terms of salary expense. Because labor is one of health care's greatest operational costs, enhancing productivity will likely produce savings.

For an inpatient unit, nurses may be assigned to a fixed number of patients during all three shifts. The ratios vary depending upon the shift and patient acuity. The nurse-to-patient ratio on a medical nursing unit may be one nurse to six (1:6) patients during the day and evening shift, whereas it may be 1:8 during the night shift. The nurse-to-patient ratio may be 1:2 for all shifts on a critical care unit. Figure 11-7 and Figure 11-8 illustrate sample staffing models.

Staffing ratios and salary data are particularly important because of the cost factor. Specialty salaries fluctuate, depending upon supply and demand. When there are shortages of certain staff, the salary tends to

increase. Additionally, a health care organization may change its benefits, offering a more attractive package that includes continuing education, paid time off for education purposes, or professional membership expenses. Institutions may also look for alternative ways to supplement or deliver services during staff shortages. This means that supplemental staff—professional agency nurses, nurses from in-house registries, or patient care technicians—may be hired at a different salary rate. It is important to note whether a unit has had historical difficulty retaining or recruiting staff. Recruitment and retention, especially attracting, interviewing, hiring, and orienting staff, require dollars. For example, it has been estimated that the turnover cost per nurse, including advertising, recruitment, orientation, and time to fill the vacancy, can equate to $65,000 (The Advisory Board Company, 1998). The average cost to educate a nurse during a 6-week orientation period is more than $5,000. Not only the salary but also benefits are frequently factored into a salary package, and they need to be included in the budget.

Unproductive Time. Unproductive time is also calculated into a budget because there has to be staff coverage when nurses or other staff members are not working. Unproductive time usually includes sick, vacation, personal, holiday, and education time. For example, Table 11-2 illustrates average number of days that a nurse at one institution may take off from work during a 12-month period. These days off may require coverage by another nurse, depending on the unit.

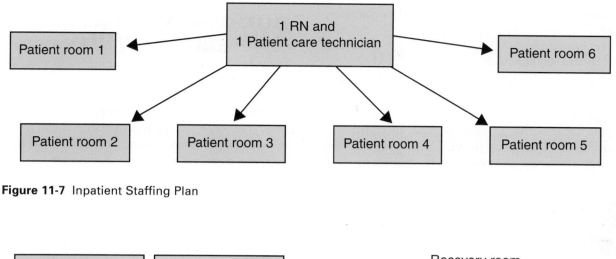

Figure 11-7 Inpatient Staffing Plan

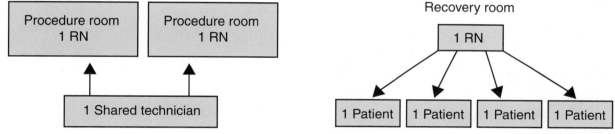

Figure 11-8 Gastrointestinal Lab Staffing Plan

TABLE 11-2	Unproductive Time
Unproductive Time	**Number of Days**
Vacation	21
Holiday	7
Sick	5
Personal	3
Education	1
Total	37

Direct and Indirect Expenses

Expenses can be further broken down into direct and indirect. **Direct expenses** are those expenses directly associated with the patient, such as medical and surgical supplies and drugs. **Indirect expenses** are expenses for items such as utilities—gas, electric, and phones—that are not directly related to patient care. Other support functions frequently charged to a department that are not specifically related to patient care delivery are housekeeping, maintenance, materials management, and finance.

Fixed and Variable Costs

Fixed costs are those expenses that are constant and are not related to productivity or volume. Examples of these costs are building and equipment depreciation, utilities, fringe benefits, and administrative salaries. Variable costs fluctuate depending upon the volume or census and types of care required. Medical and surgical supplies, drugs, laundry, and food costs often increase with the volume. Figure 11-9 shows sample worksheets used to calculate expenses.

BUDGET APPROVAL AND MONITORING

Once developed, budgets are submitted to administration for review and final approval. The approval process may take several months as the unit budgets are combined to determine the overall budget for the health care organization. Senior management, representing finance and operations, often makes the final decisions regarding acceptance of a budget.

The unit or department manager is responsible for controlling the budget. Budget monitoring is generally carried out on a monthly basis. The pur-

NET EXPENSE WORKSHEET 2003 BUDGET

DESCRIPTION	GI Lab	Medical Unit
Out Patient	8,290,564	33,450
In Patient	3,400,678	10,162,875
CORPORATE BILLING REVENUE	17,806	10,419
TOTAL OPERATING REVENUE	11,709,048	10,206,744
EXPENSES		
Salary Expense		
BUDGET REDUCTION SLALARY	0	24,932
SALARIES	1,398,630	2,098,150
SALARIES OVERTIME	219,878	142,359
PROFESSIONAL AGENCY FEE	106,608	166,456
TOTAL SALARY	1,725,116	2,431,879
TRANSPORTATION EXPENSE	4,190	3,870
TOTAL	4,190	3,870
NON-SALARY EXPENSE		
NONMEDICAL SUPPLIES		
SUPPLIES CLERICAL	12,924	8,524
PRINTED FORMS	31,486	28,854
SOAP AND CLEANING	6,092	8,950
PAPER GOOD SUPPLIES	1,192	930
FILM SUPPLY PHOTO	3,836	
PACKAGING SUPPLIES	94	
TOTAL	55,624	47,258
FOODS		
MEETING AND LUNCHEONS BANQUETS	0	495
SUNDRY FOOD ISSUES	5,872	8,990
TOTAL	5,872	9,485

MEDICAL SUPPLIES		
MEDICAL SUPPLIES	1,480,840	865,872
DIAG TEST CTR/IONIC CONTRST	2,798	
SUTURES	4,064	
DRUG SUPPLIES	120,120	569,088
IV & IRRIGATION SOLUTIONS	13,994	11,431
IV & IRRIGATION SETS	56,280	30,649
MEDIA	48	
PHLEBOTOMY SUPPLIES	680	
LAB GLASSWARE & INSTRUM	3,948	
LABORATORY SUPPLIES	156	
CHEMICALS	158	
TOTAL	1,683,086	1,477,040
TOTAL SUPPLIES	1,744,582	1,533,783
PURCHASE SERVICES		
PURCHASED SERVICES	41,436	15,678
TOTAL	41,436	15,678
UTILITIES		
TELEPHONE CHARGES-Long Distance	1,480	1,500
TELEPHONE CHARGES	13,608	15,238
TOTAL	15,088	16,736
OTHER EXPENSES		
CONTINUING ED	6,715	4,127
AUDIO VISUAL	500	0
TRAVEL EXPENSE	6,120	5,100
DISCOUNTED PARKING	190	150
MISCELLANEOUS	730	500
SM FIXTURES & EQUIPMENT	728	410
EQUIP RENTAL GENERAL	1,342	1,071
COPY MACHINE EXPENSES	13,440	6,424
BOOK LIBRARY	250	320
SUBSCRIPTION MAGAZINE	200	150
REPAIR REPL PARTS EQUIP	1,070	125
REPAIRS & REPL PARTS MED EQUIP	146,498	
FILM PROCESSING EXPENSE	220	
TOTAL	178,003	18,377
TOTAL NON-SALARY EXPENSE	1,983,299	1,588,446
TOTAL EXPENSE	3,708,415	4,020,343
TOTAL NET EXPENSES	1,983,299	1,588,446

Figure 11-9 Net Expense Worksheet (Adapted with permission of Northwestern Memorial Hospital, Chicago, IL)

pose of monitoring is to ensure that revenue is generated consistent with projected productivity and standards. Organizations often recognize a flexible budget, which allows for adjustments if the volume or census increases or decreases. If the volume increases, it is likely that expenses will increase. If the volume decreases and expenses increase, then the manager needs to determine what actions are necessary to control or bring costs down. Many organizations require managers to complete a budget variance report, which is a tool used to identify when categories are out of line, to identify the need for corrective action. Figure 11-10 illustrates a variance report.

The entire health care team is responsible for ensuring that expenses are kept within the budgeted amount and that the volume or census is maintained. The manner in which this is accomplished depends on the organization. Some institutions request that budget dashboards (see Figure 11-11) be developed reflecting departmental activity at a glance. Variance reports or dashboards may be posted so that all staff members have an opportunity to review the budget and participate in any improvement needed.

Staff can meet to discuss implementation or reinforcement of strategies that can positively affect the budget (Yoder-Wise, 1998; Elser & Nipp, 2001). Following are examples of such strategies:

	Budget	Actual	% Variance	Comments/Action
Revenue				
Inpatient				
Outpatient				
Other				
List all line items over or under budget				
Expenses				
Salary				
Full-time equivalent employees (FTEs)				
Medical supplies				
Clerical supplies				
Purchase Service				
Maintenance				
Miscellaneous				

Figure 11-10 Variance Report per Cost Center

- Analyze time efficiency of staff involved in patient care.
- Understand the process for entering patient charges.
- Educate coworkers regarding the charging process.
- Plan for supplies needed for every patient encounter and consciously eliminate unnecessary items.

- Learn how a department is reimbursed for services delivered, identifying covered and excluded expenses.
- Input charges in a timely manner.
- Discuss quality and cost differences in supplies with other staff and management.
- Evaluate staff and equipment downtime.
- Analyze cause of schedule delays, canceled cases, and extended procedure times.

Year to Date					
Volume/Access					
Department	Cost Center	Volume Year to Date	Percentage Budget Variance	Percentage Variance from Last year	Days to Next Appointment/ Available Bed
GI Laboratory	1265	6,706	16	23	3
Medical Unit	7095	9,705	18	28	1
Patient Satisfaction					
	Overall Score		Percentile	Percentile	Results Reporting
Department	Actual	Target	Actual	Target	Average Report Turnaround Time	Reports > 24
GI laboratory	90.5	91.70	90	95	28	20%
Medical unit	89	90.00	88	92	NA	NA
Human Resources					
					Employee Performance
		Actual	Vacancies	Turnover	Staff Performance Reviews on Time
Department	Manager	FTEs Year to Date	Year to Date	Rate	> 30 Days
GI laboratory	1	33.00	0.4	8%	0
Medical unit	1	45.00	6	12%	1
Expenses					
				Supply	Productivity
		Percentage of Budget Compared to Actual	Percentage Variance from Budget Year to Date	Variance from Budget Year to Date	Variance from Last Year
Department					
GI laboratory	250	(5.00)	11.00	unfavorable	unfavorable
Medical unit	118	8.00	12.00	favorable	unfavorable
Capital Budget					
Line Items	Number	Year	Budgeted	Expensed	Balance
GI lab					
7 Video endoscopes	10002895	2001	112,550.00	109,389.19	14,226.00
Endoscopy travel cart	30256409	2001	2,750.00	0.00	32,750.00
Scopes	89756452	2001	38,255.00	35,225.00	1,199.00
Comments					
Financial improvement plan ongoing in GI lab: Interventional charges have been adjusted and cost reduction/inventory control is being explored with materials management.					
Medical nursing unit has achieved highest overall patient satisfaction goal. Multidisciplinary conferences are being held every other day to focus on patient care issues.					

Figure 11-11 GI Laboratory and Medical Unit Dashboard (Adapted with permission of Northwestern Memorial Hospital, Chicago, IL)

- Explore new products with vendor representatives and network with colleagues who have tried both new and modified products.
- Reduce the length of stay by troubleshooting early.
- Assist staff in organizational planning.
- Enhance productivity through rigorous process improvement.
- Post overtime and high/low productivity analysis.
- Explore how time and motion studies may increase efficiencies by identifying gaps or duplication in effort.
- Ensure that staff have the right tools and that the tools are ready when needed.
- Analyze patient supplies and review cost per patient encounter (e.g., chemotherapy administration, dialysis, insertion of indwelling or peripheral catheter).
- Track various steps in patient care that are time consuming or problematic for a unit (e.g., communication from front desk to recovery room, staff response to patient call lights, number of staff responding to an emergency code).
- Acquire a working knowledge of how a department/unit monitors financial and quality indicators, and participate in the development of action plans to increase patient satisfaction or to create the "best patient experience."

- latory influences, and strategic initiatives. Additionally, it is helpful to understand the department's scope of service, goals, and history.
- During the budget preparation phase, it is important to examine the individual nursing or hospital department or section thoroughly. Hospital systems are frequently divided into sections, departments, or units to compartmentalize them for organizational purposes. These subsections or units, commonly called cost centers, are used to track financial data.
- Organizations typically use history or past performance as a baseline of experience and data to better understand activity in a department or unit.
- Once background data have been gathered, the development of the budget can follow. This includes projecting revenue and expenses.
- Expenses are determined by identifying the cost associated with the delivery of service. Expenditures are resources used by an organization to deliver services and may include labor, supplies, equipment, utilities, and miscellaneous items.
- Once developed, budgets are submitted to administration for review and final approval. The approval process may take several months as the unit budgets are combined to determine the overall budget for the health care organization.

KEY CONCEPTS

- Nurses play an integral role in the development, implementation, and evaluation of a unit or department budget.
- If nurses are not conscious of revenue and expenses, then deviation from financial performance will occur.
- Overall, organizational performance is dependent upon the insight and skills of staff members regarding patient care quality and financial outcomes.
- There are several types of budgets that hospitals use to help with future planning and management. These include operational, capital, and construction budgets.
- The budget preparation phase is one of data gathering related to a variety of elements that influence an organization, including demographic information, competitive analysis, regu-

KEY TERMS

accounting	indirect expenses
capital budget	operational budget
construction budget	profit
cost centers	revenue
dashboard	variable costs
direct expenses	variance
fixed costs	

REVIEW QUESTIONS

1. An operational budget accounts for
   A. the purchase of minor and major equipment.
   B. construction and renovation.
   C. income and expenses associated with daily activity within an organization.
   D. applications for new technology.

2. Revenue can be generated through
    A. billable patient services.
    B. donations to service organizations.
    C. use of generic drugs.
    D. messenger and escort activities.

3. Cost centers are used to
    A. develop historical and demographic information.
    B. track expense line items.
    C. plan for strategic growth and movement.
    D. track financial data within a department or unit.

4. The purpose of monitoring a budget is to
    A. keep expenses above budget.
    B. maintain revenue above the previous year's budget.
    C. ensure revenue is generated monthly.
    D. generate revenue and control expenses within a projected framework.

5. Productivity can be measured by
    A. number of beds in a hospital.
    B. reimbursement rates for services rendered.
    C. past performance and history regarding revenue.
    D. volume of services delivered.

REVIEW ACTIVITIES

1. Look around your clinical agency. Do you see any dashboards? What do they reveal about your agency?

2. Using the tables in this chapter as a guideline, construct a competitive analysis of one or more of the agencies in your community.

3. Using the zero-based budgeting figure in this chapter, construct an analysis of one of the clinical procedures in your agency.

EXPLORING THE WEB

- Go to the site for the Joint Commission on Accreditation of Healthcare Organizations. What information did you find there?
  www.jcaho.org
- Review the site for the American Organization of Nurse Executives. Was the information helpful?
  www.aone.org

- Review these sites for helpful information. What did you find there?
  Healthcare Financial Management Association:
  www.hfma.org
  American College of Healthcare Executives:
  www.ache.org
  The Advisory Board Company:
  www.advisory.com
  Centers for Medicare and Medicaid Services:
  www.cms.hhs.gov
  Agency for Healthcare Research and Quality:
  www.ahcpr.gov
  Food and Drug Administration: *www.fda.gov*

REFERENCES

The Advisory Board Company. (1998). *Reversing the flight of talent: executive briefing.* Washington, DC: Nursing Executive Center.

Elser, R., & Nipp, D. (2001). Worker designed culture change. *Nursing Economic$, 19*(4) 161–163, 175.

Grohar-Murray, M. E., & DiCroce, H. R. (1997). *Leadership and management in nursing.* Stamford, CT: Appleton & Lange.

Joint Commission on Accreditation of Healthcare Organizations. (2001). *Comprehensive accreditation manual for hospitals (CAMH): The official handbook.* Oakbrook Terrace, IL: Author.

Nelson, B. (1997). *1001 ways to energize employees* (pp. 30, 66, 151). New York: Workman Publishing.

Norton, D., & Kaplan, R. (2001). *The strategy-focused organization: How balanced scorecard companies thrive in the new business environment.* Boston: Harvard Business School Press.

Sullivan, E. J. & Decker, P. (Eds.). (1997). *Effective leadership and management in nursing: Key skills in nursing management* (pp. 90–104). Menlo Park, CA: Addison Wesley.

Yoder-Wise, P. (1998). *Leading and managing in nursing.* (2nd ed., pp. 226–243). St. Louis, MO: Mosby.

SUGGESTED READINGS

Barnum, B., & Kerfoot, K. (Eds.). (1995). *The nurse as executive. The nursing division budgeting* (4th ed., pp. 188–198). Gaithersburg, MD: Aspen.

Camp, R. C. (1989). *Benchmarking: The search for industry best practices that lead to superior performance.* Milwaukee, WI: ASQC Quality Press.

Carruth, A., Carruth, P., & Noto, E. (2000). Nurse managers flex their budgetary might. *Nursing Management, 31*(2). 16–17.

DiJerome, L., Dunham-Taylor, J., Ash, K., & Brown., R. (1999). Evaluating cost center productivity. *Nursing Economic$, 117*(6). 334–340.

Dixon, N. M., (2000). *Common knowledge: How companies thrive by sharing what they know.* Boston: Harvard Business School Press.

Garvin, D. (2000). *Learning in action: A guide to putting the learning organization to work.* Boston: Harvard Business School Press.

Iowa Intervention Project. (2001). Determining cost of nursing instrumentations: A beginning. *Nursing Economic$, 19*(4) 146–160.

Jones, K. R. (1999). The capital budgeting process. *Seminars for Nurse Managers, 7*(2), 55–56.

Katzenbach, J. R. & Smith, D. K. (1992). *The wisdom of teams: Creating the high-performance organization.* Boston: Harvard Business School Press.

Keeling, B. (2000). How to establish a position and hours budget. *Nursing Management, 31*(3), 26–27.

Marrelli, T. M. (1997). *The nurse manager's survival guide: Practical answers to everyday problems* (2nd ed.). St. Louis, MO: Mosby.

Robnett, M., & Schaub-Rimet, A. (1999). *Nursing administration: Managing patient care financial skills for department managers* (pp. 293–312). Stamford, CT: Appleton & Lange.

CHAPTER 12

Effective Staffing

Anne L. Bernat, RN, BSN, MSN, CNAA

High quality nursing care should be the goal of every nurse, educator and manager. High quality to me means care that is individualized to a particular patient, administered humanely and competently, comprehensively and with continuity. Primary nursing is one means of accomplishing that quality of care.

(Marie Manthey, 1980)

OBJECTIVES

Upon completion of this chapter, the reader should be able to:

1. Discuss utilization of patient classification systems data by the staff nurse and the nurse manager.

2. Develop a staffing pattern for a critical care unit with 10 patients.

3. Evaluate staffing effectiveness on an inpatient unit using two patient outcomes.

4. Compare and contrast models of care delivery.

5. Discuss the role of a case manager versus a unit staff nurse.

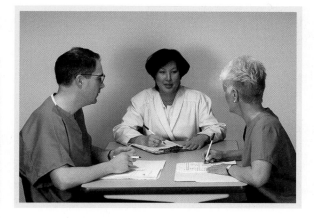

You are a new nurse manager of a 30-bed medical unit that uses primary nursing as the care delivery model. You have 40 employees who work full and part time with vacancies for 8 additional full-time staff. The current schedule does not accommodate any twelve-hour shifts. You have 5 long-term staff members who threaten to leave if they are forced to work 12-hour shifts. You have interviewed several new graduates who will come to work for you only if you offer them 12-hour shifts.

How can you accommodate the needs of both groups of staff?

What effect will the 12-hour shifts have on your care delivery model?

The ability of a nurse to provide safe and effective care to a patient is dependent on many variables. These variables include the knowledge and experience of the staff, the severity of illness of the patients, the amount of nursing time available, the care delivery model, care management tools, and organizational supports in place to facilitate care. This chapter will explore these factors, how they affect planning for staffing, and the results of staffing plans. By the end of this chapter you will understand how to plan staffing and measure the effectiveness of a staffing plan. You will also be able to articulate the models of care delivery that are applicable to your environment and patient population.

DETERMINATION OF STAFFING NEEDS

Nurse staffing has varied widely since the inception of nursing as a profession. Nursing staffing has ranged from one nurse to many soldiers, as in Florence Nightingale's time, to today when you may see one nurse to one patient in a critical care area. In today's rapidly changing health care environment, many variables must be considered in determining nurse staffing requirements. The effectiveness of the staffing pattern is only as good as the planning that goes into its preparation. The following key budget concepts and issues need to be reviewed and assessed when building or assessing a staffing pattern.

Core Concepts

Gaining an understanding of the key terms—full-time equivalents (FTEs), productive time, nonproductive time, direct and indirect care, and nursing hours per patient day (NHPPD)—is necessary to understand staffing patterns.

FTEs

A **full-time equivalent** (FTE) is a measure of the work commitment of a full-time employee. A full-time employee works 5 days a week or 40 hours per week for 52 weeks a year. This amounts to 2,080 hours of work time (Figure 12-1).

A full-time employee who works 40 hours a week is referred to as a 1.0 FTE. A part-time employee who works 5 days in a 2-week period is considered a 0.5 FTE. The FTE calculation is used to mathematically describe how much an employee works (Figure 12-2). Understanding FTEs is essential when moving from a staffing pattern to the actual number of staff required.

FTE hours are a total of all paid time. This includes worked time as well as nonworked time. Hours worked and available for patient care are designated as **productive hours**. Benefit time such as vacation, sick time, and education time is considered

| 5 days per week | × | 8 hours per day | = | 40 hours per week |
| 40 hours per week | × | 52 weeks per year | = | 2,080 hours per year |

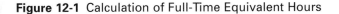

Figure 12-1 Calculation of Full-Time Equivalent Hours

1.0 FTE = 40 hours per week or five 8-hour shifts per week

0.8 FTE = 32 hours per week or four 8-hour shifts per week

0.6 FTE = 24 hours per week or three 8-hour shifts per week

0.4 FTE = 16 hours per week or two 8-hour shifts per week

0.2 FTE = 8 hours per week or one 8-hour shift per week

Figure 12-2 FTE Calculation for Varying Levels of Work Commitment

nonproductive hours. When considering the number of FTEs you need to staff a unit, you must count only the productive hours available for each staff member. Available productive time can be easily calculated by subtracting benefit time from the time a full-time employee would work (Figure 12-3).

In this case, a full-time registered nurse (RN) would have 1,848 hours per year of productive time available to care for patients.

Employees who work with patients can be classified into two categories: those who provide direct care and those who provide indirect care. **Direct care** is time spent providing hands-on care to patients. **Indirect care** is time spent on activities that are patient related but are not done directly to the patient. Documentation, time consulting with people in other health care disciplines, and time spent following up on outstanding issues, are good examples of indirect care. Even though RNs, licensed practical nurses (LPNs), and unlicensed assistive personnel (UAP) engage in indirect care activities,

the majority of their time is spent providing direct care, therefore they are classified as direct care providers. Nurse managers, clinical specialists, unit secretaries, and other support staff are considered indirect care providers because the majority of their work is indirect in nature and supports the work of the direct care providers.

Nursing Hours per Patient Day

Nursing hours per patient day (NHPPD) is a standard measure that quantifies the nursing time available to each patient by available nursing staff. For example, a nursing unit that has 20 patients at a given point during a 24-hour period, usually the midnight census, and 5 nursing staff each shift would calculate into 6 nursing hours per patient day. NHPPD reflect only productive nursing time available (Figure 12-4). This measure is useful, in quantifying nursing care, to both nurses and financial staff in an organization.

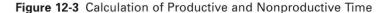

Vacation time	15 days	or	120 hours
Sick time	5 days	or	40 hours
Holiday time	6 days	or	48 hours
Education time	3 days	or	24 hours
Total nonproductive time		=	232 hours

2,080 − 232 = 1,848 hours of productive work time available for each staff member with these benefits.

Figure 12-3 Calculation of Productive and Nonproductive Time

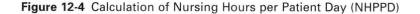

20 patients on the unit

5 staff × 3 shifts = 15 staff

15 staff each working 8 hours = 120 hours available in a 24-hour period

120 nursing hours ÷ 20 patients = 6.0 NHPPD

FTE = 8 hours per week or one 8-hour shift per week

Figure 12-4 Calculation of Nursing Hours per Patient Day (NHPPD)

Patient Classification Systems

To assess how many staff are needed at any given time, it is necessary to determine what the patients' needs are. A patient classification system (PCS) is a measurement tool used to articulate the nursing workload for a specific patient or group of patients over a specific period of time. The measure of nursing workload that is generated for each patient is called the patient acuity. Classification data can be used to predict the amount of nursing time needed based on the patient's acuity. As a patient becomes sicker, the acuity level rises, meaning the patient requires more nursing care. As a patient acuity level decreases, the patient requires less nursing care. In most patient classification systems, each patient is classified using weighted criteria that then predict the nursing care hours needed for the next 24 hours. Criteria reflect care needed in bathing, mobilizing, eating, supervision, assessment, frequent observations, and so on. In most cases, patients are classified once a day. The ideal PCS produces a valid and reliable rating of individual patient care requirements, which are matched to the latest clinical technology and caregiver skill variables (Malloch & Conivaloff, 1999). These systems are generally applied to all inpatients in an organization. Systems to classify outpatients have been less prevalent because outpatients tend to be more stable and similar in care needs. There are two different types of classification systems: factor and prototype.

Factor System

The factor system uses units of measure that equate to nursing time. Nursing tasks are assigned time or are weighted to reflect the amount of time needed to perform the task. These systems attempt to capture the cognitive functions of assessment, planning, intervention, and evaluation of patient outcomes along with written documentation processes. There are many factor systems that have been home grown or built for a specific organization. There are also many factor systems available for purchase on the open market. This is the most popular type of classification system because of its ability to project care needs for individual patients as well as patient groups. The time assigned or the weighted factor for different nursing activities can be changed over time to reflect the changing needs of the patients or hospital systems.

Advantages and Disadvantages. In the factor type of system, data are generally readily available to managers and staff for day-to-day operations. These data provide a base of information against which one can justify changes in staffing requirements. A disadvantage to this system type is the ongoing workload for the nurse in classifying patients every day. There are also documented problems with classification creep, whereby acuity levels rise as a result of misuse of classification criteria. These systems do not holistically capture the patient's needs for psychosocial, environmental, and health management support. And finally, these systems calculate nursing time needed based on a typical nurse. When a nurse is a novice, he may take longer to perform activities than the average nurse or more experienced nurse. If a majority of staff are novices, the recommended nursing time needed will be lower than the actual time needed based on the actual expertise of the staff.

Prototype System

The prototype system allocates nursing time to large patient groups based on an average of similar patients. For example, specific diagnostic-related groups (DRGs) have been used as groupings of patients to which a nursing acuity is assigned based on past organizational experience. DRGs are patient groupings established by the federal government for reimbursement purposes. DRGs are sorted by patient disease or condition. This model assumes that, on average, this will reflect the nursing care required and provided. The data are then used by hospitals in determining the cost of nursing care and negotiating contracts with payers for specific patient populations.

Advantages and Disadvantages. The distinct advantage of this system is the reduction of work for the nurse because she is not required to classify patients daily. A major disadvantage of this system is that there is no ongoing measure of the actual nursing work required by individual patients. There are also no ongoing data to monitor the accuracy of the preassigned nursing care requirements. This type of system is much less common than the factor system.

Next Generation of Classification Systems

The next generation of patient classification systems is under development. A new model has been implemented at Providence St. Peter Hospital in Olympia, Washington, that identifies seven domains of patient care needs for nurse intervention. The seven domains are cognitive status, self-care ability, emotional/social/spiritual well-being, family information needs/support status, treatments and interventions, interdisciplinary coordination, and transitions. In addition, the system evaluates four selected patient care outcomes: clinical condition, knowledge of disease condition/process, self-care management, and healthy behaviors. These indicators are measured each shift by the staff as part of the shift assessment. The model attempts to move away from tasks to indices that measure the professional components of nursing care and patient outcome (Malloch & Conivaloff, 1999). In addition, this system attempts to consider the expertise of the nurse in determining nursing time required.

Utilization of Classification System Data

Patient classification data are valuable sources of information for all levels of the organization. On a day-to-day basis, acuity data can be utilized by staff and managers in planning nurse staffing over the next 24 hours. Acuity data and NHPPD are concrete data parameters that are used to educate staff on how to adjust staffing levels. For example, for an acuity range of 1.0 to 1.10, the RN staffing should be five RNs on days. For an acuity of 1.10 to 1.15, the RN staffing on days should be six RNs. Experienced staff have the knowledge to manage staffing to acuity given the information, boundaries, and authority to do so. In many organizations, a central staffing office monitors the census and acuity on all units and deploys nursing resources to the areas in most need using the classification system data and recommended staffing levels. The manager reviews the results of staffing over the past 24 to 48 hours to adjust staffing performance to patient requirements. At the unit level, acuity data are also essential in preparing month-end justification for variances in staff utilization. If your average acuity has risen, then there should be an expected rise in NHPPD to accommodate the increased patient needs.

At an organization level, acuity data have been used to cost out nursing services for specific patient populations and global patient types. This information is also very helpful in negotiating payment rates with third-party payers such as insurance companies to ensure that reimbursement reflects nursing costs. In most organizations, the classification or acuity data are also used in preparation of the nursing staffing budget for the upcoming fiscal year. The data can be benchmarked with other organizations to lend credence to any efforts to change nursing hours. Finally, patient acuity data and NHPPD can be used to develop a staffing pattern. Patient classification and NHPPD data provide an enormous amount of information that serves a multitude of needs.

Considerations in Developing a Staffing Pattern

Developing a staffing pattern is a science and an art. The following sections will consider other areas in addition to the acuity data and NHPPD just discussed. Each of these areas should be reviewed and the findings incorporated into development of the staffing pattern.

Benchmarking

Benchmarking is a management tool for seeking out the best practices in one's industry so as to improve performance (Swansburg, 1996). In developing a staffing pattern that leads to a budget, it is important to benchmark your planned NHPPD against other organizations with similar patient populations. Purchased patient classification systems often offer acuity and NHPPD benchmarking data from around the country as part of their system. This kind of data can be helpful in establishing a starting point for a staffing pattern or as part of justification for increasing or reducing nursing hours. Caution must be used, however, because each organization has varying levels of support in place at the unit level for the nurse. For example, a nursing unit that has dietary aides from the dietary department distribute and pick up meal trays would need less nursing time than a unit that had no external support for this activity. Factors such as these contribute significantly to differences in hours of care from one organization to another.

Regulatory Requirements

Generally speaking, there are few regulatory requirements related to nurse staffing. This is changing, however, as the nursing shortage heightens. California has mandated nurse staffing levels in Emergency Departments and critical care units. Several other states have legislation pending. There is considerable controversy within the nursing profession over this issue. There are nurses who are adamant that they need to be protected by law with stipulated staffing levels. There are nurse leaders who are concerned that the mandated staffing levels would soon become the maximum staffing levels rather than the minimum.

The Joint Commission on Accreditation of Healthcare Organizations (JCAHO) surveys hospitals on the quality of care provided. The JCAHO does not mandate staffing levels but does assess an organization's ability to provide the right number of competent staff to meet the needs of patients served by the hospital (Joint Commission on Accreditation of Healthcare Organizations, 2000). Part of this assessment will be how often you staff to the requirements of your staffing pattern and how you evaluate the effectiveness of your staffing pattern. If your staffing pattern calls for four RNs for 20 patients, the JCAHO will assess how often you meet your own standards by having a nurse for every 5 patients. As a rule, you should investigate the state and federal regulations related to your patient population for any regulated staffing requirements.

Skill Mix

Skill mix is another critical element in nurse staffing. Skill mix is the percentage of RN staff to other direct care staff, LPNs, and Unlicensed Assistive Personnel (UAP). For example, in a unit that has 40 FTEs budgeted, with 20 of them being RNs and 20 FTEs of other skill types, the RN skill mix would be 50%. If the unit had 40 FTEs, with 30 of them being RNs, the RN skill mix would be 75%. The skill mix of a unit should vary according to the care that is required and the care delivery model utilized. For example, in a critical care unit, the RN skill mix will be much higher than in a nursing home where the skills of an RN are required to a much lesser degree. It is important to note that RN hours of care are more costly than those of lesser skilled workers, but there is evidence that RNs are a very productive and efficient type of labor. As nurses become more scarce, it will become even more important to evaluate the patient care required and who can perform necessary functions. For instance, if many patients require feeding, an unlicensed assistive person may be most appropriate. A note of caution: As you consider skill mix, you need

to clearly understand what activities each level of staff can engage in within the scope of practice in your state. In some states, UAP may catheterize patients if they have received training and are competent. In other states, UAP may not perform this function regardless of their training and expertise.

Staff Support

Another important factor to consider in developing a staffing pattern is the supports in place for the operations of the unit or department. For instance, does your organization have a systematic process to deliver medications to the department or do unit personnel have to pick up patient medications and narcotics? Does your organization have staff to transport patients to and from ancillary departments? The less support available to your staff, the more nursing hours have to be built into the staffing pattern to provide care to patients. Nursing areas such as critical care that have a significant amount of equipment to track and supply may benefit greatly from adding a materials coordinator. This kind of support for staff allows staff to spend their precious available time with patients rather than looking for equipment or supplies. An additional important unit-based need is secretarial support. If the unit has admissions, discharges, and transfers, it makes sense to provide unit secretarial support for the peak periods of the day. In intensive care units (ICUs), unit secretaries are commonly scheduled around the clock to provide support for the unit staff as well as for other disciplines.

Historical Information

As you consider the many variables that affect staffing, it helps to ask the following questions: What has worked in the past? Were the staff able to provide the care that was needed? How many patients were cared for? What kind of patients were they? How many staff were utilized and what kind of staff were they? This kind of information can help to identify operational issues that would not be apparent otherwise. For example, in an older part of a facility, there may not be a pneumatic delivery tube system, a system that is available in most other parts of the facility. Because it is generally available, you may overlook its absence. But its absence means a significant amount of time will be required to collect needed items, affecting the staffing pattern you develop. It would also be important to review any data on quality or staff perceptions regarding the effectiveness of the previous staffing

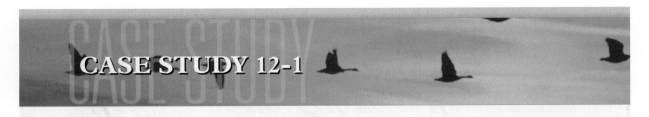

CASE STUDY 12-1

You are the manager of a critical care unit that has 12 beds. The nurse-to-patient ratio is budgeted at one nurse to two patients. Medical-surgical beds are not available for your patients who have improved. Your state does not mandate nurse-to-patient ratios. Of the 12 patients in your unit, 4 are well enough to go to a general-floor bed. On the medical-surgical units, the nurse-to-patient ratio is one RN to six patients. You are planning staffing for the next two shifts.

What factors should you consider? After consideration of key factors, what is your plan for staffing? What would you communicate to your staff?

pattern. This information will allow you to calculate previous NHPPD and outcomes for comparison to your staffing plan. History is a valuable tool that we often overlook as we plan for the future.

Establishing a Staffing Pattern

A **staffing pattern** is a plan that articulates how many and what kind of staff are needed by shift and day to staff a unit or department. There are basically two ways of developing a staffing pattern. It can be generated by determining the required ratio of staff to patients; nursing hours and total FTEs are then calculated. It can also be generated by determining the nursing care hours needed for a specific patient or patients and then generating the FTEs and staff-to-patient ratio needed to provide that care. In most cases, you would use a combination of methods to validate your staffing plan. We will start with development of a plan from the staff-to-patient ratio.

Inpatient Unit

An **inpatient unit** is a hospital unit that is able to provide care to patients 24 hours a day, 7 days a week. Establishing a staffing pattern for this kind of unit utilizes all the data discussed in the previous areas. Using data from all your sources, you can build a staffing pattern that you believe will meet the needs of the patients, the staff, and the organization. Utilizing a staffing pattern template, plot out the number and type of staff needed during the week and

weekend for 24 hours a day for the number of patients you expect to have (Figure 12-5). In this example, the number and type of staff are delineated as well the additional FTEs for weekend coverage, orientation and education, and benefited time.

For example, on a 24-bed medical unit, you expect to have, on average, 22 patients per day. The ratio of one RN to six patients and one UAP for every twelve patients works well from 7 A.M. to 7 P.M. From 7 P.M. to 7 A.M., the ratio can go to one RN to eight patients. Two UAPs are needed from 7 P.M. to 11 P.M. and then one UAP from 11 P.M. to 7 A.M. This would generate a total of 124 hours per day. The average number of patients on this unit is 22. To calculate the NHPPD see Figure 12-6.

In this example, the number of care hours available would be 5.63 NHPPD.

As you can see, the staffing pattern drives the NHPPD. The more staff available per patient, the higher the NHPPD. Cost is associated with hours of care available and skill mix. There are staffing patterns with many hours of care available, but they may be lower-cost FTEs. The key is to have the right number and skill level of caregiver available to ensure safe, effective, and appropriate care.

To develop a staffing pattern using NHPPD, you would start with a target NHPPD. If your target NHPPD were 8, for example, and you expected to have 22 patients on your 24-bed unit, you would multiply 8 NHPPD times 22 patients to get 176 productive hours needed every day. Dividing 176 by 8-hour shifts worked by an FTE gives you 22 FTEs needed per day.

STAFFING PATTERN AND PLAN

UNIT:_____

COST CENTER:_____   ADC BUDGET: [____]   ADC WD: [____]

TYPE OF SERVICE:_____   NHPPD BUDGET: [____]   ADC WE: [____]

ADC: [____]

SKILL	ON DUTY WEEKDAYS				ON DUTY WEEKENDS			WEEKEND-FTE CAL. (x .4)				7 DAY WKD TOTAL
	DAY	EVE	NIGHT	TOTAL	DAY	EVE	NIGHT	DAY	EVE	NIGHT	TOTAL	
DIRECT												
ANM												
RN												
LPN												
PCA												
NA												
OTHER 1												
SUB TOT												
INDIRECT												
NM												
CNS												
ANM												
NUR												
NUR												
SR. NUR												
MISC.												
NA I												
PSA												
OTHER 3												
SUB TOT												
TOTALS												

WEEKDAY NHPPD: WEEKEND NHPPD: AVG NHPPD [____]
DIRECT NHPPD: [____]   DIRECT NHPPD: [____]
INDIRECT NHPPD: [____] INDIRECT NHPPD: [____]

Figure 12-5 Staffing Pattern Template (Courtesy of Albany Medical Center, Albany, NY)

Determining the Number of FTEs Needed to Meet the Staffing Pattern

You have determined a staffing pattern for your unit. The staffing pattern calculates the number of FTEs needed per day, but it did not add hours for benefited time off or for days off for staff. You must now calculate the amount of additional staff that will be needed to provide for days off and benefit time. Direct caregivers will need to be replaced, but some other support staff may not need to be replaced for days off or benefited time off. Managers typically are not replaced on days off. Noting that each 8-hour shift for a FTE is equal to 0.2 FTE, to provide coverage for 2 days off a week multiply the number of

Skill	Day	Evening	Night	Total
Direct				
ANM				
RN	4	3.5	3	10.5
LPN				
Tech				
UAP	2	2	1	5
Subtotal				

10.5 staff × 8-hour shifts = 84 hours

5 staff × 8-hour shifts = 40 hours

Staff hours available per day = 124 hours

124 hours ÷ 22 patients per day = 5.63 hours of NHPPD

124 hours ÷ 8 hour shifts = 15.5 FTEs to fill the staffing pattern

Figure 12-6 Staffing Plan for a 24-Bed Medical Unit

staff needed per day by a 0.4 FTE. In the example in Figure 12-6, 15.5 FTEs per day multiplied by 0.4 FTE would be an additional 6.2 FTEs to cover 2 days off per week for a total of 21.7 FTEs.

The next step would be to provide additional FTEs for coverage for benefited time away from work. This includes vacations, educational time, orientation time, and so on. The amount of time away from work varies by organization. If every employee receives 2 weeks of vacation a year and 2 conference days, this would equate to 1,984 hours of productive time per FTE (2,080 possible hours minus 96 hours). Total FTE hours divided by 1,984 hours gives you the total FTEs needed to provide coverage. In the previous example, 21.7 FTEs multiplied by 2,080 hours equals 45,136 hours, and 45,136 hours divided by 1,984 would be 22.75 FTEs or 1.05 additional FTEs to ensure that there are staff available to work when other staff are taking benefited time off. This then means that a total of 22.75 FTEs are needed to staff this 24-bed unit.

Determining the FTEs Needed to Staff an Episodic Care Unit

An **episodic care unit** refers to a unit that sees patients for defined episodes of care; dialysis or ambulatory care units are good examples. In these

units, patients tend to be more homogenous and have a more predictable path of care. Determining staffing needs for an episodic unit starts with an assessment of the hours of care required by the patients. Using a dialysis unit as an example, to care for 16 patients receiving treatments, you determine you need four RNs for all 12 hours the unit is open, or 48 hours of RN care per day. The unit is open 12 hours a day, 6 days a week, or 312 days a year; 48 hours per day multiplied by 312 days = 14,976 total hours. As in the previous example, calculation of FTEs needed to provide coverage for productive hours can be done by dividing the total number of hours needed by the actual number of productive hours an employee would work. This method provides coverage for days off and benefited time for direct caregivers. Using our productive FTE hours of 1,848 from Figure 12-3 divided into the 14,976 hours required equates to a total of 8.10 RN FTEs.

The same calculation can be applied to other caregivers. In this same example, if two technicians were required for 12 hours a day of operation, that would mean

2 × 12 = 24 hours needed per day, and 24 × 312 days = 7,488 total hours needed.

The benefit package for technical staff is not as rich as the RN package. Their vacation is 10 days or 80 hours per year, which increases their productive time to 2,000 hours per year; 7,488 divided by 2,000 = 3.74 technical FTEs. Any staff members who do not require coverage would simply be added to the overall FTEs for the unit as a 1.0 FTE. This might apply to a secretary, social worker, or nurse manager, who support the unit but are not necessary to replace on their days off and benefited time off.

SCHEDULING

Scheduling of staff is the responsibility of the nurse manager. She must ensure that the schedule places the appropriate staff on each day and shift for safe, effective patient care. There are many issues to consider as you schedule your staff; the patient type and acuity, the number of patients, the experience of your staff, and the supports available to the staff. The combination of these factors should guide the number of staff scheduled on each day and shift. These factors must be reviewed on an ongoing basis as patient types and patient acuity drive different patient needs and staff expertise.

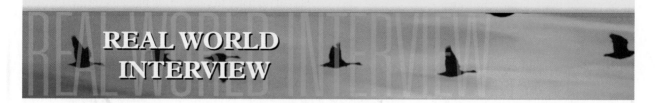

Given the need for staffing and financial accountability, I used spreadsheet software to improve the development of staffing patterns in our facility. We had been using a pencil and paper template for managers to use to develop staffing patterns. This manual template concentrated on the weekday staffing needs and applied an overall factor to calculate weekend and benefit time. The FTE number provided did not address orientation and education needs for any of the staff or benefit needs for the weekend staff. Although these staffing patterns were used to project the number of FTEs needed and the distribution of employees to staff the nursing unit, they were not used to drive the budgeted quota for the unit.

Using a computer software program, I developed a spreadsheet template the managers could use to accurately project FTEs needed to meet the staffing pattern. This computerized approach allows for weekday and weekend staffing to be considered independently considering any differences in census or direct NHPPD. A benefit time factor, tailored to our organization's specific benefit package for each skill level, was used to calculate the number of FTEs needed to staff for benefit time. Benefit time was now calculated for weekday and weekend staffing, coverage for a 24/7 operation. Additionally, an orientation and education factor is used to calculate the FTEs needed to provide coverage. For the first time, benefited time off and orientation time were built into each unit's staffing pattern. Additionally, direct and indirect NHPPD are automatically calculated as the staffing pattern is changed, and the calculated FTE needs can be compared to the current budgeted quota for variances. I also worked with Finance to use this template as the basis for a Budgeted Quota Sheet, which is used during the budget process for determining the unit quota for the next year, a quota that now includes benefited time off and orientation time.

One of the biggest assists has been the ability of the nurse managers to use the template for what-if scenarios. When they are planning for a census or patient program change, FTE needs can be quickly calculated and compared to their current budgeted quota. This tool has become part of our business planning process.

Overall, this template has been accepted as a valid management tool, has standardized inclusion of nonproductive time into FTE budgets, and has given managers a simple tool to develop new staffing patterns. It has also helped in raising the accountability of managers to develop workable staffing patterns that they can be held accountable to.

Barbara Leafer, RN, BS
Fiscal Administrator for Patient Care

Patient Need

Patients' nursing needs are measured by the patient classification system. Patient classification systems, however, do not tell you when the nursing activity will take place over the next 24 hours. In addition to planning for the acuity of the patients, the staffing pattern must support having staff working when the work needs to be done. A good example of this would be an oncology unit in which chemotherapy and blood transfusions typically occur on the evening shift. In this scenario, staffing in the evening may need to be higher than for other shifts to support these nurse-intensive activities. As patient types change, so do patients' needs and staffing requirements. Adding a population of step-down patients from the ICU would likely require additional FTEs on a medical-surgical unit. Any time patient populations change, staffing and NHPPD should be assessed.

Experience and Scheduling of Staff

Each nurse is different regarding her knowledge base, experience level, and critical thinking skills. A novice nurse takes longer to accomplish the same task than an experienced nurse. An experienced RN can handle more in terms of workload and acuity of patients. If your area requires special skills or competencies of your staff, you would also want to plan for additional nursing hours, so that staff with the special skills are scheduled when the patient care need may arise. Remember, the underlying principle of good staffing is that those you serve come first. This may dictate some undesirable shifts, but your responsibility is to ensure that there are appropriate numbers and kinds of staff on hand to care for the patients you serve. Staff are plotted out across a staffing sheet (Figure 12-7).

Staff members should be scheduled for the number of days for which they are committed: 5 days a week for a full-time employee and less for part-time employees as determined by their hiring commitment. When staff are hired, there is an agreement between the manager and the employee as to the shift, schedule, and work commitment. The scheduled days should be assigned so that there are an even number of staff available across the week. Typically, the spread of FTEs across the 24-hour period falls within the following guidelines: days 33% to 50%, evenings 30% to 40%, and nights 20% to 33%. The spread should be based on patient need. ICUs typically have a more even spread. Less acute units in which the majority of

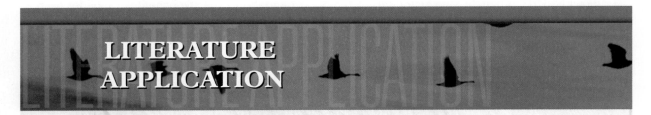

LITERATURE APPLICATION

Citation: Buerhaus, P. I. (2000, May/June). Why are shortages of hospital RNs concentrated in specialty care units? *Nursing Economic$, 18*(3), 111–117.

Discussion: In this study of the nursing shortage in hospital special care units, Dr. Buerhaus utilized data from federal databases to review trends in the nursing workforce and prospects for a future nursing shortage. Significant findings included far fewer young people choosing nursing as a career and the expansion of career opportunities for women. The lack of young people entering the profession will cause the nursing workforce to continue to age at a rapid pace, 3.4 years over the next 10 years. In addition, it can be expected that as the current workforce ages and retires, the number of RNs will remain in 2020 roughly what it was in 2000, causing ongoing nursing shortages, primarily in intensive care units (ICUs) and operating rooms (ORs). ICUs employ younger RNs than other hospital settings. The author notes that it was not until the 1970s that ICUs became prevalent in hospitals and students had rotations in these areas. It is also noted that the challenging and stimulating environment in ICUs attracts younger RNs. On the other hand, operating rooms have a large proportion of older diploma-prepared RNs working in them. Prior to the 1970s, the majority of RNs received their education in hospital-based, 3-year diploma programs, which offered students significantly greater exposure to all hospital clinical areas. The author theorizes that the RN shortage in ICUs is due to the decreasing number of young nurses coming into the profession. The shortage in OR nurses is a reflection of older RNs retiring or reducing work schedules and also the reduction of diploma programs in hospitals.

Implications for Practice: It is clear that there is and will continue to be a nursing shortage for the next decade. In addition to devising global strategies to draw more people into the nursing profession, it is imperative for managers and nurse leaders to create environments that retain staff. This includes planning staff schedules that nurses find compatible with their personal lives. As the nursing workforce ages, we must also take measures to make accommodations for the older worker, including technology to simplify work and physical plant changes to make the work less physically taxing.

	Monday 04	Tuesday 05	Wednesday 06	Thursday 07	Friday 08	Saturday 09	Sunday 10	Monday 11	Tuesday 12	Wednesday 13	Thursday 14	Friday 15	Saturday 16	Sunday 17
Melinda	D		D	D		D	D	D		D	D	D		
Jason		8.00 1900			N	N	N	D	8.00 1900		D			
Eileen	12.00 0900		12.00 0900		D	12.00 0900	12.00 0900	12.00 0900		12.00 0900	D	N		
Susan	8.00 1100	8.00 1100		E	E	E		vac		8.00 1100	E	E	E	
Barbara	D	14.00 2400	13.00 2400	13.00 2400	D				14.00 2400	13.00 2400	13.00 2400		D	D
Rosemary	D	D	D	D		E			D	N	N		E	
Robert	N	N	N	N			N	N	N	N	N			N
Jacqueline	E	E	E		E		E		E	E	E	E		E
Marcella		D		D	D	D	D		D			D		
Sara	E			E	8.00 0800		E	E			E	8.00 0800		E
Gary		E	E		E	N		E	E	E		12.00 1500		
Cynthia	N	N	N		N	P	P	N	N	P		P	N	
Toni	8.00 0730	8.00 0730	8.00 0730	8.00 0730	8.00 0730			8.00 0730	8.00 0730		8.00 0730	8.00 0730		

The 1st number in a square is the number of hours scheduled, the second number is the shift start time in military time.

Standard Work Assignments

D 0700–1500
E 1500–2300
N 2300–0700
A 0700–1900
P 1900–0700

Figure 12-7 Excerpt from Schedule for an Emergency Department Showing Great Variation in Shift Design

patient activity occurs during the daylight hours typically have less night percentage of FTEs.

Shift Variations

To attract and retain employees, organizations offer traditional schedules and flexible schedules to meet organizational and employee needs.

Traditional Staffing Patterns. Traditional staffing patterns are generally 8-hour shifts, 7 A.M. to 3:30 P.M., 3 P.M. to 11:30 P.M., and 11 P.M. to 7:30 A.M. A full-time employee works ten 8-hour shifts in a 2-week period. The start time of 8-hour shifts may vary by organization or by business unit and patient need. For example, Emergency Departments are typically busiest during the evening into the night hours. An 8-hour shift for the ED may be 7 P.M. to 3 A.M. to cover the peak activity times. Once you have determined what numbers of staff are necessary, it is important to attempt to schedule staff in a way to meet their needs. Some prefer to work long stretches to have several days off in a row. Others prefer to work short stretches.

New Options in Staffing Patterns. As the nursing shortage deepens, there will be an increasing need to develop schedules that meet the needs of both the patients and the worker. In recent years there have been more new options in scheduling to meet both of these needs. Twelve-hour shifts have become very popular across the country. In many organizations, employees can work 35 hours per week and get full-time benefits. In this situation, a nurse could work three 12-hour shifts per week and have 4 days off and be full time. Another popular option is weekend programs. Weekend program staff work two 12-hour shifts every weekend and are paid a rate that would make the 24 hours of work equal to 40 hours of work during the week. Some of these programs

include full-time benefits as well. The purpose of this kind of program is to improve weekend staffing and allow full-time staff members who usually work 26 weekends a year to work fewer weekends for staff retention purposes.

Impact on Patient Care. Any time you implement a scheduling plan, it is critical to assess what the effect will be on the care of patients. For example, workweeks made up of three 12-hour shifts have in many units disrupted continuity of care. This is especially true when the 12-hour shifts are not scheduled together. To mediate this impact, 12-hour staff can be paired so that the patient has the same pair of nurses every day for 3 days, and then the patient can be transitioned to a new pair of 12-hour staff. Units that have short patient lengths of stay may have fewer continuity problems than units with longer lengths of stay. When implementing weekend programs, you must ensure that there are always staff scheduled who are familiar with the patients and the events that have transpired previously.

Financial Implications. New staffing patterns or program changes may have significant financial implications. Because of the nursing shortage, there are a number of new programs being put into place to recruit staff and encourage staff to work more hours. Weekend programs are more expensive than traditional staffing patterns because of the high rate of hourly pay, but they are a recruitment and retention tool for nursing leadership. For example see the financial impact of the weekend program referred to earlier (Figure 12-8).

To implement a similar program or other new programs, collaboration with the finance and human resources department of the organization is necessary. This collaboration must be used to develop a financial analysis to measure the dollar and human resource impact of the program.

Weekend staff working at $35 an hour × 24 hours = $840 per weekend
Regular staff working at $20 an hour × 24 hours = $480 per weekend
Difference in cost = $360 per weekend

Six weekend staff members at $360 would cost $2,160 more than regular staff per weekend; $2,160 × 52 weekends a year would cost $112,320 more than regular staff annually.

Figure 12-8 Annual Cost of a Weekend Program for One Nursing Unit

Self-Scheduling

Self-scheduling is a process in which staff on a unit collectively decide and implement the monthly work schedule (Dearholt & Feathers, 1997). One of the issues that drives nurses from their place of employment is scheduling (Hill-Popper, 2000). Self-scheduling has been implemented to boost staff morale by increasing staff control over their work environment through self-governance activities (Dearholt & Feathers, 1997). It provides opportunities for staff to increase communication among themselves and promotes empowerment and professional growth. This form of scheduling provides maximum flexibility for staff and serves to increase their sense of ownership and shared responsibility in ensuring that their respec-

tive work areas are adequately staffed (Shullanberger, 2000). To ensure that patient care needs are met, there must be structure to a self-scheduling program.

Boundaries of Self-Scheduling. To implement self-scheduling, responsibilities and boundaries need to be established that clearly state expectations of staff. This is best done by a unit committee, made up of staff, that reports to the nurse manager. It is important to spell out the roles and responsibilities of all—the unit-based committee, the chairperson if there is one, the staff, and the manager. Generic boundaries need to be established regarding fairness, fiscal responsibility, evaluation of the self-scheduling process, and the approval process. Table 12-1 spells

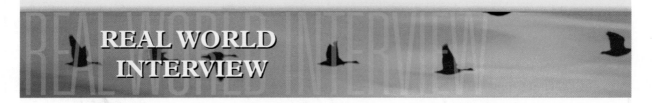

REAL WORLD INTERVIEW

As a manager of an intensive care unit, I can say that self-scheduling has greatly increased my staff's satisfaction with their schedules. I think the biggest factor in the success of our process was the initial buy-in from the staff. Before implementing, staff were surveyed to assess their commitment to making the process work. I was looking for 60% to 75% staff buy-in before implementation and found greater than 70%. A second critical factor was having clear guidelines for the process. These included time lines for how and when staff can sign up for time and how time off is prioritized.

During implementation, we learned many things. One key factor was that staff needed to have confrontation and negotiation skills in order for this process to work. Inevitably there were situations when someone had to change their schedule. When confrontation and negotiation didn't take place, there were periods of short staffing and patient care needs not being met. We also learned that this is a time-consuming process. It takes about 16 hours per month for the self-scheduling committee to put the schedule together.

Another key element I found was the manager had to maintain accountability for staffing. I meet with the scheduling committee regularly and oversee the orientation of new staff to the self-scheduling process. I sign off on every schedule to ensure that the schedule maintains appropriate staffing levels at all times. I found that I needed to identify trends that may be affecting staffing and assist the staff in addressing the trends. I also work with the staff on the implementation of any new program that affects the schedule. The weekend program is a good example of this. I worked with the staff to ensure there were appropriate guidelines for staff receiving a reduced weekend commitment. And finally, the most important role I play is to be very clear about the expectations for all—the committee, the staff, and myself. This scheduling process has been one of the most positive quality of worklife efforts for my staff.

Rob Rose, BSN, MSN
Nurse Manager, Cardiopulmonary Surgery Intensive Care Unit

out specific issues that must be addressed. During the self-scheduling process, the unit staff should be included and educated as to the guidelines as they are being developed. For this process to be successful, all staff members must understand the process, their responsibilities, and the effect of their decisions on staffing. All personnel must also be committed to providing safe staffing on all shifts for their patients.

EVALUATION OF STAFFING EFFECTIVENESS

Many patient outcomes are driven by the available hours of care delivered and the competence of staff

delivering the care. The nurse manager and the organizational nurse leader have the ongoing responsibility to monitor the effectiveness of the staffing pattern. To ensure objectivity, staffing outcomes must be delineated, measured, and reviewed.

Patient Outcomes and Nurse Staffing

The American Nurses Association (Lichtig, Knaug, Rison-McCoy, & Wozniak, 2000) commissioned two studies to determine whether there was a relationship between nurse staffing and patient outcomes. The results of these studies did confirm there is a relationship. Specifically, one study found five patient outcomes showing a consistent significant relationship

TABLE 12-1 *Issues to Be Spelled Out in Self-Scheduling Guidelines*

1. Scheduling period: Is the scheduling period 2-, 4-, or 6-week intervals?
2. Schedule time line: What are the time frames for staff to sign up for regular work commitment, special requests, overtime, and per diem workers?
3. Staffing pattern: Will 8- or 12-hour shifts be used?
4. Weekends: Are staff expected to work every other weekend? If there are extra weekends available, how are they distributed?
5. Holidays: How are they allocated?
6. Vacation time: Are there restrictions on the amount of vacation during certain periods?
7. Unit vacation practices: How many staff from one shift can be on vacation at any time?
8. Requests for time off: What is the process for requesting time off?
9. Short-staffed shifts: How are shifts that are short staffed handled?
10. On call, if applicable: How do staff get assigned or sign up for on call time?
11. Cancellation guidelines: How and when do staff get canceled for scheduled time if they are not needed?
12. Sick calls: What are the expectations for calling in sick, and how are these shifts covered?
13. Military/National Guard leave: What kind of advance notice is required?
14. Schedule changes: What is the process for changing one's schedule after the schedule has been approved?
15. Shifts defined: What are the beginning and endings of available shifts?
16. Committee time: When does the self-scheduling committee meet and for how long?
17. Seniority: How does it play into staffing and request decisions?
18. Staffing plan for crisis/emergency situations: What is the plan when staffing is inadequate?

with nurse staffing. The outcomes found to be affected by nurse staffing are length of stay and incidence of pneumonia, postoperative infections, pressure ulcers, and urinary tract infections. These outcomes are negatively affected when nurse staffing or the skill mix is inadequate. Tracking these outcomes over time will give you data to judge whether your staffing pattern is adequate or inadequate.

Nurse Staffing and Nurse Outcomes

In the previous section, we reviewed outcome measures for patients directly affected by staffing. In addition to patient outcomes, nurse outcomes should also be measured. Your staff's perception of the adequacy of staffing should be tracked. There should be the

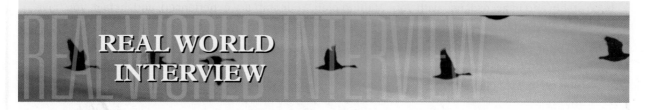

REAL WORLD INTERVIEW

We have developed a nursing practice quality scorecard. The scorecard is a tool to display data on our three organizational priorities: mission, customer orientation, and cost-effectiveness. By looking at measures in all three arenas, we can see how we are doing in these areas. We also can see if changes made in one arena positively or negatively affect the other measures. To look at nursing's mission for nursing practice, we track and trend several of the American Nurses Association national indicators. We track medication errors, patient falls, restraints, nosocomial pressure ulcers, and urinary tract infections. For customer satisfaction, we measure overall satisfaction with nursing care provided and how well patients' pain was controlled. For cost-effectiveness, we track nursing hours per patient day. All of these measures are tracked and trended on control charts every 3 months. The specific data is trended, and measures that are greater than 2 standard deviations of the target are identified as potential points to be reviewed for identification of opportunities for improvement.

One of the areas we chose to target for improvement was medication errors. It became evident that the most prominent reason for medication errors was delayed and omitted medications. Further investigation proved that the procedures for obtaining medications were unclear and outdated. We have written new procedures to specify responsibilities of the nursing staff and the pharmacy staff. We are now monitoring our rate of medication errors to see if our changes have made any improvement in the error rate.

Another example of use of the scorecard was in review of our pressure ulcer rate. We found there was an increase in the incidence of pressure ulcers in October 2000.

In review of causes, we found that the reporting system had been revised to include all stages of skin breakdown. Since the reporting change, we have seen an increase in the number of pressure ulcers reported. This is a positive change as we now have accurate data on which to target our improvement efforts.

Lessons that we have learned in the development of the scorecard is that we needed to set improvement targets earlier in the process to push the search for opportunities for improvement. We also learned that many of these measures are not well defined and therefore benchmarking to other organizations is difficult. We continue to strive for further improvement and utilize the scorecard to measure our success and look for opportunities for improvement. Reviewing nursing outcome data for the entire nursing division has been a powerful tool to ensure that care provided is meeting expected outcomes, and it allows us to benchmark our outcomes to other organizations.

Louann Villani, RN, BSN
Nursing Quality Specialist

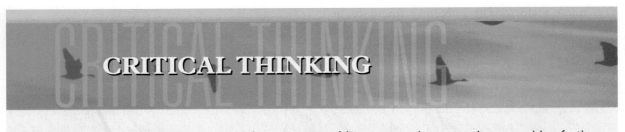

CRITICAL THINKING

Recently, you have been able to access data on your unit's pressure ulcer rates. In researching further, you uncover that your unit's rates are significantly higher than those of other units. Your staffing has been stable and in accordance with your staffing plan. Your staff are experienced, and, in fact, you have the longest tenured staff in the hospital.

Why are your pressure ulcer rates higher than other units? What would you do?

ability for staff to communicate both in written and verbal form regarding staffing concerns. Nurses have the obligation to report to their supervisor their concerns regarding staffing, and every manager has the responsibility to follow up on staffing issues identified by staff. Formalizing this communication process says that you take the issues seriously and gives you data to act on. In addition, actual staffing compared to recommended staffing should be tracked. This will identify changes in patient acuity and give you clues to other staffing issues. Medication errors is another measure that has been linked with inadequate NHPPD. When resources are scarce, data are imperative to drive needed changes. The outcomes of ineffective staffing patterns and nursing care can be devastating to both patients and staff.

MODELS OF CARE DELIVERY

To ensure that nursing care is provided to patients, the work must be organized. A care delivery model organizes the work of caring for patients. Over the history of nursing, there have been many models of care delivery. The decision of which care delivery model is used is based on the needs of the patients and the availability of competent staff in the different skill levels. The model of care delivery utilized is often determined by the nurse leader and applied across an organization. Managers have the responsibility to implement models and evaluate the outcomes in their area. Staff have the responsibility to engage in the implementation and evaluation process. Each model has strengths and weaknesses that should be considered when deciding which to implement. Several different care delivery models are explored in the following sections.

Case Method

The case method is the oldest model for nursing care delivery. As nurse training programs began to turn out educated nurses, these nurse were found working in the homes of the sick, taking care of one individual patient. In this model of care, the nurse has one patient that he cares for exclusively. Total patient care is the modern-day version of the case method.

Total Patient Care

In total patient care, the nurse is responsible for the total care for her patient assignment for the shift she is working. The RN has several patients that she is responsible for. She may have some support from LPNs or UAP, but they are not assigned to a specific group of patients. The RN's patient assignment may change from day to day.

Advantages and Disadvantages

The advantage of total patient care and the case method for the patient is the consistency of one individual caring for patients for an entire shift. This enables the patient, nurse, and family to develop a relationship based on trust. This model provides a higher number of RN hours of care than other models. The nurse has more opportunity to observe and monitor progress of the patient. A disadvantage may be that the nurse may not have the same patients from day to day and therefore looks at the patient on a shift-by-shift basis rather than on a continuum of care. Another disadvantage is that these models utilize a high level of RN nursing hours to deliver care, and, in most cases, this level of RN intensity is not warranted. These models of care delivery are more costly than other models of delivery.

Functional Nursing

This model of care delivery became popular during World War II when there was a significant shortage of nurses in the United States. This method allowed LPNs and UAP to take on tasks that were previously carried out by the RN in the case method. **Functional nursing** divides the nursing work into functional units that are then assigned to one of the team members. In this model, each care provider has specific duties or tasks they are responsible for. For instance, a typical division of labor for RNs is medication nurse or admission nurse and so on. Decision making is usually at the level of the head nurse or charge nurse (Figure 12-9).

Advantages and Disadvantages

In this model, care can be delivered to a large number of patients. This system utilizes other types of health care workers when there is a shortage of RNs. Patients are likely to have care delivered to them in one shift by several staff members. To a patient, care may feel disjointed. A risk of this model is that patients become the sum of the tasks of care they require rather than an integrated whole.

Team Nursing

During World War II, multilevel training programs were developed to teach auxiliary personnel how to perform simple care and technical procedures. In the military, these trained workers were called corpsmen. Outside of the military, there were 1-year programs developed to teach technical nursing care. On-the-job training programs were established to produce what would today be called nursing assistants. The model of team nursing was developed after the war in an effort to utilize these trained workers and to ease the shortage of nurses that most hospitals were experiencing.

Team nursing is a care delivery model that assigns staff to teams that then are responsible for a group of patients. A unit may be divided into two teams, and each team is led by a registered nurse. The team leader supervises and coordinates all the care provided by those on his team. The team is most commonly made up of LPNs and UAP, but occasionally there is another RN. Care is divided up into the simplest components and then assigned to the appropriate care provider. In addition to supervision duties, the team leader also is responsible for provid-

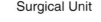

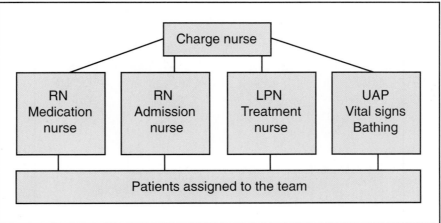

Figure 12-9 Functional Nursing Model

ing professional direction to those on his team regarding the care provided (Figure 12-10).

A **modular nursing** delivery system is a kind of team nursing that divides a geographic space into modules of patients, with each module cared for by a team of staff led by an RN. The modules may vary in size, but typically there is one RN with an LPN and nursing assistant to make up the team. In this case, the RN is responsible for the overall care of the patients in her module.

Advantages and Disadvantages

In team nursing and modular nursing, the RN is able to get work done through others, but patients often receive fragmented, depersonalized care. Communication in these models is complex. There is shared responsibility and accountability, which can cause confusion and lack of accountability. These factors contribute to RN dissatisfaction with these models. These models require the RN to have very good delegation and supervision skills.

Primary Nursing

Primary nursing is a care delivery model that clearly delineates the responsibility and accountability of the RN and designates the RN as the primary provider of care to patients. Primary nursing is a form of the case model that consists of four elements. These are allocation and acceptance of individual responsibility for the decision making to one individual; assignments of daily care by the case method; direct person-to-person communication; and one person operationally responsible for the quality of care administered to patients on a unit 24 hours a day, 7 days a week (Manthey, 1980). Patients are assigned a primary nurse, who is responsible for developing with the patient a plan of care that is followed by other nurses caring for the patient. Nurses and patients are matched according to needs and abilities. Patients are assigned to their primary nurse regardless of unit geographic considerations. In the primary nursing model, the role of the head nurse changes to one of leader by empowering the staff RNs to be knowledgeable about their patients and to direct the care of their primary patients. The primary nurse has the authority, accountability, and responsibility to provide care for a group of patients. There are associate nurses who care for the patient when the primary nurse is not working. There will be several associate nurses for each patient (Figure 12-11).

Advantages and Disadvantages

An advantage of this model is that patients and families are able to develop a trusting relationship with

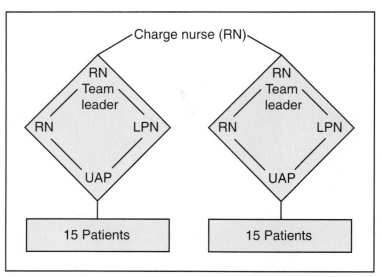

Medical Unit

Figure 12-10 Team Nursing Model

Oncology Unit

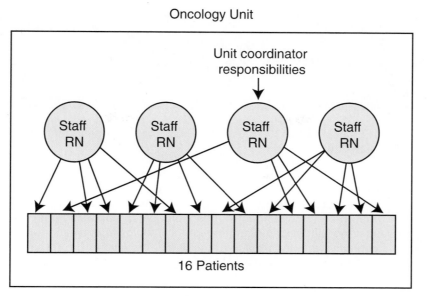

Figure 12-11 Primary Nursing Model

the nurse. There is defined accountability and responsibility for the nurse to develop a plan of care with the patient and family. There is a holistic approach to care, which facilitates continuity of care rather than a shift-to-shift focus. Nurses, when they have adequate time to provide necessary care, find this model professionally rewarding because it gives the authority for decision making to the nurse at the bedside. Disadvantages include a high cost because there is a higher RN skill mix. The person making out the assignments needs to be knowledgeable about all the patients and the staff to ensure appropriate matching of nurse to patient. With no geographical boundaries within the unit, nursing staff may be required to travel long distances at the unit level to care for their primary patients. Nurses often perform functions that could be completed by other staff. And finally, nurse-to-patient ratios must be realistic to ensure there is enough nursing time available to meet the patient care needs.

Patient-Centered or Patient-Focused Care

Patient-centered care or patient-focused care is designed to focus on patient needs rather than staff needs. In this model, required care and services are brought to the patient. In the highest evolution of this model, all patient services are decentralized to the patient area, including radiology and pharmacy services. Staffing is based on patient needs. In this model, there is an effort to have the right person doing the right thing. Care teams are established for a group of patients. The care teams may include other disciplines such as respiratory or physical therapists. In these teams, disciplines collaborate to ensure that patients receive the care they need. Staff are kept close to the patients in decentralized work stations. For example, on a rehabilitation unit, physical therapists may be members of the care team and work at the unit level rather than in a centralized physical therapy department (Figure 12-12).

Advantages and Disadvantages

The pros of the system are that it is most convenient for patients and expedites services to patients. But it can be extremely costly to decentralize major services in an organization. A second disadvantage is that some staff have perceived the model as a way of reducing RNs and cutting costs in hospitals. In fact, this has been true in some organizations, but many other organizations have successfully used the patient-centered model to have the right staff available for the needs of the patient population.

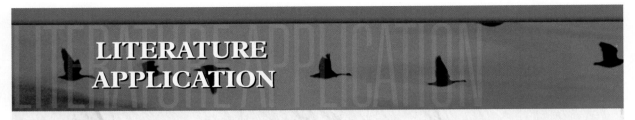

LITERATURE APPLICATION

Citation: Aiken, L. H., Sloane, D. M., & Sochalski, J. (1998). Hospital organization and outcomes. *Quality in Healthcare, 7*(4), 222–226.

Discussion: This was a comparative study of patient outcomes, nurse outcomes, and organizational variables. Thirty-nine magnet hospitals were each compared to five hospitals that most closely resembled the attributes of the respective magnet hospital. In the study, magnet hospitals had significantly lower mortality rates than their matched control hospitals. When nurse staffing was used as a variable, the magnet hospital mortality was no longer significantly lower, indicating that lower mortality rates in the magnet hospitals were not a result of nurse staffing levels. The researchers then looked at other organizational attributes and found that both nurse and patient outcomes were better in units in which nurses had autonomy in decision making, control over practice, and good relations with physicians.

Implications for Practice: This research showed that outcomes for both patients and staff are not driven solely by staffing levels. The organizational structure in which nurses work also has a significant effect on the nurses' ability to care for patients and their satisfaction with the work environment. Managers must ensure there is appropriate staffing, but the organizational structure and care delivery model that support nurse autonomy, control over practice, and good physician relationships are powerful variables that contribute to positive outcomes for both patients and staff.

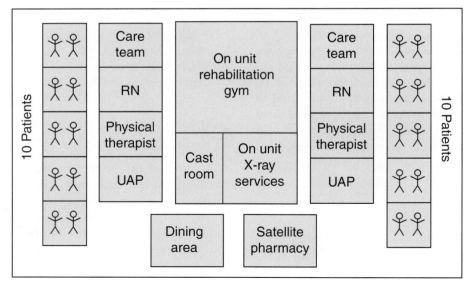

Figure 12-12 Patient-Centered Care Model

Differentiated Practice

Differentiated nursing practice is a care delivery model that sorts the roles, functions, and work of registered nurses according to some identified criteria, commonly education, clinical experience, and competence (Baker et al., 1997). This model of care delivery emerged in the mid-1980s as a way of articulating the difference in practice of RNs. Educational preparation is grouped into associate degree in nursing (ADN), bachelor of science in nursing (BSN), and master of science in nursing (MSN) as a hierarchy. Nursing competencies are generally measured in three arenas: technical skills, communication skills, and management of care or leadership skills. Pilot implementation projects have shown some positive outcomes from this model. To illustrate how this model works, review the Real World Interview below.

Advantages and Disadvantages

Differentiated practice allows nurses to work in specialized roles for which they were educated, leading to greater career satisfaction, and provides appropriate recognition and rewards across the continuum of nurses' care ("Differentiated nursing practice in all

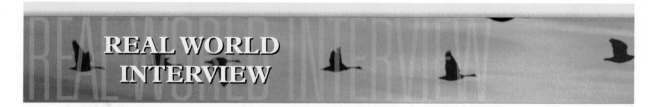

REAL WORLD INTERVIEW

In our organization, we have implemented a model of differentiated practice. Our purpose was to match individual competencies with job descriptions to maximize an individual's skills. In our model, there is one staff nurse title, but there are job descriptions and performance expectations based on the nurse's level of education, associate degree, bachelor's degree, or master's degree. Pay is based on level of education and performance. Performance expectations were developed for each education level and organized using the nursing process as a framework. The nursing process statements for each level of education reflect nursing practice from novice to expert. In this model, all nurses may participate in activities like discharge planning, but the performance expectations for a master's-prepared nurse would be different than for a diploma-prepared nurse. Each nurse has an individual performance plan that assists the nurse to meet established performance expectations and to develop and meet individual goals. This performance plan is developed annually by the staff nurse with their nurse manager.

The outcomes of this model have been improved job satisfaction and reduced turnover of the nursing staff. We have noted that more staff have engaged in formal education and are accessing educational opportunities within the organization. Some of the lessons we learned were that we had to look at people as individuals. Staff did not fit into neat categories. We learned that there was fear among the nursing administrative ranks regarding how the staff would react to a differentiated practice model. In reality, the staff accepted the model and the message that everyone has value and brings different skills to the workplace. The goal of the model was to maximize those two things. In communicating to the staff, hierarchy of any sort in the model was minimized.

In retrospect, I would spend more time up front with the managers and other leadership staff. It is key that leadership staff have a complete understanding of the model, how to communicate the key elements of the model, and how to implement the model at the unit level. Even though this was a significant culture change for our organization, the outcomes for the staff have been positive and well worth the efforts put forth.

Kathleen Brodbeck, RN, MSN
Vice President for Patient Care

care settings" 1995). A disadvantage is that nurses who have gained experience and who have the knowledge and capability to function beyond their original education may not be recognized. These staff may be disenfranchised by a model that does not factor in the learning that takes place outside of the academic setting. In addition, organizations that have established minimal educational requirements for RN positions may have difficulty recruiting staff with the requisite credentials.

Patient Care Redesign

In the 1990s, there was significant pressure to reduce health care costs. Hospitals bore the brunt of this pressure. During this decade, patient care redesign was an initiative to redesign how patient care was delivered. Those organizations that undertook redesign with the mission to maintain or improve quality of care while reducing costs had better outcomes than organizations that redesigned with the intent to reduce costs alone. In organizations looking only to reduce costs, unlicensed assistive personal were hired and trained to assist the registered nurses without review of the RN care required. Unfortunately, in many cases, the RN hours of care available did not match the patient need for RN hours and resulted in many frustrated nurses and patients. Nurse leaders must be responsible when implementing a care delivery model. The care delivery model has enormous effect on the care that patients receive, the satisfaction of patients and staff, and the cost to the organization.

CARE DELIVERY MANAGEMENT TOOLS

In the 1980s and 1990s, there were initiatives to improve care and reduce costs, many of which had positive effects. In 1983, the federal government established diagnostic-related groups (DRGs) as a payment system for hospitals. In DRGs, the national average length of stay (LOS) for a specific patient type was used to determine payment for that grouping of patients. LOS refers to the number of days a patient is hospitalized from day of admission to day of discharge. In DRGs, all hospitals were paid the same amount for caring for a DRG patient group regardless of the LOS of the specific patient. This

prompted initiatives in hospitals to reduce LOS and reduce hospital costs. Hospitals were able to benchmark their LOS for specific patient populations against a national database published through the Medicare DRG system. As hospitals looked for opportunities to reduce costs through reduction in the LOS, clinical pathways and case management surfaced as significant strategies.

Clinical Pathways

Clinical pathways were a major initiative to come out of the efforts to reduce LOS and are widely used to enhance outcomes and contain costs within a constrained length of stay (Lagoe, 1998). Clinical pathways are care management tools that outline the expected clinical course and outcomes for a specific patient type. Clinical pathways take a different form in each organization that develops them. Typically they are pathways that outline the normal course of care for a patient. Pathways are often done by day, and for each day expected outcomes are articulated. It is the expected outcomes that patient progress is measured against. In some facilities, pathways have physician orders incorporated into the pathway to facilitate care. In some organizations, the pathways include multidisciplinary orders for care, including orders from nursing, medicine, and other allied health professionals such as physical therapy and dietary services. This serves to further expedite care for patients. Figure 12-13 provides an excerpt from a clinical pathway that identifies expected outcomes.

These pathways can be used by physicians, nurses, and case managers to care for the patient and measure the patient's progress against expected outcomes. Any variance in outcome can then be noted and acted upon to get the patient back on track. Some organizations have up to 60 pathways implemented.

Advantages and Disadvantages

By articulating the normal course of care for a patient population, clinical pathways are a powerful tool for managing care. They are very instructive for new staff, and they save a significant amount of time in the process of care. In most cases, the implementation of a clinical pathway will improve care and shorten the length of stay for the population on the

Clinical Pathway: Lower Extremity Revascularization
Page 21 of 22

ADDRESSOGRAPH

DAILY ANTICIPATED OUTCOMES

POD2	Date/Time /Init When met	POD3	Date/Time /Init When met	POD4	Date/Time /Init When met	POD5	Date/Time /Init When met
Patient rates pain 0-2 on pain scale 0-10 using po analgesia.		Graft signal present with doppler		Graft signal present with doppler		Graft signal present with doppler	
Graft signal present with doppler.		Incisional edges will be approximated without drainage.		Able to participate in self-care and adjunct therapies.		Ambulates independently	
Patient will verbalize knowledge of plan of care, testing and treatment.		Site of invasive devices without signs of infection.		Patient viewed diet video.		Patient/significant other will verbalize understanding of activity/diet restrictions, medication use, wound management.	
Ambulate in hall Q I D		Ambulates in hall qid.				Completed nutrition post test.	
Tolerates po solids		Patient/significant other will describe appropriate problem solving skills to decrease anxiety.					
Voiding without difficulty		Rehab referral started: _yes _no					
		Family support available at discharge, specify _____ _____					

TO BE KEPT IN PROGRESS NOTE SECTION OF CHART AT ALL TIMES.

Figure 12-13 Example of a Clinical Pathway (Excerpt) (Courtesy of Albany Medical Center, Albany, NY)

pathway. Pathways also allow for data collection of variances to the pathway. The data can then be used to look for opportunities for improvement in hospital systems and in clinical practice.

An issue with development of pathways is that some physicians perceive pathways to be cookbook medicine and are reluctant to participate in their development. Physician participation is critical.

Development of multidisciplinary pathways also requires a significant amount of work to gain consensus from the various disciplines on the expected plan of care. For patient populations that are non-standard, pathways are less effective because the pathway is constantly being modified to reflect the individual patient's needs.

Case Management

Case management is a second strategy to improve patient care and reduce hospital costs through coor-dination of care. Typically a case manager is responsible for coordinating care and establishing goals from preadmission through discharge (Del Togno-Armanasco, Hopkin, & Harter, 1995). In the typical model of case management, a nurse is assigned to a specific high-risk patient population or service, such as cardiac surgery patients. The case manager has the responsibility to work with all disciplines to facilitate care. For example, if a postsurgical hospitalized patient has not met ambulation goals according to the clinical pathway, the case manager would work with the physician and nurse to determine what is

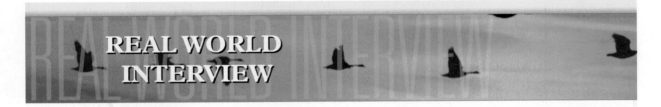

REAL WORLD INTERVIEW

In my role as a case manager, I work exclusively with the pediatric population at our hospital. I facilitate the care of patients while they are in the hospital and plan for their home care needs. Our main goal is to ensure that there is a safe transition between hospital and home. As an example of how this goal is achieved, we have met with the cardiac surgery patients and families prior to surgery to identify and proactively address insurance, equipment, or other issues that may arise during hospitalization and at discharge. We have found that patients, families, and staff find our function very helpful. For the staff RN, case managers take on the burden of complex discharge planning, which is enormously time consuming. Patients and families find it comforting to know there is someone who can help them plan for postdischarge.

As the pediatric case manager, I meet with the social worker and the RN staff on the pediatric unit weekly to go over each patient and their specific discharge and social work needs. We have found the work of the case managers and social workers to be complementary, and working together allows us to both have more information and help the patient get through our system more efficiently. All of these functions help to reduce the patient's length of stay.

As case managers, we also perform some utilization management functions for our organization. We review admission charts, assessing for evidence of meeting admission criteria that the patient's insurer will accept. In addition, we review charts daily to ensure that the patient's acuity warrants continued hospitalization. On occasion, we have to inform the patient and family that the patient's stay is no longer covered by their insurance and they will be responsible for paying the remaining portion of their hospital bill. This can be a difficult situation, and we sometimes get caught between the patient and the patient's insurer. In these cases, we sometimes refer the patients back to their insurer and sometimes we advocate for the patient to have their continued hospital stay approved.

As a case manager, I find that my diverse clinical background has enabled me to better anticipate the patient's clinical course and be proactive to support the patient's needs. This is a role that is supportive of patients, families, and staff and one I find very challenging and rewarding.

Linda Zeoli, RN
Pediatric Case Manager

preventing the patient from achieving this goal. If it turns out that the patient is elderly and is slow to recover, they may agree that physical therapy would be beneficial to assist this patient in ambulating. In other models, the case management function is provided by the staff nurse at the bedside. This works well if the population requires little case management, but if the patient population requires significant case management services, there needs to be enough RN time allocated for this activity. In addition to facilitating care, the case manager usually has a data function to improve care. In this role, the case manager collects aggregate data on patient variances from the clinical pathway. The data are shared with the responsible physicians and other disciplines that participate in the clinical pathway and are then used to explore opportunities for improvement in the pathway or in hospital systems.

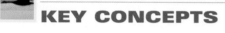

KEY CONCEPTS

- To plan nurse staffing, you must understand and apply the concepts of full-time equivalents (FTEs) and nursing hours per patient day (NHPPD).
- Patient classification systems predict nursing time required for a specific patient and then whole groups of patients; the data can then be utilized for staffing, budgeting, and benchmarking.
- Determination of the number of FTEs needed to staff a unit requires review of patient classification data, NHPPD, regulatory requirements, skill mix, staff support, historical information, and the physical environment of the unit.
- The number of staff and patients in your staffing pattern drives the amount of nursing time available for patient care.
- In developing a staffing pattern, additional FTEs must be added to a nursing unit budget to provide coverage for days off and benefited time off.
- Scheduling of staff is the responsibility of the nurse manager, who must take into consideration patient need and intensity, volume of patients, and the experience of the staff.
- Whatever staffing variations are chosen, it is critical to assess the effect on patient care and finances.
- Self-scheduling can increase staff morale and professional growth but to be successful requires clear boundaries and guidelines.

- Evaluating the outcomes of your staffing plan on patients, staff, and the organization is a critical activity that should be done daily, monthly, and annually.
- Case management and clinical pathways are care management tools that have been developed to improve patient care and reduce hospital costs.

KEY TERMS

benchmarking	nursing hours per
care delivery model	patient day
case management	patient acuity
clinical pathway	patient care redesign
diagnostic-related groups	patient-centered care
differentiated nursing	patient classification
practice	system
direct care	patient-focused care
episodic care unit	primary nursing
full-time equivalent	productive hours
functional nursing	self-scheduling
indirect care	skill mix
inpatient unit	staffing pattern
modular nursing	team nursing
nonproductive hours	total patient care

REVIEW QUESTIONS

1. Patient classification systems measure nursing workload needed by the patient. The higher the patient's acuity, the more care that is required by the patient. Which of the following statements is a weakness of classification systems?
   A. Patient classification data are useful in predicting the required staffing for the next shift and for justifying nursing hours provided.
   B. Patient classification data can be utilized by the nurse making assignments to determine what level of care a patient requires.
   C. Classification systems typically focus on nursing tasks rather than a holistic view of a patient's needs.
   D. Aggregate patient classification data are useful in costing out nursing services and for developing the nursing budget.

2. To determine the number of FTEs required for a renal transplant unit, you must review all but which of the following?
   A. Regulatory requirements from your regional, state, and federal governments
   B. The patient population care needs and the impact on your skill mix
   C. Organizational structure or supports in place to enable care providers to care for patients
   D. The chief financial officer's opinion on the number of staff needed for your unit

3. In calculating the number of FTEs needed to staff your medical-surgical unit, you must provide additional FTEs for all but which of the following?
   A. Benefited time off such as vacation and sick time
   B. Educational time for staff, including orientation of new staff
   C. Indirect patient care staff that support the operation of the direct care staff 24 hours a day
   D. Coverage for other departments that do not staff to cover their own benefited time off

4. If your RN staff members receive 4 weeks of vacation and 10 days of sick time per year, how many productive hours would each RN work in that year if they utilized all of their benefited time?
   A. 2,080 productive hours
   B. 1,840 productive hours
   C. 1,920 productive hours
   D. 1,780 productive hours

5. In building your staffing plan, which of the following would NOT be a major consideration for determining how many staff you need each day and shift?
   A. The need for your staff to have more weekends off
   B. The volume of patients that you have at different times of the day
   C. The timing and volume of nurse-intensive activities such as administration of chemotherapy and blood
   D. The skill mix of your staff and the patient care requirements throughout a 24-hour period

6. Patient outcomes are the result of many variables, one being the model of care delivery that is utilized. From the following scenarios, select which is the worst fit between patient need and care delivery model.
   A. Cancer patients cared for in a primary nursing model
   B. Rehabilitation patients cared for in a patient-centered model
   C. Medical intensive care patients being cared for in a team nursing model
   D. Ambulatory surgery patients with a wide range of illnesses being cared for using a differentiated practice model

7. The care management tools of case management and clinical pathways have led to several improvements. Which of the following would NOT be considered an outcome of these care management tools?
   A. Increased public awareness of the nurse's role in health care
   B. Length of stay reductions
   C. Reduced cost of care in many populations
   D. Identification of opportunities for improvement in care or in hospital systems

REVIEW ACTIVITIES

1. How do you know whether the outcomes of your staffing plan are positive? What measures do you have available in your organization that indicate your staffing is adequate or inadequate?

2. You are a nurse manager of a new unit for psychiatric patients. What would you consider in planning for FTEs and staffing for this unit?

3. You are a new nurse and you have increasing concerns regarding the staffing levels on your unit. You are becoming increasingly anxious each time you go to work. What would you do?

EXPLORING THE WEB

- To get more information on mandated staffing levels, go to *http://www.ana.org*. Go to staffing issues on the menu and review the legislative agenda for the ANA regarding staffing. Also review the data on the ANA's latest staff survey.

- To get more information on nursing quality measures, go to *http://www.mriresearch.org/ markets/health/health_serv/nursing.htm.* Review the quality measures.

- To get more information on case management, go to *http://www.casemanagement.com/ casemanager/reference/.* See what resources you can find for a difficult patient for whom you are caring.

REFERENCES

Aiken, L. H., Sloane, D. M., & Sochalski, J. (1998). Hospital organization and outcomes. *Quality in Healthcare, 7*(4), 222–226.

Baker, C. M., Lamm, G. M., Winter, A. R., Robbleloth, V. B., Ransom, C. A., Conly, F., Carpenter, K. C., & McCoy, L. E. (1997). Differentiated nursing practice: Assessing the state-of-the-science. *Nursing Economic$, 15*(5), 253–261.

Buerhaus, P. I. (2000, May/June). Why are shortages of hospital RNs concentrated in specialty care units? *Nursing Economic$, 18*(3), 111–117.

Dearholt, S., & Feathers, C. A.. (1997). Self-scheduling can work. *Nursing Management, 28*(8), 47–48.

Del Togno-Armanasco, V., Hopkin, L. A., & Harter, S. (1995). How case management really works. *American Journal of Nursing, 5,* 24i, 24j, 24l.

Differentiated nursing practice in all care settings. (1995). *Journal of Nursing Administration, 25*(7/8), 5, 6, 11.

Hill-Popper, M. (2000, January). *Reversing the flight of talent.* Symposium at the Nursing Executive Center annual meeting, The Advisory Board Company, Washington DC.

Joint Commission on Accreditation of Healthcare Organizations. (2000). *2000 hospital accreditation standards.* Oakbrook Terrace, IL: Author.

Lagoe, R. J. (1998). Basic statistics for clinical pathway evaluation. *Nursing Economic$, 16*(3), 125–131.

Lichtig, L. K., Knaug, R. A., Rison-McCoy, R., & Wozniak, L. M. (2000). *Nurse staffing and patient outcomes in the inpatient hospital setting.* Washington, DC: American Nurses Association.

Malloch, K., & Conivaloff, A. (1999). Patient classification systems, part 1. *Journal of Nursing Administration, 29*(7/8), 49–56.

Manthey, M. (1980). *The practice of primary nursing.* Boston: Blackwell Scientific.

Shullanberger, G. (2000). Nurse staffing decisions: An integrative review of the literature. *Nursing Economic$, 18*(3), 124–136.

Swansburg, R. C. (1996). *Management and leadership for nurse managers* (2nd ed.). Sudbury, MA: Jones & Bartlett.

SUGGESTED READINGS

A brief history of pathways: From case management plans to care maps. (1998). *Hospital Case Management, 6*(4), 67, 84, 98.

Buckingham, M., & Coffman, C. (1999). *First break all the rules—what the world's greatest managers do differently.* New York: Simon & Schuster.

DeGroot, H. A.. (1994). Patient classification systems and staffing: Part 1, problems and promise. *Journal of Nursing Administration, 24*(9), 43–51.

Delivering care, part 1: Delivery systems. (1996). *Professional Nurse, 11,* 459–463.

Falco, J., Wenzel, K., Quimby, D., & Penny, P. (2000). Moving differentiated practice from concept to reality. *Aspen Advisor for Nurse Executives, 15*(5) 6–9.

Nardone, P. L., Markie, J. W., & Tolle, S. (1995). Evaluating a nursing care delivery model using a quality improvement design. *Journal of Nursing Care Quality, 10*(1), 70–84.

Nelson, J. W. (2000). Consider this . . . Models of nursing care: A century of vacillation. *Journal of Nursing Administration, 30*(4), 156, 184.

Schneider, P. (1998). How do you measure success? *Healthcare Informatics, 15*(3), 44–48.

Scott, K. (1996). Case management: A quality process. *Topics in Health Information Management, 16*(3), 58–64.

Seago, J. A. (1999). Evaluation of hospital work redesign: Patient focused care. *Journal of Nursing Administration, 29*(11), 31–38.

Zander, K. (1996). The early years: The evolution of nursing case management. In D. L. Flarey, et al. (Eds.), *Handbook of nursing case management: Health care delivery in a world of managed care* (pp. 23–45). Gaithersburg, MD: Aspen.

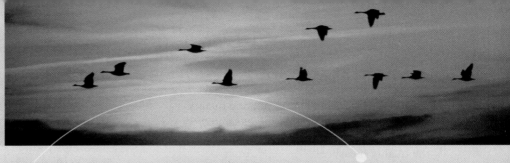

CHAPTER 13

Delegation of Nursing Care

Maureen T. Marthaler, RN, MS

When delegating a task, be sure you're clear on the nursing knowledge components of the task. (Mary Ann Boucher, instructor at Frances Payne Bolton School of Nursing)

OBJECTIVES

Upon completion of this chapter, the reader should be able to:

1. Review the history of delegation.
2. Define delegation, accountability, responsibility, authority, and assignment making.
3. Identify responsibilities the health team members can perform.
4. List the five delegation rights.
5. Identify three potential delegation barriers.
6. List six cultural phenomena that affect transcultural delegation.

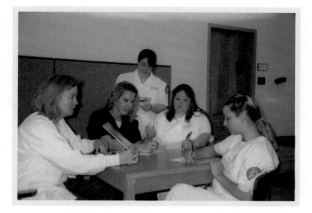

Delegation to the appropriate personnel is an important responsibility in nursing. Inappropriate delegation can be life threatening as in the following instance.

A patient was admitted to the hospital for a shunt placement to divert fluid that had been building up in her cranial vault. Her past history included a shunt insertion 6 months ago. She had surgery and was 2 days postop. She required neurological assessments to be performed at the onset of every shift and whenever necessary as indicated by a change in the patient's condition. The night nurse assessed the patient at the beginning of her shift, noting that the patient's neurologic status was fully intact. During the night, the nurse periodically checked on the patient every 2 hours but did not awaken the patient. A sitter was in the room with the patient. The sitter had assured the nurse that the patient was "doing fine." The sitter did not report that when the patient had been assisted to the bathroom initially, she had no difficulty. Upon assisting the patient a second time, the sitter noted that the patient was leaning to one side so badly that she could not stand and required help from two additional aides.

The change in the patient's condition was not reported to the nurse. The patient ended up with fluid retention in the shunt, resulting in permanent paralysis.

How could this have been prevented?

Who is accountable?

What are the responsibilities of the nurse, the sitter, and the two aides?

How could delegation have been appropriately performed in this situation?

On the National Council of State Boards of Nursing Licensure Examination (NCLEX), a student may often encounter test questions that assess the ability of the nurse to delegate care. Safeguarding patients is a number one patient care priority. To ensure that this responsibility is met, nurses are accountable under the law for care rendered by both themselves and other personnel. Multiple levels of unlicensed assistive personnel (UAP) give care to patients, including nurse aides, nurse technicians, patient care technicians, personal care attendants, unit assistants, nursing assistants, and other nonlicensed personnel. This is part of a response to changes in the structuring of health care delivery. Recent cost containment efforts have resulted in a variety of nurses being placed in new and innovative positions. This often leads UAP to be asked to consider performing duties that may not be within their scope of education and abilities. With increased opportunities to delegate care, nurses will be able to meet the duty of safe, quality care to their patients only by delegating properly. Without delegation skills, nurses caring for patients in today's health care community will not be able to complete the necessary duties, tasks, and responsibilities. They will find themselves stressed and exhausted by the many activities their nursing role requires. An inability to delegate can engender feelings of frustration, poor self-esteem, and lack of control. As nurses develop appropriate delegation skills, they become more productive and enjoy their work more.

PERSPECTIVES ON DELEGATION

As the history of nursing shows, Florence Nightingale had foresight regarding how nurses would function. Nightingale is quoted as saying, "But again, to look at all these things does not mean to do them yourself....But can you not ensure that it is done when not done by yourself" (Ulrich, 1992, p. 38). Thus, delegation in nursing formally was recognized in the 1800s with Nightingale and has continued to evolve as health care delivery models have evolved.

Today, delegation is a must for the new nurse as well as the experienced nurse. Delegating to personnel with different educational levels from a variety of nursing programs requires nurses to be vigilant in ensuring that safety is maintained for the patient.

According to Fisher (2000), delegation of certain tasks helps reduce health care costs by making more efficient use of nursing time and the facility's resources. Efficient delegation of care protects the patient and provides desirable outcomes.

DELEGATION DEFINED

Different organizations and experts define delegation in different ways. The American Association of Critical-Care Nurses (AACN) states that delegation is not a skill that is simply learned in a classroom. It requires a discussion of concerns related to delegation, and then clinical assistance or mentorship in delegation responsibilities. The process also includes discussion of how to handle situations where tasks were not accomplished when delegated (Salmond, 1994). The National Council of State Boards in Nursing (NCSBN) defines delegation as transferring to a competent individual the authority to perform a selected nursing task in a selected situation. The nurse retains accountability for the delegation (NCSBN, 1995).

All delegation involves at least two individuals as well as specifying duties to be accomplished with or through others via a transfer of authority. The authority has to be delegated along with the ability to direct others. To be effective in accomplishing goals, the individual delegating must take on the leadership role. With successful delegation, the patient's personal health needs are addressed and the nurse's professional goals are achieved. Communication techniques facilitate the delegation process for the registered nurse.

It is frustrating for registered nurses to have to accomplish all of their duties single-handedly. Many new graduate nurses become overwhelmed by the large number of duties to be learned and implemented. In nursing school, students typically perform total patient care for one or two patients. Students might occasionally ask another student to help them, or perhaps they might pitch in to help others on their unit. Rarely will they have the opportunity to delegate to another nurse or UAP. So it can be a shock to new nurses that delegation is now an expected part of their behavior. It is required in the health care setting, and the NCLEX also tests them on it.

Delegation is not meant to intimidate or isolate the new nurse. The sole purpose of delegation is to get the job done in the most efficient way utilizing appropriate resources. The job must be delegated to personnel who can handle it and who understand what the goal is. Delegation can be done to spark interest and prevent personnel from becoming bored, nonproductive, and ineffective. Finding the duties or tasks that best suit the personnel can help them feel as if they are part of the team, regardless of their position. Personnel want to feel they are making a difference in the well-being of the patient, whether through a bath, medications, or even a simple smile. To delegate, the nurse takes into account the personnel's personal and professional position within the health care team, including their ability, education, and experience as well as the patient's needs. Infection control and patient safety are high priorities in making assignments. The NCSBN developed a Delegation Decision-Making Grid that is available at its web site: *www.ncsbn.org/public/res/UAP/delegationgrid.pdf.*

ACCOUNTABILITY AND RESPONSIBILITY

The nurse is legally liable for her actions and is answerable for the overall nursing care of her patients. This is the definition of accountability. An RN is accountable for her actions and related consequences, including the initiation and follow-through of the nursing process. Nurses are also accountable for following their state nurse practice act, standards of professional practice, the policies of their health care organization, and ethical-legal models of behavior. RNs are accountable for monitoring changes in a patient's status, noting and implementing treatment for human responses to illness, and assisting in the prevention of complications. As stated by the AACN in 1995, nursing tasks that do not involve direct patient care can be reassigned more freely and carry fewer legal implications for registered nurses than delegation of direct nursing practice activities. The assessment, analysis, diagnosis, planning, teaching, and evaluation stages of the nursing process may not be delegated to UAP. Delegated activities usually fall within the implementation phase of the nursing process.

Responsibility involves reliability, dependability, and the obligation to accomplish work. Responsibility also includes each person's obligation to perform at an acceptable level—the level to which the person has been educated. For example, a nurse aide is expected to provide the patient with a bed bath. She does not administer pain medication or perform invasive or sterile procedures. After the nurse aide performs the assigned duties, she provides feedback to the nurse about the performance of the duties and the outcome of her actions. This feedback is given to the nurse within a specified time frame.

Note that feedback works two ways. It is also the registered nurse's responsibility to follow up with ongoing supervision and evaluation of activities performed by nonnursing personnel. The nurse transfers responsibility and authority for the completion of a delegated task, but the nurse retains accountability for the delegation process. Whenever nursing activities are delegated, the RN is to follow federal regulations, state nursing practice acts, state boards of nursing rules and regulations, and the standards of the hospital.

AUTHORITY

The responsibility to delegate duties and give direction to UAP places the RN in a position of authority. Authority occurs when a person who has been given the right to delegate, based on the state nurse practice act, also has the official power from an agency to delegate. According to Ellis and Hartley (2000), the concept of authority is often associated with power because authority given by an agency legitimizes the right of a manager or supervisor to give direction to others and expect that they will comply. The best working environment is one in which the personnel view authority with respect.

ASSIGNMENT MAKING

Assignment making is the process of delegating the duties and all aspects of care for a patient to individual personnel. It includes giving clear, concise directions and delegating the responsibility and the authority for the performance of the care. The RN retains accountability for the assignment. It is necessary to ensure that the education, skill, knowledge, and judgment levels of the personnel being assigned to a task are commensurate with the assignment. For example, administration of intravenous solutions to patients on a nursing unit would initially best be assigned to an RN who has received education about intravenous solutions and who has been performing these duties on a regular basis rather than to someone who has little or no experience in administering intravenous solutions. When an assignment is made, the RN should specify the expected outcome of the assignment, the time frame for completion, and any limitations on the assignment.

RESPONSIBILITIES OF HEALTH TEAM MEMBERS

The new graduate nurse may feel overwhelmed by the amount of patient care required and the lack of time to complete the care. The new graduate may be consumed by feelings of inadequacy and failure. Thoughts of not knowing how to answer the phone or find a washcloth, as well as not finding time to eat lunch, can be exhausting. All of these feelings and behaviors may be a result of trying to do it all and not asking for help. New graduate nurses may quickly realize that if they do not delegate, the patient's care will not be completed in a timely and effective manner.

The AACN (1990) suggests five factors that must be considered when delegating patient care:

1. Potential for harm to the patient
2. Complexity of the nursing activity
3. Extent of problem solving and innovation required
4. Predictability of outcome
5. Extent of interaction

Attention to these five factors will improve nursing delegation.

Nurse Manager Responsibility

The nursing manager is responsible for developing the staff members' ability to delegate. Guidance in this area is necessary because new graduates, wanting to be regarded favorably, may not ask too much of UAP. Delegation is a skill that requires practice.

The nurse manager will determine the appropriate mix of personnel on a nursing unit. The nurse manager may have personnel with a variety of skills, knowledge, and educational levels. The acuity and needs of the patients usually determine the personnel mix. From this personnel mix, the new graduate nurse will begin to identify who can best perform assigned duties. The nonnursing duties are shifted toward clerical personnel, UAP, or housekeeping personnel to make the best use of individual skills.

New Graduate Responsibility

New graduate nurses need to focus on the duties for which they are directly responsible. What duties can they delegate and to what extent? What do UAP do? What do licensed practical nurses/licensed vocational nurses (LPNs/ LVNs) do? These questions need to be answered prior to the delegation of duties. Table 13-1 includes delegation suggestions for RNs.

Registered Nurse

The registered nurse is responsible and accountable for the provision of nursing care. According to Barter and Furmidge (1994), the registered nurse is always responsible for patient assessment, diagnosis, care planning, and evaluation. Although unlicensed assistive personnel may measure vital signs, intake and output, or other patient status indicators, it is the registered nurse who analyzes this data for comprehensive assessment, nursing diagnosis, and development of the plan of care. Assistive personnel may perform simple nursing interventions related to patient hygiene, nutrition, elimination, or activities of daily living, but the registered nurse remains responsible for the patient outcome. Having UAP perform functions outside their scope of practice is a violation of the state nursing practice act and is a threat to patient safety.

Misusing UAP is a practice common to many health care settings, according to the American Nurses Association (ANA) publication *Registered Professional Nurses & Unlicensed Assistive Personnel* (1996). UAP are often asked to perform duties beyond their scope of practice. Lack of personnel and high patient acuity rates contribute to the incidences of misuse. Nurses must be alert and avoid such misuse of UAP.

UAP

The increase in numbers of UAP in acute care settings poses a degree of risk to the patient. The House of Representatives, Patient Safety Act of 1996, assists in the campaign for safe staffing levels using an appropriate skill mix. The Act ensures that every patient is assigned a registered nurse. According to the Act, UAP are to be trained to perform duties such as bathing, feeding, toileting, and ambulating patients (Figure 13-1). UAP are also expected to document and report information related to these activities. The RN will delegate to the UAP and is liable for those delegations. According to the ANA (1996), if the RN knows or reasonably believes that the assistant has the appropriate training, orientation, and documented competencies, then the RN can reasonably expect that the UAP will function in a safe and effective manner.

Reasons for using UAP in acute care settings include cost control; freeing RNs from duties,

TABLE 13-1	*Delegation Suggestions for RNs*

1. Include all personnel in the delegation process when making assignments.

2. Assess what is to be delegated and identify who would best complete the assignment.

3. Communicate the duty to be performed and identify the time frame for completion. The expectations for personnel should be clear and concise.

4. Avoid removing duties once assigned. This should be considered only when the duty is above the level of the personnel, as when the patient's care is in jeopardy because the patient's status has changed.

5. Evaluate the effectiveness of the delegation of duties, check in frequently, and ask for a feedback report on the outcomes of care delivery.

6. Accept minor variations in the style in which the duties are performed. Individual styles are acceptable as long as the duty is performed correctly within the scope of practice.

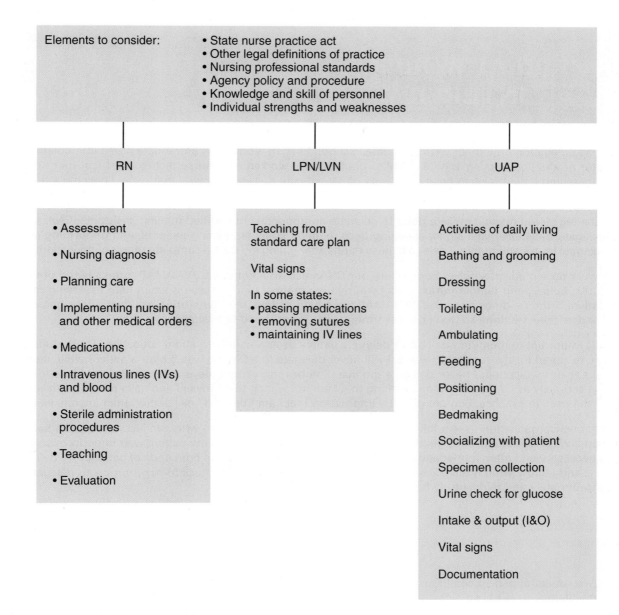

Figure 13-1 Considerations in Delegation

primarily nonnursing duties; and allowing time for RNs to complete assessments of patients and their potential responses to treatments. UAP cannot be assigned to assess or evaluate responses to treatment because that is the role of the RN. It is cheaper to have UAP perform nonnursing duties than to have nurses perform them. UAP can deliver supportive care. They cannot practice nursing or provide total patient care. The RN has an increased scope of liability when tasks are delegated to UAP. The RN must

be aware of the job description, skills, and educational background of the UAP prior to the delegation of duties.

The ANA pamphlet *Registered Professional Nurses & Unlicensed Assistive Personnel* (1996) has categorized the work duties of licensed and unlicensed personnel. The ANA states that because the RN is accountable for the delegation of nursing care activities, the following need to be considered in determining the appropriate utilization of UAP:

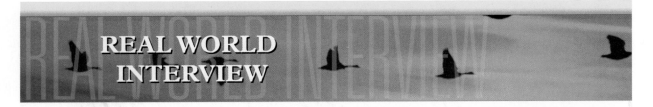

I use delegation now that I have completed school. I began working as a graduate nurse immediately after graduating nursing school. Prior to graduation, I worked as a nurse technician. I feel that I do understand how it feels to be at both ends of patient care delivery. I vowed that when I became a registered nurse, I would delegate appropriately and fairly to others.

As a registered nurse, I make a point to delegate appropriately to certified nursing assistants (CNAs). I delegate duties like vital signs, changing beds, bathing patients, feeding patients, and performing an accurate intake and output. I delegate these things after giving my CNA a complete report of my patients.

I work on a medical-surgical floor where our CNAs use an automated DYNAMAP to take blood pressures, pulses, and temperatures. I will take my own manual blood pressure when I am assessing my patient if the readings from the DYNAMAP were high or low. My CNAs bring me their vital signs as soon as they are done so that I can determine what more I need to evaluate.

It is important to mention that I never delegate patient assessments or patient education. These duties are reserved for the registered nurse. I will never delegate to a CNA to watch over a patient while they take their medication. I never delegate the insertion or removal of Foleys. I do believe my CNAs take me seriously as I do not delegate anything that I am not willing to do myself and have not done myself in the past. In essence, I do not give the impression that I am "beyond" or "better" than anyone else.

I get concerned when I see a fellow nurse walk out of a patient's room who has just requested a bedpan and go to find a CNA to get him that bedpan. I would never make my patient wait to perform such a necessary and often immediate task. Like I said earlier, I have been on both ends of patient care delivery, and I know what it feels like to be unappreciated. So far, I have stuck to my promise to delegate appropriately and fairly. I truly believe my CNAs would agree.

Shelly A. Thompson
New Graduate Nurse

- Assessment of patient condition
- Capabilities of the UAP
- Complexity of the nursing task
- Amount of supervision the RN will be able to provide
- Available staff assigned to accomplish the unit workload

Licensed Practical/Vocational Nurse

Licensed practical/vocational nursing caregivers who have undergone a standardized training and competency, and licensing evaluation are licensed practical nurses/licensed vocational nurses (LPNs/LVNs). Even though LPNs/LVNs are able to perform duties

and functions that UAP are not allowed to do, LPNs/LVNs are held to a higher standard of care and are responsible for their actions. Common LPN/LVN duties include the duties of the UAP plus teaching from a standard care plan and, in some states, passing medications and so forth. The RN is still primarily responsible for overall patient assessment, nursing diagnosis, planning, implementation, and evaluation of the quality of care delegated. Table 13-2 (National Council of State Boards of Nursing, Inc., 1995) lists five rights of delegation to be considered.

When considering delegating the right task to the right person, check the state nurse practice act, the policy and procedures of the agency, and job descriptions of all staff involved (e.g., LPN, UAP, RN, and so on). Also consider the training and

TABLE 13-2	*Five Rights of Delegation*

1. The right task

2. Under the right circumstances

3. Using the right person

4. With direction and communication

5. With the right supervision

competence of all staff. Is the task being delegated by the right person to the right person? Is this a task that can be delegated by a nurse?

When considering the right circumstance, determine whether the staff members understand how to do a procedure safely and correctly, and whether the action requires staff competency to be documented.

When considering the right person, ascertain whether the patient is stable with predictable outcomes and whether it is legally acceptable to delegate to this person, keeping in mind the setting and available resources.

When considering the right direction and communication, be sure the RN communicates the task with clear directions and that the steps of the task, and expected outcomes are carefully spelled out.

When considering the right supervision, be sure the RN answers all staff members' questions and is available to solve problems as needed. UAP should report task outcomes and the patient's response to the RN who delegated the task. Thus, appropriate supervision and evaluation are maintained. The RN provides follow-up monitoring, intervention, feedback, evaluation, teaching, and guidance to the staff in an ongoing fashion.

DIRECT DELEGATION VERSUS INDIRECT DELEGATION

According to the ANA, direct delegation is usually verbal direction by the RN delegator regarding an activity or task in a specific nursing care situation. Indirect delegation is performed using an approved listing of activities or tasks that have been established in the policies and procedures of the health care institution or facility.

The use of good professional judgment is vital when making the decision to delegate. Direct delegation gives the RN the opportunity to communicate clearly the duty to be completed, what to expect while completing the duty, and what the RN expects. Personnel then should be given the chance to clarify the duty.

The process of indirect delegation begins at a variety of levels. The nurse manager prepares a list of duties that can be delegated. The list includes those duties that are delegated from nurse manager to RN, RN to UAP, RN to LPN/LVN, nurse manager to unit secretary, RN to unit secretary, and so on. The duties are listed according to the hospital policy. The types of duties delegated reflect the ability of the UAP to complete the duties in a timely manner, according to their education and experience.

Underdelegation

Personnel in a new job role, such as nurse manager, RN, or nursing graduate, often underdelegate. Believing that older, more experienced staff may resent having someone new delegate to them, a new nurse may simply avoid delegation. Or, the new nurse may seek approval from other staff members by demonstrating her capability to complete all assigned duties without assistance. In addition, a new nurse may be reluctant to delegate because she does not

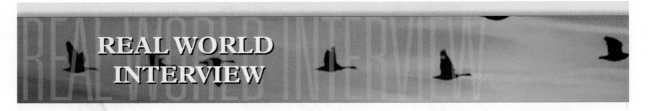

Upon evaluating delegation on several, varied nursing units, I arrive at one conclusion; we as professional nurses just do not do it well. There is the exception, of course, that being the individual who has developed an outstanding ability to delegate nearly all of his or her responsibilities to others in an authoritative or diplomatic manner with the recipients either loving or hating it.

Part of the problem may lie with the job description, that black-and-white document that delineates a role in great detail right up to the final statement of "inclusive of duties as assigned." The latter statement is too vague and the delegated task should be clearly stated somewhere in the job description.

On a nursing unit, it generally falls on the charge nurse to function in the assigning and delegating role. For this role, he or she is often criticized, most frequently behind the scenes, though occasionally they are blasted right out in the open. "What do you mean I am getting the next admission; I already have gotten two!" At best, one becomes apprehensive when assigning *anything*, from an admission to cleaning up the break room. I wonder, if that is the fate of the charge nurse, just how well would one expect the staff RN to delegate?

Perhaps our failures with delegation stem from our predominantly female, motherly gender. Moms can do it! Moms can do it all. Often, Mom finds the route of least resistance: "It's just easier to do it myself!" It is the same thing with RNs; RNs can do it, RNs can do it all.

I believe that the fine art of delegation needs to be taught more in the educational process, along with the concept of teamwork. The team is hindered when we become ineffective at delegation. The challenges in contemporary health care are tremendous, only to become even more challenging in the future. We as professional nurses would do well to acquire advanced skills in delegation, team building, and diplomacy, for these skills will become tools of survival in the very near future.

Suzanne Kalweit, RN, MS
Charge Nurse

know or trust individuals on her team or is not clear on the scope of their duties or what they are allowed to do. New nurses can become frustrated and overwhelmed if they fail to delegate appropriately. They may fail to establish appropriate controls with staff or fail to follow up properly; they may fail to delegate the appropriate authority to go with certain responsibilities. Perfectionism and a refusal to allow mistakes can lead a new nurse in over her head in patient care responsibilities. More-experienced staff members can help new personnel by intervening early on and assisting in the delegation process, and by clarifying responsibilities.

OVERDELEGATION

Overdelegation of duties can also place the patient at risk. Delegating duties inappropriate for personnel to perform because they have been inadequately educated is dangerous. The liability resting on the RN who has delegated professional duties to UAP is clear. This inappropriate delegation is against the state nurse practice act. The reasons for overdelegation are numerous. Personnel may feel uncomfortable performing a duty with which they are unfamiliar and may depend too much on a superior. They may be unorganized, or inclined to avoid responsibility or

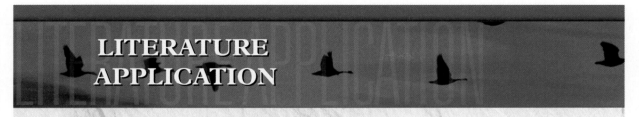

LITERATURE APPLICATION

Citation: Hansten, R., & Washburn, M. (2001, March). Delegating to UAPs: Making it work. *NurseWeek*, 21–23.

Discussion: With the declining enrollment in nursing schools, the United States and other countries have resorted to filling in the gaps with UAP. Partnering with UAP and working effectively in a team-based system, RNs can improve patient care outcomes. Coercing UAP to perform tasks beyond their capabilities, however, creates risk for the patient and nurse. It is important to remember the "rights of delegation." Even Florence Nightingale stated more than 100 years ago, "Let whoever is in charge keep this simple question in her head, not how can I always do this right thing myself, (but) how can I provide for this thing to always be done?" (Ulrich, 1992, p. 38).

Implications for Practice: It is important for nurses to delegate correctly to ensure safe patient care.

immerse themselves in trivia. Overdelegating duties can overwork some personnel and underwork others, creating resentment among colleagues.

TRANSCULTURAL DELEGATION

Nurses and patients come from diverse cultural backgrounds. Transcultural delegation is the process of having personnel perform duties with this cultural diversity taken into consideration. Poole, Davidhizar, and Giger (1995) suggest there are six cultural phenomena to be considered when delegating to a culturally diverse staff: communication, space, social organization, time, environmental control, and biological variations.

Communication

Communication, the first cultural phenomenon, is greatly affected by cultural diversity in the workforce. Elements of communication, including dialect; volume; use of touch; context of speech; and kinesics, such as gestures, stance, and eye behavior, all influence how messages are sent and received (Poole, Davidhizar, & Giger, 1995). For example, if a nurse were talking to UAP in a loud voice, it could be inter-

preted as anger. However, the nurse may be from a cultural background whose members always speak loudly—she may not be angry at all. Alternately, a nurse, because of cultural upbringing, may speak in a quiet, nondirective way that could be wrongly perceived as lacking authority. All nursing programs teach basic communication skills. These skills are the basis of delegation.

Space

Cultural background influences the space that individuals maintain between themselves. Some cultures prefer physical closeness while other cultures prefer more distance to be maintained between people. Ineffective delegation can take place when an individual's space is violated. Some delegators stand too close when speaking. Conversely, some members of a group may feel left out if they are not sitting close to the delegator. They may not feel included or important.

Social Organization

In different cultures, the social support in a person's life varies from support in one's own family to support from collegial relationships with the staff. If staff look to other staff for social support, those staff will

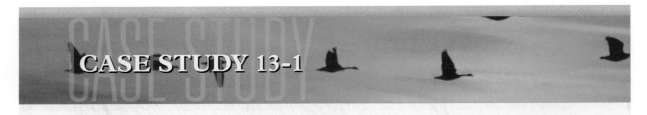

CASE STUDY 13-1

A new nursing graduate, Sandy, has been assigned to work with Luke, a UAP, and five patients. Sandy introduces herself to Luke and asks him what types of patient care he usually performs. He tells Sandy that he gives baths and takes vital signs. Sandy asks Luke to get all of the vital signs and give them to her written on a piece of paper. She asks Luke if he documents them. He states that he does document them.

Later that morning, Dr. Kent is making rounds on his patients, two of whom are Sandy's patients. He asks Sandy for the most recent vital signs. She then asks Luke for the vital signs on all the patients. Luke tells her he has not taken them yet. Dr. Kent then asks Sandy to get the vitals herself. By the time Sandy returns with the vital signs, Dr. Kent has gone and has written orders she cannot read.

There are several factors in this delegation situation that should have been handled differently. Can you name any?

Do you think the new graduate was ready to delegate to the UAP? Why?

Were the duties delegated appropriate for the UAP?

have difficulty fulfilling any tasks delegated to them that could threaten their social organization.

Time

Another cultural phenomenon affecting delegation is the concept of time. How often have you heard people say, "They are on their own time schedule"? Some people tend to move slowly and are often late, whereas other people move quickly and are prompt in meeting deadlines.

Poole, Davidhizar, and Giger (1995) describe different cultural groups as being either past, present, or future oriented. Past-oriented cultures focus on their tradition and its maintenance. For example, these cultures invest time into preparation of food that is traditional even though the food can be bought prepared in a store. Present-oriented cultures focus on day-to-day activities. For example, our present-oriented culture works hard for today's wages and does not plan for the future. Future-oriented cultures worry about what might happen in the future and prepare diligently for a potential problem, perhaps financial or health related. A nurse delegator should always be aware of duties to be completed and their deadline so that appropriate personnel can achieve their responsibilities in a timely fashion. Otherwise, people who meet deadlines in a timely fashion may be frustrated by those who do not.

Environmental Control

Poole, Davidhizar, and Giger (1995) define environmental control as people's perception of their control over their environment. This is also called internal locus of control. Some cultures place a heavier weight on fate, luck, or chance, believing, for example, that a patient is cured from cancer based on chance. They may think the health care treatment had something to do with the cure but was not the sole cause of it. How personnel perceive their control of the environment may affect how they delegate and perform duties. Personnel with an internal locus of control are geared toward taking more initiative and not requiring assistance in decision making. They believe in taking action and not relying on fate. Personnel with an external locus of control may wait for fate to determine their actions.

Biological Variations

The sixth and final cultural phenomenon is biological variations. Biological variations are the biopsychological differences between racial and ethnic groups. These biopsychological variations include physiological differences, physical stamina, and susceptibility to disease. Such factors need to be considered. For example, it would be problematic if the care of a comatose patient who weighs more than 300 pounds and needs frequent turning were delegated to a small nurse who cannot physically handle the patient. Perhaps this patient should be assigned to two nurses. A nurse who is pregnant would not be assigned to this patient because of the potential injury to the baby and nurse. Likewise, a pregnant nurse would not be assigned to a patient with radium implants because of the risks that the radium poses to the baby and mother. Biological variations must be considered, for the sake of both the health care providers and the patient.

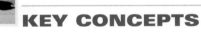

KEY CONCEPTS

- Delegation is a practiced and learned behavior.
- The RN must have a clear definition of what constitutes the scope of practice of all personnel.
- The five rights of delegation are the right task, the right circumstance, the right person, the right direction and communication, and the right supervision and evaluation.
- Accountability is when the nurse is legally liable for her actions and is answerable for the overall nursing care of her patients.
- Responsibility involves reliability, dependability, and the obligation to accomplish work. Responsibility also includes each person's obligation to perform at an acceptable level.
- Authority occurs when a person who has been given the right to delegate based on the state nurse practice act also has the official power from an agency to delegate.
- The RN is accountable for the delegation and performance of all nursing duties.
- There are several potential barriers to good delegation.
- Transcultural delegation is encouraged to provide a patient with optimal care.

KEY TERMS

accountability
authority
delegation
responsibility

REVIEW QUESTIONS

1. Which of the following statements about RNs and UAP is true?
   A. UAP and RNs have equal responsibilities.
   B. UAP are responsible for all patient care.
   C. RNs are less accountable for patient care when UAP are assisting.
   D. The RN provides patient care, delegating to other RNs or UAP as necessary.

2. If a nurse has difficulty completing nursing duties on schedule, a transcultural phenomenon to be considered is
   A. biological variations.
   B. time.
   C. space.
   D. social organization.

3. Which of the following is an inappropriate task for an LPN/LVN?
   A. Taking vital signs on a new patient
   B. Completing an Accucheck and reporting it to the RN
   C. Completing a pain assessment that the UAP identified as being changed from an earlier assessment
   D. Discharging the patient after teaching has been completed by the RN

4. If a patient being discharged requires teaching reinforced, the most appropriate caregiver to perform this would be
   A. a unit secretary.
   B. an LPN/LVN.
   C. a CNA.
   D. UAP.

5. Which patient is most appropriate to assign to the UAP for basic care?
   A. Patient with acute peritonitis
   B. Patient with stable congestive heart failure
   C. New postop acute appendectomy patient
   D. Recent head injury patient

REVIEW ACTIVITIES

1. To determine what your scope of practice is, call your state nurses association for information on your state's laws and regulations.

2. Read the study in the April 14, 1999, *Journal of the American Medical Association*, by Dr. Peter Pronovost and colleagues at the John Hopkins University. They found that a decreased ICU nurse-patient ratio during the day or evening was associated with increased ICU days and increased hospital length of stay. Could some of this high acuity patient care be safely delegated?

3. Observe delegation procedures at your institution. Is transcultural delegation considered? If so, which phenomena have you observed?

4. Take an informal survey of UAP in the institution in which you are having your clinical practicum. Ask them what duties they are assigned. Ask them whether there are any duties with which they are not comfortable. Discuss your findings.

5. Have you had any clinical opportunities to delegate duties? Identify to whom and what you delegated and discuss how it affected the patient and your work. What would you do differently next time?

EXPLORING THE WEB

- Log on to *http://www.aacn.org* and go to Clinical Practice. Click on Public Policy and find the advisory team member of your state. Note what policies, if any, consider delegation of care to UAP and LPNs.

- The state of California is the first state to require all its licensed hospitals to meet fixed nurse-to-patient ratios. Log on to the California Nurses Association Web site at *http://www.calnurse.org/* to identify the particulars of this bill.

- Log on to *http://www.nursingworld.org*, the American Nurses' Association (ANA) site, to view safety and quality of care issues.

REFERENCES

American Association of Critical Care Nurses (AACN). (1990). *Delegation of nursing and non-nursing activities in critical care: A framework for decision making.* Irvine, CA: Author.

American Nurses Association (ANA). (1996). *Registered professional nurses and unlicensed assistive personnel,* 2d ed. Washington, DC: American Nurses Publishing.

Barter, M., & Furmidge, M. L. (1994). Unlicensed assistive personnel: Issues relating to delegation and supervision. *Journal of Nursing Administration, 24*(4), 36–40.

Boucher, M. A. (1998). Delegation alert. *American Journal of Nursing, 98*(2), 26–32.

Ellis, J. R., & Hartley, C. L. (2000). *Managing and coordinating nursing care.* Philadelphia: Lippincott.

Fisher, M. (2000). Do you have delegation savvy? *Nursing2000, 30*(12), 58–59.

Hansten, R., & Washburn, M. (2001, March). Delegating to UAPs: Making it work. *NurseWeek,* 21–23.

National Council of State Boards of Nursing. (1995, December). Delegation: Concepts and decision-making process. *Issues,* 1–2.

Poole, V., Davidhizar, R., & Giger, J. (1995). Delegating to a transcultural team. *Nursing-Management, 26*(8), 33–34.

Pronovost, P. J., Jenckes, M., Dorman, T., Garrett, E., Breslow, M. J., Rosenfeld, B. J., Lipsett, P. A., & Bass, E. (1999). Care of the critically ill. *Journal of the American Medical Association, 281,* 1310–1317.

Salmond, S. (1994). *Perceived effectiveness of models of care using clinical nursing assistants.* Pitman, NJ: National Association of Orthopedic Nurses.

Ulrich, B. (1992). *Leadership and management according to Florence Nightingale.* Norwalk, CT: Appleton & Lange.

SUGGESTED READINGS

Barter, M., & McLaughlin, F. E. (1997). Registered nurse role changes and satisfaction with unlicensed assistive personnel. *Journal of Nursing Administration, 27*(1), 29–38.

Bellack, J. P., & O'Neil, E. H. (2000). Recreating nursing practice for a new century: Recommendations and Implications of the Pew Health Professions Commission's Final Report. *Nursing and Health Care Perspectives, 21*(1), 14–21.

Benner, P. (1984). *From novice to expert: Excellence and power in clinical nursing practice.* Menlo Park, CA: Addison-Wesley.

Bernreuter, M. E., & Cardona, M. S. (1997). Survey and critique of studies related to unlicensed assistive personnel from 1975 to 1997, part I. *Journal of Nursing Administration, 27*(6), 24–29.

Blouin, A. S., & Brent, N. J. (1995). Unlicensed assistive personnel: Legal considerations. *Journal of Nursing Administration, 25*(11), 7–8.

Burns, J. P. (1998). Performance improvements with patient service partners. *Journal of Nursing Administration, 28*(1), 31–37.

Canadian Nurses Association. (1995). *Policy statement: Necessary support for safe nursing care.* Ottawa: Author.

Canavan, K. (1997, May). Combating dangerous delegation. *American Journal of Nursing, 97*(5), 57–58.

Gordon, S. (1997). What nurses stand for. *Atlantic Monthly, 279*(2), 80–88.

Johnson, S. (1996). Teaching nursing delegation: Analyzing nurse practice acts. *The Journal of Continuing Education in Nursing, 27,* 52–58.

Parkman, C. A. (1996, September). Delegation: Are you doing it right? *American Journal of Nursing 96*(9), 43–48.

Parsons, L. C. (1997). Delegation decision-making. *Journal of Nursing Administration, 27*(2), 47–52.

Princeton Research Survey Associates. (1996). *Nursing and the quality of patient care: 1996 survey.* Princeton, NJ: Author.

Shindul-Rothschild, J., Berry, D., & Long-Middleton, E. (1996, Nov.). Where have all the nurses gone? Final results of our Patient Care Survey. *American Journal of Nursing, 11,* 25–39.

Smith, J. (1998, July). RNs and UAPs: Not much difference? *RN, 62*(7), 37–38.

Zimmerman, P. G. (1996, February). Use of unlicensed assistive personnel: Anecdotes and antidotes. *Journal of Emergency Nursing, 22*(1), 42–48.

Zimmerman, P. G. (1996, June). Delegating to assistive personnel. *Journal of Emergency Nursing, 22*(3) 206–212.

Zimmerman, P. G. (1997, May). Delegating to unlicensed assistive personnel. *Nursing, 27*(5), 71.

CHAPTER 14

First-Line Patient Care Management

Kathleen Fischer Sellers, PhD, RN

OBJECTIVES

Upon completion of this chapter, the reader should be able to:

1. Define first-line patient care management.
2. Discuss elements of strategic planning—philosophy, mission, vision.
3. Define nursing shared governance.
4. Identify Benner's concepts of novice, advanced beginner, competent, proficient, and expert nursing practice.
5. Identify accountability-based care delivery systems.
6. Identify measures of a unit's performance.

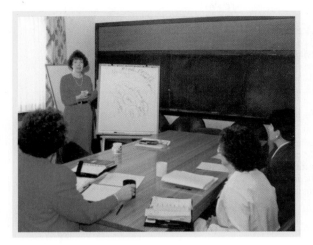

A first-line patient care manager has been informed that there are plans to merge the acute care surgical unit that she manages with an ambulatory surgery unit that currently cares for patients requiring 24-hour observation. As a visionary first-line patient care manager with a great depth of experience, she has been recommended to oversee the development of the new work unit. The institution believes the creation of this new unit will enhance revenue, staff productivity, and continuity of patient care. Therefore, resources are available to design and staff the new work unit in a manner that is congruent with the institution's mission with the understanding that the investment will bring added value to the organization.

What structures and processes have to be put in place?

What care delivery system would you put in place?

How would you ensure the competency and continued professional growth of new staff?

What outcomes would you hope to achieve? Within what time frames?

First-line patient care management utilizes the nursing process to plan, implement, and evaluate the outcomes of care for populations of patients rather than individual patients. First-line patient care management is akin to conducting a large orchestra. Like the conductor, the first-line patient care manager leads or coordinates a team of diverse individuals with varied talents and expertise toward a common goal (MacGregor-Burns, 1979). The orchestra creates beautiful music. The patient care team provides an outcome of quality, cost-effective patient care.

Successful first-line patient care management requires governance structures, patient care delivery processes, and measures of the outcomes of care delivery. These must be consistent with the mission and vision of the organization and are built on a philosophy of professional practice. First-line patient care management built on the tenets of professional nursing practice requires a structure of shared decision making or shared governance between nursing management and clinical nursing staff. Such a framework creates an environment in which the processes of patient care delivery demand an accountability-based system such as primary nursing, patient-focused care, or case management. In such an environment, the outcomes of care delivery, clinical quality, access, service, and cost can regularly be evaluated.

UNIT STRATEGIC PLANNING

Strategic planning is a process designed to achieve goals in dynamic, competitive environments through the allocation of resources (Andrews, 1990).

Assessment of External and Internal Environment

As outlined in Figure 14-1, strategic planning involves clarifying the organization's philosophical values; identifying the mission of why the organization exists; articulating a vision statement; and then conducting an environmental assessment, or SWOT analysis, which examines the Strengths, Weaknesses, Opportunities, and Threats of the organization. This information provides data that then drive the development of 3- to 5-year strategies for the organization. Tactics are then created and prioritized. Finally, goals and objectives are concretized into annual operating work plans for the organization. This same process is used for unit or departmental strategic planning.

Development of a Philosophy

A **philosophy** is a statement of beliefs based on core values—inner forces that give us purpose (Yoder-Wise, 1999). A unit's mission and vision are most

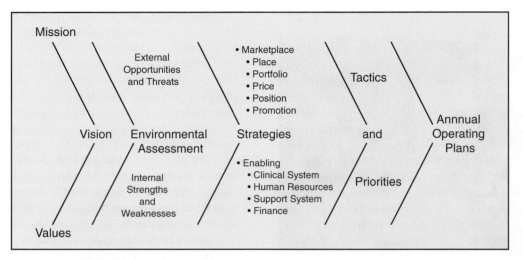

Figure 14-1 Bassett Healthcare Strategic Planning Framework (Developed by Gennaro J. Vasile, PhD, FACHE, Bassett Healthcare)

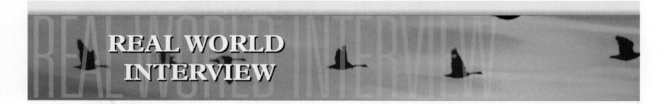

REAL WORLD INTERVIEW

At our academic health science center, leaders in the organization, board members who represent the community, and customer stakeholders develop the strategic plan. Once the strategic plan is developed, it is published and reviewed at a centerwide management meeting. It is then reviewed in divisional meetings and presented to staff through unit staff meetings. This is where the voice of the chief nursing officer has the most impact. I essentially interpret the rationale for the corporate strategic plan to my staff and glean their reactions. I then communicate the staff's feedback to the corporate level.

Articles are also published in our organizational newsletter for all staff describing the plan and addressing points of clarification. Each division and department then undertakes the process of developing divisional and department plans that support the strategic plan. For example, in the strategic plan a few years ago, it was articulated that our academic center would become a major cardiac center with a state-of-the-art cardiac catheterization laboratory. The department of cardiac services then included development of a state-of-the-art cardiac catheterization laboratory into its plan.

Anne L. Bernat, RN, MSN, CNAA
Chief Nursing Officer

authentic if they are developed based on the philosophy or core beliefs of the work team (Wesorick, Shiparski, Troseth, & Wyngarden, 1997). Core beliefs may be complex as those expressed in Table 14-1. Or they can be short statements developed from a staff brainstorming session, such as "patient centered," "partnering," "healing environment," and the like. A

unit's core beliefs or values are then incorporated into the unit's mission and vision statements.

Mission Statement

A **mission** is a call to live out something that matters or is meaningful (Wesorick et al., 1997). An orga-

TABLE 14-1	Core Beliefs

- Quality exists where shared purpose, vision, values, and partnerships are lived.

- Each person has the right to health care, which promotes wholeness in body, mind, and spirit.

- Each person is accountable to communicate and integrate his/her contribution to health care.

- Partnerships are essential to plan, coordinate, integrate, and deliver health care across the continuum.

- Continuing to learn and think in different ways is essential to improve health.

- A healthy culture begins with each person and is enhanced through self-work, partnerships, and systems supports.

From "Mission and Core Beliefs," by B. Wesorick, *CPMRC Connections ... for Continuous Learning*, December 2000, 3, p. 3.

nization's mission reflects the purpose and direction of the health care agency or a department within it.

Covey (1990) states, "An organizational mission statement—one that truly reflects the shared vision and values of everyone within that organization—creates a unity and tremendous commitment" (p. 139). For the unit mission statement to have the greatest effect, all members of the unit work team should participate in its development.

Questions to be answered by the group charged with development of the unit mission include the following:

- What do we stand for?
- What principles or values are we willing to defend?
- Who are we here to help?

There are three elements to a unit mission statement:

1. A mission statement is no longer than a couple of sentences.

2. It states the unit's purpose using action words.
3. It should be simple and from the heart. (Jones, 1996)

Mission statements are so broad that often units adopt the organization's mission statement, as the surgical unit of Bassett Healthcare did. The mission statement shown in Figure 14-2 is that of both the organization and the unit.

Vision Statement

The unit vision statement reflects the organization's vision. A unit vision statement then exemplifies how the mission and vision of the unit will be actualized within the organization's mission and vision.

Following are four elements of a vision:

1. It is written down.
2. It is written in present tense, using action words, as though it were already accomplished.
3. It covers a variety of activities and spans broad time frames.

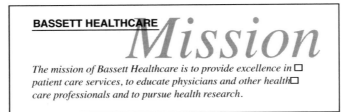

Figure 14-2 Bassett Healthcare Mission Statement (Courtesy Patricia Roesch, BS, RN, Bassett Healthcare)

4. It balances the needs of providers, patients, and the environment. This balance anchors the vision to reality. (Wesorick et al., 1997)

The surgical unit vision statement in Table 14-2 exemplifies the core values of the unit: patient centered, partnering, healing environment, and knowledge. The written statement tells the reader the work of the unit, why it is done, how, and for what reasons. In short, it delineates how the unit fulfills its mission.

Goals and Objectives

The next step in the strategic planning process is for the work unit to develop broad strategies that span the next 3 to 5 years and then develop annual goals and objectives to meet each of these strategies. A goal is a specific aim or target that the unit wishes to attain within the time span of 1 year. An objective is the measurable step to be taken to reach a goal.

THE STRUCTURE OF PROFESSIONAL PRACTICE

In an organization in which professional nursing practice is valued, strategic initiatives are developed and implemented most effectively through a structure of shared governance and shared decision-making between management and clinicians.

Shared Governance

Shared governance is an organizational framework grounded in a philosophy of decentralized leadership that fosters autonomous decision making and professional nursing practice (Porter-O'Grady, 1992). Shared governance, by its name, implies the allocation of control, power, or authority (governance) among mutually (shared) interested vested parties (Stichler, 1992).

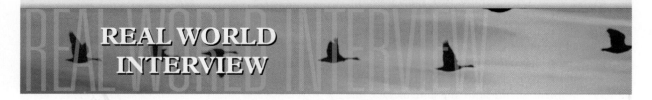

REAL WORLD INTERVIEW

We plan every year, but I'd say we look at our unit philosophy based on our core values and reevaluate the strategic plan every 2 to 3 years. We had three core values that guided us, and then this year, with all the external pressures, we added a fourth. We keep these core values in the forefront when we do our annual planning. The process we used to develop and reevaluate the core values was really very powerful and staff driven.

SPAN—Staff Planning Action Network—is our unit-based shared governance organization. SPAN met and developed draft mission and vision statements from our philosophy, which is based on our current core values—patient centered, partnering, and healing environment. They then transcribed these draft statements onto three flip charts and for 15 minutes per shift circulated these terms throughout the unit and got staff's reaction and feedback to the statements. Revisions were made from the feedback received. These were then presented at a staff meeting. What was emerging from the feedback was a focus on the need for continuing education and training related to the rapidly changing environment. So we added a fourth value—knowledge.

Our unit philosophy, stemming from our core values, is what we believe in. We've expanded these core values into a vision statement that demonstrates what it is to practice on this unit.

Pat Roesch, BSN, RN
First-Line Patient Care Manager

TABLE 14-2 *Surgical Unit Vision Statement*

The work we do: Affects the outcomes that patients desire in their pursuit of wellness.

Why we do it: To provide a healing environment in which an individual's physical, mental, emotional, and spiritual well-being will be nurtured.

Who we are: Practicing within partnering relationships that communicate respect while recognizing and valuing diversity.

How we do it: By committing to continued learning. Our knowledge fosters our growth; our mentoring nurtures our practice. (Roesch, 2000)

In most health care settings, the vested parties in nursing fall into two distinct categories: (1) nurses practicing direct patient care such as staff nurses and (2) nurses managing or administering the provision of that care such as managers. In shared governance, a nursing organization's management assumes the responsibility for organizational structure and resources. Management relinquishes control over issues related to clinical practice. In return, staff nurses accept the responsibility and accountability for their professional practice.

Unit-based shared governance structures are most successful if there is an organization-wide structure of shared governance in place that unit-based functions can articulate with. Organizational shared governance structures are usually council models that have evolved from preexisting nursing or institutional committees. In a council structure, clearly defined accountabilities for specific elements of professional practice have been delegated to five main arenas: clinical practice, quality, education, research, and management of resources (Porter-O'Grady, 1992). Figure 14-3 illustrates a shared governance model.

Clinical Practice Council

The purpose of the clinical practice council is to establish the practice standards for the work group. Often this council or committee is a unit-level committee that works in conjunction with the organizational committee accountable for determining policy and procedures related to clinical practice. Evidence-based practice fostered by research utilization initiatives ensures that practice standards are developed based on the state of the science of clinical practice and not merely on tradition.

Quality Council

The purpose of the quality council is twofold: (1) to credential staff and (2) to oversee the unit quality management initiatives. In the role of credentialing staff, this committee is responsible for interviewing potential staff and reviewing their qualifications, or credentials. It then makes recommendations regarding hiring. The quality committee also serves as the body that reviews staff credentials on an ongoing basis and makes recommendations regarding promotion.

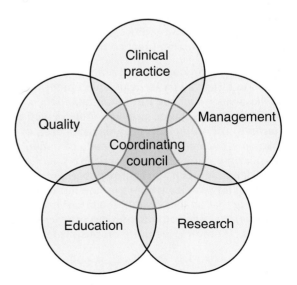

Figure 14-3 A Shared Governance Model

Quality management initiatives for which the council is responsible can include review of indicators of the unit's overall clinical performance, such as medication errors, patient falls, family satisfaction, and response time in answering call lights. At times, a unit will also participate in an organizational disease management study looking at the care of a specific patient population such as patients with diabetes.

Education Council

The purpose of the education council is to assess the learning needs of the unit staff and develop and implement programs to meet these needs. This council usually works closely with organizational education and training departments. Unit orientation programs and training programs related to new clin-

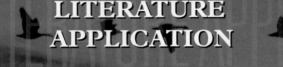

LITERATURE APPLICATION

Citation: Sellers, K. F. (1996). *The meaning of autonomous nursing practice to staff nurses in a shared governance organization: A hermeneutical analysis.* Unpublished doctoral dissertation, Adelphi University, Garden City, New York.

Discussion: Sellers conducted a study looking at autonomous nursing practice in an acute care hospital that was part of an integrated rural health network in upstate New York. She wished to know the impact of implementing a shared governance structure on autonomous nursing practice. She reviewed recent literature (Ludemann & Brown, 1989; Welsch & LaVan, 1981; Westrope, Vaughn, Bott, & Taunton, 1995) that had found that this model fostered recruitment and retention of nurses. However, she was interested in its effect on the autonomous practices of nurses in a hospital setting.

Sellers found that autonomous nursing practice was an everyday occurrence and to some extent had always existed within this organization. However, it had not always been recognized and legitimized by the larger organizational culture. Therefore, there had not always been the opportunity for the staff nurses to practice authentically, that is, with recognition. In the past, when the nursing organization was more traditional and centralized, autonomous nursing practice was informal. Often actions were performed at the risk of receiving an administrative reprimand. Despite this potential threat, autonomous actions were performed because they were appropriate actions to take for the patient. The catalyst for autonomous nursing practice had always been patient advocacy or doing what is right for the patient.

Today, autonomous nursing practice within the context of a shared governance organization manifests itself in everyday patterns of action determined by decisions that staff nurses make themselves based on knowledge gained from their experience. These actions are determined through the process of collaboration and shared decision making with colleagues within and outside the profession. These patterns of action include everyday practices of responding to patients' clinical needs and coordinating systems of care to meet the needs of patients. There is recognition of these patterns of action by the larger community. These practices are legitimized in collaboratively negotiated, written protocols and standards. As such, the shared governance culture has created the opportunity for legitimate or authentic nursing practice within the nursing organization of this hospital setting. The findings of this study indicate that as this institution shifted from a hierarchial nursing organization to a shared governance culture, the autonomous nursing practices of staff nurses were recognized, acknowledged, and legitimated. Therefore, the autonomous professional identity of nursing is now valued in this organization.

Implications for Practice: A culture of shared governance on a nursing unit helps develop the autonomous professional identity of nursing.

ical techniques and new equipment are examples of programs sponsored by the education council.

Research Council

At the unit level, the research council advances research utilization with the intent of incorporating research-based findings into the clinical standards of unit practice. Research utilization is the process of staff critiquing available research literature and then making recommendations to the practice council so that clinical policies and procedures can be based on evidence-based research findings. The research council may also coordinate research projects if advanced practice nurses are employed at the institution.

Management Council

The purpose of the management council is to ensure that the standards of practice and governance agreed upon by unit staff are upheld and that there are adequate resources to deliver patient care. The first-line patient care manager is a standing member of this council. Other members include the assistant nurse managers and the charge or resource nurses from each shift.

Coordinating Council

Shared governance structures also include a coordinating council. The purpose of the coordinating council is to facilitate and integrate the activities of the other councils. This council is usually composed of the first-line patient care manager and the chairpeople of the other councils. This council usually facilitates the annual review of the unit mission and vision and develops the annual operational plan (Sellers, 1996).

Unit-based shared governance structures may be less diverse. Often some of the councils are combined into one council, for example, education and research. Or a council may contain subcommittees whose purposes are to perform very specific tasks, for example, credential and promote staff or recruit and retain staff. Unit-based structures are varied, with the primary purpose being to empower staff by fostering professional practice while meeting the needs of the work unit.

ENSURING COMPETENCY AND PROFESSIONAL STAFF DEVELOPMENT

Professional practice through the vehicle of shared governance requires competent staff. Competency is defined as possession of the required skill, knowledge, qualification, or capacity (*Webster's Encyclopedic Unabridged Dictionary,* 1996) and is best determined in practice by a group of one's peers. Alspach (1984) defines competency as a determination of an individual's capability to perform to defined expectations (p. 656). Competency of professional staff can be ensured through credentialing processes developed

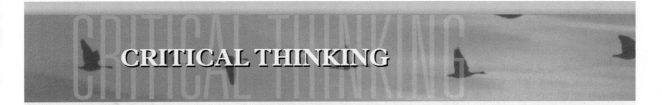

CRITICAL THINKING

As a nurse practicing in a shared governance organization, you remember a decade ago when the organization decentralized, made a commitment to nursing professional practice, and implemented shared governance. Everywhere you went, people were talking about it and displaying posters and other signs of nursing's importance to the organization. That was 6 years ago, before managed care and all the changes and before this latest nursing shortage. Now you do not hear people talking about it so much. You wonder, does professional practice still exist? How can you tell? How does your organization compare with other organizations that do not have shared governance? Is it possible that professional practice has become the culture and so there is no need to talk about it anymore?

around a clinical or career ladder staff promotion framework. A **clinical ladder** acknowledges that staff members have varying skill sets based on their education and experience. As such, depending on skills and experience, staff members may be rewarded differently and carry differing responsibilities for patient care and the governance and professional practice of the work unit.

Benner's Novice to Expert

Benner's (1984) model of novice to expert provides a framework that, when developed into a clinical or career promotion ladder, facilitates professional staff development by building on the skill sets and experience of each practitioner. Benner's model acknowledges that there are tasks, competencies, and outcomes that practitioners can be expected to have acquired based on five levels of experience.

Benner's model of novice to expert is based on the Dreyfus and Dreyfus (1980) model of skill acquisition applied to nursing. There are five stages of Benner's model: novice, advanced beginner, competent, proficient, and expert. Novice nurses are recognized as being task oriented and focused. Once they have mastered most tasks required to perform their ascribed roles, they move on to the phase of advanced beginner. The nurse who can demonstrate marginally acceptable independent performance illustrates the advanced beginner.

A competent nurse is one who has been in the same role for two to three years. These nurses have developed the ability to see their actions as part of the long-range goals set for their patients. The conscious, deliberative planning that is characteristic of this skill level helps achieve efficiency and organization.

Proficient nurses characteristically perceive situations as wholes rather than a series of tasks. They develop a plan of care and then guide the patient from point A to point B. They draw on their past experiences and know that in a typical situation, a patient must exhibit specific behaviors to meet specific goals. They realize that if those behaviors are not demonstrated within a certain time frame, then the plan needs to be changed.

The experts are those nurses who intuitively know what is going on with their patients. Their expertise is so embedded in their practice that they have been heard to say, "There is something wrong with this patient. I'm not sure what is going on, but you had better come and evaluate them." Not heeding the call derived from the intuitive sense of an expert nurse has resulted in a patient's cardiac arrest. These expert nurses often seek advanced education and become clinical specialists.

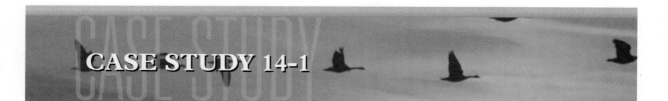

CASE STUDY 14-1

You are a competent nurse who is a member of the credentialing committee of the quality council. A fellow peer has presented his credentials for review in hopes of being promoted to the next level on the clinical ladder. You review the packet and make the recommendation that he be promoted. However, at the credentialing committee meeting, it is revealed that the first-line patient care manager and the individual's preceptor, another member of the committee, have not recommended promotion.

You wonder if your colleague is aware that there were concerns about his performance.

Are there guidelines and standards that you are not aware of that have not been met?

What is the next course of action for the committee?

What should your response be at this meeting?

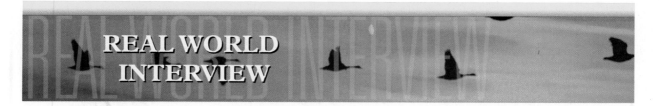

REAL WORLD INTERVIEW

There are five levels of our clinical ladder, which is similar to Benner's novice to expert model. The RNIs or novices are the new graduates and people in orientation. The experts are the clinical specialists. A lot of them have also become nurse practitioners so that the organization can receive some reimbursement for their patient care services. This is a good thing because otherwise I'm afraid we wouldn't have these expert nurses anymore. They are the true mentors for nursing staff, especially when you are working with a very complex or difficult patient situation.

Staff nurses also mentor each other. During orientation, your preceptor guides you along the path from RN I to RN II. When you decide you'd like to advance to RN III, you can choose another mentor. RN IIIs provide much more clinical leadership for staff and for the overall unit. I decided I was ready to be promoted to that level when other staff consistently were coming to me for clinical guidance and with patient care questions. Now, as an RN III, I am the chairperson of our unit-credentialing committee, which is part of the quality council of our shared governance model.

Our clinical ladder uses a portfolio as the main tool to evaluate the nurse's readiness to advance. When you are an RN I in orientation, you are first introduced to the idea of a portfolio and how to put it together. It is difficult at first, as people do not know what is expected. However, after that first time when you are promoted from an RN I to an RN II, it becomes easier. You just build on what is already in the portfolio.

A portfolio should include the following:

Licenses
Your resume
Letters of reference
Evaluations
Clinical documentation of patient care
Validations for competencies related to technical
  skills (medication administration, IV therapy)

Examples of participation in development
  of the team plan of care
Exemplars
CEU certificates
Presentations
Publications

The portfolio tells the story of your practice. When a group of people are ready for promotion, the members of the credentialing committee meet. We review the portfolios and make recommendations related to advancement. The nurse manager is a member of this committee. She always reviews the portfolio and gives us her feedback even if she is unable to attend the credentialing meeting. I enjoy reading the exemplars the best. Exemplars are mini-stories that paint the pictures of each nurse's practice, and they are all so different.

Stacey Conley, RN, BS
Staff Nurse

The Colorado Differentiated Nursing Practice Model (Figure 14-4) builds on the work of Benner (1984) regarding career ladder stages. Stage I is characterized as the entry/learning stage. Stage II is characterized by the individual who competently demonstrates acceptable performance adapting to time and resource constraints. Stage III is characterized by the individual who is proficient. And stage IV is characterized by the individual who is an expert. The stages in this model are specifically defined by behaviors that are consistently exhibited or practiced over a defined period of time.

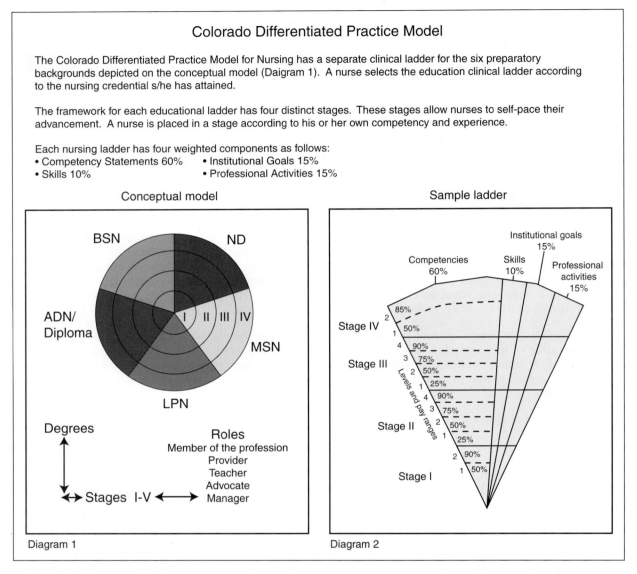

Colorado Differentiated Practice Model

The Colorado Differentiated Practice Model for Nursing has a separate clinical ladder for the six preparatory backgrounds depicted on the conceptual model (Daigram 1). A nurse selects the education clinical ladder according to the nursing credential s/he has attained.

The framework for each educational ladder has four distinct stages. These stages allow nurses to self-pace their advancement. A nurse is placed in a stage according to his or her own competency and experience.

Each nursing ladder has four weighted components as follows:
• Competency Statements 60%   • Institutional Goals 15%
• Skills 10%   • Professional Activities 15%

Conceptual model

Sample ladder

BSN   ND

ADN/ Diploma   I II III IV

MSN

LPN

Degrees

Roles
Member of the profession
Provider
Teacher
Advocate
Stages I-V   Manager

Diagram 1

Competencies 60%   Skills 10%   Institutional goals 15%   Professional activities 15%

Stage IV   2 85%   1 50%
Stage III   4 90%   3 75%   2 50%   1 25%
Levels and pay ranges   4 90%   3 75%
Stage II   2 50%   1 25%
Stage I   2 90%   1 50%

Diagram 2

Figure 14-4 Colorado Differentiated Nursing Practice Model (Courtesy Marie E. Miller, Colorado Nursing Task Force)

THE PROCESS OF PROFESSIONAL PRACTICE

Ongoing professional staff development is part of the regular performance feedback that staff can expect to receive from the first-line patient care manager or the credentialing committee. The first-line patient care manager also provides ongoing professional development of staff in their daily interactions on the unit and identifies projects and activities that meet a staff member's readiness for leadership development and advancement.

Situational Leadership

The leadership framework developed by Hersey and Blanchard (1993), when combined with an individual's position on a clinical/career ladder, is useful to the first-line patient care manager in discerning the best approach to take in developing the potential of staff members. **Situational leadership** maintains

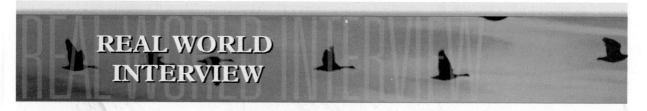

REAL WORLD INTERVIEW

I have a particularly touching story to tell you. D.T. was a 44-year-old man who was admitted from our ear, nose, and throat clinic with a large mass at the base of his tongue. Upon arrival on the unit, the patient appeared very anxious, not knowing what he would face in the next few days. The patient and his wife had been told that he would end up having a tracheostomy placed. This was quite a shock to their systems. They were both feeling overwhelmed with the situation.

As it happened, I was present for every major event that occurred with this family during that admission. I can recall the day when the patient was told that the mass was cancerous. He and his family were devastated. I went in to talk with the family and proceeded to tell them I could not begin to imagine what they must be going through, but that if they needed to talk, I was a good listener. I could tell that they very much appreciated that.

During the next few days, the family began to accept what was going on and we began working together to teach them all they needed to know about tracheostomies and how to care for them. D.T. and his wife learned quickly how to be independent with tracheostomy care. In the coming days, the patient underwent a feeding tube placement so that he could get some nutrition. I taught him and his wife how to care for the feeding tube and how to hang tube feedings. They learned so quickly that toward the end of the hospital stay, they were doing all his care independently. The patient was informed that he would need to undergo radiation and chemotherapy. In preparation for the treatment, the patient needed to have a complete dental extraction. Considering all that D.T. and his wife went through in such a short amount of time, they both responded quite well to the situation.

Upon discharge, I set the patient up with Lifeline (an emergency response service), nursing services, and equipment for the tracheostomy and tube feedings. This was no easy task because they did not have much money and their insurance company was quite difficult to deal with. As their primary nurse, I literally spent days on the phone in preparation for their discharge. It was quite challenging but rewarding when all was accomplished. It was both a happy and a sad day when the patient and his wife were discharged. Since the patient has left, I have kept in touch through writing, and in person when he has been readmitted to the medical floor for his chemotherapy treatment. I am glad to report that thus far D.T. is doing well.

This was a particularly touching experience for me. This family was very special to me, and I am glad for the opportunity I had to get to know them and be a special part of their lives. As an unknown author says, in the end, we will not remember the years we spent nursing, we will only remember the moments.

Stacey Conley, RN, BS
Staff Nurse

that there is no one best leadership style, but rather that effective leadership lies in matching the appropriate leadership style to the individual's or group's level of task-relevant readiness. Readiness is how able and motivated an individual is to perform a particular task. A basic assumption of situational leadership is the idea that a leader should help followers grow in their readiness to perform new tasks as far as they are able and willing to go. This development of followers is accomplished by adjusting leadership behavior through four styles along the leadership curve.

According to Hersey and Blanchard's (1993) model, individual followers with low task readiness, such as novice nurses, require a telling style on the part of the leader. They need to be told what to do and be given strong direction if they are to be successful and productive. As these followers grow in readiness, the leader should shift to a selling style, with more positive reinforcement and socioemotional support.

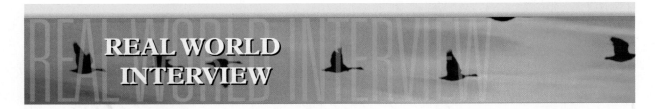

REAL WORLD INTERVIEW

I am an acute care inpatient case manager. I'm a member of an interdisciplinary patient care team. My role is multifaceted, with three broad areas of responsibility: utilization management, variance tracking, and complex discharge planning. Utilization management is the process of monitoring the usage of inpatient resources. The hospital purchases nationally developed criteria. These criteria set the standards for admission and continued inpatient stays. Many of the insurance companies use the same or similar criteria. Every admission is reviewed to determine whether or not the patient met the criteria to be admitted. Concurrent reviews are done to determine if the continued stay criteria is being met. I also meet daily with the team to review each patient. We discuss the patient's current health care status, the plans for the day, and attempt to project tentative discharge dates. After 3 years, many of the doctors have learned the value of these meetings. By taking 15 to 20 minutes each morning to meet and discuss our patients, we have decreased the length of stay and have developed a forum to discuss potential utilization concerns. Many of the insurance companies call daily to get clinical information on their clients. I spend much of my day talking with them, attempting to justify why the patient requires inpatient care. Some of the companies can be nitpicky and cost driven.

The reviews and daily rounds are important to the variance tracking I do. I attempt to identify delays in service, unnecessary usage of inpatient resources, and ways to improve outcomes. The variance data will help the hospital identify ways to improve how they do business.

In the hospital where I work, the primary or staff nurse is responsible for the development of the patients' discharge plan. They will develop this plan with the patient and arrange for equipment, transportation, and home care services. During the patient's stay, if it is determined that the patient has more complex needs, I will become involved in the discharge arrangements. Sometimes my involvement will be to get needed equipment or services approved by the third-party payer. I have spent hours on the phone with the insurers, advocating for patients with complex needs, then spent time convincing the patient's physician to write letters of justification for the care that they deem necessary. Once I successfully got approval for a bariatric lift for a 600-pound woman who was bed bound. This lift enabled her to go home with her family and avoid nursing home placement.

In addition to assisting with complex home discharges, I also work with patients that have needs such as posthospital rehabilitation or skilled nursing facility placement. With the help of the other members of the team, I am able to present the options to the patient and their family. Together we discuss the options, how these options are paid for, and arrange for their placement in a rehabilitation or a skilled nursing facility.

I enjoy my role as case manager. It has evolved a great deal in the 3 years I've been in this position. I look forward to its continued development.

Cynthia Whispell, BSN, RN
Nursing Case Manager

Once individuals reach higher levels of readiness, as a proficient or expert nurse, the leader should respond by decreasing control. The leader moves first to a participatory style characterized by a high degree of relationship with staff and a lower need to give task direction, and then, with expert staff the leader moves to a style of delegating, communicating a sense of confidence and trust because highly competent individuals respond best to greater freedom.

Individuals' readiness to learn and accept new tasks may change for a variety of reasons. When first-line managers discern a change, they must readjust their style of interaction with the nurse—moving forward or backward through the leadership curve—and provide the appropriate level of support and direction to facilitate that individual's continued development, productivity, and success as a member of the patient care team. Development of staff based on their innate readiness to accept new tasks and responsibilities facilitates their promotion along a continuum of novice to expert and ensures a professional patient care team that is able to consistently deliver accountability-based patient care.

Accountability-Based Care Delivery

Accountability-based care is essential in today's value-driven workplace. Individuals who are accountable are, by definition, able to report, explain, or justify their actions (*Webster's Encyclopedic Unabridged Dictionary,* 1996). Accountability is about achieving outcomes and is the foundation for evaluation. (Porter-O'Grady, 1995). The following care delivery systems are built on the tenet of accountability to the patients who are the receivers of nursing care. As such, they provide systems or processes of care congruent with professional practice.

Primary Nursing

Primary nursing is a system of care that was founded in the 1960s at a time when nurses were searching for more independence and autonomy in their practice. In a **primary nursing** model, one nurse is accountable for the care a patient receives during a given episode of care. She functions through associate nurses during the hours of the day when she is not present in the workplace. Communications occur through a written plan of care. The primary nurse assumes responsibility for the patient's admission to the site of care, development of the care plan, major communications with other care providers, and overseeing the patient's discharge to home or to another level of care. The hallmark of primary nursing is that one nurse maintains 24-hour accountability for a specific patient's care. In this model, the role of the first-line patient care manager is to manage the staff not the patient care, ensure that systems work for the caregivers, and ensure that caregivers work for their patients.

The advantages of primary nursing include continuity of patient care, as well as nurse and patient satisfaction. Primary nursing is, however, an expensive system of care delivery because it requires a higher proportion of registered nurses. As such, in

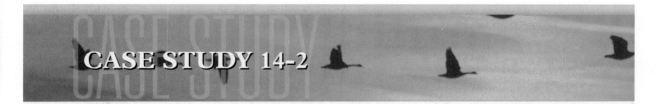

CASE STUDY 14-2

You are a primary nurse working as part of the interdisciplinary orthopedic team. You notice that there are an increasing number of diabetic patients being admitted for elective total hip surgery. Because the length of stay is so short and your team has such a surgical focus in caring for patients, their underlying chronic diseases have not been a focus on the unit. However, you are aware that the larger organization is beginning to evaluate how different populations of patients, such as diabetics, are cared for across the continuum of care.

What should you do to improve care for your patients?

recent years health care delivery systems have had difficulty continuing to support the model.

Patient-Focused Care

Patient-focused care is a model of differentiated nursing practice that emphasizes quality, cost, and value (Reisdorfer, 1996). In this model, the first-line patient care manager assumes an expanded role. She assumes accountability to manage nurses and staff from other departments, such as staff from radiology, physical therapy, and so on. Her focus is more sophisticated. It has expanded to include overseeing the coordination of all care activities required by patients and their support systems.

Case Management

Nursing case management is another accountability-based care delivery system that evolved in the late 1980s and early 1990s in response to spiraling health care costs. The primary goal of case management is to deliver high-quality patient care in the most cost-effective way by managing human and material resources. Other goals are to manage the delivery of care within a given time frame, to decrease length of stay for inpatient care, to ensure appropriate utilization of services and resources, to improve continuity of care, to standardize the care delivered for a given diagnosis, and to improve patient outcomes from a given episode of care (Satinsky, 1995). Nursing case management has used critical paths, Care Mapping (Zander, 1995), and interdisciplinary care protocols to achieve its objectives. The indicators of care embedded in these tools are used to measure the outcomes of care delivery.

MEASURABLE QUALITY OUTCOMES

An important component of first-line patient care management is regular evaluation of a unit's performance to ensure that the outcomes of care delivery are meeting the objectives of professional practice as outlined in the unit's annual operational plan. The development of process improvement measures in today's health care organizations is driven by the multiple domains of quality required by the Joint Commission on Accreditation of Healthcare Organizations (JCAHO) (*www.jcaho.org*) and now the National Council for Quality Assurance (NCQA)

(*www.ncqa.org*), the credentialing organization that certifies managed care organizations.

Unit-Based Performance Improvement

To develop a comprehensive unit-based quality improvement program to meet the requirements of today's competitive, value-driven health care system, the first-line patient care manager should track outcomes from four domains: access, service, cost, and clinical quality (G. Vasile, Cooperstown, NY, Bassett Healthcare, personal communication, August 16, 2000). See Figure 14-5 for the inpatient surgical unit 2000 performance improvement plan.

Outcomes of unit quality improvement programs can be succinctly displayed using the Quality Compass (Nelson, Mohr, Batalden, & Plume, 1996). The Bassett Quality Compass in Figure 14-6 measures quality from four domains: functional status, clinical outcomes, cost and utilization, and patient satisfaction. This Quality Compass depicts the outcomes of an organization-wide disease management asthma study prior to an asthma disease management intervention. The Compass tells us that functionally 30% of the population has moderately severe asthma and that the majority of asthmatics have little documented teaching in use of a peak flow meter or metered-dose inhalers (MDIs), which is the current standard of care. More than 30% of the patient visits for asthma are urgent visits, indicating that a large portion of the asthma population will benefit from the disease management intervention of increased patient teaching and development of individual specific asthma care plans. The Quality Compass provides a framework to guide the development of a unit-based quality improvement program and provides a tool with which to present the outcomes of quality improvement in the succinct visual format of an executive summary.

The first-line patient care manager is the fundamental operations person in the health care system. Successful orchestration of a patient care unit in today's health care system is achieved through vision-driven professional practice. Implementing this vision is achieved through a unit governance structure of shared decision making, an accountability-based patient care delivery system, and regular evaluation of performance based on the tenets of performance improvement.

2000 PERFORMANCE IMPROVEMENT PLAN

As part of Bassett's commitment to quality, the Surgical Unit will strive to improve performance through a cycle of planning, process design, performance measurement, assessment and improvement. There will be ongoing assessment of important aspects of care and service and correction of identified problems. Problem identification and solution will be carried out using a systematic intra- and interdepartmental approach organized around patient flow or other key functions, and in concert with the approved visions and strategies of the organization. Priorities for improvement will include high risk, high volume and problem-prone procedures.

The Surgical Unit will:

• promote the Plan-Do-Check-Act methodology for all performance improvement activities
• provide staff education and training on integrated quality and cost improvement
• collect data to support objective assessment of processes and contribute to problem resolution

In identifying important aspects of care and service, the Surgical Unit will select performance measures in the following operational categories:

A. Clinical Quality
1. Patient safety

• Patient falls
• Indicator: # of patient falls per month/# of patient days with upper control limits set by the research department based on statistical deviation

• Medication and IV errors
• Indicator: # of patient IV/medication errors per month/# of patient days with upper control limits set by the research department based on statistical deviation

• Restraint use
• Indicator: % of compliance with policy for use of restraints and overall rate of restraint use

2. Pressure ulcer prevention
• Indicator: Rates of occurrence-quarterly tracking report

3. Surveillance, prevention and control of infection
• Indicator: Infection control statistical report of wound and catheter associated infections
• Indicator: Quarterly monitoring of compliance with standards for Acid Fast Bacilli (AFB) room use; evidence of staff validation in AFB practice

4. Employee safety
• Injuries resulting from
• Back and lifting-related injuries
• Morbidly obese patients
• Orthopedic patients
• Indicators: # of injuries sustained by employees and any resultant workmen's compensation (Human Resources quarterly report)
• 100% competency validation in lifting techniques and back injury prevention
• Respiratory fit testing
• Indicator: competency record of each employee

5. Documentation by exception
Indicators:
• 100% validation of RN/LPN staff
• Monthly chart audit (10% average daily census or 20 charts) meeting compliance with established standards

B. Access:
• Maintenance of the 30 minute standard for bed assignment of ED admissions
• Indicator: Quarterly review of ED tracking record

C. Service:
Patient Satisfaction
Indicator: Patient Satisfaction Survey: 90% or above response to, "Would return", and "Would recommend"

D. Cost:
• Nursing staff productivity will remain at 110% of target of 8.5 worked hours per adjusted patient day within a maximum variance range of 10%

For each of the above performance measures, this performance improvement plan will:

• address the highest priority improvement issues
• require data collection according to the structure, procedure and frequency defined
• document a baseline for performance
• demonstrate internal comparisons trended over time
• demonstrate external benchmark comparisons trended over time
• document areas identified for improvement
• demonstrate that changes have been made to address improvement
• demonstrate evaluation of these changes; document that improvement has occurred or, if not, that a different approach has been taken to address the issue

The Inpatient Surgical Unit will submit biannual status reports to the Bassett Improvement Council (BIC) through the Medical Surgical Quality Improvement Council (MSQIC).
I

Approved by:_____**Date:**_____

(Chief or Vice President)

Figure 14-5 Inpatient Surgical Unit, 2000 Performance Improvement Plan (Courtesy Patricia Roesch, BS, RN, Bassett Healthcare)

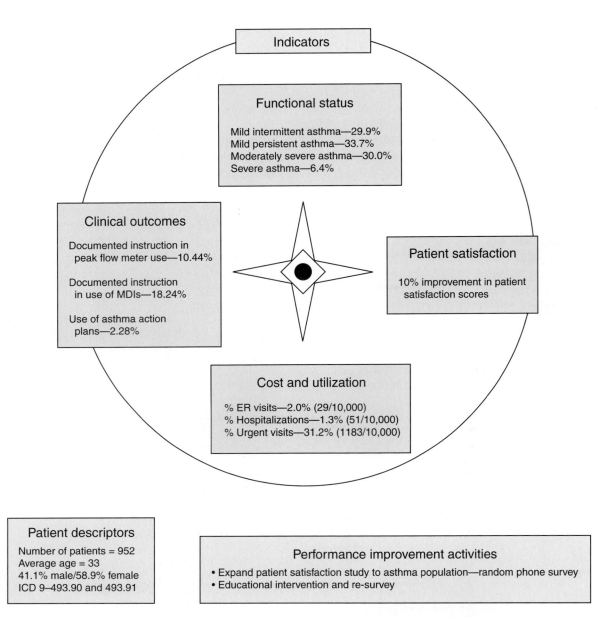

Figure 14-6 Bassett Healthcare Quality Compass (Courtesy Kathleen F. Sellers, PhD, RN, Bassett Healthcare)

![icon] **KEY CONCEPTS**

- Successful orchestration of a patient care unit in today's health care environment is achieved through vision-driven professional practice.
- Strategic planning is a process that is designed to achieve goals in dynamic, competitive environments through the allocation of resources (Andrews, 1990).

- Shared governance is an organizational framework grounded in a philosophy of decentralized leadership that fosters autonomous decision making and professional nursing practice.
- A clinical/career promotional ladder provides a framework that facilitates professional staff development by building on the skill sets and experience of each practitioner.
- Situational leadership maintains that there is no one best leadership style but rather that effective

leadership lies in matching the appropriate leadership style to the individual's or group's level of task-relevant readiness.

- Individuals who are accountable are, by definition, able to report, explain, or justify their actions.
- Accountability-based care delivery systems include primary nursing, patient-focused care, and case management.
- A comprehensive unit-based quality improvement program should include outcomes that are tracked from four domains: access, service, cost, and clinical quality.

KEY TERMS

case management
clinical ladder
goal
mission
objective
patient-focused care

philosophy
primary nursing
shared governance
situational leadership
strategic planning

REVIEW QUESTIONS

1. Shared governance
   A. is an accountability-based care delivery system.
   B. is a tested framework of organizational development.
   C. is a competency-based career promotion system.
   D. implies the allocation of control, power, or authority (governance) among interested parties.

2. The five levels of a clinical promotion ladder built on Benner's theoretical framework include all of the following EXCEPT
   A. proficient.
   B. competent.
   C. orientee.
   D. expert.

3. Case management, patient-focused care, and _____ are accountability-based nursing care delivery systems.
   A. functional nursing
   B. team nursing

   C. primary nursing
   D. case finding

4. In developing a unit-based Quality Compass, all the following areas are usually considered EXCEPT
   A. patient satisfaction.
   B. cost.
   C. administrative satisfaction.
   D. clinical outcomes.

REVIEW ACTIVITIES

1. You have been asked by your first-line patient care manager to participate on a performance improvement team looking at care of the diabetic patient. What areas other than clinical quality will you evaluate? Identify indicators for each area to measure. What it is you are seeking to improve?

2. You have been practicing now for 3 years. This summer you have been precepting a new graduate. He is having difficulty mastering changing a sterile dressing. You must give him feedback. You are uncertain on how to do this most effectively and wonder if you are part of the reason he is having difficulty. Review situational leadership. At what level of readiness is this new graduate? Has your leadership style been appropriate for that level of experience and motivation?

3. You have been practicing as a new graduate for a little over a year. You are feeling more confident about your clinical practice and think you might want to expand your leadership experience. Your unit governance framework is shared governance. Review the common councils of shared governance. Given your education and experience, which council would you like to join?

EXPLORING THE WEB

- You have been asked by your nurse manager and members of the credentialing committee to revamp the current clinical promotion ladder so that it more clearly differentiates and rewards nurses for their education level as well as expertise. Go to *http://www.uchsc.edu/ahec/ cando/nursing/diffpractice97.htm*

What does the University of Colorado's clinical ladder incorporate that yours does not?

- Go to the magnet hospitals site (*http://www.ana.org/ancc/magnet.htm*) and see whether there is information there that would help your organization foster professional nursing practice. Striving for magnet hospital designation increases an organization's ability to recruit and retain nurses.

- Go to *http://www.nursingsociety.org*. This site provides weekly literature updates from Sigma Theta Tau International, the nursing profession's honor society. What new books and periodicals are available that may be helpful to you in your practice?

REFERENCES

Alspach, J. (1984). Designing a competency-based orientation for critical care nurses. *Heart and Lung, 13,* 655–662.

Andrews, M. (1990). Strategic planning: Preparing for the 21st century. *Journal of Professional Nursing, 6*(2), 103–112.

Benner, P. (1984). *From novice to expert.* Menlo Park, CA: Addison-Wesley.

Clifford, J., & Horvath, K. J. (1990). *Advancing professional nursing practice: Innovations at Boston's Beth Israel Hospital.* New York: Springer.

Covey, S. R. (1990). *The seven habits of highly effective people.* New York: Fireside.

Dreyfus, S. E., & Dreyfus, H. L. (1980). *A five stage model of the mental activities involved in directed skill acquisition.* Unpublished report supported by the Air Force Office of Scientific Research, USAF (Contract F49620-79-C-0063), University of California at Berkeley.

Hersey, R. E., & Blanchard, T. (1993). *Management of organizational behavior.* Edgewood Cliffs, NJ: Prentice-Hall.

Jones, L. B. (1997). *The path: Creating your mission statement for work and for life.* New York: Hyperion.

Ludemann, R. S., & Brown, C. (1989). Staff perceptions of shared governance. *Nursing Administration Quarterly, 13*(4), 49–56.

MacGregor-Burns, J. (1979). *Leadership.* New York: Harper & Row.

Nelson, E., Mohr, J. J., Batalden, P. B., & Plume, S. K. (1996, April). Improving health care, part 1: The clinical value compass, *Journal of Quality Improvement, 22*(4), 243–258.

Porter-O'Grady, T. (1992). *Implementing shared governance: Creating a professional organization.* St. Louis, MO: Mosby-Year Book.

Porter-O'Grady, T. (1995). *The leadership revolution in health care.* Gaithersburg, MD: Aspen.

Reisdorfer, J. T. (1996). Building a patient-focused care unit. *Nursing Management, 27*(10), 38, 40, 42, 44.

Roesch, P. (2000, October). Surgical unit practice. *Nursing Matters, 7*(3), 1. Bassett Healthcare, Cooperstown, NY.

Satinsky, M. A. (1995). *An executive guide to case management strategies.* Chicago: American Hospital.

Sellers, K. F. (1996). *The meaning of autonomous nursing practice to staff nurses in a shared governance organization: A hermeneutical analysis.* Unpublished doctoral dissertation, Adelphi University, Garden City, New York.

Stichler, J. F. (1992). A conceptual basis for shared governance. In N. D. Como & B. Pocta (Eds.), *Implementing shared governance: Creating a professional organization* (pp. 1–24). St. Louis, MO: Mosby.

Webster's encyclopedic unabridged dictionary of the English language (2nd ed.). (1996). New York: Random House.

Welsch, H., & LaVan, H. (1981). Inter-relationships between organizational commitment and job characteristics, job satisfaction, professional behavior, and organizational climate. *Human Relations, 24*(12), 1079–1089.

Wesorick B., Shiparski, L., Troseth, M., & Wyngarden, K. (1997). *Partnership council field book: Strategies and tools for co-creating a healthy work place.* Grand Rapids, MI: Practice Field.

Westrope, R. A., Vaughn, L., Bott, M., & Taunton, R. L. (1995, December). Shared governance: From vision to reality. *Journal of Nursing Administration, 25*(12), 45–54.

Yoder-Wise, P. S. (1998). *Leading and managing in nursing* (2nd ed.). St. Louis, MO: Mosby.

Zander, K. (1995). *Managing outcomes through collaborative care: The application of care mapping and case management.* Chicago: American Hospital.

SUGGESTED READINGS

Aiken, L. H., Havens, D. S., & Sloane, D. M. (2000, March). The magnet nursing services recognition program. *American Journal of Nursing, 100*(3), 26–35.

Bell, C. (1996). *Managers as mentors.* San Francisco: Berrett-Koehler.

Bridges, W. (2000). *Managing transitions: Making the most of change.* New York: Perseus Books Group.

Hirsh, S. K., & Kummerow, J. M. (1990). *Introduction to type in organizations.* Palo Alto, CA: Consulting Psychologists Press.

Kaplan, R. S., & Norton, D. P. (2001). *The strategy focused organization.* Boston, MA: Harvard Business School.

Loverage, C., & Cummings, S. H. (1996). *Nursing management in the new paradigm.* Gaithersburg, MD: Aspen.

Manion, J. (1996). *Team based health care organizations.* Gaithersburg, MD: Aspen.

McClure, M. L., Poulin, M. A., Sovie, M. D., & Wandelt, M. A. (1983). *Magnet hospitals.* Kansas City, MO: American Nurses Publishing.

Myers, I. B. (1993). *Introduction to type.* Palo Alto, CA: Consulting Psychologists Press.

Sellers, K. F., Hargrove, B., & Jenkins, P. (2000). Asthma disease management programs improve clinical and economic outcomes. *MEDSURG Nursing, 9*(4), 201–203, 207.

Senge, P. (1990). *The fifth discipline.* New York: Doubleday.

Senge, P. (1994). *The fifth discipline fieldbook* (p. 49). New York: Doubleday.

Silvetti, C., Rudan, V., Frederickson, K., and Sulivan, B. (2000, April). Where will tomorrow's nurse managers come from? *Journal of Nursing Administration, 30*(4) 157–159.

Wesorick, B. (1998). *The way of respect in the workplace* (p. 15). Grand Rapids, MI: Practice Field.

Zemke, R., Raines, C., & Filipczak, B. (2000). *Generations at work: Managing the clash of veterans, boomers, xers and nexters in your workplace.* New York: AMACOM.

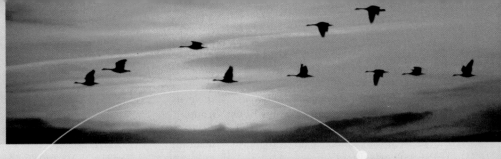

CHAPTER 15

Patient Teaching

Paul Heidenthal, MS

OBJECTIVES

Upon completion of this chapter, the reader should be able to:

1. Identify five major steps of a teaching methodology.
2. Explain three components of the analysis phase of teaching.
3. Discuss at least two major theories of learning style.
4. Explain the major learning domains.
5. State the four components of a behavioral objective.
6. Explain the relationship between terminal and enabling objectives.
7. Discuss the importance of Gagne's key learning events in planning a teaching session.
8. Name two forms of evaluation and explain the goals of each.
9. Construct behavioral objectives for a teaching session.
10. Create a lesson plan for a teaching session.

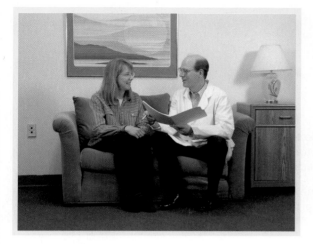

Your patient, Mr. Abado, age 50, has just been diagnosed with diabetes. He is anxious and verbalizes his concerns to you. His mother died from diabetes and he wants to be sure that he understands how to take care of himself and prevent diabetic complications. You are busy with all your patients, yet you want to teach him about his diet, medication, and exercise needs.

How can you help Mr. Abado?

How will you develop a teaching plan?

Patient teaching is an inherent part of the nursing process. Teaching is a tool through which nurses bolster patients' self-care abilities by providing patients with information about specific disease processes, treatment methods, and health-promoting behaviors.

Patient teaching is also a legal component of the nursing process. In most states, teaching is a required function of nurses. Patient teaching is also mandated by several accrediting bodies, such as the Joint Commission on Accreditation of Healthcare Organizations (2002). The American Hospital Association's *Patient's Bill of Rights* (1972) also calls for the patient's understanding of health status and treatment approaches.

INFORMAL AND FORMAL PATIENT TEACHING

Patient teaching occurs informally and formally. Informal teaching can be as basic as exchanging infor-

mation during a conversation with the patient. Formal teaching is planned, structured, and directed toward specific topics and goals. Formal teaching also contains evaluation, which measures the patient's success in retaining and applying information.

INDIVIDUAL AND GROUP TEACHING

The nurse provides teaching in an individual or group setting. Individual patient teaching frequently occurs in a clinical environment, often when an individual is facing the immediate impact of a specific health care situation. The term *patient teaching* may also be a misnomer in many of these situations because the nurse may be teaching the patient's family members or health care providers along with or instead of the patient. Even when others are involved, however, the focus of the teaching usually remains on the needs of an individual patient.

While most patient teaching occurs on an individual basis, nurses are increasingly becoming involved in teaching on a group level. As hospitals and other health care organizations adopt a proactive approach to health care, they are increasingly reaching out to the community, providing informational seminars and wellness classes that address common health care situations or emphasize preventive behavior.

METHODOLOGY

Whether conducted in an individual or group setting, the teaching process is more effective when it follows a structured, standardized approach. Such an approach is called a methodology. The methodology presented in Table 15-1 contains five major steps in the development and delivery of formal teaching.

Analysis

The first step in developing any teaching is to perform an analysis, to define the type of teaching needed. The nurse should analyze three major elements:

- Context
- Learner
- Content

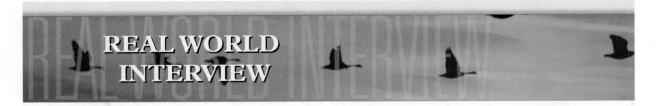

I had severe pain in my right foot, around the middle toe area. The diagnosis was Morton's neuroma. The nurse explained how it developed, how the doctor would remove it, and, most importantly, what the aftereffects would be. I've never had the aftereffects explained to me; I never even thought to ask!

To me this represents quality care. The nurse told me what to expect. The majority of my non-health care friends and myself don't even know enough to think of the questions. I really appreciated this information.

Tessie Dybel
Patient

TABLE 15-1	*Teaching Development Methodology*			
Analysis	**Design**	**Development**	**Implementation**	**Evaluation**
• Context	• Objectives	• Format	• Environment	• Learner
• Learner	• Sequence Content	• Strategies	• Learner	• Teaching
• Content		• Media	• Presentation	
		• Lesson plan	• Content	

Context Analysis

The context consists of the situational context in which the teaching need arose and the instructional context in which the teaching will occur.

 The situational context is the situation that creates the need for learning. For example, is the patient facing a particular health care procedure such as a heart operation? Has the patient expressed concerns over an existing or potential health care condition such as diabetes? Does the patient have multiple diagnoses such as a diabetic patient facing a heart operation?

 The instructional context refers to the conditions under which teaching will occur. In what environment will teaching be presented? Is it a health care facility, a home, a community environment, or some other setting? How will this affect the ability to provide and access resources? How will it affect the nurse's ability to effectively control the teaching environment? How will it affect the patient's attention and motivation?

 The instructional context also includes the time for teaching: when will the teaching occur and how long will the nurse have? Will it occur too early or too late to be useful to the patient? Is the amount of time planned for teaching adequate? Is the amount of time flexible or is it fixed such as 1 hour allotted at a community center for giving a course on diabetes management?

Learner Analysis

The nurse should also conduct a learner analysis (Figure 15-1). **Learner analysis** is the process of identifying the learner's unique characteristics and

Patient name _____
Any other learners? ☐ No ☐ Yes If yes, list names and affiliation with patient. _____   _____ _____   _____
Diagnosis _____
Patient/learner gender ☐ Male ☐ Female
Cultural/religious/lifestyle factors that may affect teaching? ☐ No ☐ Yes If yes, describe. _____
Patient/learner's primary language ☐ English ☐ Spanish ☐ Other _____ Translation/assistance needed? ☐ No ☐ Yes
Is patient/learner ☐ Child ☐ Adolescent ☐ Adult ☐ Elderly
Any limitations to patient/learner learning? Cognitive ☐ No ☐ Yes Describe _____ Physical ☐ No ☐ Yes Describe _____ ☐ Auditory ☐ Visual ☐ Tactile ☐ Pain ☐ Discomfort Emotional ☐ No ☐ Yes Describe _____
Literacy: Can patient/learner read at an appropriate level for the teaching materials? ☐ No ☐ Yes If no, alternate materials needed? ☐ No ☐ Yes
Are there any other factors that may affect patient/learner teaching? ☐ No ☐ Yes If yes, please describe _____
Has patient/learner had previous health care experience with this topic? ☐ No ☐ Yes Previous teaching on this topic? ☐ No ☐ Yes Describe _____
Describe any known information about patient/learner learning styles/preferences _____

Figure 15-1 Learner Analysis (Individual Session)

needs and the ways in which these can influence the teaching process. This is an important consideration, especially in the individualized teaching that occurs in nursing. Understanding the patient's unique characteristics and needs helps the nurse develop teaching that is relevant and effective.

While at one level people can be said to be similar, at another level they are all unique. Even though teaching is based on a standard methodology, it is also a human interaction, and its success is influenced by the unique personalities of the people involved. Understanding the patient's unique characteristics may not guarantee success in teaching, but it can contribute to its effectiveness. The patient-centered and empathetic traits inherent in the nursing process can help nurses develop personal understanding and awareness of their patients.

The first question facing the nurse is, Is the patient the learner? If not, who is?

In most cases, the learner will in fact be the patient. However, in some cases, the patient may be unable or unwilling to participate in the learning process. In other instances, there may be other learners in addition to the patient, such as family members, legal guardians, or others, who may make health care decisions for the patient. Family members or significant others may not directly participate in the patient's health care but, with the patient's permission, may require or desire information nonetheless. Learners may be caregivers who, whether related or not, will be participating in the patient's care.

Demographics. After identifying the learners, the nurse can analyze specific characteristics of the

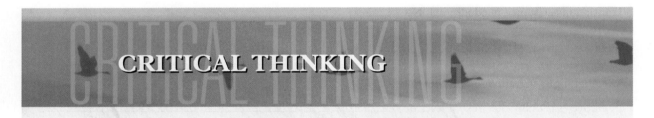

CRITICAL THINKING

You work on a nursing unit that cares for cancer patients. Many of these patients are in constant pain. How can you teach patients who are in pain? How can you reduce the stress of these patients and increase the likelihood of their retaining your teaching? Is it possible to teach these patients? Who else can you involve in their patient teaching?

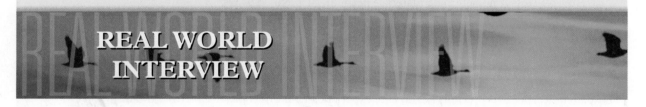

REAL WORLD INTERVIEW

My husband, Ted, was ill with cancer and developed a wound on his leg. The nurses cared for the leg wound while Ted was in the hospital. When they wanted to discharge him from the hospital, the nurse from the wound clinic taught me to how to do the dressing. She showed me how to clean it and apply ointment and a dressing to it. Then, she had me change the dressing. I felt comfortable doing it and I was happy they taught me. The nurse said I was doing a good job. At home, the visiting nurse asked me, "Are you comfortable doing this?" I was happy as I felt I could do it as well as they could.

Florence Lebryk
Patient's Wife

learners. This analysis helps the nurse identify unique needs of the learners and develop teaching that addresses those needs.

Various demographic characteristics can influence a learner's response to the health care and learning environments. These factors include:

- Cultural background
- Language
- Age
- Education
- Health care background
- Physiological condition

The nurse's major goal is to identify characteristics that may indicate how the patient may respond to teaching. Some of these are physical such as pain or physical discomfort that will affect the patient's concentration. Others may be psychosocial such as cultural beliefs that influence the patient's ideas about health care—for example, reliance on folk remedies. Cultural factors may also influence how a patient reacts to the nurse during a teaching session. Culturally influenced suspicion of or deference to health care staff may prevent the patient from effectively communicating with the teacher. Recent theories (Strauss & Howe, 1991) even suggest that people born in a common generation, such as baby boomers or Generation Xers, may share similar values and attitudes, which they carry with them throughout life. These common traits may have implications for the way they approach learning.

The nurse may not be able to identify all of these characteristics prior to the teaching session. However, the more the nurse knows about the patient, the more the nurse can develop teaching that effectively incorporates the patient's unique characteristics and needs.

Learning Styles. A **learning style** is a particular manner in which a learner responds to and processes learning. Traditional teaching often has expected the learner to adjust to the teaching style of the instructor rather than vice versa. In recent decades, this attitude has changed, and educational researchers and the educational community have come to agree on a principle that many people have always espoused: People learn differently.

The different ways in which people learn are still being determined and debated. Several theories of learning style exist, though they typically fall into one of three categories: perception, information processing, and personality (Conner & Hodgins, n.d.).

Perception. Perception theories emphasize the way in which people's senses affect learning. For example, some learners easily retain information when they can see or visualize it. Others retain best when they hear information. Still others learn best through physical action or involvement. Examples of perception theories include the Visual-Auditory-Kinesthetic (VAK) Model (Rose, 1985), shown in Table 15-2, and Gardner's Multiple Intelligences (Gardner, 1993), shown in Table 15-3.

Information Processing. Information processing theories emphasize different styles of thinking. Does the learner prefer concrete facts or abstract theory, reflective observation or direct experience? An example is the Kolb Experiential Learning Style (Kolb, 1984), shown in Figure 15-2 (see page 308).

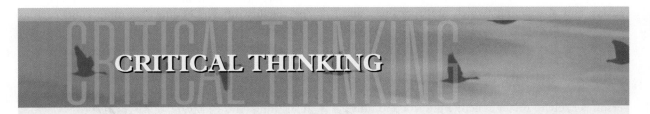

CRITICAL THINKING

Think about how you learn. How would you describe your own learning style? When you develop teaching, does your teaching reflect your own learning preferences, or does it reflect the learning style of the patient? Look at a recent teaching session you observed. What changes would you make so that it addresses a different learning style?

TABLE 15-2	**Rose's Visual–Auditory–Kinesthetic (VAK) Model of Learning**	
Style	**Design**	**Description**
Visual learner	Learn best when they see; prefer graphic images and written text	• Use charts, graphs, pictures, diagrams, and so on. • Include outlines, handouts, and other material for reading and note taking. • Allow plenty of empty space in materials for learner to take notes, draw diagrams, and so on. • Preview and review teaching content visually, through flip charts, outlines, or other visual means. • Include both textual and graphic versions of information within material.
Auditory learner	Learn best when they hear and say	• Present material verbally. • Include verbal preview and review of material. • Involve learner through verbal questions and answers, discussion. • Include verbal activities, such as brainstorming, discussion, and quiz show activities that require verbal response.
Kinesthetic learner	Learn best when they touch and move	• Use activities to get learners up and moving. • Use music and color during presentation (these stimulate senses). • Whenever possible, physically demonstrate learning and have learner physically practice it. • Provide frequent breaks during presentation so learners can get up and move around. • Provide toys, models, equipment, or other objects learners can touch. • For complex tasks, have learners visualize physically performing the task.

Compiled from *Accelerated Learning*, by C. Rose, 1985, New York: Dell.

In Kolb's theory, there are four major thinking styles: sensing and abstracting (which are opposites) and doing and watching (also opposites). An individual's style combines two of these styles, with one dominating. For example, a person whose style combines sensing and watching, with sensing dominant, is described by Kolb as a reflector personality. Such a person is likely to prefer concrete information rather than abstractions, prefers social situations to solitary ones, and judges performance by external measures rather than by personal criteria. Educationally, this person would probably learn best in an interactive group setting in which performance expectations are clearly stated and information is specific and factual.

Personality. Personality theories emphasize how personality differences affect learning. Traits such as introversion or extroversion, preference for rational objectivity or instinctive "gut feeling" affect the individual's learning. An example is a theory based on the Myers-Briggs Personality Dichotomies (Table 15-4), which in turn are based on personality theories of Carl Jung (Briggs Myers, & Myers, 1995).

This theory suggests that personality is made up of four complementary sets of traits: extroversion-introversion, sensing-intuition, thinking-feeling, and judging-perceiving. Within each of these sets, there is a sliding scale, so to speak. For example, on the extroversion-introversion scale, 1 might be com-

TABLE 15-3	Gardner's Multiple Intelligences	
Type	**Characteristics**	**Teaching Considerations**
Verbal—linguistic	Responds to rhythms and patterns of words, whether written or oral	Prefers activities that involve listening, speaking, writing
Logical—mathematical	Responds to reasoning, logic, recognition of patterns and structures	Prefers activities that involve abstract symbols, formulas, numbers, problem solving
Musical	Responds to pitch, melody, rhythm, and tone	Prefers activities that involve audio, musical rhythms, tonal patterns, melodic sound
Spatial	Responds to two- and three-dimensional visual representations	Prefers using or creating graphics and models, "visualizing" abstract information
Bodily—kinesthetic	Responds to physical movement and activity (sports, dancing)	Prefers activities involving physical movement and gestures
Interpersonal	Responds to social interactions and relationships	Prefers group activities or other situations that involve human interaction or collaboration
Intrapersonal	Responds to personal, inner emotions to understand self and others	Prefers activities that use introspection, processing emotions, reflection
Naturalist	Responds to intricacies and subtleties of patterns and relationships in nature	Prefers activities that provide involvement in the natural world (plants, animals, other natural phenomena)

Compiled from *Frames of Mind,* by H. Gardner, 1993, New York: Basic Books.

pletely extroverted, 10 completely introverted, and 5 equally both. In most cases, one or the other usually dominates. Through testing, an individual can be identified as one of 16 possible types, based on the person's score in each of the four areas. The personality type is identified by a four-letter indicator. For example, an INTJ would be an introvert-intuitive-thinking-judging personality. An ESFP would be an extrovert-sensory-feeling-perceiving personality. In the theories of Jung and Myers-Briggs, each personality type has specific characteristics that affect the individual's approach to life experiences, including learning. Extroverts prefer to interact with people; introverts prefer to be alone. Thinking personalities prefer an objective, unwavering approach; feeling personalities are more likely to bend the rules if they think it makes people happy.

Such personality differences can affect the way individuals approach and engage in a learning experience.

Knowledge of patient learning style is significant because it directly influences the nurse's choices when it comes to selecting teaching strategies and media. For example, if the patient is a visual learner, using graphics and charts is a logical teaching choice.

If at all possible, the nurse should make an effort to identify and understand the patient's learning style because this knowledge can significantly affect the teaching process.

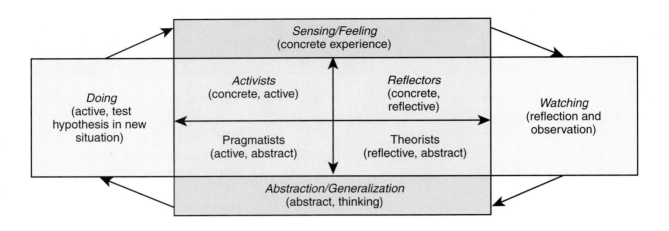

Figure 15-2 Kolb's Experiential Learning Style. Compiled from *Experiential Learning,* by D. A. Kolb, 1984, Englewood Cliffs, NJ: Prentice-Hall/TPR.

Knowledge of patient demographics and learning style is more useful in individual patient teaching, for which teaching can be tailored to a specific individual. Such tailoring is usually not possible in group teaching because members of the group will have a variety of characteristics. Rather than tailor group teaching to one style or characteristic, the nurse will need to incorporate teaching methods that address various styles and characteristics.

Content Analysis

During context analysis, the nurse determines the overall type of information that teaching should address, such as information about diabetes. Learner analysis helps the nurse understand patient characteristics and learning styles and how they might influence teaching strategies.

During content analysis, the nurse begins to drill down and identify more specific information

TABLE 15-4	*Myers-Briggs Personality Dichotomies*			
Extroversion	Prefer interaction with people, conversation; learn when explaining to others or selves	vs.	Introversion	Reflective, focus on inner thoughts; think more than talk; need to establish frameworks for information they learn; see global view
Sensing	Rely on senses; detail oriented, prefer facts; prefer linear, structured presentation	vs.	Intuition	Seek patterns and relationships in information; rely on hunches; learn by discovery, prefer big picture or framework
Thinking	Prefer analysis and logic when making decisions; stress objectivity and fairness; want clear goals and objectives; want their learning expectations stated in clear, precise, and concrete terms	vs.	Feeling	Oriented toward human values and needs when making decisions; stress empathy and harmony; enjoy group exercises
Judging	Decisive, goal-oriented; value action and planning	vs.	Perceiving	Curious, adaptable, spontaneous; process-oriented rather than goal-oriented; continually gather information; may be pursuing many goals simultaneously; may learn better when given small and frequent tasks and deadlines

Compiled from *Gifts Differing,* by I. Briggs Myers and P. B. Myers, 1995, Palo Alto, CA: Davies-Black.

that teaching should address. For example, a person needing to learn diabetic self-management may need to learn the following:

- Understanding of diabetes and its effects
- How to obtain and interpret a blood sugar reading
- How to manage diabetes through diet and exercise
- Knowledge of diabetic medications, their effects and side effects, specifically the medications that the patient will use
- How to administer insulin injections or other forms of medication
- How to determine when to contact health care staff

The nurse must also determine what information is essential to the teaching session. While there may be a wealth of information available for a topic, all the available information may not be necessary information. Some of it may be irrelevant, redundant, or nonessential.

A typical rule of thumb in choosing content for teaching is to distinguish between need to know versus nice to know. Need-to-know information can further be identified as common and critical. Teaching should address information the patient must commonly use, such as how to obtain and interpret a blood sugar reading, and information the patient must know to address or avoid critical situations, such as how to administer an insulin injection. Any information that does not fall into these categories is considered

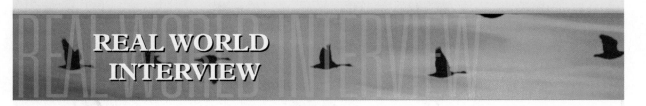

REAL WORLD INTERVIEW

I recently experienced a burning sensation in my chest and tried to relieve the pain by taking several Tums tablets. The sensation decreased slightly, but the Tums did not relieve the pain totally. I called my family doctor for advice, and his suggestion was to go to the Emergency Room. They admitted me to the hospital and scheduled me to take a stress test the next day. Electrocardiograms and blood samples were taken throughout the balance of the day and through the night. They indicated that things were not quite right. An angiogram the next morning showed a 90% blockage in one artery and 60% blockage in a second artery. An angioplasty with a stent was performed on the artery with 90% blockage. The second artery was not cleared. My care at the hospital was excellent. The nurses, doctors, and staff were very caring. They taught me what I needed to know about my heart attack and the need to follow a prescribed diet and exercise rehabilitation program. I appreciate the excellent care and teaching I received.

Steve Manich
Patient

nonessential and can be classified as nice to know, for example, the history of diabetes management in the United States. Nice-to-know information can be shared with the patient if there is time and the patient has mastered essential information, but it has a lower priority in the teaching session.

In health care, such information may already be dictated by health care standards. Therefore, nurses will find that many content decisions may have already been made. However, there may still be additional information that can potentially be included. The nurse must analyze such information and determine whether it fits in the teaching situation.

Learning Domains

The goal of teaching is not just dispensation of knowledge but change in behavior. This is especially true in health care.

Learning theory suggests that learning can be classified into taxonomies, or **learning domains**, each based on the major type of learning involved.

Each taxonomy is organized into a hierarchy that progresses from simple to complex behaviors. These behaviors can be observed and measured. This means that the nurse does not just present infor-

mation to a patient and hope that the patient has learned and mastered it, but that the nurse can document behavioral changes by measuring the patient's performance at appropriate levels. The nurse can also examine what types of behavior the information represents: acquiring knowledge, gaining skill, or changing attitude.

Educators have identified three domains of learning:

1. Cognitive (Bloom & Krathwohl, 1956)
2. Psychomotor (Simpson, 1971)
3. Affective (Krathwohl, Bloom, & Masia, 1999)

The **cognitive domain** is centered on knowledge, or what the learner knows (Table 15-5).

The **psychomotor domain** is centered on skill, or what the learner does (Table 15-6).

The **affective domain** is centered on attitude, or what the learner feels/believes (Table 15-7).

The emerging pattern of behaviors sets the stage for the design phase of teaching development, in which the nurse translates the behaviors into objectives, develops teaching topics corresponding to the objectives, and arranges those topics into a structured topic sequence. This provides an organized, structured framework on which to build an effective teaching session.

| | TABLE 15-5 | *Taxonomies of Learning: Cognitive Domain* | |

Level	Description	Actions
Knowledge	Recalls information	Define, describe, identify, know, label, list, name, recall, recognize, select, state
Comprehension	Understands meaning of information, as demonstrated by the ability to restate the information in the learner's own words	Comprehend, convert, defend, distinguish, estimate, explain, generalize, give example of, interpret, paraphrase, rewrite, summarize, translate
Application	Uses information in a new situation	Apply, change, compute, construct, demonstrate, discover, manipulate, modify, predict, prepare, produce, relate, solve
Analysis	Separates information into component parts to understand the overall structure	Analyze, break down, compare, contrast, diagram, deconstruct, differentiate, discriminate, distinguish, identify, illustrate, outline, relate, select, separate
Synthesis	Puts information together to form a new meaning or structure	Categorize, combine, compile, compose, create, devise, design, generate, modify, organize, plan, rearrange, reconstruct, reorganize, revise, summarize
Evaluation	Makes judgments about the value of ideas	Appraise, compare, conclude, contrast, criticize, critique, defend, evaluate, explain, interpret, justify, support

Compiled from *Taxonomy of Educational Objectives, Handbook 1,* by B. S. Bloom and D. Krathwohl, 1956, Boston: Addison-Wesley.

Design

The purpose of the design phase is for the nurse to organize and structure the content identified in the analysis phase. The nurse accomplishes this by establishing objectives and by sequencing content.

Establishing Behavioral Objectives

The behaviors identified in content analysis are now translated into behavioral objectives. A **behavioral objective** states a specific and measurable behavior that should result from the teaching session. Behavioral objectives define what the nurse will teach, thereby providing the skeleton of the teaching session. They also provide the basis for patient evaluation because the success of patient learning is gauged by whether the patient achieves these objectives.

The essential component of a behavioral objective is a performance, specifically one that can observed and measured. For example, the following is a behavioral objective: "List the major bones of the human skeleton from head to toe."

However, this statement leaves some elements undefined. Who is doing the listing? The person(s) who performs the behavior is the *audience*.

This objective also does not state how well the person should perform the objective. Is 20% accuracy acceptable, or 50%, or 80%? The *degree* identifies how well the behavior is performed.

When we add audience and degree to the objective, it reads this way: "The patient will list the major bones of the human skeleton from head to toe, with 100% accuracy."

TABLE 15-6	*Taxonomies of Learning: Psychomotor Domain*	

Level	Description	Actions
Perception	Observes behaviors involved in a performance	Choose, describe, detect, differentiate, distinguish, identify, isolate, relate, select
Set	Demonstrates readiness to perform; understands steps in a task, adopts physical posture to perform the task	Begin, display, explain, move, proceed, react, show, state
Guided response	Imitates performance and refines it through trial and error, practice	Copy, trace, follow, react, reproduce, respond
Mechanism	Performs task comfortably	Assemble, calibrate, construct, dismantle, fasten, fix, manipulate, measure, mend, mix, organize
Complex overt response	Performs task skillfully and automatically (increased proficiency, accuracy, and coordination)	Same as for Mechanism, but adverbs/adjectives indicate increase in speed or accuracy of performance
Adaptation	Alters performance to adapt to new situations	Adapt, alter, change, rearrange, reorganize, revise, vary
Origination	Creates an original skill	Arrange, build, combine, compose, construct, create, design, initiate, make, originate

Compiled from "Educational Objectives in the Psychomotor Domain," by E. Simpson, in *Behavioral Objectives in Curriculum Development,* edited by M. Kapfer, 1971, Boston: Educational Technology.

These three elements—audience, performance, degree—should always be present in an objective.

There is a fourth, optional component of an objective. It is called the condition. The condition indicates any restrictions or specific requirements involved in performing the behavior. For example: Given a color photograph of the skeletal system and a pad of paper to write on, the patient will list the major bones of the human skeleton from head to toe, with 100% accuracy. In this example, the condition is the phrase *given a color photograph and a pad of paper to write on.*

One way to remember the components of an objective is to think of the ABCD method: A = Audience, B = Behavior, C = Condition, and D = Degree (Table 15-8).

It is up to the nurse to determine how detailed objectives should be. The important consideration is that they indicate a behavior that can reasonably be observed and measured.

Terminal and Enabling Objectives. When developing teaching, the nurse often begins with a primary goal for the session—for example, the patient will demonstrate diabetic self-care. As the nurse develops objectives, a hierarchy of objectives may evolve, much like an outline or a hierarchical organization chart. Certain primary behaviors, each supporting the session goal, become evident. A terminal objective identifies a major behavior that contributes to achievement of the overall session goal. Terminal behaviors may in turn be achieved through the performance of related, secondary behaviors. An enabling objective identifies a secondary behavior that contributes to, or enables, achievement of terminal objectives.

Table 15-9 illustrates this concept of terminal and enabling objectives.

The emerging objectives will suggest the teaching topics for the session. If topics do not match up

---

TABLE 15-7 *Taxonomies of Learning: Affective Domain*

Level	Description	Actions
Receiving/attending	Displays attention, willingness to listen	Ask, choose, describe, follow, give, identify, locate, name, select, use
Responding	Displays active participation, willingness, motivation	Answer, assist, aid, comply, conform, discuss, help, label, perform, practice, present, read, recite, report, select, tell, write
Valuing	Shows acceptance, preference, and commitment for the value	Complete, demonstrate, differentiate, explain, follow, form, initiate, invite, join, justify, propose, read, report, select, share, study
Organization	Organizes and prioritizes values through contrasting them, resolving value conflicts, and developing a personal value system	Adhere, alter, arrange, combine, complete, defend, explain, formulate, generalize, identify, integrate, modify, order, organize, propose, relate, synthesize
Characterization (internalizing values)	Exhibits a value system that drives the individual's behavior	Act, discriminate, display, influence, modify, perform, practice, propose, qualify, question, revise, serve, solve, verify

Compiled from *Taxonomy of Educational Objectives, Handbook 2,* by D. Krathwohl, B. S. Bloom, and B. B. Masia, 1999, Boston: Addison-Wesley.

TABLE 15-8 *Components of a Behaviorial Objective*

Audience	Behavior	Condition	Degree
Who will perform the behavior	What the performer will do	What limitations or other conditions will be placed on the performance	What degree of measurement will be used to determine successful performance
The patient	*Will identify the major valves of the heart*	*Using the anatomical heart chart provided by the teacher*	*With an accuracy of 100%*

to objectives, or vice versa, this indicates a potential problem in the teaching session.

Objectives also dictate the items for learner evaluation. Each evaluation item should correspond to an objective. If the nurse is creating objectives for performances that are not relevant or necessary to evaluate, the nurse should examine those objectives and eliminate them.

Sequencing Content

As the nurse analyzes content and develops objectives, the main topics within the teaching session and the order in which they appear become clearer. The nurse should then choose a specific topic-sequencing structure. In many situations, there will be only one choice, such as when teaching a procedure in the

TABLE 15-9	Example of Session Goal, Terminal Objectives, and Enabling Objectives

Session goal: The patient will be able to demonstrate diabetic self-care.

Terminal objective 1: Perform an accurate blood sugar reading.	Terminal objective 2: Develop a diabetic behavior management plan.	Terminal objective 3: Perform insulin self-administration.
Enabling objectives: • Identify equipment for taking a blood sugar reading. • Demonstrate the procedure for taking a blood sugar reading. • State the acceptable range of blood sugar level.	Enabling objectives: • Identify symptoms of hypoglycemia and hyperglycemia. • List foods that can raise blood sugar levels. • Discuss ADA diet plan. • Develop a regular exercise plan.	Enabling objectives: • Identify equipment necessary for insulin self-administration. • Discuss medication and method of administering. • Demonstrate correct method for administering insulin injection.

CASE STUDY 15-1

Mr. Albee, a 68-year-old male, has been your patient since he was admitted 2 days ago with diabetes. He has been unable to control his blood sugar with oral medication. His physician has ordered insulin injections for him. You gave him his first injection this morning and plan to begin teaching him how to give himself injections today. How will you approach Mr. Albee? Who else will you involve in his teaching? How will you develop a teaching plan for Mr. Albee?

order in which the steps are performed. In other situations, no one sequence is obvious, and the nurse has various options from which to choose.

Table 15-10 describes common sequencing structures.

Development

In the design phase, the nurse essentially determines what objectives teaching should accomplish and what information will support those objectives. During the development phase, the nurse clarifies how to teach by determining what strategies and resources to use.

Format

Modern educators have come up with various formats for teaching. One of the most common is Gagne's nine events of instruction (Gagne, 1985), described in Table 15-11. This provides an effective framework for conducting the teaching session.

Any teaching session should incorporate certain effective elements.

Repetition. There is an old adage in adult training: Tell them what you're going to tell them; tell them what you want to tell them; tell them what you just told them.

TABLE 15-10	Common Sequencing Structures

Type	Characteristics
Chronological	Information is arranged in time sequence, based on the sequential occurrence of events. Typically used for teaching history.
Procedural (step by step)	Presents the steps in a procedure in the order in which they are performed.
Categorical	Information is organized into categories that are related to the primary topic. Allows the nurse to develop an arbitrary, but logical, structure when the information does not fit any of the other structures described here.
Topical	Patient is immediately placed in the middle of a topical problem or issue. Teaching may then address how the issue originated and the concerns surrounding its resolution.
Parts to whole; whole to parts	Presents the parts, then shows how they relate to the whole, or presents the whole, then talks about each part.
General to specific; specific to general	Similar to the above; presents the "big picture" first, then presents details. Or presents details first, then shows how they fit into the big picture.
Problem to resolution	Presents a problem/situation, then presents the topics involved in its resolution.
Known to unknown; unknown to known	Known to unknown begins with patient's existing information/experience and uses it as a bridge to new, unknown information. Unknown to known presents unfamiliar information, later showing its connection to what the patient already knows.
Theoretical to practical; practical to theoretical	Presents the theory, then demonstrates how it is used. Or shows practical applications of information, then presents the theory.
Simple to complex; complex to simple	Begins with information that is easier to present or easier for the patient to learn, then moves to more difficult information. Or presents the most complex material first, then progresses to easier information.

Based on *Designing Powerful Training,* by M. Milano and D. Ullius, 1998, San Francisco: Jossey-Bass.

In other words, preview information, present the information, then review information. Previewing information allows the patient to understand what is to come and mentally prepare, much like providing a road map of an upcoming trip. It also provides a framework so that when information is presented, the patient knows where he is in the process. Finally, review provides the patient with an opportunity to organize the information and reinforce the learning. Therefore, repetition provides one of the most effective methods of teaching and should be incorporated into the teaching as much as possible.

Interaction. Learning works best when there is interaction between patient and teacher and when the patient is involved. Constant conversation with and questioning of the patient stimulates interaction and involvement. So does incorporating activities throughout the teaching session.

Presentation, Performance, Practice. The nurse can incorporate repetition, as well as interaction, into teaching through a format of presentation, performance, and practice. The nurse presents material to the patient, the nurse performs a

TABLE 15-11	*Gagne's Nine Events of Instruction*

Event	Explanation
1. Gain attention.	Engage the learner and stimulate interest and motivation.
2. Inform learner of objective.	Stating objectives establishes the expectations for the learner and provides an opportunity to preview the content of the teaching event.
3. Stimulate recall of prerequisite learning.	Try to relate the content to previous learning or experience. This provides the learner with a familiar context in which to approach learning.
4. Present stimulus materials.	Present the content.
5. Provide learning guidance.	Perform/demonstrate the learning for the learner or in conjunction with the learner.
6. Elicit performance.	Have the learner practice or demonstrate the learning.
7. Provide feedback.	Help the learner refine learning by providing feedback and suggestions.
8. Assess performance.	Evaluate learner performance in terms of the learning objectives.
9. Enhance retention and transfer.	Review learning and encourage learner to use learning in new situations.

Compiled from *The Conditions of Learning and the Theory of Instruction,* by R. Gagne, 1985, New York: Holt, Rinehart & Winston.

demonstration either alone or along with the patient, and then the patient practices the performance, either independently or with nurse observation. This format allows the patient to repeat and reinforce learning while also increasing the patient's interaction with the nurse and active involvement in the learning.

Variety. A certain amount of variety in teaching maintains the patient's interest. Using different approaches and media can add variety to the teaching session. However, don't overdo variety because too much can break continuity and confuse the patient.

Strategies

Although Gagne's events provide a structure for the overall teaching session, they do not prescribe how teaching will occur at the topic level. At this level, teaching can take various forms, commonly called strategies. Examples of teaching strategy include lecture, group discussion, and role play, to name just a few. The number and types of strategies the nurse chooses depend on several factors such as the type of content being taught, the patient's learning style, the nurse's own comfort level with various strategies, the resources available, the teaching environment, and so on. The nurse may use a single teaching strategy throughout the session or may vary strategy from topic to topic. Strategy may also be influenced by the teaching event; that is, it may be different during presentation and performance.

The nurse has wide latitude in selecting teaching strategies, but the nurse should choose strategies that are most effective in meeting the patient's learning needs.

Media

Equally important to consider are the resources to be used during the teaching event. Resources consist of various media such as written, visual, audio, video, computer-based, or other material, or combinations of these materials. As in selecting teaching strategy, a single medium may be used throughout the event, or several may be used, depending on such factors as content type, teaching strategy, patient learning style, teacher preference, or the limitations of what is available. The nurse has several options but should make decisions based on the idea of what would be best for the patient's learning.

The nurse must consider two categories of media for patient teaching—media to be used during teaching and media to be provided to the patient for reference. Because the latter is likely to be used outside the presence and supervision of the nurse, it is especially important that it be appropriate for the patient to use.

Media Evaluation and Selection. When possible, the nurse should use media resources that are already available. This frees the nurse from the task of creating materials and allows for more time to be devoted to developing and managing the teaching event. However, the nurse must examine available materials and determine whether they are truly suitable for use in teaching.

The nurse should look at several factors. Is the content presented in the material appropriate for the patient's needs? Is it accurate? Is the material of suitable quality; for example, is the audio understandable, is video of appropriate visual quality, are graphics understandable, is text readable or at the appropriate reading level? Is the source reliable; for example, does information on a web site come from a reputable and verifiable source?

Materials Development. Preferably, the nurse should use existing materials when developing a teaching session. In many situations, the nurse's organization will have existing materials and encourage their use. In other situations, the nurse may have greater freedom in selecting teaching materials.

In some situations, the nurse may find that no materials exist or existing materials are not appropriate for the content to be taught. The nurse may need to create materials, either to augment existing materials or to fill a void. Keep in mind that creating materials can be both a creative and a frustrating endeavor.

Lesson Plan

So far, the nurse has analyzed teaching content, designed behavioral objectives, organized the sequence of content, established the overall format of teaching, and selected appropriate teaching strategies and materials. All these decisions will be reflected in the lesson plan. A **lesson plan** is a document that provides the blueprint for the teaching session. (See Table 15-12 for a sample lesson plan.) It provides the necessary information for the nurse or other teacher to conduct the teaching session.

Implementation

During the implementation phase, the nurse actually conducts the teaching. The lesson plan defines the objectives, topics, strategies, and materials needed for the session. Using this plan, the nurse begins the teaching session.

However, the best-laid plans often change in the face of reality. When the nurse actually begins the teaching session, various factors will affect the success of the session. Some of these factors are highly controllable, others less so. Some of the more influential factors are environment, patient condition, nurse teaching skills, and nurse communication skills.

Environment

The environment in which the teaching will occur can have a major impact on the effectiveness of teaching. Before beginning to teach, the nurse should evaluate physical environment factors such as lighting, temperature, and sound quality. Also consider the patient's privacy needs, interior or exterior distractions, and the environment's ability to support the teaching session, for example, whether there are enough electrical outlets for equipment. Some of these situations may be outside the nurse's control; therefore, the nurse may have to quickly adapt the teaching session to compensate. In other situations, the nurse may need to relocate to another environment.

Learner

The nurse must also assess whether the learner's or patient's condition at the time of the teaching event

TABLE 15-12 *Sample Lesson Plan*

Lesson Plan Title: Diabetic Self-Management

Patient	Juan Abado
Presenter	John Reilley, RN
Setting	Patient's hospital room
Brief patient/learner summary	Patient is a 50-year-old English-speaking Hispanic male, college graduate, newly diagnosed with diabetes and unfamiliar with the self-injection process. No other learners involved. No physical limitations to learning. Mild anxiety about self-injection, but high motivation. Initial interview suggests preference for learning through visual means.
Overall goal	The patient will understand and demonstrate diabetic self-care.
Objectives	After completing the session, the patient will be able to do the following:

- Perform an accurate blood sugar reading
  - Identify equipment for taking blood sugar reading
  - Demonstrate the procedure for taking a blood sugar reading
  - State the acceptable range of blood sugar level

- Develop a diabetic behavior management plan
  - Identify symptoms of hypoglycemia and hyperglycemia
  - List foods that can raise blood sugar levels
  - Discuss the ADA diet plan
  - Develop a regular exercise plan

- Administer insulin self-injection
  - Identify equipment necessary for insulin self-injection
  - Discuss insulin and method for self-injection
  - Demonstrate correct procedure for insulin self-injection

Topic outline (excerpt)

Time: 1 minute

Preview
In this session, we will learn about diabetes and three major elements of diabetic self-care:
- Monitoring blood sugar
- Developing appropriate diet and exercise
- Insulin self-injection

Time: 3 minutes

Objective: Identify equipment for taking a blood sugar reading

Topics:
1. Importance of taking a blood sugar reading
2. When/how often to take a blood sugar reading
3. Equipment for taking a blood sugar reading
   a. Accu-Check and similar machines
   b. Interpretation strips

Strategy: Lecture and demonstration/return demonstration

Medium: Handout—*Monitoring Blood Sugar*

(continues)

Table 15-12 *(continued)*

Time: 10 minutes	Objective: Demonstrate the procedure for taking a blood sugar reading

Topics:
1. How to put the interpretation strip in the machine
2. How to disinfect the finger
3. How to stick the finger
4. How to apply the blood to the interpretation strip
5. How to interpret the results

Strategy: Presentation of video and discussion with patient; nurse demonstration followed by patient demonstration

Medium: Equipment—Accu-Check machine and interpretation strips; video segment—*Taking a Blood Sugar Reading*; handout—*Monitoring Blood Sugar*

(Continue with this format for each objective in the session. Each segment lists the objective, the related topics to be covered, the teaching strategy used, and the presentation medium. It is also helpful to indicate the estimated amount of time needed to conduct each segment.)

Time: 3 minutes

Review

(In this segment, the nurse reviews the major objectives and topics covered in the session. This is also a useful time for asking the patient whether there are any topics he is unsure of or has further questions about.)

Strategies for retention/transfer

(In this segment, the nurse indicates any methods for helping the patient apply the teaching to future situations.)

Have patient perform own blood sugar tests four times daily during remaining time in hospital.

Evaluation

(This segment can take the form of a behavioral checklist, in which the nurse checks off that the patient has acceptably performed the behavior, or specific evaluation items, such as questions or other forms of evaluation. The example below contains samples of each.)

Identifies equipment for taking blood sugar reading   ☐ Yes   ☐ No

Demonstrates the procedure for taking a blood sugar reading
   ☐ Yes   ☐ No

Blood sugar readings are taken using an Accu-Check machine and

_____ .

Before sticking the finger, you should
A. put the blood on the strip.
B. read the blood sugar results.
C. disinfect the finger.
D. close your eyes.

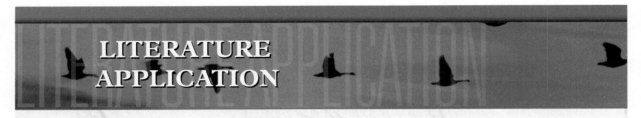

LITERATURE APPLICATION

Citation: Bruccoliere, T. (2000). How to make patient teaching stick. *RN, 63*(2), 34–38.

Discussion: Bruccoliere's article discusses a number of physiological conditions that may affect a patient's learning. These are conditions you can look for when conducting a learner assessment. Her article also provides suggestions for how to address these conditions during teaching. You can incorporate and expand on these suggestions when you plan your teaching. The article contains an insert titled "How Learning Occurs," which describes four stages of adult learning.

Implications for Practice: Knowledge of the four stages of adult learning will be helpful to nurses in planning short-term and long-term patient education.

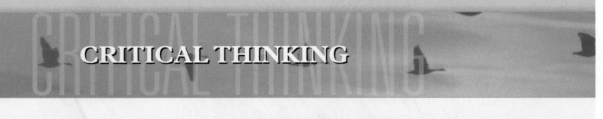

CRITICAL THINKING

You are caring for a patient with lung cancer. She is having a difficult time stopping smoking. Even though all her cigarette packs state that smoking can cause lung cancer, she has not been able to stop. How would you approach this patient? Is it possible to teach her to stop smoking? What factors decrease her chances of stopping? What factors increase her likelihood of stopping?

may affect learning, and be prepared to adapt accordingly. The patient's condition can be affected by physical factors, such as discomfort or pain, and by psychological factors, such as anger, depression, or anxiety. Any of these factors can seriously affect the patient's ability to participate in teaching. The nurse must decide how to address these factors or whether to postpone teaching until a more appropriate time.

Presentation and Content

An effective nurse-teacher must bring certain qualities to the teaching event. While every individual will have varying degrees of talent in each area, nurse-teachers must constantly be aware of these qualities and strive to exhibit them in the teaching event. These qualities include the following:

- Content knowledge: The nurse need not be an expert on a topic but must be able to demonstrate knowledge to the patient.
- Teaching experience: The nurse must be able to come across as an experienced and professional teacher.
- Communication: The nurse should be able to communicate clearly and at a professional level.
- Intelligence: The nurse must be intelligent and able to grasp the complexities of the content.
- Adaptability: The nurse must be able to adapt to changes in the teaching content and format and be able to adapt to unforeseen changes in the teaching session.
- Patience: The nurse must be patient and caring with learners.
- Self-confidence: The nurse must be able to continue forward in the face of numerous changes

and frustrations and maintain a poised and professional manner when interacting with learners.

- Self-direction: The nurse must be able to assume initiative, identify needs, and solve problems. The nurse must be able to work independently without supervision.
- Interactive: The nurse must enjoy dealing with people and interacting with them, while also being able to handle work with difficult people when necessary.
- Organization: The nurse must be able to organize tasks and information and work efficiently.

Communication Skills

While communication can be viewed as another teaching skill, it is more significant than all others in producing successful teaching. Both verbal and non-verbal communication skills are essential to effective teaching.

As much as possible, the nurse should maintain a professional speaking voice:

- Tone should be calm and reassuring yet authoritative.
- Volume should be appropriate enough that the patient can hear.
- Pace should be appropriate enough for the patient to hear and process information.
- Avoid the use of fillers, such as "um," "you know," and so on.
- Speak clearly and with correct grammar.
- Speak in an active voice.

The nurse should also be careful about use of health care terminology. The patient is not likely to have the same familiarity with health care concepts and terms. Avoid using technical terminology if possible, or take the time to explain terms to the patient. If using such terminology, use terms consistently to avoid confusing the patient. However, do not talk to the patient in condescending terms.

Listening skills are critical for good teaching. The nurse must constantly watch and listen to the patient, looking for cues as to the patient's reaction to the teaching. The nurse must involve the patient in learning and look for opportunities to clarify, support, encourage, and incorporate patient responses. This further involves the patient in the learning process and increases patient motivation.

Body language says a lot about the nurse's level of interest and motivation. The nurse should maintain a professional appearance during the teaching event. Eye contact, use of hands, movement, and distance between nurse and patient all send messages about the nurse's attitude toward the teaching event.

Evaluation

Evaluation is the process of determining the effectiveness of teaching. There are two major concerns of evaluation:

- Learner evaluation: Did the patient learn what the patient was supposed to learn?
- Teaching evaluation: Was the teaching presented in an effective manner?

Learner Evaluation

What to evaluate is determined by the objectives. There should be a direct correlation between the objectives established for the teaching and the learner evaluation that occurs during the teaching.

The following demonstrates an objective and the related evaluation item.

Objective: Identify three medications for the treatment of diabetes.

Evaluation item: List three medications for the treatment of diabetes.

Evaluation can take many forms. Asking the learner to recall information, answer questions, perform procedures, solve relevant problems, analyze a situation, or construct a plan of action are all forms of learner evaluation. The nurse should choose evaluation events based on how effectively they reflect the associated learning objective, how realistically the patient can be expected to perform the evaluation, and how practically the nurse can observe and measure successful performance. If possible, the nurse may also want to consider the patient's learning style when planning learner evaluation. For example, if the patient is more of an auditory learner, questions can be posed verbally rather than in written form.

The nurse must also remember that the purpose of evaluation is to validate that the patient has effectively processed and adopted the learning. The purpose of learner evaluation is not to produce devious questions that defeat the patient. Many patients feel anxious at any event that has the slightest hint of "testing." The nurse can reduce patient anxiety by presenting evaluation in the context of a review of the teaching. If the patient is having trouble with certain topics, the nurse can revisit those topics or, if conditions make that approach impractical, provide additional resources or referrals to the patient.

Teaching Evaluation

Teaching evaluation is concerned with whether the teaching event itself was effectively constructed and presented. It is often helpful for the nurse to examine the teaching event, not only to identify areas for improvement but also to identify and reinforce those elements that were effective.

Teaching evaluation can involve feedback from the nurse-teacher, the patient, and/or third-party observers. Measurement can be formal or informal and can involve verbal or written feedback.

Table 15-13 identifies some of the elements that can be examined in teaching evaluation.

While the nurse's health care organization may mandate that some of these factors be evaluated, the nurse has considerable leeway in determining what to

---

TABLE 15-13 *Teaching Evaluation*

Possible Areas for Teaching Evaluation

Patient learning	Did the patient learn the appropriate content, as indicated by such tools as learner evaluation results and follow-up observations? Were learner evaluation items appropriate and reliable?
Patient satisfaction/comfort	Was the patient satisfied with the content presented? With the effectiveness of the presenter? Did the patient feel that questions were addressed appropriately?
Environment	Was the environment conducive to learning? Were there distractions from inside or outside the room? Was lighting appropriate? Room temperature?
Design	Were the objectives appropriate? The topics? The order of sequence?
Knowledge	Did the materials and/or teacher reflect adequate knowledge of the content?
Organization	Was the information well organized?
Accuracy	Was the information presented accurate?
Relevance	Was information presented not relevant to the patient's situation? Or was relevant information missing?
Delivery	Were teaching strategies effective? Materials?
Pacing	Did teaching move too fast or too slow? Were demonstrations at a pace the patient could follow? Was the patient given enough time for practice?
Variety	Was there too much of one type of activity? Not enough variety in teaching methods or presentations? Too much variety, creating a sense of confusion?
Involvement	Was there enough patient involvement? Was there a lack or shortage of activities and/or practice time?
Communication	Did the nurse communicate clearly and effectively with the patient?
Focus	Did the materials and/or teacher stay on the topics?
Assistance	Did the teacher provide enough assistance? Did the materials provide cues or explanations to assist the user in completing activities?

evaluate and how to evaluate. However, the nurse should bear in mind that ongoing evaluation and improvement of the teaching process will provide patients with a rewarding and qualitative learning experience.

Patient teaching is an inherent component of the nursing process, as well as a rewarding experience for the nurse and the patient. The nurse can provide a professional and gratifying learning situation through application of a structured approach to the design, development, and delivery of teaching.

learned, and teaching evaluation, which measures how well the teaching was conducted.

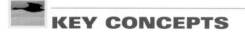

KEY TERMS

affective domain
behavioral objective
cognitive domain
enabling objective
evaluation
learner analysis

learning domains
learning style
lesson plan
methodology
psychomotor domain
terminal objective

KEY CONCEPTS

- A standard teaching methodology contains five major phases: analysis, design, development, implementation, and evaluation.
- Analysis consists of context analysis, learner analysis, and content analysis.
- Learners have unique learning styles; some learners respond better to some teaching situations than others.
- All learning can be classified under three domains: cognitive, psychomotor, and affective.
- Each learning domain contains a hierarchy of behaviors.
- The design phase consists of establishing objectives and sequencing content.
- Behavioral objectives measure performance of behaviors.
- Behavioral objectives consist of an audience, behavior, condition (optional), and degree.
- Behavioral objectives form the skeleton of the teaching session.
- Teaching content is sequenced based on its relation to objectives and on common sequencing structures.
- The development phase consists of establishing format, selecting strategies and media, and finalizing the lesson plan.
- The lesson plan documents the objectives, content, sequence, strategies, media, and evaluation methods of the teaching session.
- The implementation phase consists of conducting teaching. Effective implementation requires attention to the environment, learner, presentation, and learning content.
- The evaluation phase consists of learner evaluation, which measures how well the patient

REVIEW QUESTIONS

1. A person who learns best when teaching involves movement and tactile experience demonstrates which learning style?
   A. Visual
   B. Auditory
   C. Kinesthetic
   D. Activist

2. Which learning domain involves changes in the learner's feelings and beliefs?
   A. Cognitive
   B. Psychomotor
   C. Affective
   D. Reflective

3. Which of the following forms of analysis is concerned with the situation that created the need for teaching and with the conditions under which teaching will occur?
   A. Context analysis
   B. Learner analysis
   C. Content analysis
   D. Teaching analysis

4. Which of these is NOT a component of a behavioral objective?
   A. Audience
   B. Barrier
   C. Condition
   D. Degree

5. According to Gagne, how many events of instruction are present in teaching?
   A. Four
   B. Five
   C. Seven
   D. Nine

REVIEW ACTIVITIES

1. Identify a patient teaching project that you can develop for one of your patients. Develop a lesson plan for this patient. Are your objectives in one, two, or three domains of learning?

2. Identify a patient in a clinical unit who needs teaching. Are there any learner characteristics that would affect the teaching for this patient? How would you adjust the teaching to address these characteristics?

3. Look at Table 15-13, which lists areas for teaching evaluation. What means would you use to evaluate these items? Are there other items that you think should be evaluated? For each item, what would you do to improve performance if necessary?

EXPLORING THE WEB

- Look at the following sites and take the tests to determine your learning style:
  http://www.metamath.com/multiple/multiple_ choice_questions.cgi
  http://www.mxctc.commnet.edu/clc/survey.htm

  Do you think the tests accurately predicted your learning styles? Ask a few friends to take the tests and see how they react. If their styles are different, discuss with them how they prefer to learn.

- Go to the Keirsey web site:
  http://www.keirsey.com

  Complete and score a simplified version of the MBTI. Then go to the link that describes your preferences and potential areas for growth. Do these seem accurate? Have a fellow team member or your first-line patient care manager complete the same questionnaire.

  Share your types and the interpretations with each other.

  Do you agree with the interpretation?

  Given your preferences, do you see why you work well together? Does knowing your preference style help you understand why there are some areas of tension when relating to or working with each other?

  In what areas might communication between you be difficult?

  (The ethics of MBTI state that the sharing of one's type with each other is a personal decision.) MBTI first helps us understand ourselves, and then each other. What other applications of the MBTI can you think of?

- The following sites provide more information on instructional design and adult learning:
  tip.psychology.org/theories.html
  http://www.nwlink.com/~donclark/hrd/sat.html
  seamonkey.ed.asu.edu/~mcisaac/disted/final98/ finallj.html

  Which of these is most helpful to you in developing patient education? Which would you recommend to others who are creating patient education?

- The following sites provide on-line health information for consumers:
  http://www.mayoclinic.com
  http://www.webmd.com
  http://www.allhealth.com
  http://dir.yahoo.com/Health/

  How useful are these sites? How accurate is the information they provide? Would any of them be useful to incorporate in patient teaching? Go to the following site and note the criteria it lists for evaluating consumer health web sites. Using these criteria, how would you evaluate the sites? Are there any other criteria you would add? *http://www.viterbo.edu/personal pages/faculty/Jkanderson/PTEAssignment.html*

- Not all your patients will be adults. Go to *http://www.healthteacher.com*. Look at the lesson plans provided there. Would these be useful in patient teaching for children?

- The following sites represent major health organizations in the United States. What kind of information do these sites contain that would be useful in patient teaching? How would you evaluate these sites in comparison to the consumer sites listed previously?

American Dietetic Association:
http://www.eatright.org

American Diabetes Association:
http://www.diabetes.org

American Heart Association:
http://www.americanheart.org

American Cancer Society:
http://www.cancer.org

National Institute of Health: *http://www.nih.gov*

- Can you find any sites that relate specifically to patient teaching by nurses? Can you find web sites for foreign or international health care organizations? What kind of information do they provide?

REFERENCES

American Hospital Association. (1972). *A patient's bill of rights.* Chicago: Author.

Bloom, B. S., & Krathwohl, D. (1956). *Taxonomy of educational objectives: Handbook I: Cognitive domain.* Boston: Addison-Wesley.

Briggs Myers, I., & Myers, P. B. (1995). *Gifts differing.* Palo Alto, CA: Davies-Black.

Bruccoliere, T. (2000). How to make patient teaching stick. *RN, 63*(2), 34–38.

Conner, M., & Hodgins, W. (n.d.). *Learning styles.* Last updated February 20, 2002, from http://www.learnativity.com/learningstyles.html.

Gagne, R. M. (1985). *The conditions of learning and the theory of instruction* (4th ed.). New York: Holt, Rinehart, & Winston.

Gardner, H. (1993). *Frames of mind: The theory of multiple intelligences* (10th anniversary edition). New York: Basic Books.

Joint Commission on Accreditation of Healthcare Organizations. (2002*). Comprehensive accreditation Manual for Hospitals: The official handbook.* Chicago: Author.

Kolb, D. A. (1984). *Experiential learning: Experience as the source of learning and development.* Englewood Cliffs, NJ: Prentice-Hall/TPR.

Krathwohl, D. R., Bloom, B. S., & Masia, B. B. (1999). *Taxonomy of educational objectives: Handbook 2: Affective domain.* Boston: Addison-Wesley.

Milano, M., & Ullius, D. (1998). *Designing powerful training.* San Francisco: Jossey-Bass.

Rose, C. (1985). *Accelerated learning.* New York: Dell.

Simpson, E. (1971). Educational objectives in the psychomotor domain. In M. Kapfer (Ed.), *Behavioral objectives in curriculum development.* Englewood Cliffs, NJ: Educational Technology.

Strauss, W., & Howe, N. (1991). *Generations: The history of America's future, 1584 to 2069.* New York: Morrow.

SUGGESTED READINGS

American Society for Training and Development. (1995). *Info-line: Basic training for trainers, vols. 1–3.* Alexandria, VA: Author.

Kemp, J. E. (1977). *Instructional design: A plan for unit and course development* (2nd ed.). Belmont, CA: Fearon-Pitman.

Kemp, J. E., Morrison, G. K., & Ross, S. M. (1994). *Designing effective instruction.* New York: Merrill.

Knowles, M. (1984). *The adult learner: A neglected species* (3rd ed.). Houston, TX: Gulf.

Mager, R. (1975). *Preparing instructional objectives* (2nd ed.). Belmont, CA: Fearon-Pitman.

Rothwell, W. J., & Kazanas, H. C. (1992). *Mastering the instructional design process: A systematic approach.* San Francisco: Jossey-Bass.

Smith, P. L., & Ragan, T. J. (1993). *Instructional design.* New York: Macmillan.

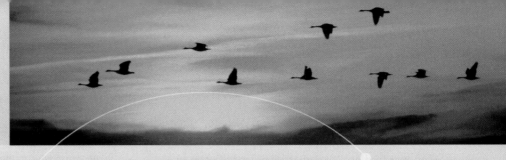

CHAPTER 16

Change and Conflict Resolution

Margaret M. Anderson, EdD, RN, C, CNAA

OBJECTIVES

Upon completion of this chapter, the reader should be able to:

1. Define change from personal, professional, and organizational perspectives.
2. Identify the change theorists.
3. Discuss the concept of the learning organization.
4. Identify driving and restraining forces of change within a structured setting context.
5. Discuss change strategies.
6. Discuss the role and characteristics of a change agent in the change process.
7. Utilize the change process to plan, implement, and evaluate a change project.
8. Identify conflict situations.
9. Identify steps in the conflict resolution process.

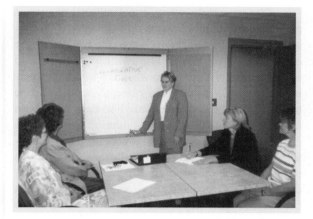

Mary has been a nurse manager for five years. In that time, she has had five supervisors. In addition, she has had to introduce three different methods of care delivery on her unit and has experienced two corporate mergers resulting in changes in corporate culture and mission. Mary just completed her bachelor of science in nursing (BSN) degree and wonders whether she can make it through another change. She raises her head, looks in a mirror, and says to herself, "Of course I can. Change is inevitable and ever-present. The opportunities another change presents are exciting and pervasive." With that, Mary puts on a smile, walks out the office door, and greets her staff.

What do you think Mary is feeling?

How should Mary go about introducing yet another change to her staff?

In health care, is change inevitable, pervasive, and exciting?

This chapter is designed to introduce the concepts of change and conflict resolution. Change is an inevitable and frequent occurrence in health care and life. Technology, biomedical discoveries, and advances in disease treatment and medications cause revolutions in the treatment and course of illness. These advances also make changes in wellness and health promotion rapid and sweeping. Along with change, conflict is also inevitable. The resolution of that conflict is necessary for the good of the patient and the organization. While conflict in itself is not bad, unresolved conflict can thwart the efforts of the best-intentioned change agent and cause stagnation and tension in a work team. This chapter will help to alleviate the anxiety surrounding change and conflict as well as teach the importance of embracing change and confronting conflict. Change is frightening only if one is not a part of it or has no input into

it. The staff nurse has a responsibility to provide input, even if it is not invited, and to become involved in the planning and implementation of change. Equally important is the evaluation of change. Evaluating honestly and making necessary modifications are as important to the success of a change project as the planning and orderly implementation. If nothing else is learned, learn to embrace change as an opportunity to improve patient care and to advance the profession of nursing. Look at conflict resolution as an opportunity to learn something new or as the opportunity to persuade others.

CHANGE

There are many definitions of change, and there are many types of change. For simplicity, **change** can be defined as "making something different from what it was" (Sullivan & Decker, 1997, p. 6). The outcome may be the same, but the actions performed to get to the outcome may be different. For instance, because of road closures, how one gets to work may have to change. The goal of getting to work remains the same, but the method may be different, perhaps by bus rather than automobile or by use of a different route. In the professional nursing setting, new patient admission forms may necessitate a different method of assessing the patient or change the number of people involved in the admission process. Rather than one registered nurse conducting the entire admission process, the process may be broken down so that individuals with different skill levels conduct parts of the process. The goal is still the admission of the patient to a unit; how it is done may be different. Most change is implemented for a good or reasonable purpose. Most organizational change is planned, and most change is purposeful (Sebastian, 1999). If employees do not understand the reason behind change, they should ask.

For purposes of discussion, **personal change** is a change made voluntarily for one's own reasons, usually for self-improvement. This may include changing one's diet for health reasons, taking classes for self-improvement, or removing oneself from a destructive or unhealthful environment or situation. **Professional change** may be a change in position or job such as obtaining education or credentials that will benefit one in a current position or allow one to be prepared for a future position. Professional change is often planned and involves extensive change in both personal and professional lives. While either personal or professional change may be stressful, if it is voluntary and carries intrinsic or extrinsic rewards, it is often considered important and worth the stress.

Organizational change is the type of change that often causes the most stress or concern. Sometimes there is a lot of preparation and prior discussion. Sometimes it is a surprise to the employees and causes a great deal of consternation and stress. Organizational change is usually planned, and the purpose is generally to improve efficiency, or to improve financial standing, or for some other organizational reason. Change is planned to meet organizational goals (Sebastian, 1999).

Unfortunately, when organizational change is planned, the employees are often the last to know what the anticipated change is but are frequently the ones most affected by it. The staff nurse is expected to implement the new care delivery system, but he may also be the last one to know about the change until it is to be implemented. For example, in an organization in which primary nursing has been the care delivery system for several years, the implementation of modified team nursing is a major change in philosophy and thinking. If proper care and planning of the change process is not used, the staff will resist the change and make the implementation much more stressful than necessary.

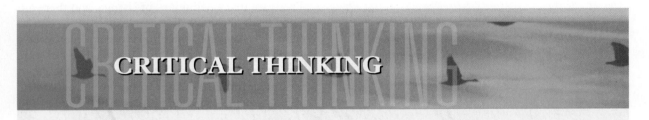

CRITICAL THINKING

Think about a time you were determined to make a personal change in your life. What emotions did you experience? Did you have support for this change? Did you set a realistic goal for yourself?

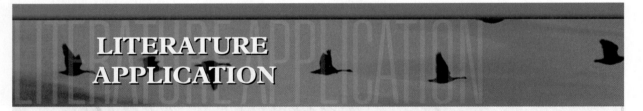

LITERATURE APPLICATION

Citation: Ingersoll, G. L., Kirsch, J. C., Merk, S. E., & Lightfoot, J. (2000, January). Relationship of organizational culture and readiness for change to employee commitment to the organization. *Journal of Nursing Administration, 30*(1), 11–20.

Discussion: This is a research article on employees' commitment to the organization and readiness for change. It discusses the relationship of organizational culture and readiness for change to employee commitment to the organization. The authors found that employee readiness for change often lagged behind the need for change within the organization.

Implications for Practice: Both employers and employees should recognize that change is inevitable. In these times of rapid health care change, employee readiness and commitment are important, but they cannot be the deciding factor in whether to change. The employer must change to keep up with the economic climate. The employee has a responsibility to change as necessary to help the employer maintain fiscal health.

Traditional Change Theories

The change theories discussed here are Lewin's Force-Field Model (1951), Lippitt's Phases of Change (1958), Havelock's Six-Step Change Model (1973), and Rogers' Diffusion of Innovations Theory (1983). These are classic change theories and are based on Lewin's original model.

Lewin's model has three simple steps. The steps are unfreezing, moving to a new level, and refreezing. Unfreezing means that the current or old way of doing is thawed. People begin to be aware of the need for doing things differently, that change is needed for a specific reason. In the next step, the intervention or change is introduced and explained. The benefits and disadvantages are discussed, and the change—the move to a new level—is implemented. In the third step, refreezing occurs. This means that the new way of doing is incorporated into the routines or habits of the affected people. While these steps sound simple, the process of change is, of course, more complicated (Lancaster, 1999).

Lippitt's Phases of Change are built on Lewin's model. Lippitt defined seven stages in the change process. These steps include (1) diagnosis of the problem, (2) assessment of the motivation and capacity for change, (3) assessment of the change agent's motivation and resources, (4) the selection of progressive change objectives, (5) choosing an appropriate role for the change agent, 6) maintenance of the change once it has been started, and (7) termination of the helping relationship. Lippitt emphasized the participation of key personnel and the change agent in designing and planning the intended change project. Lippitt also emphasized communication during all phases of the process (Sullivan & Decker, 2001).

Havelock designed a six-step model of the change process. This model is based on Lewin's model, but Havelock included more steps in each stage. The planning stage includes (1) building a relationship, (2) diagnosing the problem, and (3) acquiring resources. This planning stage is followed by the moving stage, which includes (4) choosing the solution, and (5) gaining acceptance. The last stage, the refreezing stage, includes (6) stabilization and self-renewal. Havelock emphasized the planning stage. He believed that resistance to change can be overcome if there is careful planning and inclusion of the affected staff. Havelock also believed that the change agent, the person responsible for planning and implementing the change, encouraged participation on the part of the people. The more the people affected by the change participate in the change, the more they are likely to make the change successful and to support the necessity for the change (Sullivan & Decker, 2001).

In 1983, Rogers published his Diffusion of Innovations Theory. Though based on Lewin's model, this theory is much broader in scope and approach. He developed a five-step innovation/decision-making process. Rogers believes that the change can be rejected initially and then adopted at a later time. He believes that change is a reversible process and that initial rejection does not necessarily mean the change will never be adopted. This also works in reverse—the change may initially be adopted and then rejected at a later time. Rogers' approach emphasized the capriciousness of change. In his theory, timing and format take on new meaning and importance—as the time involved in change implementation grows longer, the more the change process takes on a life of its own and the original change and reasons for it may be lost. The change process must be carefully managed and planned to ensure that it survives mostly intact. Table 16-1 is a comparison chart of these change models.

The theories described in Table 16-1 are linear in nature, meaning they more or less proceed in an orderly manner from one step to the next. This linearity and the fact that they are all based on Lewin's theory make them similar in complexity and in use. These theories work well for low-level, uncomplicated change. They do not work well in highly complex and nonlinear situations. Health care organizations are very complex and require more sophisticated theories of change.

Emerging Theories of Change

There are two often-used and emerging theories of change that are much more complex in breadth and depth than the theories previously discussed. These theories are the chaos theory and the learning organization theory. Thietart and Forgues (1995) state that "organizations are potentially chaotic" (p. 19). Chaos theory hypothesizes that chaos actually has an order. That is, although the potential for chaos appears to be random at first glance, further investigation reveals some order to the chaos. Health care organizations

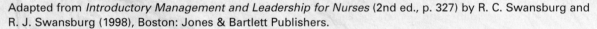

TABLE 16-1	Comparison Chart of Change Theories and Their Uses			
Theorist and Year	Lewin (1951)	Lippitt (1958)	Havelock (1973)	Rogers (1983)
Title of Model	Force-Field Model	Phases of Change	Six-Step Change Model	Diffusion of Innovations Theory
Steps in Model (The steps in the models are spaced to indicate their correlation to Lewin's model.)	1. Unfreeze	1. Diagnose problem 2. Assess motivation and capacity for change 3. Assess change agent's motivation and resources	1. Build relationship 2. Diagnose problem 3. Acquire resources	1. Awareness
	2. Move	4. Select progressive change objective 5. Choose appropriate role of change agent	4. Choose solution 5. Gain acceptance	2. Interest 3. Evaluation 4. Trial
	3. Refreeze	6. Maintain change 7. Terminate helping relationship	6. Stabilization and self-renewal	5. Adoption

Adapted from *Introductory Management and Leadership for Nurses* (2nd ed., p. 327) by R. C. Swansburg and R. J. Swansburg (1998), Boston: Jones & Bartlett Publishers.

have experienced chaos at times in the past 10 to 15 years. Chaos theory would say that this is normal. Most organizations go through periods of rapid change and innovation and then stabilize before chaos erupts again. Even though each chaotic occurrence is similar to the one that occurred before, each is different. The political, scientific, and behavioral components of the organization are different from before, so the chaos looks different. Order emerges through fluctuation and chaos. Thus, the potential for chaos means that the organization must be able to organize and implement change quickly and forcefully. There is little time for orderly linear change.

Leaders in these organizations are expected to act quickly and be flexible to meet the challenge of the potentially chaotic forces. Theoretically, the organization should be able to respond more quickly and intensely to the chaos because of its repetitive nature even though the forces causing the chaos are different and make the chaos appear differently (Menix, 1999).

Peter Senge (1990) first described learning organization theory. Learning organizations demonstrate responsiveness and flexibility. Senge believed that because organizations are open systems, they could best respond to unpredictable changes in the environment by using a learning approach in their interactions and interdisciplinary workings with one another. The whole cannot function well without a part regardless of how small that part may seem. For example, a well-equipped stove cannot work without a source of electricity or gas. It does not matter how new, innovative, or energy efficient the stove is, it cannot function without an energy source. An example in health care is that the billing department cannot submit an accurate bill to the insurance company without the cooperation of the nurse, nurse assistant, or central supply clerk. If the patient is not charged appropriately for items used, then the biller cannot prepare an accurate bill. Without the proper bill, the organization cannot be paid for the actual services and supplies used. The learning organization understands these interrelationships and responds quickly to improve relationships. This may be through dialogue or team problem solving, but all parties must understand what is at stake for cooperation to occur.

Senge has developed five disciplines that he believes are necessary for organizations to achieve the "learning organization status" to deal effectively with chaos. These disciplines are systems thinking, personal mastery, mental models, building shared vision, and team learning. Senge defines disciplines as the "critical and interrelated elements that compose a grouping that can only function effectively when all elements are present, linked and interacting" (Menix, 1999, p. 78). In the learning organization, each individual has something to offer that melds with what others have to offer to determine the right steps to take in sorting out the causes of chaos and responding positively to it. The goals of the organization and individual are mutually related so that quick response to chaos occurs, with positive results for both the organization and individual. The key to development of Senge's five disciplines is two-way communication or open discussion and dialogue (Menix, 1999). Most experts agree that few, if any, health care organizations have evolved to the learning organization status. While this is a goal to work toward, health care itself has not evolved to the point of quick reaction to chaos and a rapidly changing environment.

The Change Process

Planned change in the work organization is not much different from planned change on a personal level. The major difference is that more people are involved, the scale is larger, and more opinions must be considered. There are three basic reasons to introduce a change: (1) to solve a problem, (2) to improve efficiency, and (3) to reduce unnecessary workload for some group (Marquis & Huston, 2000). To plan change, one must know what has to be changed. Change for the sake of change is unnecessary and stressful (Bennis, Benne, & Chin, 1969).

Steps in the Change Process

The change process can be related to the nursing process. Using the nursing process as a model, the first step in the change process is assessment.

Assessment. In assessment, one identifies what the problem is or the opportunity for improvement through change by collecting and analyzing data. The data collection and analysis should be from several sources: structural, technological, and people. A structural problem is one of physical space or the configuration of physical space. For instance, a medical-surgical unit in a hospital may move to the space vacated by the old obstetrics unit. The problem may be that the space is large enough but it is not configured so that it is conducive to the care of medical-surgical patients. Assessment of structural components may include examination of the location of elevators, supply stations, patient charts, telephones, call lights, and other physical or structural components. Structural components often mandate how the work is done or the process of doing the work. Poor structural configuration may require the work team to perform extra steps to accomplish its goals. Technological problems may include a lack of wall outlets for necessary equipment, poorly situated computer locations, and lack of computer system interface ability. Sometimes, technology lags behind the goals of a work team and therefore slows down the team. The team spends more time troubleshooting technology than in providing care. People problems may include personnel with inadequate training to accomplish the goals, unwillingness to meet the goals, lack of commitment to the organization, or lack of understanding for the need for change.

Assessment data are collected from internal and external sources. Lewin identified forces that were supportive of as well as barriers to change. He called these driving and restraining forces. If the restraining forces outweigh the driving forces, then the change must be abandoned because it cannot succeed. Driving and restraining forces include political issues, technology issues, cost and structural issues, and people issues. The political issues include the power groups in favor of or against the proposed change. This may include physicians, administrators, civic and community groups, or state and federal regulators. The technology issues include whether to update old equipment, computer systems, or methods for accounting for supply use. Cost and structural issues include the costs, desirability, and feasibility of remodeling or building new construction for the change project. People issues include the commitment of the staff, their level of education and training, and their interest in the project. The most common people issue is fear of job loss or fear of not being valued. It bears repeating that if the restraining forces outweigh the driving forces, then the change will not succeed and it should be abandoned or rethought.

During data analysis, potential solutions may be identified, sources of resistance may come to light, determination of strategies may become apparent, and some areas of consensus may become evident. Statistical analysis is an important component of analysis. This should be done whenever possible to provide persuasive information in favor of the change, especially if meeting cost or mission objectives is the issue. The goal of data analysis is to support the need to change and offer data to support the potential solution selected. The people who are potentially going to be most affected by the change need to be involved in the assessment, data collection, and data analysis. They have a vested interest in the change and must not only support the change but also be willing to implement change (Bennis, Benne, Chin, 1969).

Planning. The next step is to plan. In this step, it is determined who will be affected by the change and when change will occur. All the potential solutions are examined. The driving and resisting forces are again examined and strategies determined for implementing the change. The target date for implementation and the outcomes or goals are clearly delineated and stated in measurable terms. Again, the most successful plan for change is one in which the individuals who will be most affected are involved, satisfied, and committed.

It is also important to include in the plan how the change will be implemented, although this may require modification as the implementation begins.

For instance, how many work groups or units will implement the change at once? Will the change implementation be staggered from month to month or week to week? Will the supports necessary to manage the change go into effect first? Just how will this change be implemented? Finally, the overall plan includes plans for evaluation. It is crucial that evaluation be built in. Expected outcomes must be identified in measurable terms, and the plan to evaluate those outcomes and a timetable for evaluation must be evident. Unevaluated change will not succeed.

Implementation of Change Strategies. Bennis, Benne & Chin. (1969) identified three strategies to promote change in groups or organizations. Different strategies work in different situations. The power or authority of the change agent has an impact on the strategy selected. Most change agents use a variety of strategies to promote successful change. The power-coercive strategy is very simple—"do it or get out." This is a strategy based on power, authority, and control. This is a strong indication of the political clout of the change agent. There is very little effort to encourage participation of employees, and there is little concern about their acceptance or resistance to the proposed change. Sullivan and Decker (2001) use the federal government's decision to impose prospective payment on Medicare hospital clients as an example of the power-coercive strategy—no discussion, simply, this is what will be. This group of strategies is generally reserved for situations in which resistance is expected but not important to the power group.

The second group change strategy is normative-reeducative. This strategy is based on the assumption that group norms are used to socialize individuals. This strategy focuses on using the individual's need for satisfying social relationships in the workplace. Very few individuals can withstand social isolation or rejection by the work group. Compliance and support for a change are garnered by focusing on the perceived loss of social relationships in the workplace. While some resistance to change may be expected, this strategy assumes people are interested in preserving relationships and will go along with the majority.

The third group of strategies is rational-empirical. This group assumes that humans are rational people and will use knowledge to embrace change. It is assumed that once the self-interests of a group are evident, the group will see the merit in a change and embrace that change. Knowledge and training are the components used to encourage compliance with change. This is a very successful strategy when little resistance is anticipated. Table 16-2 summarizes the strategies for change.

Evaluation of Change. In the evaluation step, the effectiveness of the change is evaluated according to the outcomes identified during the planning step. Evaluation is the most overlooked step, although it is considered by some experts to be the most important step. Usually, not enough time is allowed for the change to become effective or stable. This is a grave error. The time intervals for evaluation should be identified and allowed to elapse before modifications are made and declarations of failure are asserted. A certain period of confusion and turmoil accompanies all changes, whether large or small. If the outcomes are achieved, then the change was a success. If not, then some revision or modification may be necessary to achieve the outcomes that were anticipated.

Stabilization of Change. Once effectiveness is determined, then stabilization of the change is completed. The project is no longer a pilot or experiment but is a part of the culture and function of the organization. While there is no magical time frame for stabilization to occur, it should be encouraged as soon as possible to make the change project complete. Often, reevaluation is planned after the first 6 months or year of implementation to ensure that stabilization of the change has occurred.

TABLE 16-2	Strategies for Change
Strategy	**Description**
Power-coercive approach	Uses authority and threat of job loss to gain compliance with change.
Normative-reeducative approach	Uses social orientation and the need to have satisfactory relationships in the workplace as a method of inducing support for change. Focuses on the relationship needs of workers.
Rational-empirical approach	Uses knowledge as power base. Once workers understand the organizational need for change or understand the meaning of the change to them as individuals and the organization as a whole, they will change.

REAL WORLD INTERVIEW

One of the things I have learned about change is that fear of the change is worse than the change itself. Now I concentrate on getting my staff to focus on what will be the same, and what will be different will be better. This decreases the fear.

Joy Churchill, RN
Team Leader

CRITICAL THINKING

Consider one of the changes you have experienced in a personal or work setting. Was there any plan for evaluation of the change? Was any thought given to making some modification in the change when it was obvious the change could not be implemented as designed? What could have been done differently?

Responses to Change

People do have responses to change. The most typical response to change is resistance. Humans like order and familiarity; they enjoy routine and the status quo. It is most common for humans to resist change. The more the relationships or social mores are challenged to change, the more resistance there is to change. Marquis and Huston (2000) point out that nurses are more likely to accept a change in an intravenous pump rather than a change in who can administer the intravenous fluid. This suggests that the social mores of a group are more important than technology in a change. The social mores dictate the roles and responsibilities of groups of workers such as registered nurses, licensed practical nurses, nurse aides, and so on. Registered nurses are often less concerned with technology and more concerned with maintaining traditional roles and responsibilities.

There are several factors that affect resistance to change. The first is trust. The employee and employer must trust that each is doing the right thing and that each is capable of producing successful change. In addition to capability, predictability is important. The employee wants a predictable work environment and security. When change is introduced, then that predictability—and, therefore, capability—begins to come into question (Duck, 1993). Another factor is the individual's ability to cope with change. Silber (1993) points out four factors that affect an individual's ability to cope with change:

1. Flexibility for change, that is, the ability to adapt to change
2. Evaluation of the immediate situation, that is, if the current situation is unacceptable, then change will be more welcome

3. Anticipated consequences of change, that is, the impact change will have on one's current job
4. Individual's stake or what the individual has to win or lose in the change, that is, the more individuals perceive they have to lose, the more resistance they will offer.

Change is a scary prospect if one has not had much experience with change or if one has had negative experiences with change. It is important to help individuals remember that change is inevitable and ever present. Developing an attitude of embracing and accepting change is desirable.

Bushy (1992) has identified six behavioral responses to planned change. These are usually apparent in every health care facility and every nursing unit. These behavioral responses are as follows:

1. Innovators: Change embracers. Enjoy the challenge of change and often lead change.
2. Early adopters: Open and receptive to change but not obsessed with it.
3. Early majority: Enjoy and prefer the status quo but do not want to be left behind. They adopt change before the average person.
4. Late majority: Often known as the followers. They adopt change after expressing negative feelings and are often skeptics.
5. Laggards : Last group to adopt a change. They prefer tradition and stability to innovation. They are somewhat suspicious of change.
6. Rejectors: Openly oppose and reject change. May be surreptitious or covert in their opposition. They may hinder the change process to the point of sabotage.

Other responses to change have been identified. These include grieving, denial, anger, depression, and bargaining (Marquis & Huston, 2000). Regardless of the importance and necessity of change, the human response is very important and cannot be dismissed. So often, in one's zeal to respond to a need, the change agent forgets that the human side of change must be dealt with. People have a right to their feelings and a right to express them. The important point is the change agent helps people respond and then move on to the goal of implementing the change. Gently but firmly, people must be guided toward acceptance.

The Change Agent

Throughout this discussion of change, the term **change agent**, has been used instead of manager, leader, or administrator. The change agent is one who is responsible for implementation of a change project. This person may be from within or outside an organization. She may be a leader or manager. She may be a leader or manager because she is an innovator and therefore likely to enjoy change. This is the person who is ultimately responsible for the success of the change project, large or small. The role of the change agent is to manage the dynamics of the change process. This role requires knowledge of the organization, knowledge of the change process, knowledge of the participants in the change process, and understanding of the feelings of the group undergoing change. Probably the most important role of the change agent is to maintain communication, momentum, and enthusiasm for the project while still managing the process. Table 16-3 summarizes the roles and characteristics of the change agent.

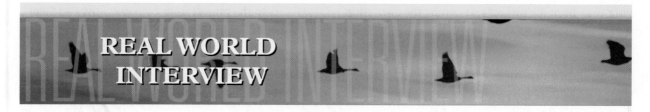

REAL WORLD INTERVIEW

Change is all about growing and developing, but the change agent or nurse manager has to be honest and truthful. Once he or she lies to us, then trust is destroyed and the change will surely fail. It's okay to not have the answer or not to be able to give the answer, but don't lie about it.

Caron Martin, RN
Staff Nurse

TABLE 16-3 — Roles and Characteristics of the Change Agent

- Leader of change process
- Manages process and group dynamics
- Understands feelings of group experiencing the change
- Maintains momentum and enthusiasm
- Maintains vision of change
- Communicates change, progress, and feelings
- Knowledgeable about the organization
- Trustworthy
- Respected
- Intuitive

The recipients of change must trust the change agent's interpersonal skills to provide information and manage change but also the agent's personal integrity and honor as an honest, principled individual. The executives in the organization must trust that the change agent will accomplish the established goals, given the proper support. The change agent will also have to recognize that those developing the project have some definite inclusion concepts that must be folded into the vision for success. Inclusion concepts are those ideas or concepts that the affected parties believe are absolutely necessary for their peace of mind or moral value. When these concepts are included, people feel ownership and value—a piece of them or their idea is in the plan.

Finally, the change agent must use some intuition during the evaluation steps so that he can bow out of the change, and those affected can accept ownership. This is a matter of timing and insight into when the staff is ready to accept and incorporate the change as its own. Bennis (1989) warns that not stepping away from the project and cutting the ownership bonds means that it is the change agent's project for many years to come, even after the change agent might leave the organization. During evaluation, the change agent must support modifications and revisions that help transfer project ownership.

Change Agent Strategies

Following are some strategies the change agent can use in managing the process:

1. Begin by articulating the vision clearly and concisely. Use the same words over and over. Constantly remind people of the goals and vision.
2. Map out a tentative time line and sketch out the steps of the project. Have a good idea of how the project should go.
3. Plant seeds or mention some ideas or thoughts to key individuals from the first step through the evaluation step so that some idea of what is expected is under consideration.
4. Select the change project team carefully. Make sure it is heavily loaded with those who will be affected and other experts as needed. Select a variety of people. For example, an innovator, someone from the late majority group, a laggard, and a rejector are probably good to include. These people provide insight into what others are thinking.
5. Set up consistent meeting dates and keep them. Have an agenda and constantly check the time line for target activities.
6. For those not on the team but affected by the project, give constant and consistent updates on progress. If the change agent does not, someone on the project team will, and the change agent wants to control the messages.
7. Give regular updates and progress reports both verbally and in writing to the executives of the organization and those affected by the change.
8. Check out rumors and confront conflict head on. Do not look for conflict, but do not back away from it or ignore it.
9. Maintain a positive attitude and do not get discouraged.
10. Stay alert to political forces both for and against the project. Get consensus on important issues as the project goes along, especially if policy, money, or philosophy issues are involved. Obtain consensus quickly on major issues or potential barriers to the project from both executives and staff.
11. Know the internal formal and informal leaders. Create a relationship with them. Consult them often.
12. Having self-confidence and trust in oneself and one's team will overcome a lot of obstacles. (Lancaster, 1999)

As has been reiterated over and over, change is an inevitable part of life and will continue to affect the health care system for several years to come. It is important to maintain an attitude that change is preferable to stagnation. This will help leaders to identify opportunities for change and embrace those changes for a better quality work life or for better care for the patient. Nothing can ever stay the same for long.

CONFLICT

An important part of the change process is the ability to resolve conflict. Conflict resolution skills are leadership and management tools that all registered nurses should have in their repertoire. Conflict itself is not bad. Conflict is healthy. It, like change, allows for creativity, innovation, new ideas, and new ways of doing things. It allows for the healthy discussion of different views and values and adds an important dimension to the provision of quality patient care.

Conflict can occur in almost any situation about almost anything. Conflict can arise over a matter as trivial as the size of an earring allowed in the dress code or as serious as who the final authority is on a patient care policy. Without some conflict, groups or work teams tend to become stagnant and routinized. Nothing new is allowed to penetrate the "way we have always done it" mentality. The change agent and the nurse manager quickly become targets if they introduce new ideas or new systems of operating.

There are a variety of definitions of conflict. Conflict can be defined as two or more parties holding differing views about a situation (Tappen, 2001); or as differences in beliefs, values, goals, priorities, and so on (Keenan & Hurst, 1999); or as the consequence of real or perceived differences in mutually exclusive goals, values, ideas, and so on within one person or among groups of two or more (Sullivan & Decker, 2001). As can be surmised from these definitions, conflict can be defined as a disagreement about something of importance to each person involved. Not all disagreements become conflicts, but all disagreements have the potential for becoming a conflict, and all conflicts involve some level of disagreement. It is the astute manager who can determine which disagreements might become conflicts and which ones will not. This discussion of conflict resolution does not include professional communication skills. These are discussed elsewhere in this book.

Sources of Conflict

Whenever there is the opportunity for disagreement, there is a potential source of conflict. The common sources of conflict in the professional setting include disputes over resource allocation or availability, personality differences, differences in values, threats from inside or outside an organization, cultural differences, and competition. In recent years, organizational, professional, and unit goals have served as a major source of conflict. Nurses frequently see financial goals and patient care goals as being in direct conflict with one another. In many organizations, this is the most frequently mentioned source of emotionally charged conflict (Sullivan & Decker, 2001).

Sources of conflict in personal arenas include differences in values, threats to security or well-being, financial problems, and cultural problems. Family relationships are often sources of conflict because of the complexity of these relationships.

Types of Conflict

There are three broad types of conflict: intrapersonal, interpersonal, and organizational. Intrapersonal conflict occurs within the individual. For example, if Marilyn is not granted her requested day off, she may have internal conflict about whether to call in sick or to take the day off without pay or to go to work. Or Marilyn may have conflict about priorities: should she attend her daughter's softball game or write her paper for school?

An interpersonal conflict may be between two people or between groups or work teams. There may be disagreement in philosophy or values, or policy or procedure. It may be a personality conflict; for example, two people just rub each other the wrong way. This type of conflict is not unusual in the work situation. People new to a team may bring ideas with them that are not totally acceptable to the members in place. Individuals who transfer from one unit to another often stir up a certain amount of conflict over processes and procedures. For example, the nurse transferring from the intensive care unit (ICU) to the coronary care unit (CCU) may be comfortable with one way of making assignments and then try to encourage his new peers to adopt that methodology without sharing the rationale for why his way is better.

Organizational conflict is at times a healthy way of introducing new ideas and encouraging creativity. Competition for resources, organizational cultural differences, and other sources of conflict help organizations identify areas for improvement. Conflict helps organizations identify legitimate differences among departments or work teams based on corporate need or responsibility. When organizational conflict is highlighted, corporate values and differences are aired and resolved.

The Conflict Process

In 1975, Filley suggested a process for conflict resolution that is widely accepted. In this process, there are five stages of conflict: (1) antecedent conditions, (2) perceived and/or felt conflict, (3) manifest behavior, (4) conflict resolution or suppression, and (5) resolution aftermath. In Filley's model, conflict and conflict resolution follow a specific course. The process begins with specific preexisting conditions called antecedent conditions. As the situation develops, conflict is perceived or felt by the involved parties. This triggers a response or manifest behavior.

The conflict is either resolved or suppressed, leading to the development of new feelings and attitudes, and may create new conflicts. Conflict resolution is vital in change. The antecedent conditions that Filley suggests may or may not be the cause of the conflict, but they certainly move the disagreement to the conflict level. The sources of these conditions include those discussed earlier: disagreement in goals, values, or resource utilization. Other issues may also serve as antecedent conditions such as the dependency of one group on another. For instance, the nursing department is dependent on the pharmacy department to provide drugs for the nursing unit in a timely fashion. The goals and priorities of pharmacy and nursing may be different at the time the nurse requests the drugs and so a source of disagreement arises. If the circumstances for disagreement continue, a conflict will develop. According to Sullivan and Decker (1997), goal incompatibility is the most important antecedent condition to conflict.

Meaning of the Conflict

Conceptualization of the meaning of a conflict develops when individuals form an idea or concept of what the conflict is about, such as a conflict over control, professional standards, values, goals, and so on. Each party may or may not be aware of the other's conceptualization of the meaning of the conflict, but the parties do have what they believe is a clear concept of the conflict in their own mind. To determine the accuracy of the beliefs about the conflict, both parties need to sit down and determine the existence and nature of the conflict and the reasons it exists. According to Keenan and Hurst (1999), people may disagree on four aspects of a conflict. These include facts, goals, methods of goal achievement, and the values or standards used to select the goals or methods. This means that the actual facts of the dispute may be in question, the goals each side wishes to achieve may not be the same, the means of achieving the agreed-upon goal may not be acceptable to one side or the other, or values may be in dispute. Once the nature of the conflict or the points of disagreement are known, then resolution can begin.

The actions taken to resolve conflict can take many forms. There may be movement toward resolution by discussion of the conflict, or someone in power may take steps to end the conflict or at least suppress it, or there may be a decision on the part of one or both parties to do nothing to resolve the conflict. Failure to successfully resolve the conflict leads to more frustration and a further heightening of the conflict. Communication breaks down and conflict spreads to the pettiest of issues. Once a conflict is apparent, some sort of successful resolution must occur. People simply do not get over it and move on. It is a source of friction and pain that must be resolved.

Conflict Resolution

There are essentially seven methods of conflict resolution. These methods dictate the outcomes of the conflict process. While some methods are more desirable or produce more successful outcomes than others, there may be a place in conflict resolution for all the methods, depending on the nature of the conflict and the desired outcomes. Table 16-4 is a summary of these methods, highlighting some of their advantages and disadvantages. The five techniques most commonly acknowledged are avoiding, accommodating, competing, compromising, and collaborating. The other techniques are negotiating and confronting.

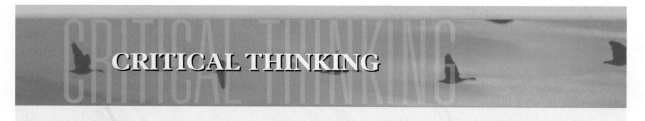

CRITICAL THINKING

Recall a time of conflict in your life. Looking at it with a different perspective, what antecedent conditions led to the conflict? What was the core of the conflict? Were personal goals or values at stake? How would you look at the same conflict now?

TABLE 16-4	Summary of Conflict Resolution Techniques	
Conflict Resolution Technique	**Advantages**	**Disadvantages**
Avoiding—ignoring the conflict	Does not make a big deal out of nothing; conflict may be minor in comparison to other priorities	Conflict can become bigger than anticipated; source of conflict might be more important to one person or group than others
Accommodating—smoothing or cooperating. One side gives in to the other side	One side is more concerned with an issue than the other side; stakes not high enough for one group and that side is willing to give in	One side holds more power and can force the other side to give in; the importance of the stakes are not as apparent to one side as the other; can lead to parties feeling "used" if they are always pressured to give in
Competing—forcing; the two or three sides are forced to compete for the goal	Produces a winner; good when time is short and stakes are high	Produces a loser; leaves anger and resentment on losing sides
Compromising—each side gives up something and gains something	No one should win or lose but both should gain something; good for disagreements between individuals	May cause a return to the conflict if what is given up becomes more important than the original goal
Negotiating—high-level discussion that seeks agreement but not necessarily consensus	Stakes are very high and solution is rather permanent; often involves powerful groups	Agreements are permanent, even though each side has gains and losses
Collaborating—both sides work together to develop optimal outcome	Best solution for the conflict and encompasses all important goals to each side	Takes a lot of time; requires commitment to success
Confronting—immediate and obvious movement to stop conflict at the very start	Does not allow conflict to take root; very powerful	May leave impression that conflict is not tolerated; may make something big out of nothing

Avoiding is a very common technique. The parties involved in the conflict ignore it, either consciously or unconsciously.

Accommodating is often called smoothing or cooperating. In this technique, one side of the disagreement decides or is encouraged to accommodate the other side by ignoring or sidestepping their own feelings about the issue. This is often done when the stakes are not all that high and the need to move on is pressing. Frequent use of this method, however, can lead to feelings of frustration or being used—one person is "used" to get the cooperation of another.

Competing is a conflict resolution technique that produces a winner and loser. The concept is that there is an all-out effort to win at all costs. This technique may be used when time is too short to allow other techniques to work or when a critical, though unpopular, decision has to be made quickly. This is often called forcing because the winner forces the loser to accept his stance on the conflict.

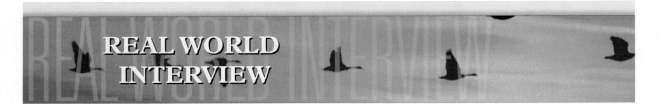

REAL WORLD
INTERVIEW

One of the biggest errors a leader can make is to assume everything is okay. The leader who ignores conflict is not a leader but an avoider. Like the ostrich, hiding won't make it go away.

Sally Dessner, RN
Nurse Executive

Some authorities see negotiation and compromise as the same; others see them as separate. *Compromising* is a method used to achieve conflict resolution in situations in which neither side can win and neither side should lose. Compromise is rampant in our society and is useful for goal achievement when the stakes are important but not necessarily critical. Compromise is often seen as appeasement—each side gives up something and each side gains something. Compromise is a good technique for minor conflicts or conflicts that cannot be resolved satisfactorily for both sides. Both parties win and lose.

Negotiating requires careful communication techniques and highly developed skills. The optimum solution for the conflict may not be reached, but each side has some wins and some losses. The term *negotiation* is often used in reference to collective bargaining or politics. It is, however, a very useful technique for conflict resolution at all levels. Negotiating is used when the stakes are considerably higher or when

return to the conflict cannot occur. Return to the conflict may not be possible for a variety of reasons, such as a union contract, permanent change in policy or governance, or career or life changes. The idea of negotiation is that each party will gain something, so general agreement is reached, but consensus—that is, agreement in concept—is not necessarily the goal.

According to Lewicki, Hiam, and Olander (1996), there are five basic approaches to negotiating: collaborative (win-win), competitive (win at all costs), avoiding (lose-lose), accommodating (lose to win), and compromise (split the difference). These five approaches to negotiation are influenced by the importance of maintaining the relationship relative to the importance of achieving one's desired outcomes (Figure 16-1).

Collaborating occurs in conflict resolution when both sides work together to develop the optimal outcome. It is a creative endeavor designed to find the best solution to the conflict so that all of the per-

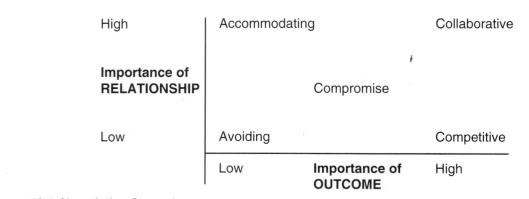

		Accommodating	Collaborative
High			
Importance of RELATIONSHIP		Compromise	
Low		Avoiding	Competitive
		Low	**Importance of OUTCOME**	High

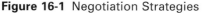

Figure 16-1 Negotiation Strategies

ceived important goals are achieved. This technique requires both sides to seek a permanent acceptable solution to the conflict so all parties feel their goals or objectives have been achieved.

One other technique used in conflict resolution is *confronting*. This technique heads off conflict as soon as the first symptoms appear. Both parties are brought together, the issues are clarified, and some outcome is achieved.

Success of the techniques presented here depends on several factors. The importance of the issue in the conflict to the various sides has an enormous impact on the technique selected and the degree of success that will be achieved. Conflict resolution is never really permanent because new issues will always arise. The trick for the leader/manager is to determine what conflicts require intervention and what techniques stand the best chance of success. If one technique does not work, try another. Conflicts should be suppressed or avoided only under special circumstances that are dependent on the issues involved and the importance of the issues to the parties. Keep in mind that little problems become big problems later if the stakes are high and the issue is important to someone.

Strategies to Facilitate Conflict Resolution

Open, honest, clear communication is the key to successful conflict resolution. The nurse manager/leader and all parties to the conflict must agree to communicate with one another openly and honestly. Courtesy in communicating is to be encouraged. This includes listening actively to the other side.

The setting for the discussions for conflict resolution should be private, relaxed, and comfortable. If possible, external interruptions from phones, pagers, overhead speakers, and personnel should be avoided or kept to a minimum. The setting should be on neutral territory so that no one feels overpowered. The ground rules, such as not interrupting, who should go first, time limits, and so on, should be agreed upon in the beginning. Adherence to ground rules should be expected.

In the conflict resolution process, it is expected that both sides in the conflict will comply with the results. If one party cannot agree to comply with the decisions or outcomes, there is no point to the process. In this case, disciplinary action should be

considered if the employee is function or interfering with goa. rare cases of noncompliance or agreed-upon conflict resolution, should seek expert legal counsel w tion. In most conflicts, the parties ѕ ... ... will-ing to comply with the results, and the outcomes prove to be positive. A tool for assessing conflict is identified in Figure 16-2. This tool can be used to determine interpersonal or intergroup conflict within an organization and whether a given conflict is functional or dysfunctional.

Leadership and Management Roles

Marquis and Huston (2000) have identified some leadership and management roles in conflict management. Leadership roles include the role modeling of conflict resolution methods as soon as the conflict is evident. This strategy demonstrates awareness of and works to resolve intrapersonal or interpersonal conflict and sets the goal of conflict resolution so that both parties win. The leader also works to lessen the perceptual differences of the conflicting parties about the conflict and tries to encourage each side to see the other's view. The nurse manager/leader assists the conflicting parties to identify techniques that may resolve the conflict and accepts differences between the parties without judgment or accusation. The leader fosters open and honest communication.

The manager role includes the creation of an environment conducive to conflict resolution. The manager uses his authority to solve conflicts including the use of competition for immediate or unpopular decisions. The manager facilitates conflict resolution in a formal manner when necessary. The manager competes and negotiates for available resources for unit needs when necessary. He can compromise unit goals when necessary to achieve another more important unit goal. The manager negotiates consensus or compliance to conflict resolution outcomes or goals. While the roles of leader and manager often appear in the same person, the leadership roles in conflict resolution are often more important to resolution and compliance. The manager has formal power that can be used when necessary, but it should be reserved for truly unresolvable or important issues.

Interpersonal or intergroup?

1. Who?
   - Who are the primary individuals or groups involved? Characteristics (values; feelings; needs; perceptions; goals; hostility; strengths, past history of constructive conflict management; self-awareness)?
   - Who, if anyone, are the individuals or groups that have an indirect investment in the result of the conflict?
   - Who, if anyone, is assisting the parties to manage the conflict constructively?
   - What is the history of the individuals' or groups' involvement in the conflict?
   - What is the past and present interpersonal relationship between the parties involved in the conflict?
   - How is power distributed among the parties?
   - What are the major sources of power used?
   - Does the potential for coalition exist among the parties?
   - What is the nature of the current leadership affecting the conflicting parties?

2. What?
   - What is (are) the issues(s) in the conflict?
   - Are the issues based on facts? Based on values? Based on interests in resources?
   - Are the issues realistic?
   - What is the dominant issue in the conflict?
   - What are the goals of each conflicting party?
   - Is the current conflict functional? Dysfunctional?
   - What conflict management strategies, if any, have been used to manage the conflict to date?
   - What alternatives in managing the conflict exist?
   - What are you doing to keep the conflict going?
   - Is there a lack of stimulating work?

3. How?
   - What is the origin of the conflict? Sources? Precipitating events?
   - What are the major events in the evolution of the conflict?
   - How have the issues emerged? Been transformed? Proliferated?
   - What polarizations and coalitions have occurred?
   - How have parties tried to damage each other? What stereotyping exists?

4. When/Where?
   - When did the conflict originate?
   - Where is the conflict taking place?
   - What are the characteristics of the setting within which the conflict is occurring?
   - What are the geographic boundaries? Political structures? Decision-making patterns? Communication networks? Subsystem boundaries?
   - What environmental factors exist that influence the development of functional versus dysfunctional conflict?
   - What resource persons are available to assist in constructive conflict management?

Functional or dysfunctional?	**YES**	**NO**
Does the conflict support the goals of the organization?	[ ]	[ ]
Does the conflict contribute to the overall goals of the organization?	[ ]	[ ]
Does the conflict stimulate improved job performance?	[ ]	[ ]
Does the conflict increase productivity among work group members?	[ ]	[ ]
Does the conflict stimulate creativity and innovation?	[ ]	[ ]
Does the conflict bring about constructive change?	[ ]	[ ]
Does the conflict contribute to the survival of the organization?	[ ]	[ ]
Does the conflict improve initiative?	[ ]	[ ]
Does job satisfaction remain high?	[ ]	[ ]
Does the conflict improve the morale of the work group?	[ ]	[ ]

A yes response to the majority of the questions indicates that the conflict is probably functional. If the majority of responses are no, then the conflict is most likely a dysfunctional conflict.

Figure 16-2 Guide for the Assessment of Conflict

CONFLICT MANAGEMENT AND CHANGE

Conflict management and resolution are important parts of the change process. Change can often threaten individuals and groups, so conflict is an inevitable part of the process. It is important to keep in mind that some conflicts resolve themselves, so the change agent should not be too quick to jump into an intervention mode. Figure 16-3 provides a guide for assessment of the level of conflict. If the level of conflict is too high, the nurse manager must apply conflict resolution strategies.

Is conflict too low?	YES	NO
Is the work group consistently satisfied with the status quo?	[ ]	[ ]
Are no or few opposing views expressed by work-group members?	[ ]	[ ]
Is little concern expressed about doing things better?	[ ]	[ ]
Is little or no concern expressed about improving inadequacies?	[ ]	[ ]
Are the decisions made by the work group generally of low quality?	[ ]	[ ]
Are no or few innovative solutions or ideas expressed?	[ ]	[ ]
Are many work-group members "yes-men"?	[ ]	[ ]
Are work-group members reluctant to express ignorance or uncertainties?	[ ]	[ ]
Does the nurse manager seek to maintain peace and group cooperation regardless of whether this is the correct intervention?	[ ]	[ ]
Do the work-group members demonstrate an extremely high level of resistance to change?	[ ]	[ ]
Does the nurse manager base the distribution of rewards on "popularity" as opposed to competence and high job performance?	[ ]	[ ]
Is the nurse manager excessively concerned about not hurting the feelings of the nursing staff?	[ ]	[ ]
Is the nurse manager excessively concerned with obtaining a consensus of opinion and reaching a compromise when decisions must be made?	[ ]	[ ]

A yes response to the majority of these questions can be indicative of a too-low conflict level in a work group.

Is conflict too high?	YES	NO
Is there an upward and onward spiraling escalation of the conflict?	[ ]	[ ]
Are the conflicting parties stimulating the escalation of conflict without considering the consequences?	[ ]	[ ]
Is there a shift away from conciliation, minimizing differences, and enhancing goodwill?	[ ]	[ ]
Are the issues involved in the conflict being increasingly elaborated and expanded?	[ ]	[ ]
Are false issues being generated	[ ]	[ ]
Are the issues vague or unclear?	[ ]	[ ]
Is job dissatisfaction increasing among work-group members?	[ ]	[ ]
Is the work-group productivity being adversely affected?	[ ]	[ ]
Is the energy being directed to activities that do not contribute to the achievement of organizational goals (e.g., destroying opposing party)?	[ ]	[ ]
Is the morale of the nursing staff being adversely affected?	[ ]	[ ]
Are extra parties getting dragged into the conflict?	[ ]	[ ]
Is a great deal of reliance on overt power manipulation noted (threats, coercion, deception)?	[ ]	[ ]
Is there a great deal of imbalance in power noted among the parties?	[ ]	[ ]
Are the individuals or groups involved in the conflict expressing dissatisfaction about the course of the conflict and feel that they are losing something?	[ ]	[ ]
Is absenteeism increasing among staff?	[ ]	[ ]
Is there a high rate of turnover among personnel?	[ ]	[ ]
Is communication dysfunctional, not open, mistrustful, and/or restrictive?	[ ]	[ ]
Is the focus being placed on nonconflict relevant sensitive areas of the other party?	[ ]	[ ]

A yes response to the majority of these questions can be indicative of a conflict level in a work group that is too high.

Figure 16-3 Guide for the Assessment of Level of Conflict

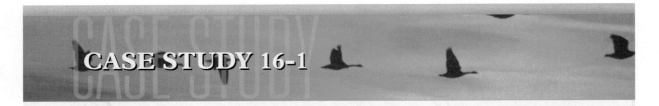

CASE STUDY 16-1

Jane's staff was about 3 weeks into the latest change in care delivery when one of the staff nurses, Linda, returned from maternity leave. Linda tended to be negative about change, but she had terrific clinical skills and often served as a preceptor for new staff. Jane knew that if she could control Linda's tendency toward the negative, then not too much would happen to get the change off course. Linda's first words to Jane were "Whose brilliant idea is this? I do not want to work with Kathy. She is an idiot." Jane smiled and said, "Welcome back, Linda. We have missed you. How is the baby? Got any pictures?"

What do you think Jane should do to help Linda adjust to the change? Should Jane explore Linda's feelings about Kathy? Which is most stressful for Linda, the change or working with Kathy? Should Jane have done something to prepare Linda for this change and her assignment to work with Kathy?

KEY CONCEPTS

- Change is inevitable, exciting, and anxiety provoking.
- Change is defined as making something different from what it was.
- Major change theorists include Lewin, Lippitt, Havelock, and Rogers.
- Senge's model of five disciplines describes the learning organization. This model describes organizations undergoing continuous and unrelenting change.
- The change process is similar to the nursing process.
- Strategies for change include the power-coercive approach, the normative-reeducative approach, and the rational-empirical approach.
- The change agent is an important part of the change process. The change agent is responsible and accountable for the project.
- Conflict is a normal part of any change project.
- Conflict comes from many sources, including value differences, fear, and goal disagreement.
- The techniques for conflict resolution include avoiding, accommodating, compromising, competing, negotiating, confronting, and collaborating.
- There are several strategies for conflict resolution. Clear, open communication is key.
- Conflict can move the change process along if it is handled well. Conflict can stop the change

process if it is handled poorly or allowed to get out of control.

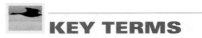

KEY TERMS

change
change agent
conflict
organizational change
personal change
professional change

REVIEW QUESTIONS

1. What is the most desirable conflict resolution technique?
   A. Avoiding
   B. Competing
   C. Negotiating
   D. Collaborating

2. What is the most common source of conflict in today's health care organization?
   A. Goals
   B. Values
   C. Resource allocation disputes
   D. Competition

3. The change agent and the person responsible for conflict resolution have what characteristic in common?
   A. Secretive and willful
   B. Trustworthy and a good communicator

C. Ambitious and avoiding

D. Powerful and dictatorial

REVIEW ACTIVITIES

1. Select a change project that either you have personally achieved or you have experienced in a clinical situation, and discuss with your classmates how you felt and how the change agent maintained momentum and enthusiasm for the project. If this is a personal change, how did you maintain enthusiasm?

2. Recall a conflict with which you have been involved in the clinical situation. Discuss each of the methods of conflict resolution identified in the chapter. Identify which ones would have worked. Did the conflict ever get resolved? How?

3. Discuss with a nurse manager how she determines whether a conflict is occurring and what steps she takes to bring it out in the open. Share the information with your classmates.

4. Discuss with a nurse manager how he feels about constant change on a personal level. How did he present an impending change to the staff? Did he use any of the techniques discussed in this chapter? Was the change successful?

EXPLORING THE WEB

- Look up this journal and describe its purpose. Would this journal be useful to the new nurse manager? A new nurse? Anyone else in health care?

  Journal of Conflict Resolution: *http://www. ingenta.com/isis/browsing/allissues%3fjournal= infobike://sage/j22*

REFERENCES

Bennis, W. (1989). *On becoming a leader.* Reading, MA: Addison-Wesley.

Bennis, W., Benne, K., & Chin, R. (Eds.). (1969). *The planning of change* (2nd ed.). New York: Holt, Rinehart, Winston.

Bushy, A. (1993). Managing change: Strategies for continuing education. *The Journal of Continuing Education in Nursing, 23,* 197–200.

Duck, J. D. (1993, November/December). Managing change: The art of balancing. *Harvard Business Review,* 109–118.

Filley, A. C. (1975). *Interpersonal conflict resolution.* Glenview, IL: Scott, Foresman.

Havelock, R. G. (1973). *The change agent's guide to innovation in education.* Englewood Cliffs, NJ: Educational Technology.

Ingersoll, G. L., Kirsch, J. C., Merk, S. E., & Lightfoot, J. (2000, January). Relationship of organizational culture and readiness for change to employee commitment to the organization. *Journal of Nursing Administration, 30*(1), 11–20.

Keenan, M. J., & Hurst, J. B. (1999). Conflict: The cutting edge of change. In P. S. Yoder-Wise, *Leading and managing in nursing* (2nd ed.) (pp. 318–334). St. Louis, MO: Mosby.

Lancaster, J. (1999). *Nursing issues in leading and managing change.* St. Louis, MO: Mosby.

Lewicki, R. J., Hiam, A., & Olander, K. W. (1996). *Think before you speak.* New York: John Wiley & Sons.

Lewin, K. (1951). *Field theory in social science.* New York: Harper & Row.

Lippit, R., Watson, J., & Westley, B. (1958). *The dynamics of planned change.* New York: Harcourt, Brace.

MacFarland, G., et al. (1984). *Nursing leadership and management.* Clifton Park, NY: Delmar Learning.

Marriner-Tomey, A. (2000). *Guide to nursing management and leadership* (6th ed.). St. Louis, MO: Mosby Company.

Marquis, B. L., & Huston, C. J. (2000). *Leadership roles and management functions in nursing: Theory applied* (3rd ed.). Philadelphia: Lippincott.

Menix, K. D. (1999). Leading change: Nurse manager as innovator. In P. S. Yoder-Wise, *Leading and managing in nursing* (2nd ed.) (pp. 73–89). St. Louis, MO: Mosby.

Rogers, E. M. (1983). *Diffusion of innovations* (3rd ed.). New York: Free Press.

Sebastian, J. G. (1999). Organizational change and the change process. In J. Lancaster, *Nursing issues in leading and managing change.* St. Louis, MO: Mosby.

Senge, P. M. (1990). *The fifth discipline: The art and practice of the learning organization.* New York: Doubleday.

Shortell, S. et al. (1994). *Health Care Management—Organization Design and Behavior* (3rd ed.). Clifton Park, NY: Delmar Learning.

Silber, M. B. (1993, September). The "C"s in excellence: Choice and change. *Nursing Management, 24*(9), 60–62.

Simms, L. et al. (2000). *The Professional Practice of Nursing Administration* (3rd ed.). Clifton Park, NY: Delmar Learning.

Sullivan, E. J., & Decker, P. J. (2001). *Effective leadership & management in nursing* (5th ed.). Menlo Park, CA: Addison-Wesley.

Swansburg, R. C., & Swansburg, R. J. (1998). *Introductory management and leadership for nurses* (2nd ed.). Boston: Jones and Bartlett.

Tappen, R. M. (2001). *Nursing leadership and management: Concepts and practice* (4th ed.). Philadelphia: F. A. Davis.

Thietart, R. A., & Forgues, B. (1995). Chaos theory and organizations. *Organization Science, 6*(1), 19–31.

SUGGESTED READINGS

Bennis, W., & Nanus, B. (1985). *Leaders: The strategies for taking charge.* New York: Harper & Row.

Curtin, L. L. (1995, March). Blessed are the flexible". . . . *Nursing Management, 26*(3), 7–8.

Entine, J., & Nichols, M. (1997, January/February). Good leadership: What's its gender? *Female Executive,* 50–52.

Heim, P. (1995). Getting beyond "she said, he said." *Nursing Administration Quarterly, 19*(2), 6–18.

Johnson, S. (1998). *Who moved my cheese?* New York: G.P. Putnam.

Jost, S. G. (2000). An assessment and intervention strategy for managing staff needs during change. *Journal of Nursing Administration, 30*(1), 34–40.

Kotter, J. P. (1996). *Leading change.* Boston: Harvard Business School Press.

McFarland, G., Leonard, H., & Morris, M. (1984). *Nursing leadership and management.* New York, NY: Wiley.

Marriner-Tomey, A. (2000). *Guide to nursing management and leadership* (6th ed.). St. Louis, MO: Mosby.

McDaniel, R. R. (1997). Strategic leadership: A view from quantum and chaos theories. *Health Care Management Review, 22*(1), 21–37.

Rosswurm, M. A., & Larrabee, J. H. (1999). A model for change to evidence-based practice. *Image: Journal of Nursing Scholarship, 31*(4), 317–322.

Schweikhart, S. B., & Smith-Daniels, V. (1996). Reengineering the work of caregivers: Role redefinition, team structures, and organization redesign. *Hospital & Health Services Administration, 41*(1), 19–36.

Simms, L. M., Price, S. A., & Ervin, N. E. (2000). *The professional practice of nursing administration* (3rd ed.). Clifton Park, NY: Delmar Learning.

Zukowski, B. (1995). Managing change—before it manages you. *Medical Surgical Nursing, 4*(4), 325–326.

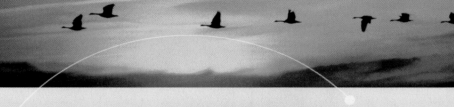

CHAPTER 17

Power

Terry W. Miller, PhD, RN

Significant progress has occurred over the years toward advancing nursing's presence, role, and influence in the development of health care policy. However, more nurses need to learn how to identify issues strategically; work with decision makers; understand who holds the power in the workplace, communities, state and federal level organizations; and understand who controls the resources for health care services. (Stephanie L. Ferguson, 2001)

OBJECTIVES

Upon completion of this chapter, the reader should be able to:

1. Define the concept of power.
2. Identify the various sources of power, i.e., coercion, reward, legitimacy, expertise, reference, information, and connection.
3. Recognize power at a personal level, a professional level, and an organizational level.
4. Describe how a nurse's perception of power affects patient care.
5. Describe the association of connection power and relationships.
6. Explain why nurses are faced with a paradox within the context of information power.

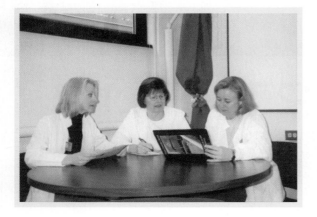

Nurse Pat, who just finished her orientation, is working with a patient for whom a surgical consult has been written. The unit clerk and a long-time nurse on the unit remark that Dr. Killian, the physician doing the surgical consultation, should be named Dr. Killjoy because she humiliates new nurses to try to put them in their place. Based on previous reports by other nurses on the unit, Pat knows Dr. Killian has the reputation of being demeaning and inappropriately demanding when interacting with new nurses. Two hours later, Dr. Killian appears on the unit and asks to see the nurse who did the surgical admission sheet.

    What would you do if you were Pat?
    How would you approach Dr. Killian?

Effective nurses are powerful. They show objectivity, creativity, and knowledge throughout their practice and regardless of their work setting. They have and exert power by understanding the concept of power from multiple perspectives; they then use this understanding to motivate others; accomplish organizational goals; and provide safe, competent care. Yet the nursing profession has been criticized for not accepting this fact and for not knowing enough about the power that nursing holds.

Nurses have struggled with the concept of power throughout the profession's history. Many outside the profession continue to challenge the nurse's role in wielding power at any level, including the bedside. Much of the challenge to the nurse's power can be linked directly to nursing being a predominantly female occupation. In many cultures, a majority of people subscribe to the notion that women do not need and should not have power (Mason, Talbott, & Leavitt, 1993). However, nursing has a rich history,

with many of its leaders overcoming the prejudicial challenges confronting them. This chapter will discuss power and how nursing power affects patient care.

DEFINITIONS OF POWER

Power has been defined in multiple ways, some not so positive. Commonly, **power** is described as the ability to create, get, and use resources to achieve one's goals. If the goals are self-determined, there is an implication of even greater power than if the goals are made by or with others. Power can be defined at various levels: personal, professional, or organizational. Power, regardless of level, comes from the ability to influence others or affect others' thinking or behavior.

Power at the personal level is closely linked to how an individual perceives power, how others perceive the individual, and the extent to which an individual can influence events. Nurses who feel empowered at a personal level are likely to manifest a high level of self-awareness. They are more likely to understand nursing as a profession because it represents a group to which they belong. They also understand the structure and operations of health care because it represents their work environment.

People who are perceived as experts in health care have a significant amount of authority and influence, which makes them more effective than those not perceived as experts. There are at least two ways to wield the influence of an expert. The first way is to be introduced and promoted to a group as an expert, which validates one's expertise; the second way is to actually become an expert based on knowledge, skills, and abilities that are consistently demonstrated in practice settings. Remarkably, nurses are often reluctant to be identified as experts to patients, physicians, administrators, some nurses, other health care workers, and the public in general. This lack of awareness must be addressed if the nursing profession is to achieve the status and degree of empowerment it seeks. Disch (2000) stated, "In today's health care environment, what is valued, preserved, and receives resources is that which is visible" (p. 189).

The personal power of nurses is evident in the decisions they make on a daily basis about how their lives and work are organized to accomplish what they want and obtain what they need for themselves and their patients. The more nurses believe they can influence events through personal effort, the greater their sense of power. Many accept the idea that if individuals believe they can make a difference and influence events in their lives, they are likely to participate actively in trying to get what they want. This participation will make them feel more powerful even if their efforts are not all that successful. Similarly, if individuals believe themselves to be powerless to influence events and do not even try to exert any influence, they will feel even more powerless (Rowland & Rowland, 1997).

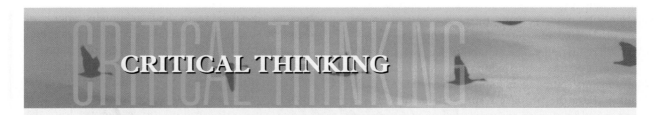

CRITICAL THINKING

The work and contributions of some nurses are so significant that they change the world. To be effective, these nurses define themselves as something far more powerful than what others may want them to be. When we ignore the relevance and significance of nursing history, we discount the contributions nurses have made to improve the lives of others. Our lack of historical awareness empowers others to discount nursing. Ultimately, we limit our own future as nurses by hindering our potential for making even greater contributions to the future of health care.

Can you name two nurses who represent powerful figures in modern history and tell why their contributions are so significant? See Exploring the Web in this chapter.

Can you identify some obstacles they experienced because they were nurses?

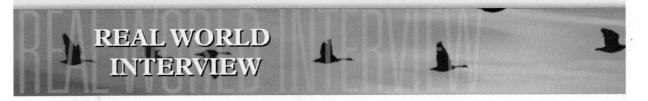

REAL WORLD INTERVIEW

I try not to use power in an authoritarian manner in the pain management clinic that I manage. Instead, I attempt to get people to move without them necessarily knowing they are being helped. I think that power at the bedside is a personal thing. Confidence, authenticity, and genuineness are qualities I most value and see as empowering nurses in practice. I feel that the middle manager in nursing gets power by developing staff, building self-confidence on a personal level, and delegating authority in a way that supports others. In higher levels of management I found, through my military experience, that the best leaders almost give power away with the caveat that the persons are being delegated to represent the leader and are accountable for the decisions they make. I believe that the tighter a person holds onto power, the less powerful she or he becomes. I also believe that nurses run the risk of losing power when they look for power outside nursing to direct them. New graduates should seek experiences and input from a variety of people and glean what they can from each experience. It is somewhat like a smorgasbord. Ultimately, the new nurse has to decide what she or he wants because there is no one answer or approach to power. No one really has *the* answer; instead, they have *an* answer.

Nancy Safranek, MSN, RN
RN Director, OPS, PACU, SP, PMC

POWER AND ACCOUNTABILITY

Nurses have a professional obligation not to view power merely as a negative concept so that they may avoid power struggles and those who seem to savor power. Effective nurses view their ability to understand and use power as a significant part of their responsibilities to patients, their coworkers, the nursing profession, and themselves.

Traditionally, accountability has been considered one of the major hallmarks of the health care professions. Nursing is a profession and, as such, nurses have the primary responsibility for defining and providing nursing services. Yet some nurses appear to have a difficult time understanding the underlying accountability that comes with this powerful claim. Inherent in the role of the nurse are professional accountability and direct responsibility for decisions made and actions rendered.

SOURCES OF POWER

Most researchers agree that the sources of power are diverse and vary from one situation to another. They also agree that these sources of power are a combination of conscious and unconscious factors that allow an individual to influence others to do as the individual wants (Fisher & Koch, 1996). Articles and textbooks about nursing administration, educational leadership, and organizational management commonly include references to the work of Hersey, Blanchard, and Natemeyer (1979), an expansion of the power typology originally developed by French and Raven in 1959 (cited in Hersey, Blanchard, & Natemeyer, 1979). The typology helps nurses understand how different people perceive power and subsequently relate to others in the work setting and in attempts to achieve their goals. Power is described as having a basis in expertise, legitimacy, reference (charisma), reward, coercion, or connection. More recently, another power source—information—has been added to the typology (Wells, 1998). Generally speaking, nurses exert influence derived from one or a combination of these power sources.

Power derived from the knowledge and skills nurses possess is referred to as **expert power**. There are, however, special considerations to keep in mind about expertise and power. The geometric explosion of knowledge has made expertise more valuable, and technological advances for accessing information have enabled more people to acquire expertise on any given subject. Knowing more about a subject than others, combined with the legitimacy of holding a position, gives an individual a decided advantage in any situation. But the less acknowledged that experts are in a group, the less effective their expert powers become. Visible reciprocal acknowledgment of expertise among group members balances power and enhances productivity, whereas lack of reciprocal acknowledgment has the opposite effect. Combining expertise with high position is most powerful if the person consistently demonstrates expertise.

Legitimate power is power derived from the position a nurse holds in a group, and it indicates the nurse's degree of authority. The more comfortable nurses are with their legitimate power as nurses, the easier it is for them to fulfill their role. Nurses in legitimate positions are expected to use what authority they have and may be punished for not doing so. Sometimes, too little legitimacy or authority is delegated to nurses who are given the responsibility for leading. People generally follow legitimate leaders with whom they agree. Although legitimacy is a significant part of influence and control, it is not universally effective and is not sufficient as one's only source of power.

Power derived from how much others respect and like any individual, group, or organization is referred to as **referent power**, or charismatic power. Nurses who are trusted and respected by others are most able to exert influence over them. People want to agree with and follow referent leadership. Such leaders tend to be charismatic, and followers often rationalize or explain away any incongruent behaviors to maintain their high level of trust in the referent. It is erroneous to assume that only people who are less intelligent than the charismatic or referent leader will follow that leader. The referent leader who inspires trust and confidence also makes other people feel valuable.

The ability to reward or punish others, as well as to create fear in others to influence them to change their behavior, is commonly termed **reward power and coercive power**. Meaningful rewards exist other than money, such as formal recognition before one's nursing peers at an awards ceremony. The manner in which rewards are distributed is important. Rewards seldom motivate as effectively as a vision that unifies the members of the group, thus reward power is an uncertain instrument for long-term change. Rewards are not likely to permanently change attitudes. Withholding rewards or achieving a goal by instilling fear in others often results in resentment.

People who have the ability to administer punishment or take disciplinary actions against others have coercive power. This type of power is often considered the least desirable tactic to be used by people in positions of authority. Typically, people do not enjoy being coerced into doing something other than what they choose to do, and often perceive punishment as humiliating.

The extent to which nurses are connected with others having power is called **connection power**. Leaders can dramatically increase their influence by understanding that people are attracted to those with power and their associates. As a new nurse, when you go to the office of the director of nursing services or the vice president for patient care services, do not forget that the clerical workers in the outside office have relationships with their boss—thus they have connection power. If you try to go around them and take their power lightly, and insult or patronize them, you have risked your own power base in relation to the director or vice president. Similarly, if a nurse bypasses a person who is directly responsible for a situation, the attempted circumvention reflects negatively on the nurse. Nurses should work to resolve issues at the appropriate level before they take their concerns to a higher level of authority. Nurses are expected to understand the structure and policies of the organizations in which they provide services.

Nurses who influence others with the information they provide to the group are using **information power**. Regardless of a nurse's leadership style, information plays an increasingly critical role. Legitimate power, reward power, and coercive power tend to be bestowed on individuals by their organizations. They tend to be effective only for a short period of time unless they are accompanied by another form of power, such as information power. Information power is especially important because, to be functional, health care teams and organizations require accurate and timely information that is shared. To be seen by others as having information power, nurses must share knowledge that is both accurate and useful. Information sharing can improve patient care, increase collegiality, enhance organizational effectiveness, and

strengthen one's professional connections. See Table 17-1 for a summary of the different types of power.

Effective nurses use the sources of power covered thus far: expertise, legitimacy, reference, reward, coercion, connection, and information. They have the ability to combine referent (charismatic) power and expert power from a legitimate power base, adding carefully measured portions of reward power and little or preferably no coercive power (Fisher & Koch, 1996). These leaders gather and use information in new and creative ways. They understand that power should be a means to accomplish a goal instead of a goal in itself.

PERSONAL ORIENTATION AND THE INTERNET

In the simplest terms, a person's desire for power, whether it is for impact, strength, or influence, takes one of two forms. The first form is an orientation toward achieving personal gain and self-glorification. The second form is an orientation toward achieving gain for others or the common good. Orientation to power as corruptive or evil is reflected in the 19th century quote attributed to Lord Acton: "All power corrupts, but absolute power corrupts absolutely" (Bothamley, 1993). People having this orientation tend to believe that those wielding or afforded power ultimately should not have power because of their potential to misuse it, that people desiring power should not be trusted because their motivation for acquiring power is inherently wrong—they want power for personal gain at any cost.

Many believe the Internet will level the playing field of power for all humanity. The free flow of information will empower nurses and other people, that is, all those who have access to the Internet and have the ability to use it effectively.

EMPOWERMENT AND DISEMPOWERMENT

Empowerment is a popular term in the nursing literature related to management, leadership, and politics. Authors describing empowerment usually view it as something positive or highly desirable to be aspired to, advocated for, or attained. Kelly (Kelly &

TABLE 17-1	*Principles for Understanding and Using Different Types of Power*

Concept	How it works
Expertise (Fisher & Koch, 1996)	Power derived from the knowledge and skills nurses possess is referred to as expert power. The greater nurses' proficiency in performing their role, the greater their expert power.
Legitimacy (Fisher & Koch, 1996)	Legitimacy as a nurse is based on several factors. These include licensure, academic degrees, certification, experience in the role, and title/position in the institution.
Referent (charisma) (Fisher & Koch, 1996)	Referent power is based on the admiration, trust, and respect that people feel toward an individual, group, or organization. The referent person has the ability to inspire confidence. In any situation, strong referent leaders are considered people of great vision, which may or may not be the reality.
Reward and coercive	The ability to reward or punish others as well as to create fear in others to influence them to change their behavior is commonly termed reward power and coercive power.
Connection	Both personal and professional relationships are part of a nurse's connections. People who are strongly connected to others, both personally and professionally, have enhanced resources, capacity for learning and information sharing, and increase their overall sphere of influence. Teamwork, collaboration, networking, and mentoring are some of the ways in which nurses can become more connected and therefore more powerful.
Information (Bower, 2000)	Information power is based on the information that any person can provide to the group. Authoritarian leaders attempt to control information. Charismatic leaders provide information that is seductive for many people. Information leaders provide a sense of stability with the use and synthesis of information. If one knows how to get it and what to do with it, the greatest power may be in information.

Joel, 1996) defined empowerment as the "process by which we facilitate the participation of others in decision making and take action within an environment where there is an equitable distribution of power" (p. 420).

Nurses empower themselves and others in many ways. At the most basic level, they empower others because they perceive them to be powerful. If an individual, a group, or an organization is perceived as being powerful, that perception can empower that individual, group, or organization. Some health care provider groups are viewed as more powerful than others because of the alliances they have formed with associations such as the American Medical Association (AMA), known to be powerful. Similarly, nurses disempower themselves if they see nurses or nursing as powerless.

Role of the Media

People who work in the media recognize the relationship between power and perception. Those who work in advertising, marketing, and public relations understand how media can be used to create or change perceptions. They have long recognized that the public's perception can be created or changed through advertising and marketing campaigns, damage control, timely press releases, and well-orchestrated media events.

The way the media present nursing to the public will empower or disempower nursing. Nurses have not been able to consistently use the media as effectively as other more powerful occupational groups. To date, the media have failed to recognize nursing as one of the largest groups in health care. It is hoped

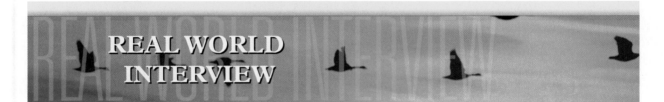

CRITICAL THINKING

Are you interested in becoming the best nurse possible? Do you enjoy meeting and associating with people who are successful? Do you feel most comfortable when you are in control over personal situations? Do you feel uncomfortable when you have little or no influence over the actions of others? Responding yes to these questions suggests that you have motives for personal achievement, being affiliated with others, and having power. **Achievement** (accomplishment of goals through effort), **affiliation** (associations and relationships with others), and power are interrelated from a behavioral perspective. All three can be positive attributes of one's personality, or they can lead to highly destructive behavior. Affiliation and power needs are predominantly interpersonal, whereas the need for achievement is predominantly intrapersonal, that is, motivated by one's personal conviction that one is capable and competent. People with high achievement needs tend to rely on themselves to get things done. They activate their intrapersonal motivation. Consequently, they expend a high degree of energy and focus on improving their personal skills and learning new things. Depending on their past experiences and current interests, nurses engage in a variety of behaviors that reflect their needs for achievement, affiliation, or power. Can you name two occupations that are associated with having a high level of motivation in terms of achievement, affiliation, and power? (Modified and updated from Grasha, 1978; 1995.)

REAL WORLD INTERVIEW

Ms. Cox is 38 years old and has been hospitalized four times. She underwent surgery this past spring and has encountered nursing care and nurses in various roles throughout the health care system. Ms. Cox is articulate and reflective, having earned a degree in English and holding a position at a selective liberal arts university as an admissions counselor. She states, "I don't think nurses know they are powerful .... Nurses can take on more than they think they can. They have the power to change the system in which they work. Yet I see nurses as the most overworked, underpaid, and underachieving professions also. There is so much more they could be doing if they didn't spend so much time railing against the machine. They are telling the wrong people—each other—that they are frustrated. They should be telling the ones with real power, or, better yet, more of them should become the ones in power. Instead, they suffer with each other and stay angry. It appears almost passive-aggressive how nurses deal with power. My concern is that it can affect patient care in such a negative way. Believe me when I say patients value nurses, but the people writing the paycheck for nurses must value nurses. Patients need nursing far more than they need anything else. The better nurses that have cared for me have been instrumental in my healing. Beyond knowing when I need medication or doing some procedure, it is the smile, the touch, and the well-placed word of encouragement that has gotten me through. This is where nurses have power because no one but a real nurse can provide it. It comes from the heart."

Audrey Cox
Patient

that the media's presentation of the rapidly growing nursing shortage over the next decade will improve the public's perceptions of nursing as a career and human service. The media need to show nurses as decision makers, coordinators of care, and primary care providers as well as order followers in health care. Too often the media has presented a stereotypical, insignificant view of nurses, and too often nurses fail to view nursing as the honorable profession it is. One strategy for empowering nursing would be to employ the media to create a stronger, more powerful image of nursing. That would require more nurses to become active participants in some formal part of their profession—the American Nurses Association (ANA), the National League for Nursing (NLN), or one of the nursing specialty organizations.

A PLAN FOR PERSONAL EMPOWERMENT

Understanding power helps the novice nurse to become more effective, to make better decisions, and to better help others. Understanding power from a

variety of perspectives is not just important for nurses professionally, it is important for them personally as well. It allows nurses to gain more control of their work lives and personal lives. There are three ways to imagine the future: (1) what is possible, (2) what is probable, and (3) what is preferred. A nurse who wants to experience a preferred future should think about what is happening to her as a person and as a nurse, what possibilities she faces as a person and as a nurse, and what she is going to do about it.

POWER AND THE LIMITS OF INFORMATION

Even if nurses could fully trust the completeness and accuracy of information they have in their practice, they would have insufficient data. "There is no end to information just as there is no end to what we could know about something" (Wells, 1998, p. 29). To make good decisions, nurses must be able to gather enough information and realistically interpret its value, as well as share and apply information in a

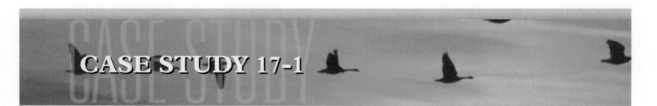

CASE STUDY 17-1

Maria and Haley work on the same nursing unit in a large, metropolitan hospital. Both predominantly work the evening shift and have less than 1 year's experience since graduating from nursing school. Maria has been offered increasingly difficult patient assignments, given charge duties, and recently was selected for a 2-week leadership training program. Haley has not adapted as well and has withdrawn from what was once a close relationship with Maria. Haley seeks consolation with the nurses she and Maria claimed they would never emulate. Haley takes her breaks and eats dinner with two nurses who complain that the best nurses are undervalued in the organization, yet these same nurses were not supportive of Maria or Haley or any other new nurses oriented to their unit. Maria seeks out others she perceives to be knowledgeable and more satisfied in their professional roles. She strives to participate in nonmandatory meetings as well as clinical rounds, using them as an opportunity to ask questions, thus she is beginning to increase her personal level of power by connecting with the other staff and gathering information. One night after a difficult shift, Haley accuses Maria of abandoning her, and playing up to administration and states that Maria is being used by the unit's nurse manager. Haley tells Maria that the other nurses are planning to file a complaint against the unit supervisor for selecting Maria over the nurses that have been on the unit longer to attend the leadership training program.

How should Maria react to Haley in this situation?

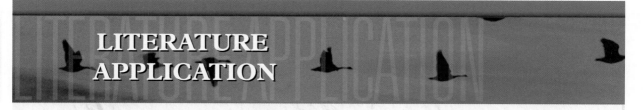

LITERATURE APPLICATION

Citation: Laschinger, H. K. S., & Wong, C. (1999). Staff nurse empowerment and collective accountability: Effect on perceived productivity and self-rated work effectiveness. *Nursing Economic$, 17*(6), 308–316.

Discussion: The findings of this survey supported empowerment, collective decision-making authority, productivity, accountability, formal and informal power, and political and social alliances in the workplace. Shared governance was criticized because authority for patient care was not shifted to nurses. The study reported that an essential strategy for fostering high-quality professional practice was creating environments to include free access for staff nurses to empowering structures and opportunities for access to information and resources, along with appropriate support. Nurses reported their accountability to each other and their contribution to the organization as moderate, their overall work effectiveness high, but their productivity lower than expected. Recommendations included essential changes in the manager role to exclude traditional control and include support for nurses in their performance.

Implications for Practice: Assumption of greater power by nurses as primary service providers necessitates far-reaching changes in organizational operations, administrative structures, budget processes, individual service planning procedures, and professional cross-disciplinary relationships. The findings of this study offer more insight into what staff nurses expected to be more effective in providing patient care services.

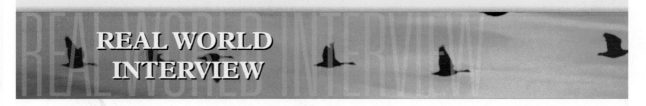

REAL WORLD INTERVIEW

Power is the ultimate responsibility to care for the patient. Our assessment and subsequent actions can determine whether a patient will live or die. I feel confident in my abilities for the future, but as a new nurse, it is difficult to feel powerful because there is so much to learn. I believe that nurses tend to perceive power as being able to stand up to those above or higher up in the work setting. I think nursing is changing for the better because of the power gained with nurses having more autonomy. There is more trust put into the nurse's judgment because women's roles in society have changed. Equal opportunity programs have created the structure to protect women and others who have been vulnerable to those in positions of greater power. I have learned that you do not have to be afraid to advocate for your patient. If you need to call the attending physician during the night, then you do it. I have come to realize that power is not abusing the people working under you. Also, to understand power, it is important to understand people's roles and where they are coming from.

Julie Bergman
New Nursing Graduate

safe, competent manner. Effective nurses understand time constraints and set priorities to ensure that what is most important receives the most attention. These nurses are willing to take the inherent risk of making a decision, while understanding there will always be more information to gather and analyze. They recognize that choosing to make no decision is a decision in itself and that information is never complete. Table 17-2 presents a framework for becoming empowered using information.

TABLE 17-2	A Framework for Becoming Empowered Using Information
Background	An empowered nurse has the ability to discover what is important information and to use it to her advantage as well as to the advantage of her patients.
Steps	• Find and maintain good sources of information. • Get involved beyond direct patient care. • Ask questions. • Listen to and analyze the answers. • Make a plan with the information acquired. • Evaluate the plan.
Information for providing care	• Assess patient's condition using relevant, objective measurements. • Consult with other nurses, physicians, and other health care workers involved in the care of your patients. • Consult with significant others, friends, and members of the patient's family.

Information for becoming more effective in the work setting	• Get involved beyond direct patient care.
	• Volunteer for committee assignments that will challenge you to learn and experience more than what is expected of you in a staff nurse role.
	• Think about the following when involved with committees:
	  1. What is the committee trying to do?
	  2. What specific information does the committee use to make decisions?
	  3. How does the committee's work apply to my practice, my colleagues, my patients, my organizational unit, and the organization as a whole?
	• Assess the strength of the information you have in relation to your patients, your colleagues, your organizational unit, the organization as a whole, and the profession of nursing.
	• Readily share information with others who will value it and use it to a good end.

Evaluation	Periodically, reexamine your plans. Did you achieve your expected outcomes? If not, why? Were there staffing problems or patient crises? Were the activities that were necessary for outcome achievement carried out? What have you learned from this evaluation that you can apply to the future?

MACHIAVELLI ON POWER

It would be naive to think that one can necessarily expect easy acceptance, understanding, or even support for what one is attempting to do. Machiavelli is reported to have said,

> There is nothing more difficult to take in hand, more perilous to conduct than to take a lead in the introduction of a new order of things because the innovation has for enemies all those who have done well under the old conditions and lukewarm defenders in those who may do well under the new. (Hanson, 2000, p. 7)

KEY CONCEPTS

- Effective nurses are powerful. They show objectivity, creativity, and knowledge throughout their practice and regardless of their work setting.
- Effective nurses have and exert power by understanding the concept of power from multiple perspectives, they then use this understanding to motivate others; accomplish organizational goals; and provide safe, competent care.
- Power has been described as the ability to create, get, and use resources to achieve one's goals.
- Power can be defined at a personal level, a professional level, and an organizational level.
- The personal and information power of nurses is evident in the decisions they make.
- Hersey, Blanchard, and Natemeyer (1979) help the nurse understand how different people perceive power by describing sources of power as coercion, rewards, legitimacy, expertise, reference, information, and connection.

KEY TERMS

achievement	legitimate power
affiliation	power
connection power	referent power
empowerment	reward power and
expert power	coercive power
information power	sources of power

REVIEW QUESTIONS

1. The most effective nurses use power
   A. in one primary way.
   B. to influence others or affect others' thinking or behavior.
   C. predominantly at an organizational level.
   D. only to gain the necessary resources to be a better nurse.

2. Power has been described in the literature
   A. consistently as a negative concept.
   B. most often as a manifestation of personal ambition.
   C. as maintained through one's position in society, a work setting, or family.
   D. in multiple ways, some not so positive.

3. When a person fears another enough to act or behave differently than he would otherwise, the source of the other person's power is called
   A. coercive power.
   B. reward power.
   C. expert power.
   D. connection power.

4. What source of power has become increasingly important because of technological innovation in the past decade?
   A. Expert power
   B. Information power
   C. Connection power
   D. Legitimate power

5. Nurses disempower themselves by
   A. facilitating the participation of others in decision making.
   B. taking action within an environment where there is an equitable distribution of power.
   C. believing they are empowered.
   D. discounting the role the media plays in the public's perception of nursing.

6. A nurse's personal power can be enhanced by
   A. collaborating with colleagues on special projects outside the work setting.
   B. developing skills that do not apply directly to patient care.
   C. volunteering to serve on organizational committees led by nonnurses.
   D. All of the above

REVIEW ACTIVITIES

1. Identify a nursing leader. Observe her and note what type of power she uses to meet her objectives.

2. Watch a television show that portrays nurses. Note how nurses use or do not use the different types of power available to them. What do you observe?

3. Observe our national leaders. What examples of the use of power do you see? Is power used in helpful or unhelpful ways? Explain.

EXPLORING THE WEB

- Which sites can you visit for information on nursing leaders and nursing history?
  http://members.tripod.com/~DianneBrownson/ history.html

- Which sites can you visit for information on power, leadership, and women?
  http://members.aol.com/douglaseby/Page6.html
  http://albie.wcupa.edu/ttrreadwell/paper20

- What site has a funny, not scholarly, synopsis of nursing power? *http://www.NursingPower.net/ nursingpower/webring.html*

- What site supports political power for patients? *http://www.healthcarereform.net*

- Which site discusses a variety of nursing resources and issues, including collective power? *http://www.nursingworld.org*

- Go to the site for the Center for Health Policy, Research and Ethics, College of Nursing & Health Science, George Mason University. Note the seminars and internships offered to nurses interested in health policy.
  http://hpi.gmu.edu

- On the Google search engine, perform a search using the term "nursing leaders."
  http://www.google.com

- Find two nurses identified on the following site: *http://dbois@distinguishedwomen.com*

REFERENCES

Bothamley, J. (1993). *Dictionary of theories*. London: Gale Research International.

Bower, F. L. (2000). *Nurses taking the lead: Personal qualities of effective leadership*. Philadelphia: Saunders.

Disch, J. (2000, July-August). Nurse executive: Make the glue red. *Journal of Professional Nursing, 16*(4), 189.

Ferguson, S. L. (2001). An activist looks at nursing's role in health policy development. *Journal of Obstetric, Gynecologic, and Neonatal Nursing, 30*(5), 546–551.

Fisher, J. L., & Koch, J. V. (1996). *Presidential leadership: Making a difference*. Phoenix, AZ: American Council on Education and The Oryx Press.

Grasha, A. F. (1978). *Practical applications of psychology*. Cambridge, MA: Winthrop.

Grasha, A. F. (1995) *Practical applications of psychology* (4th ed.). Menlo Park, CA: Addison-Wesley.

Hanson, W. (2000). We shall be transformed. *e-gov: The Next Challenge*, available at www.govtech.net.

Hersey, P., Blanchard, K., & Natemeyer, W. (1979). Situational leadership, perception and impact of power. *Group and Organizational Studies, 4*, 418–428.

Kelly, L. Y., & Joel, L. A. (1996). *The nursing experience: Trends, challenges, and transitions* (3rd ed.). New York: McGraw-Hill.

Laschinger, H. K. S., & Wong, C. (1999). Staff nurse empowerment and collective accountability: Effect on perceived productivity and self-rated work effectiveness. *Nursing Economic$, 17*(6), 308–316.

Mason, D. J., Talbott, S. W., & Leavitt, J. K. (1993). *Policy and politics for nurses: Action and change in the workplace, government, organizations and community*. Philadelphia: Saunders.

Rowland, H. S., & Rowland, B. L. (1997). *Nursing administration handbook*. Rockville, MD: Aspen.

Wells, S. (1998). *Choosing the future: The power of strategic thinking*. Boston: Butterworth-Heinemann.

SUGGESTED READINGS

American Nurses Association. (1985). *Nursing's social policy statement*. Washington, DC: American Nurses Publishing.

Benner, P. E. (2000). *From novice to expert: Excellence and power in clinical nursing practice* (Commemorative edition). Upper Saddle River, NJ: Prentice Hall.

Government Technology (any recent issue). (Available free online at www.govtech.net or by writing to Government Technology at 100 Blue Ravine Road, Folsom, CA 95630.)

    Addresses the information age and the power of information.

Hanna, L. A. (1999). Lead the way. *Nursing Management, 30*(11), 36–39.

Leddy, S., & Pepper, J. M. (1998). *Conceptual bases of professional nursing* (4th ed.). Philadelphia: Lippincott.

Short, P. M. (1998). Empowering leadership. *Contemporary Education, 69*(2), 70–72.

Spitzer, K. L., Eisenbery, M. B., & Lowe, C. A. (1998). *Information literacy essential skills for the information age.* Syracuse, NY: ERIC Clearinghouse on Information & Technology.

Strasen, L. (1987). *Key business skills for nurse managers.* Philadelphia: Lippincott.

CHAPTER 18

Time Management

Patsy L. Maloney, RN, C, MSN, EdD, CNAA

Autonomy means decision control over the kind and degree of service a client will receive. It involves a conscious decision about what will and what will not be done when there is more work than available time. Control over time use is a key aspect of professional nurse practice.

(Roxane Spitzer-Lehmann, 1996)

OBJECTIVES

Upon completion of this chapter, the reader should be able to:

1. Discuss general time management techniques.
2. Describe strategies to plan effective use of time.
3. Apply time management strategies to the reality of delivering effective nursing care.
4. Apply time management strategies to enhance personal productivity.

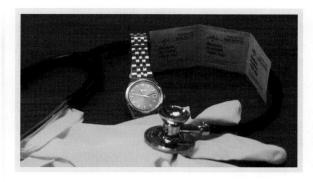

Sharon has just completed her medical-surgical orientation as a new graduate registered nurse. This evening is her first solo shift. But she is not really alone. Sharon and Carole—the other RN—and one certified nursing assistant are responsible for 12 possible patients in this section of the unit. Currently there are 10 patients in this section, but a new admission is on the way, another patient is returning from surgery, the dinner trays are arriving, and Sharon has medications to pass. Just as the dinner trays arrive, a family member runs out to Sharon and states that her mom is confused and incontinent and has pulled out her IV.

How would you react if you were Sharon? What would you do first?

Many nurses become nurses out of idealism. They want to help people by meeting all their needs. Unfortunately, most new graduates find it impossible to meet all or even most of their patients' needs. Needs tend to be unlimited while time is limited. In addition to the direct patient care responsibilities, there are shift responsibilities, charting, doctors' orders to be transcribed or checked, medication supplies to be restocked, and reports to be given.

New graduates often go home feeling totally inadequate. They wake up remembering what they did not accomplish. One young nurse shared with tears in her eyes that once, when she answered a call bell late in her shift, the patient requested a pain medication. She went to the narcotics cabinet to get the medication but was interrupted by an emergent situation. When she arrived home, she was so exhausted that she fell asleep rapidly, only to awaken with the realization that she had not returned with her patient's medication. Her guilt was tremendous. She had gone into nursing to relieve pain, not to ignore it.

Time management allows the novice nurse to prioritize care, decide on outcomes, and perform the most important interventions first. Time management skills are important not just for nurses on the job but for nurses in their personal lives as well. They allow nurses to make time for fun, friends, exercise, and professional development.

ACHIEVING MORE WITH GENERAL TIME MANAGEMENT TECHNIQUES

Time management has been defined as "a set of related common-sense skills that helps you use your time in the most effective and productive way possible" (Mind Tools, nd.-b). In other words, time management allows us to achieve more with available time. Time management requires self-examination of what pursuits are really important, analysis of how time is currently being used, and assessment of the distractions that have been siphoning time from more important pursuits.

There is a simple principle, the **Pareto principle**, which states that 20% of effort results in 80% of results, or conversely that 80% of unfocused effort results in 20% of results (Figure 18-1). The Pareto principle reminds us to focus our efforts on the most important activities to maximize the results we get.

The Pareto principle, formulated by Vilfredo Pareto in the late 1800s, was invoked by the total quality management (TQM) movement as a strategy for balancing life and work (Fryxell, 1997; Graham, 1998; Koch, 1999). Effective time management requires that a shift be made from unfocused efforts that require 80% of time for achieving 20% of desired results to one of planned and focused efforts that use only 20% of time or effort to achieve 80% of desired results.

If time management is so easy, why do so many people continue at a crazy, hurried pace? There are

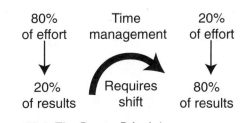

Figure 18-1 The Pareto Principle

several possible explanations for this. They do not know about time management, they think they do not have time to plan, they do not want to stop to plan, or they love crises (Mind Tools, n.d.-b).

Shift to an Outcome Orientation

The first step in any time management strategy is to shift to an outcome or results orientation, not a task orientation. Long-term goals must be determined, and it is best to break down these long-term goals into achievable outcomes that are the steps toward long-term goals. Long-term goals cannot be achieved overnight. Long-term goals and outcomes should be written down and should remain flexible. There may come a time when the outcome is no longer realistic or should be shifted to a more realistic goal as circumstances change (Reed & Pettigrew, 1999).

Analysis of Time

Analysis of time use is the first step in developing a plan to effectively use time. Nurses cannot possibly know how to better plan time without knowing how they currently use time. When keeping track of time, it is important to consider the value of a nurse's time as well as the use of the time.

Value of Nursing Time

Nurses often undervalue their time. Consider salary and benefits. Benefits are frequently forgotten, but they raise employer costs by 15% to 30% of salary. If a nurse is making $18 an hour, benefits add $2.70 to $5.40 to the hourly cost of a nurse's time. The value of nursing time in this example, excluding what the organization is paying in workers' compensation and payroll taxes, is $20.70 to $23.40 an hour. The organization has also invested in nurse recruitment, orientation, and development. Nursing time is an expensive commodity. Keeping this in mind will be invaluable when considering work that can be delegated to personnel who receive less compensation or when considering spending time on completing a task that does not support achieving an outcome.

Use of Time

Numerous studies have shown how nurses use their time. Most studies have been done on acute care nurses because they comprise the majority of nurses. Only 30% to 35% of nursing time is spent on direct patient care (Scharf, 1997). Twenty-five percent of a nurse's time is spent on charting and reporting, and the remainder of time is spent on admission and discharge procedures, professional communication, personal time, and providing care that could be provided by unlicensed personnel, such as transportation and housekeeping (Upenieks, 1998). Urden and Roode (1997) summarized various work sampling studies to show that RNs spend 28% to 33% of time on direct patient care, defined as activities performed in the presence of the patient or family; 42% to 45% of time on indirect care activities, which include all activities done for an individual patient but not in the patient's presence; 15% on unit-related activities, which include all unit general maintenance activities; and 13% to 20% on personal activities, which include activities that are not related to patient care or unit maintenance.

Given such a distribution of nurses' time, shifting the use of time could have a major impact on outcomes (Tappen, 2001). If nonnursing activities could be performed by nonnursing personnel instead of nurses, about 48 minutes per nurse per shift could be redirected toward essential nursing responsibilities (Prescott, Phillips, Ryan, & Thompson, 1991).

How do you use your time? Memory and self-reporting of time have been found to be unreliable. Nurses are often unaware of the time spent socializing with colleagues, making and drinking coffee, snacking, and other nonproductive time. Self-reporting of time is not recommended for estimating the total number of activities or the average time an activity takes to complete (Burke, Mckee, Wilson, Donahue, Batenhorst, & Pathak, 2000).

An **activity log** is a time management tool that can assist the nurse in determining how time is used. The activity log (Figure 18-2) should be used for several days. Behavior should not be modified while keeping the log. The nurse should record every activity, from the beginning of the shift until the end, as well as periodically note feelings while doing the activities—alert, energetic, tired, bored, and so on. Review of this log will illuminate time use as well as time wasted. Analysis of the log will allow the separation of essential professional activities from activities that can be performed by someone else (Grohar-Murray & DiCroce, 1997; Sullivan & Decker, 2001). You can also use this log to monitor your personal activities.

Name of activity	Beginning and ending time	Outcome desired [prevention of complications, improved health, and so on]	Feelings [alert, energetic, tired, bored, and so on]	Would it be better done by someone else? Who? [LPN, nursing assistant, housekeeper, other]
Work-related (medication administration, vital signs, bed making, patient transport, and so on):				
Personal (exercise, meal, rest, specific chore, travel, and so on):				

Figure 18-2 Nursing Activity Log

After completing the nursing activity log for at least three shifts, a nurse needs to consider all activities that have been completed, how much time each activity took, what was achieved by performing the activities, and whether the activities could have been done by someone else. When considering these questions, ask how would the Pareto principle apply? Has 80% of the effort resulted in 20% of the outcome achievement? If the activities have not achieved the desired outcomes, the nurse needs to focus on priorities.

STRATEGIES TO PLAN EFFECTIVE USE OF TIME

To plan effective use of time, nurses must understand the big picture, and decide on achievable outcomes.

Understand the Big Picture

Before priorities are set, the big picture must be examined. No nurse works in isolation. Nurses should know what is expected of their coworkers, what is happening on the other shifts, and what is happening beyond the unit. If nurses know what is expected of their coworkers, they can offer assistance during coworkers' busy times and in turn receive assistance during their own busy times. If the previous shift was stressed by a crisis, a shift may not get started as smoothly (Hansten & Washburn, 1998). If areas outside of the unit are overwhelmed, someone might be moved from one unit to assist on the overwhelmed unit elsewhere in the hospital. When nurses take the big picture into consideration, they are less likely to be frustrated when asked to assist others on their unit or others on other units in the hospital. They can also build into their time management plan the possibility of giving and receiving assistance.

Decide on Optimal Desired Outcomes

When nurses begin their shifts, they need to decide what optimal outcomes can be achieved. Optimal outcomes are the best possible objectives to be achieved given the resources at hand.

Once nurses have decided on optimal outcomes, they must consider what can and should be achieved given less-than-optimal circumstances and limited resources. These circumstances could include a rough start to a busy shift; personnel late, absent, or uncooperative; and a patient crisis. It is hard for nurses to give themselves permission to do less-than-optimal work, but sometimes achievement of reasonable outcomes is the best that can be expected (Hansten & Washburn, 1998). Reasonable outcomes are objectives that can and should be achieved given less-than-optimal circumstances and limited resources.

Do First Things First

To decide what is reasonable to accomplish, a nurse has to come to terms with the resources that are available and the outcomes that must be achieved. If someone has called in sick and no replacement is available, it might be unreasonable for a nurse to plan to reinforce teaching or discuss the home environment with a patient scheduled to leave the next day. However, there would be no question that interventions that prevent life-threatening emergencies or save a life when a life-threatening event occurs are priorities. They must be done no matter how short the staffing. It is imperative that nurses protect their patients and maintain both patient and staff safety as well as perform the activities essential to the nursing and medical care plans (Hansten & Washburn, 1998).

First Priority: A Life-Threatening or Potentially Life-Threatening Occurrence

Life-threatening conditions include a patient at risk to himself or others and a patient whose vital signs and level of consciousness indicates potential for respiratory or circulatory collapse (Hansten & Washburn, 1998). A patient whose condition is life threatening is the highest priority and requires monitoring until transfer or stabilization. Life-threatening conditions can occur at any time during the shift and may or may not be anticipated.

Second Priority: Activities Essential to Safety

Activities that are essential to safety include those responsibilities that ensure the availability of life-saving medications and equipment and that protect patients from infections and falls. They include asking for assistance or providing assistance during two-people transfers, or turning and movement of heavy patients (Hansten & Washburn, 1998).

Third Priority: Activities Essential to the Plan of Care

Activities that are essential to the plan of care are activities that lead to the outcomes that relieve symptoms or lead to healing. They are the activities that, if omitted, will hinder the patient's recovery. These activities include nutrition and medication administration, ambulation, positioning, and so on.

Covey, Merrill, and Merrill (1994) developed another way of setting priorities. Activities are classified as urgent or not urgent, as important or not important. If an activity is neither important nor urgent, then it becomes the lowest priority.

Some activities that are often thought of as important may not be. Sometimes laboratory data, vital signs, and intake and outputs are ordered to be monitored more frequently than the status of the patient indicates. Frequent monitoring of these parameters may make no significant difference in patient outcomes. When nurses begin their shifts, they should question the activities that make no difference in outcomes (Hansten & Washburn, 1998). If a physician orders these activities, a nurse should work to get the order changed. If there is a nursing order that does not make a difference, the nurse should change it. Nurses should give priority to the activities that they know are going to make a difference in patient outcomes.

APPLICATION OF TIME MANAGEMENT STRATEGIES TO THE DELIVERY OF CARE

Once priorities are set, nurses know which are the most important activities to accomplish first. Time management strategies can be used in all areas of care delivery to maximize the effectiveness of the nurse's time and minimize lost time and efforts.

Estimate Activity Time Consumption

Nurses need to estimate how much time each activity will take, and plan accordingly. The previously discussed activity log may help estimate how much time many activities will take. Perhaps Mr. B tends to need more time for medication administration than other patients do, so the wise nurse will save Mr. B's medication administration until last. By estimating the time of activities, nurses can schedule the best time to perform activities. Nurses may notice when passing 6 P.M. medications that water pitchers are empty and juice cups dry. Scheduling the nursing assistant to fill water pitchers and pass refreshments prior to medication administration will be a prudent response to such an observation.

proficient

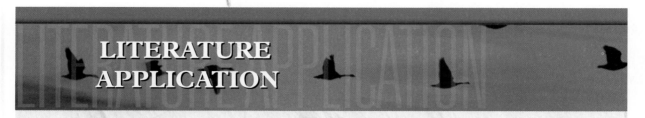

LITERATURE APPLICATION

Citation: Benner, P. (1984). *From novice to expert: Excellence and power in clinical nursing practice* (pp. 151–161). Menlo Park, CA: Addison-Wesley.

Discussion: Patricia Benner's work is a classic. It addresses issues faced by beginning nurses who struggle with time management issues and explains how expert nurses deal with time management using contingency planning.

Benner's study of how nurses cope with staffing shortages found that nurses who continuously respond to the challenge of each situation frequently end up feeling that they fail to meet their patients' needs in a timely manner. They lack two important sources of job satisfaction—interpersonal connection and a sense of accomplishment and competency that comes from meeting patients' needs when they need it. Nurses who work successfully and who consistently deal with a heavy workload develop a system of contingency planning that allows them to meet their patients' needs in a timely manner. This contingency planning includes rapidly assessing patient needs and setting and shifting priorities. They continuously evaluate routine standards and procedures. Standard priorities include attending to radically abnormal vital signs, signs and symptoms of respiratory or circulatory compromise, intravenous medications running dry, and intravenous medication administration. But even these priorities can be shifted when a patient on the unit actually is in a crisis. Expert nurses learn to anticipate and prevent periods of extreme workload within a shift.

Implications for Practice: This study emphasizes the importance of new nursing graduates learning to prioritize care and finding the human connection and a sense of competency and accomplishment in their work. Benner quotes a nurse who left nursing because of the lack of time to truly care for his patients. Often nurses leave practice before they develop time management skills that allow them to prioritize care and develop shift contingency plans.

Create an Environment Supportive of Time Management and Patient Care

Often in the frenzy of giving care, nurses forget the obvious. Where are the linens, supplies, medications, and so on located? Are there optimal locations? Is stocking things a priority in order to make them available? Do nurses really stop and think before going to a patient's room with pain medications or for a treatment?

How many trips does one treatment take? It should take only one trip, but if a nurse hurries in and leaves something at the nurse's station, then he will have to return to retrieve it. How many times do nurses count narcotics that have not been used in months? These are simple things that take time. The nurse should give consideration to all aspects of the unit environment and get together with coworkers to make a difference. Are specialty carts needed to become more efficient and effective?

Shift Report as a Tool for Effective and Efficient Care

Before a plan is made for the shift, the shift report at best can lead to a smooth and effective start to the shift. At worst it can leave the oncoming shift members with inadequate or old data on which to base their plan. There are several ways to give the end of shift report—a face-to-face meeting, audiotaping, and walking rounds (Table 18-1).

Whether the report is conducted face to face, via audiotape, or through walking rounds, informa- tion has to be transmitted to allow for the effective and efficient implementation of care. If the outgoing

TABLE 18-1   *Change of Shift Reports: Advantages and Disadvantages*

Method of Shift Report	Advantages	Disadvantages
Face-to-face report	• Nurses get clarification and can ask questions. • Nurse giving report has actual audience and tends to be less mechanical. • Nurses are more likely to give pertinent information than they would give to a tape recorder.	• It is time consuming. • It is easy to get sidetracked and gossip or discuss nonpatient-related business. • Both oncoming and departing nurses are in report. • Patients are not included in planning.
Audiotaped report	• Report is brief due to lack of interruptions by questions and comments. • Departing shift tapes report for oncoming shift prior to arrival of new shift workers. • Previous shift can provide care while oncoming shift gets report.	• Variables in the taping process such as the quality of tape and machine, the clarity and diction of the nurse who is recording, and the hearing of the oncoming shift can interfere with the communication. • It is difficult to get questions answered. The nurse must find the caregiver after report to ask questions. • Information is taped earlier in the shift and may no longer be accurate. • There is sometimes not enough information given due to the tendency of person talking into tape recorder to read from kardex instead of explaining about patient.
Walking rounds	• Provides the prior shift and incoming shift staff the opportunity to observe the patient while receiving report. Staff can address any assessment or treatment questions. • Information is accurate and timely. • Patient is included in the planning and evaluation of care. • Accountability of outgoing care provider is promoted. • Patient views the continuity of care. • Incoming shift makes initial nursing rounds. • Departing nurse can show assessment and treatment data directly to oncoming nurse.	• It is time consuming. • There is a lack of privacy in discussing patient information.

nurse fails to cover all pertinent points, the oncoming shift must ask for the appropriate information. See Table 18-2 for a tool for taking and giving reports.

Formulate and Write the Shift Action Plan

Having received pertinent information from the shift report, nurses can consider the big picture; decide on optimal and reasonable outcomes; and set priorities based on life-threatening conditions, safety considerations, and activities essential to safety and the plan of care. The nurse can then formulate a shift action plan, a written plan that sets the priorities for the shift and makes assignments to team members (Figure 18-3). Assignments should include specific reporting guidelines and deadlines for accomplishment of the tasks. Some nurses will prefer to take report directly on the shift action plan rather than using a separate tool or form. The shift action plan should also identify the time an intervention should be completed.

Make Patient Care Rounds

When nurses make patient care rounds, they perform rapid assessments of each patient. The information that is gathered on rounds may change the nurses' plans. They might get information that increases the need for patient monitoring. It is important to

TABLE 18-2	Tool for Taking/Giving Report
Patient data	Room number Name Sex Physician
Diagnoses	Primary and secondary Nursing and medical
Patient condition	Current vital signs Oxygen saturation Pain score Skin condition Ambulation Signs/symptoms of potential complications
New orders	New orders or changes in treatment/teaching plan
Expected shift outcomes	Priority outcomes for one or two nursing diagnoses Patient learning outcomes
Plans for discharge	Expected date of discharge Referrals needed Progress toward self-care and readiness for home
Care support	Availability of family or friends to assist in ADL/IADL (activities of daily living/instrumental activities of daily living)
Priority interventions	Interventions that must be done this shift

From *Nursing Documentation: Charting, Recording, and Reporting* (p. 217), by E. T. Eggland and D. S. Heinemann, 1994, Philadelphia: Lippincott. Adapted with permission.

Room Name	Patient Description	Special Needs	Assignment * All to report outcomes to Mary, RN at 8:30 PM -Report abnormals stat
1. Ms. JD	68 year old female, Post-op day 1 Post shoulder repair Confused Fall risk	Up in chair at 6 PM Vitals 4 PM and 8 PM Posey Check dressings 4 PM and 8 PM Check voiding 6 PM	Mary, RN
2. Mr. DB	55 year old male diabetic Post-op day 2 Right below the knee amputee Insulin sliding scale	Accuchek 4 PM and 9 PM Up in chair 6 PM Vitals 4 PM and 8 PM Pain medication as needed	Cindy, patient care technician
3. Ms. HM	85 year old female IV-5% Dextrose in water at 125 cc/hour Alert	Up in chair 6 PM Vitals 4 PM and 8 PM	Cindy, patient care technician

Figure 18-3 Shift Action Plan (Sample)

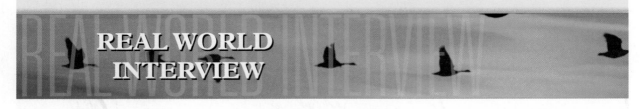

Ms. DuBose underwent elective surgery this summer. When asked about nurses and time management, she said, "The nurses that cared for me were always going back to the station to get something. It took three trips to get me my pain medication. If they had asked me when I requested the pain medication what I thought I needed, checked the order carefully, and brought the shot with an alcohol swab, they would have saved two extra trips and 30 minutes."

Ina DuBose
Patient

remember that plans are just that, plans, and have to be flexible based on ever-changing patient care needs. Times for treatments and medications may have to be changed. Often nurses believe that the times for administering medication are inflexible, yet physicians usually write medication orders as daily, twice a day, three times a day, or four times a day. These kinds of orders give nurses flexibility in administration times. Although unit policy dictates when these medicines are given, unit policy is under nursing control.

Evaluate Outcome Achievement

At the end of the shift, the nurse reexamines the shift action plan. Did he achieve the outcomes? If not, why? Were there staffing problems or patient crises? What was learned from this for future shifts?

If, at the end of a shift, the nurse did not accomplish the outcomes, she might review the shift activities to see what time wasters interfered with outcome achievement. Marquis and Huston (2000)

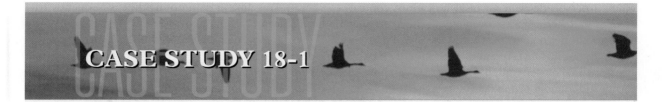

CASE STUDY 18-1

You are working the day shift on a medical-surgical unit. You are responsible for six patients with the assistance of a patient care technician. What are reasonable outcomes? Is a particular situation life threatening or potentially life threatening? Is an action essential for safety? Is an action essential to the nursing/medical plan?

1. Ms. JD is a 68-year-old who is post-op day 1 after a total shoulder replacement following a traumatic fall. She is confused and on multiple medications with a history of hypertension and multiple falls. She is anxious and frightened by the "visiting spirits."

2. Mr. DB is a 55-year-old with insulin-dependent diabetes mellitus, juvenile onset at age 12. He is post-op day 2 after a right-below-the-knee amputation. He complains of severe right leg pain. Mr. DB has a history of noncompliance with diet and sliding scale insulin administration.

3. Ms. HM is an 85-year-old patient transferred from a nursing home because of dehydration. She has vomiting and abdominal pain of unknown etiology. Intravenous hydration continues, and a workup is planned. Ms. HM is alert and oriented.

4. Mr. JK is a 35-year-old patient with a history of alcohol abuse admitted for severe abdominal pain. He is throwing up coffee-ground-like emesis.

5. Mr. AB is a 72-year-old patient who is status post cerebral vascular accident. He is to be transferred to rehabilitation. He needs his belongings gathered and a nursing summary written.

6. Ms. VG is an 82-year-old patient who is post-op 5 days after an open reduction of tibia-fibula fracture. She has a history of congestive heart failure, hypertension, and takes multiple medications. She is to be discharged to her daughter's care.

described time wasters as procrastination, inability to delegate, inability to say no, management by crisis, haste, and indecisiveness. Sullivan and Decker (2001) add interrupting telephone calls and socialization to the list. Reed and Pettigrew (1999) add complaining, perfectionism, and disorganization to the list of time wasters.

STRATEGIES TO ENHANCE PERSONAL PRODUCTIVITY

Time management applies not only to work but also to the nurse's personal life. Too often nurses feel that they have no personal life because of rotating shifts, weekend work, and stressful work experiences.

Proper time management will allow nurses to take control of both their work life and their personal life. Use a variation of the nursing activity log in Figure 18-2 to review how you spend your personal time. It will help to determine one's most energetic time of day. Activities that take focus and creativity should be scheduled at high-energy times and dull, repetitive tasks at low-energy times. Scheduling time for proper rest, exercise, and nutrition allows for quality time.

Create More Personal Time

There are three major ways to create time. One is to delegate work to others or hire someone else to do work. Another is to eliminate chores or tasks that add no value. The last way is to get up earlier in the day.

When a person delegates a task, he cannot control when and how the task is completed. Initially, it may take more time to get others to do the chore than to just do it, but this investment of time should save the investor time and energy in the future. If a chore is boring and mundane, it makes more sense to work an hour more at a job one enjoys in order to pay for someone else to do unrewarding, boring work.

Getting up 1 hour earlier in the day for a year can free up 365 hours, or approximately weeks a year, extra time that can be used to enrich life. After several days of rising an hour earlier, an individual may feel tired and respond to the fatigue by going to bed a little earlier (Mind Tools, n.d.-a). This may be a good strategy for many people, especially those who are not productive in the evening and spend time doing activities that are minimally rewarding such as watching television. If a person does not try to get to bed earlier, though, and the end result of getting up early is fatigue, the strategy is not beneficial.

Use Downtime

During any day there is time available that is seldom used, often referred to as downtime. When waiting at appointments, in lines, or for others, people often have time available to use. Wait time can sometimes be avoided by calling ahead to verify appointments and arriving no more than five minutes early. During unavoidable waits, the time can be put to good use by having reading and writing materials handy.

Traveling or commuting time is frequently frittered away. Listening to books on tapes is a good way to catch up on reading. Many libraries have a collection of books on tape. If privacy is not an issue, phone calls can be initiated and returned during commutes. But saving phone calls to make while driving can be a dangerous practice unless the car is equipped with a hands-free phone.

Sometimes it is important just to sit back and enjoy the scenery or the company. Time management principles aim at creating more enjoyable time, not filling every moment with chores.

Control Unwanted Distractions

Personal life is not immune from distractions that get in the way of accomplishing personal goals. These may include such distractions as visitors, unplanned phone calls, low priority tasks, and requests for assistance. Refer to Table 18-3.

Find Personal Time for Lifelong Learning

Finding time for lifelong learning is a struggle for recent graduates and even more-seasoned nurses.

There are ways to achieve one's dreams, work, and have a personal life. Flaherty (1998) offers tips for balancing school, family, and work in Table 18-4.

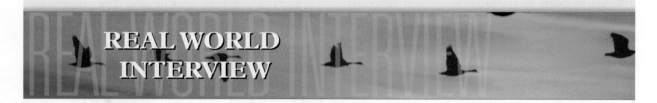

REAL WORLD INTERVIEW

Cherie, a new graduate, states that working 40 hours a week seems like a lot. "I thought I was busy in school, but I seem to have less time now that I work full time. I am struggling to prioritize my family and work. I want to find time to go to graduate school, and I don't know how I can fit it in."

Cherie McCann, RN
New Graduate

TABLE 18-3 Strategies for Avoiding Personal Time Distractions

Distraction	Strategies
Casual visitors	Make your environment less inviting. Remain standing. Remove your visitor chair. Keep a pen in your hand.
Unplanned phone calls	Use an answering machine or voice mail. Consider a humorous message. Set a time to return calls.
Unwanted/ low-priority jobs	Say no to jobs that have little value or in which you have little interest. Leave low-priority tasks undone. If an unwanted job must be done, pay or ask for assistance.
Requests for assistance	Encourage others to be more independent. Give them encouragement, but send them back to complete the job. Decisions to help should be conscious decisions, not drop-in distractions.

TABLE 18-4 Maintaining Balance in Life When Returning to School

1. Let your employer know that you are interested in returning to school. Most employers are supportive of additional education and will be flexible with your schedule. But they will continue to expect a competent, dedicated employee.

2. Develop computer skills. By using a computer, you can e-mail professors and classmates at any time. You can do on-line research. You can easily incorporate constructive criticisms into papers and build on previous work. Technology is the working student's friend.

3. Discover a flexible, educational program. Many programs offer several classes in a row on a single day, weekend and night classes, or weeklong immersion classes. Some programs offer distance learning opportunities.

4. Do not be surprised by the demands of school. Courses will be difficult and demanding of time. Remember that you have faced difficult demands and challenges before. Use the same techniques that helped you in the past.

5. Solicit support from family and friends. They can offer emotional support as well as child care.

6. Use all available resources at the school and at work. Develop mentors and role models. Establish relationships with faculty. Discover and use academic support services such as writing centers and tutors. Read syllabi and course instructions carefully.

7. Focus on the outcome. Keep the end in sight and do not give up. Take it one course at a time. Reward yourself along the way. When a course is completed, celebrate.

(continues)

Table 18-4 *(continued)*

8. Be careful of the sacrifices. You may replace some hobbies with school. But save some time for the things that are really meaningful to you and your family.

9. Manage time. Ten minutes spent on planning saves time and energy later. Keep your sense of humor.

10. Take care of yourself and your responsibilities. Set aside a day to take care of personal chores and errands.

11. If you need a break, take one. Take time to reflect on what you are accomplishing. If you are feeling overwhelmed, take only one course or take a semester off.

12. Study on the run. Taping lectures and listening to them as you commute is a great way to study on the run.

Adapted from "The Juggling Act: 10 Tips for Balancing Work, School, and Family," by M. Flaherty, *Nurseweek*, retrieved July 15, 2000, from http://www.nurseweek.com/features/98-5/juggle.html.

Returning to school is certainly a challenge, but with time management skills the return to school can result in the accomplishment of personal outcomes, a degree, and new knowledge.

KEY CONCEPTS

- General time management strategies include having an outcomes orientation, analyzing time cost and use, focusing on priorities, and visualizing the big picture.
- Shift planning begins with developing reasonable outcomes.
- Priority setting takes into account what is life threatening or potentially life threatening, what is essential to safety, and what is essential to the nursing and medical plan.
- Planning effective time use includes time estimates and environmental considerations that culminate in a shift action plan that is based on priorities.
- The shift action plan assigns activities aimed at outcome achievement within a time frame.
- There are three alternatives for shift reports: face-to-face meetings, audiotaped reports, and walking rounds.
- Implementing the shift action plan requires patient rounds and setting the times for monitoring and treatments.
- The shift action plan is evaluated at the end of the shift by determining whether optimal or reasonable outcomes have been achieved.
- Time wasters that might interfere with outcome achievement include procrastination, inability to delegate, inability to say no, management by crisis, haste, indecisiveness, interruptions, socialization, complaining, perfectionism, and disorganization.
- Time management applies to one's personal life as well as one's job.
- Quality time can be achieved by analyzing time use and energy patterns.
- Delegating and getting up 1 hour earlier can create time for individuals.
- Efficient use can be made of travel and waiting time.
- Distractions can be controlled by making your environment less inviting, by using voice mail or an answering machine, by saying no, and by encouraging others to be independent.
- It is possible to balance work, family, and school.

KEY TERMS

activity log	reasonable outcomes
optimal outcomes	shift action plan
Pareto principle	time management

REVIEW QUESTIONS

1. All of the following are general time management techniques EXCEPT
   A. allowing distractions.
   B. outcomes orientation.
   C. time analysis.
   D. focus on priorities.

2. Which of the following are strategies to plan effective time use during an 8-hour shift?
   A. Using time wasters and distractions
   B. Estimating the time of activities and developing the shift action plan
   C. Setting priorities, giving report, and evaluating outcomes
   D. Walking rounds, patient care rounds, and report

3. Today you get out of patient report late, your nursing assistant has not arrived, one of your patients is being transferred to the intensive care unit, and you are getting an admission into the bed that your transfer patient is vacating. What outcomes will you work toward for the shift?
   A. None. The situation is hopeless.
   B. Optimal outcomes. There is never an excuse not to do your best.
   C. Minimal outcomes. We can accomplish no more.
   D. Realistic outcomes. We can be safe and effective.

4. Which of the following is the most efficient and effective way to give the shift report?
   A. Audiotaped report
   B. Walking rounds
   C. Face-to-face meeting
   D. Any of the above

5. Personal productivity can be enhanced by
   A. analyzing time, getting up an hour early, delegating unwanted tasks.
   B. getting up an hour early, answering your phone, and inviting a friend in to talk.
   C. analyzing use of time, getting up early, waiting patiently.
   D. avoiding working and going to school at the same time.

REVIEW ACTIVITIES

1. For the next 3 days, complete an activity log for both your personal time and your work time. On what activities are you spending the majority of time? When is your energy level the highest? Is your energy level related to food intake?

2. What are your biggest time wasters?

3. What are your personal desired outcomes?

4. What are your distractions from outcome achievement? Develop a plan to minimize your distractions.

5. Use Table 18-2 or Figure 18-3 to organize your report.

EXPLORING THE WEB

- If you would like to find a system for managing your time, the following web sites offer electronic organizers (e.g., Casio electronic organizer, Sharp electronic organizer, Palm Pilot electronic organizer):
  http://www.casio.com
  http:// www.sharp-usa.com
  http://www.palm.com

- If you prefer a less technological time management system, the following web sites offer non-electronic organizers and systems for time management (e.g., Day-Timer, Covey, Franklin):
  http://www.daytimer.com
  http://www.covey.com
  http://www.franklin.com

- Want a free on-line calendar that you can access from anywhere?
  http://calendar.yahoo.com

- Look at all the hints and free tools on time management at the Mind Tools web site. Can you put any of the ideas to use? *http://www.mindtools.com/page5.html*

- If you find time management an impossible challenge, you can find professional assistance at the Professional Organizers web site. *http://www.organizerswebring.com/*

- Search this web site for tips on time management at work. *http://oxygen.com/money/index.html*

- What questions do you have on time management and productivity? You can find your answers at *http://www.infoworth.com/time.htm*

- Check out this University of Michigan site for time management tips as part of its stress management strategies. *http://www.umich.edu/~fasap/stresstips/contents.html*

- Take a look at the handy hints at this University of Nebraska site. Can you put any of these to use? *http://www.ianr.unl.edu/pubs/homemgt/nf172.htm*

REFERENCES

Benner, P. (1984). *From novice to expert: Excellence and power in clinical nursing practice.* Menlo Park, CA: Addison-Wesley.

Burke, T. A., McKee, J. R., Wilson, H. C., Donahue, R. M., Batenhorst, A. S., & Pathak, D. S. (2000). A comparison of time-and-motion and self-reporting methods of work measurement. *Journal of Nursing Administration 30*(3), 118–125.

Covey, S. R., Merrill, A. R., & Merrill, R. R. (1994). *First things first: To love, to learn, to leave a legacy.* New York: Simon & Schuster.

Eggland, E. T. & Heinemann, D. S. (1994). *Nursing documentation: Charting, recording, and reporting.* Philadelphia: Lippincott.

Flaherty, M. (1998). The juggling act: 10 tips for balancing work, school, and family. *Nurseweek.* Retrieved July 15, 2000, from http://www.nurseweek.com/features/98-5/juggle.html

Fryxell, D. A. (1997). The 80% solution. *Writer's Digest, 77*(5), 57.

Graham, A. (1998). The vital few, the trivial many. *Internal Auditor, 55*(6), 6.

Grohar-Murray, M. E. & DiCroce, H. R. (1997). Managing Resources. In M. E. Grohar-Murray (ed.), *Leadership and management in nursing* (2nd ed., pp. 291–315). Norwalk, CT: Appleton & Lange.

Hansten, R. I. & Washburn, M. J. (1998). *Clinical delegation skills: A handbook for professional practice.* Gaithersburg, MD: Aspen.

Koch, R. (1999). *The 80/20 principle: The secret to success by achieving more with less.* New York: Doubleday.

Marquis, B. L., & Huston, C. J. (2000). *Leadership roles and management functions in nursing: Theory and application* (3rd ed.). Philadelphia: Lippincott.

Mind Tools (n.d.-a). Creating extra hours—get up early! Retrieved September 5, 2000, from http://www.mindtools.com/tmgetup.html

Mind Tools (n.d.-b). How to achieve more with your time. Retrieved September 5, 2000, from http://www.mindtools.com/tmintro.html

Prescott, P. A., Phillips, C. Y., Ryan, J. W., & Thompson, K. O. (1991). Changing how nurses spend their time. *Image: Journal of Nursing Scholarship, 23*(1), 23–28.

Reed, C. R. & Pettigrew, A. C. (1999). Self management: Stress and time. In P. S. Yoder-Wise (Ed.), *Leading and managing in nursing* (2nd ed., pp. 185–204). St. Louis, MO: Mosby.

Scharf, L. (1997). Revising nursing documentation to meet patient outcomes. *Nursing Management, 28*(4), 38–39.

Sullivan, E. J., & Decker, P. J. (2001). *Effective leadership and management in nursing* (5th ed.) Menlo Park, CA: Addison-Wesley.

Tappen, R. M. (2001). *Nursing leadership and management: Concepts and practice.* (4th ed.) Philadelphia: F. A. Davis.

Upenieks, V. B. (1998). Work sampling: Assessing nursing efficiency. *Nursing Management, 49*(4), 27–29.

Urden, L., & Roode, J. (1997). Work sampling: A decision-making tool for determining resources and work redesign. *Journal of Nursing Administration, 27*(9), 34–41.

SUGGESTED READINGS

Axelrod, A., Holtje, J., & Holtje, J. (1997). *201 ways to manage your time better.* New York: McGraw-Hill.

Bly, R. W. (1999). *101 ways to make every second count: Time management tips and techniques for more success with less stress.* New York: Career Press.

Booher, D. (1999). Get a life by clearing the clutter. *Family Practice Management, 6*(5), 60.

Brider, P. (1992). The move to patient-focused care. *American Journal of Nursing, 92*(9), 27–33.

Brink, P. J. (2000). I'm too busy. *Western Journal of Nursing Research, 22*(4), 383.

Cericola, S. A. (2000). Time/stress management techniques. *Plastic Surgical Nursing, 20*(1), 48–49.

Dawes, B. S. (1999). Perspectives on priorities, time management, and patient care. *AORN Journal, 70*(3), 374–377.

Folan, D. (1999). *Time management, world of Irish nursing by Irish Nurses Organization.* Retrieved September 10, 2000, from http://www.ino.ie/news_detail.php3?nNewsld=1260&nCatld=215

Hemphill, B. (2000). 10 tips to beat post-travel clutter. *Nursing Management, 31*(6). 57.

Perlow, L.A. (1998). Finding time, stopping the frenzy. *Business and Health, 16*(8), 31–35.

Plasker, E. (2000). Brilliant time management strategies. *Chiropractic Journal, 14*(9), 45.

Pratt, J. (2000). Time management: The hurrier I go, the behinder I get. *Home Health Care Management and Practice, 12*(4), 61.

Shumaker, R. P (1998). A time for reflection. *AORN Journal, 68*(6), 940–942.

Smith, H. W. (1995). *The 10 natural laws of successful time and life management: Proven strategies for increased productivity and inner peace.* New York: Warner Books.

Vaccaro, P. J. (1999). Kick the procrastination habit. *Family Practice Management, 6*(7), 60.

Vaccaro, P. J. (1999). Tips for life balance and time management. *Family Practice Management, 6*(3), 66.

Watkins, D. (1999). Are you a time-management junkie? *Information Outlook, 3*(1), 34–35.

CHAPTER 19

If you always do what you've always done, you will always get what you've always gotten.

(Jay Katz, 1992)

Managing Outcomes Using an Organizational Quality Improvement Model

Mary McLaughlin, RN, MBA
Karen Houston, RN, MS

OBJECTIVES

Upon completion of this chapter, the reader should be able to:

1. Articulate major principles of quality and performance improvement (PI), including customer identification; the need for participation at all levels; and a focus on improving the process, not criticizing individual performance.

2. Describe how performance improvement affects the patient and the organization.

3. Identify how data are utilized for PI (time series data, Pareto charts).

4. Describe the difference between risk management and PI.

5. Describe how the principles of PI are implemented in the organization.

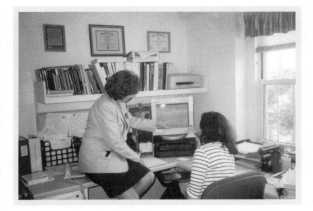

University HealthSystem Consortium (UHC), a group of about 110 academic health science centers, did a benchmark study on total hip arthroplasty. Albany Medical Center, an organization that participated in that study, noted that compared to other organizations, its average length of stay (LOS) was long (the Albany Medical Center LOS was 7.07 days; the average LOS for UHC was 5.78 days). It also noticed that the percentage of patients that used a pneumatic compression device (a device to decrease the postoperative rate of deep vein thrombosis) was 85% for UHC but only 53% for Albany Medical Center. The percentage use of indwelling catheters in total hip arthroplasty patients at Albany Medical Center (indwelling catheters are associated with an increase in postoperative urinary tract infections, or UTIs) was 53%. Although this catheter use was lower than the UHC average, the team believed it could decrease the rate further. Albany Medical Center also delivered an average of three physical therapy (PT) visits postoperatively per patient, whereas UHC's average was five visits per patient. There was also an increased cost at Albany Medical Center versus the average cost at UHC.

Albany Medical Center decided to assign an interdisciplinary team the responsibility of identifying opportunities for improvement. The team began by developing a clinical pathway based on the most recent research in this area. Using data and research, the team looked for ways to improve the patient care process. The team incorporated the best practices that they found: this meant designing into the clinical pathway increased use of the pneumatic compression device, more physical therapy, earlier catheter removal, and an earlier discharge date. To prepare the patient properly for the earlier discharge, the team added preoperative home visits to the clinical pathway. The Visiting Nurses Association would make the home visit and then make a recommendation for dis-

charge planning prior to the patient's admission. This process expedited initiation of referrals to an acute rehabilitation facility or home care following discharge, if needed. If the family home had to be rearranged to accommodate limited ambulation or stair use, these recommendations were made early in an effort to allow the family to prepare ahead of time.

The higher costs at Albany Medical Center seemed to be related to the number of prosthetic vendors. When fewer vendors are used, the volume with each vendor is higher, allowing more competitive price negotiation among vendors. The organization worked with the surgeons on the team to decrease the number of vendors to a ratio of 0.25 vendors to surgeons.

Continuous quality improvement has been shown to be a powerful tool to help make health care organizations more effective. Plsek (1993) notes that without strong, effective leadership and an infrastructure to support quality management, improvements may or may not happen, and they may quickly dissipate because of neglect and lack of integration with other activities within the organization. The improvement philosophies of quality experts such as Deming (1986) and Crosby (1989) also emphasize the commitment of management.

Quality improvement is described as both a science and an art. The science of improvement is the development of new ideas, the testing of those ideas, and the implementation of change. As Langley, Nolan, Norman, Provost, and Nolan (1996) described, W. Edwards Deming has provided an important contribution to the science of improvement. Deming's components of appreciating a system, understanding variation, and applying knowledge and psychology are fundamental improvement principles. Quality improvement is also described as an art that taps into creative, "out of the box" ideas. It is about systematically testing new ideas to improve customer care. Health care customers are patients, families, staff, and so forth. If the change is planned, measured, and does not negatively affect quality of customer care, there are limitless boundaries to what can be achieved.

Adapting the concepts of science and art in improving health care can create an enthusiasm for change and a passion for results. This chapter will discuss and provide examples of the application and implementation of quality improvement principles in a health care setting.

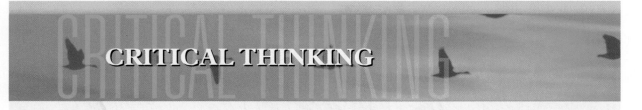

CRITICAL THINKING

Refer back to the chapter Opening Scenario. If you were a staff nurse on the orthopedic unit at Albany Medical Center, what could you do to improve the quality of care? How would you encourage the decreased use of indwelling catheters? How would you encourage the use of a pneumatic compression device?

How could you bring your ideas to other staff members without making them feel that the quality of their care was being criticized? For example, many staff members feel that catheter use is better for the patient's skin and reduces the need for assistance in ambulating the patient to the bathroom. You know that research shows indwelling catheters and decreased ambulation increase risk of complications. How do you deal with these competing positions?

What measures would you use to ensure that while you were improving some aspects of care, you were not decreasing other critical outcome measures? For example, as you decrease catheter use, what is happening to UTI and fall rates?

HISTORY OF QUALITY ASSURANCE

Consider Berwick and Plsek's red bead example (1992):

In a group of beads in a bag, there are 90 blue beads and 10 red beads. There are four workers whose job it is to take blue beads out of a bag. They cannot see what color bead they are taking. The supervisor watches to see how many red beads are pulled out of the bag. The first day, worker A has 1 red bead, worker B has 4 red beads, worker C has 3 red beads, and worker D has 2 red beads. The supervisor states that worker A has done a great job and worker B has done a terrible job. He tells them they have to improve. The beads go back in the bag and they start over the next day. This day, worker A has 4 red beads, worker B has 0 red beads, worker C has 2 red beads, and worker D has 4 red beads. The supervisor praises worker B for the improvement and yells at workers A and D for not doing a good job. The truth is these workers do not have any ability to change the number of red beads that they pull out of the bag.

This example demonstrates random variation. Using inspection in systems to reward or punish ran-

dom variation results in tampering with the system rather than quality improvement. Instead of improving the process, the tampering encourages staff to look for someone to blame rather than to change the process to improve outcomes. So the question is, how much variability do we expect? This can be calculated on a time series chart and will be discussed in more detail later in the chapter.

Quality assurance (QA) emerged in health care in the 1950s, about the same time as hospital-accrediting organizations were founded (AMC Q Series, 1998). QA began as an inspection approach to ensure that health care institutions—mainly hospitals—maintained minimum standards of care. The use of QA grew over time, as did federal and state regulatory controls. QA departments became the organizational mechanism for measuring performance against standards and reporting incidents and errors, such as mortality and morbidity rates. This approach was reactive and fixed the errors after a problem was noted. QA's methods consisted primarily of chart audits of various patient diagnoses and procedures. The method was thought to be punitive, with its emphasis on "doing it right," and did little to sustain change or proactively identify problems before they occurred. It did, however, accomplish the task of monitoring minimum standards of performance.

Total Quality Management

Total quality management (TQM), also referred to as quality improvement (QI) and **performance improvement** (PI), began in the manufacturing industry with W. Edwards Deming and Joseph Juran in the 1950s. TQM, QI, and PI are terms that are frequently interchanged. For the purposes of this chapter, **quality improvement** (QI) will be referred to as a systematic process to improve outcomes based on customers' needs. This proactive approach emphasizes "doing the right thing" for customers, and the end result of this method is to satisfy customers. This approach was integrated into the health care industry in the 1980s when cost and quality of care pressures from health maintenance organizations and other third-party payers increased along with competition for patients (AMC Q Series, 1998). Movement into QI is thought to be more an overall management approach than a single program. Integrating concepts of quality into daily organizational operations is key to successful outcomes. Table 19-1 notes the difference in focus between QA and QI.

GENERAL PRINCIPLES OF QUALITY IMPROVEMENT

Quality improvement is a structured system for creating organization-wide participation and partnership in planning and implementing continuous improvement methods to understand and meet or exceed customer needs and expectations. Quality principles include the following:

1. The priority is to benefit patients and all other internal and external customers.
2. Quality is achieved through the participation of everyone in the organization.
3. Improvement opportunities are developed by focusing on the work process.
4. Decisions to change or improve a system or process are made based on data.
5. Improvement of the quality of service is a continuous process.

Early QA literature focused on fixing problems, "doing it right," and having zero defects. Over time, a gap was found between theory and practice.

TABLE 19-1	Difference in Focus between Quality Assurance and Quality Improvement

Focus of Quality Assurance (doing it right)

1. Assessing or measuring performance
2. Determining whether performance conforms to standards
3. Improving performance when standards are not met

Focus of Quality Improvement (doing the right thing)

1. Meeting the needs of the customer
2. Building quality performance into the work process
3. Assessing the work process to identify opportunities for improved performance
4. Employing a scientific approach to assessment and problem solving
5. Improving performance continuously as a management strategy, not just when standards are not met

It was determined that quality is not about being perfect. First, it is about being better, doing things right the first time, and being better than the competition. This increases an organization's chances of survival during highly turbulent and competitive times. Second, quality is about health care professionals seeing themselves as having customers. The notion of "customer" requires major shifts in mind-set for the health care professional. The term *customer* is frequently used in business, and calling a patient a "customer" was initially thought to undermine the professional care provided to patients. Designing health care processes from the customer's point of view versus the professional's point of view is a challenge and requires changes in thinking and redesign of health care processes. Health care involves work processes in which one step leads to the next step. Improving these steps in the work process is an important part of improving care and customer satisfaction. Customer satisfaction is rooted in the way health professionals treat their patients/customers and in the quality of their outcomes. Having the goal of astounding patients with quality in every interaction is key to achieving satisfaction and loyalty. Third, quality directs health professionals to give their customers more than the basics so that customers will recommend and demand these services. This is achieved by proactively seizing opportunities to perform better, driving for quality consistently and continuously, and not waiting for a problem to be pointed out or for pressure from a competitor to improve. Improvements are sustained over time when interdisciplinary teams collaborate and decisions about change are supported by data.

The primary benefits of adopting quality concepts and principles include discovering performance issues more quickly and efficiently by looking at every problem as an opportunity for improvement; involvement of staff in how the work is designed and carried out to improve staff satisfaction; and empowering staff to identify and implement change. Increasing the customer's perception that you care by designing health care work processes to meet the customer's needs, rather than the health care provider's, and decreasing unnecessary costs from waste and rework, lost business, and not meeting regulations are also quality concepts. These quality concepts should be emphasized until they become work habits and part of an organization's daily operations.

Customers in Health Care

A customer is anyone who receives the output of your efforts. There are internal and external customers. An internal customer is anyone who works within the organization and receives the output of another employee. Internal customers include health care staff such as physicians, nurses, pharmacists, physical therapists, respiratory therapists, occupational therapists, pastoral caregivers, and so on. An external customer is anyone who is outside the organization and receives the output of the organization. The patients are external customers, but they are not the only external customers. Other external customers include private physicians, insurance payers, regulators such as the Department of Health, the Joint Commission on Accreditation of Healthcare Organizations (JCAHO), and the community you serve.

Participation of Everyone in the Organization

QI is achieved through the participation of everyone in the organization at all levels. A participation and empowerment initiative must be built by first offering employees the opportunity for appropriate involvement. An organization that encourages empowerment promotes a culture of employee ownership. In this type of culture, employees do the following:

- Take responsibility for the success or failure of an organization
- Take an active part in developing new ways of doing business and securing new customers
- Trust that their efforts are valued

A new staff member can participate in the design and improvement of daily work practices and processes on an individual, unit, or organizational level. For example, as an individual, a nurse could change the organization of her day to spend more time with patients' families. On a unit level, a nurse could work with others on the unit to change the way patient report is given to be more time efficient. On an organizational level, a nurse could suggest that the process for notifying pharmacy about a missing medication could be improved. The nurse could participate on a team to find a solution.

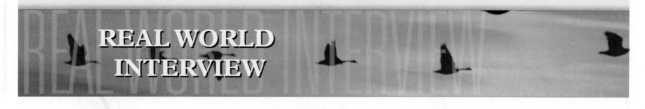

In my area of work, I feel empowered because of my expertise in my field. My decisions are made based on clinically relevant data. I believe it is important to gain support from key players who have to deal with the implementation of any change. If it relates to care of patients or improvement in documentation, I meet with the appropriate team members.

Sue Ciarmello RN
Quality Specialist

All members of the staff are encouraged to participate in quality improvement processes. These include the physician, registered nurse, physical therapist, occupational therapist, speech therapist, pharmacist, case management worker, social worker, medical technologists, and any member of the health care team who cares for the patient or contributes to the care of the patient. The goal of QI efforts, as well as the process being worked on, determines who participates on the team. For example, if you were trying to decrease the time a patient waits outside the radiology suite for a test, you would need to include the patient transportation staff, unit clerks, unit registered nurses, and radiology staff in your QI efforts. If you were trying to ensure that patients with congestive heart failure are discharged understanding the importance of weighing themselves daily, you would need the cardiac unit's registered nurse, clinical dietician, visiting nurses association staff, primary care physician, cardiologist, pharmacist, and a patient and the patient's family. The key in determining who participates is including the point-of-service staff: the workers on the front line who do the direct care involved in the work process you are trying to change. They are the people who have the most knowledge of the work process so they can look for potential areas of improvement. There should be a clearly identified way for staff to suggest improvement opportunities that they see in their day-to-day work. For example, an x-ray technologist may note steps in the process of scheduling and transporting patients that create a long wait time for x-ray testing. If a mechanism for suggesting improvement exists in the radiology

department, the technologist could suggest and test ideas for change.

Focus on Improvement of the Health Care Work Process

Improvement opportunities are focused on the process of work that the health care team delivers. A **process** is a set of causes and conditions that repeatedly come together in a series of steps to transfer inputs into outcomes (Langley et al., 1996). All work processes have inputs, steps, and outputs. An example of a work process is a patient receiving a chest x-ray. All the steps of the chest x-ray process can be measured. These steps are then reviewed, applying evidence-based principles, as appropriate to improve patient care. Steps may be eliminated or changed and then standardized so that all staff use the improved work process.

Improvement of the System

A **system** is an interdependent group of items, people, or processes with a common purpose (Langley et al., 1996). In a system, the processes as well as the relationships among the processes lead to the outcome. You can improve the outcome by examining these processes and relationships. In a system, every step of a process affects the following step. For example, if the x-ray staff members place the patient who has had a chest x-ray in the hall and call transportation to take the patient back to his room but do not

CRITICAL THINKING

In the orthopedic scenario at the start of this chapter, when the original length of stay data by nursing unit was examined, one unit had a much shorter length of stay than the other. At first there was discussion about this variance and the idea emerged of just going to the floor with the longer length of stay and fixing things there. The group members decided that rather than approach the task from this limited perspective, they would study the process as a whole and determine whether there were steps they could take to improve the process before going after the staff on the floor with the longer length of stay. Several excellent opportunities for improvement were identified, as noted previously—for example, preoperative home evaluation, increased physical therapy involvement, and shorter Foley catheter use. All these areas contributed to the process improvement, and the outcome was that both units ended up reducing their lengths of stay. These opportunities would have been lost had the group members used the data only to say that one unit was doing a bad job. They needed to review the process as a whole to improve the length of stay on both units.

How could you improve care in a patient care unit that you are familiar with? What patient care process could be improved? Who would you ask to work on the improvements with you?

consider the transportation process, they may decrease the total time a patient is in radiology but increase the patient's time in the hall waiting for transportation. You cannot improve care unless you review all the steps in the system's process.

A Continuous Process

Improvement of quality of service is a continuous process. Walter Shewhart, the director of Bell Laboratories in the mid-1920s, is credited for the concept of the cycle of continuous improvement. This concept suggests that products or services are designed and made based on knowledge about the customer. Those products or services are marketed to and judged by the customer. As the customer makes judgments, changes are made to improve the product or service (Al-Assaf & Schmele, 1997). Hence, the process of QI is continuous, because it is linked to changing customer needs and judgments.

Improvement Based on Data

Decisions to change or improve a system or process are made based on data. When someone says, "The

patients are waiting too long to return from radiology," it is time to look at the data. Review the waiting time data to see whether waiting times are increasing. The data clarify these issues. Using data correctly is important. Data should be used for learning, not for judging. It is critical to look at work processes rather than people for improvement opportunities. In the radiology example, if we jumped to the conclusion that someone was not doing his job correctly, we might criticize the transportation staff person who returned the patient from radiology. This would not foster improvement ideas. By not analyzing the process (patient has chest x-ray, is put in hall, clerk at desk calls transportation, transportation clerk pages transportation aide, and so on) and the relationships among the processes (waiting times between calls, transportation phone process, page system, and so on), we could miss finding where the real improvement opportunity lies. Perhaps it has nothing to do with the transportation person who returned the patient to the room. It may be that the actual root cause is a long delay in the paging system. Reviewing the wait time data is an example of examining the process, not the people carrying out the process.

IMPLICATIONS FOR PATIENT CARE

The implications of quality improvement for patient care can be measured by the overall value of care. Value is a function of both quality outcomes and cost. Outcomes can be a patient's clinical or functional outcomes. For example, did the patient live, can the patient go back to work? Outcomes can also be measured by patient satisfaction. For example, would the patient recommend this health care facility to someone else? Cost is the cost of both direct and indirect patient care needs. Direct cost is the cost of the care of the patient: for example, cost of medications, operating room equipment, and direct patient caregiver salaries. Indirect costs are the costs of nondirect care activities, including electricity and salaries of nondirect patient caregivers such as secretaries or human resource staff.

$$\text{Value} = \frac{\text{Quality of outcomes}}{\text{Cost}}$$

In most QI efforts, as quality is improved by standardizing care delivery processes and applying evidence-based principles, the cost of care decreases. The example in the opening scenario illustrated this. The length of stay decreased as the team found ways to standardize care and evaluate the patient prior to admission in order to plan for discharge and prepare the family. A decrease in length of stay generally translates into a decrease in costs.

METHODOLOGIES FOR QUALITY IMPROVEMENT

There are several models that outline methodologies for quality improvement. Two are reviewed here: the Plan Do Check Act (PDCA) Cycle and the FOCUS methodology. Improvement comes from the application of knowledge (Langley et al., 1996). Thus, any approach to improvement must be based on building and applying knowledge.

The Plan Do Check Act Cycle

The PDCA Cycle starts with the following three questions:

1. What are we trying to accomplish?
2. How will we know that a change is an improvement?
3. What changes can we make that will result in improvement?

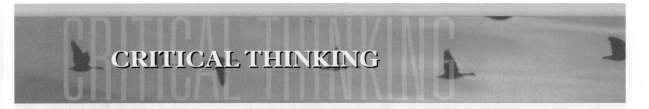

CRITICAL THINKING

The third-party payer system in the United States is complex and constantly changing. Third-party payers are the organizations that pay patients' hospital bills. They include government payers, such as Medicaid and Medicare and private payers such as health insurance companies. For example, to some payers, decreasing lengths of stay may mean decreasing payments. Other payers will pay for a patient admission using a **diagnosis-related group** (DRG) payment schedule with preset fees, regardless of the length of stay. DRG payment schedules are based on groups of patients that are medically related with respect to diagnosis, presence of a surgical procedure, age, and presence or absence of comorbidities or complications. So under this type of payment, if the patient is discharged in a short time, generally the facility will make money. If patients stay a long time, hospitals will lose money.

What do you think of these types of cost reimbursement? What can you do to keep health care costs down for your patient?

As these questions are being answered, testing needs to be done to evaluate any proposed changes. Testing is done to evaluate the effect of a proposed change and to learn about different alternatives (Figure 19-1). The goal is to increase the ability to predict the effect that one or more changes would have if they were implemented (Langley et al., 1996). The plan for testing should cover who will do what, when they will do it, and where they will do it. Using the PDCA Cycle encourages ongoing quality improvement.

The FOCUS Methodology

The FOCUS methodology describes in a stepwise process how to move through the improvement process (Figure 19-2).

F: Focus on an improvement idea. This step asks the question, "What is the problem?" During this phase, an improvement opportunity is articulated and data are obtained to support the hypothesis that an opportunity for improvement exists.

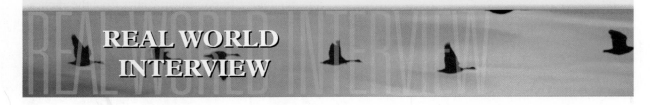

REAL WORLD INTERVIEW

In my job, I review a patient's chart and compare it to evidence-based guidelines to see if the patient's health care is being performed in the appropriate setting. I will review if the patient's care is medically necessary. If it is not, I assist the hospital case managers or physicians to move the patient to the appropriate level of care. For example, IV antibiotics can sometimes be administered at home or in another facility. When the situation at home is such that the family cannot manage it, the patient could move to a subacute facility, if available, or the patient could stay in the hospital with the hospital paid at a different rate. Documentation is critical in this type of review. An accurate clinical picture of the patient needs to be reflected in the documentation.

Marguerite Montyako, RN
Case Manager, Albany Medical Center

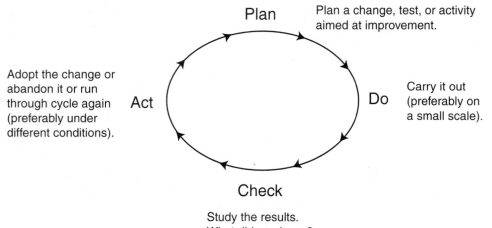

Figure 19-1 PDCA Cycle (Courtesy of Albany Medical Center, Albany, NY)

O: Organize a team that knows the process. This means identifying a group of staff members who are direct participants in the process to be examined—the point-of-service staff. A team leader is identified who will appoint team members.

C: Clarify what is happening in the current process. A flow diagram (see Figure 19-3) is very helpful for this. A detailed flowchart can be analyzed in two ways to uncover possible problems—at a macro level and at the micro level.

At the macro level, scan the flowchart for any indication that the process is broken. Red flags include the following:

- Many steps that represent quality checks or inspections for errors. When you notice too many boxes in your flow diagram describing similar steps, this could indicate rework or lack of clarity in roles.
- Areas in the process that are not well understood or cannot be defined. If the process cannot be defined well, you can be certain it is not being performed efficiently, with maximized outcomes.
- Many wait times between processes. Wait times should always be minimized to improve efficiency of the process.

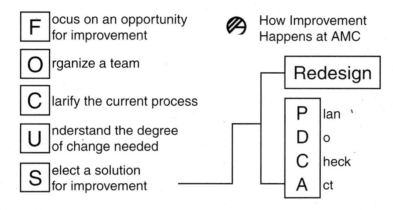

Figure 19-2 FOCUS Method (Courtesy of Albany Medical Center, Albany, NY)

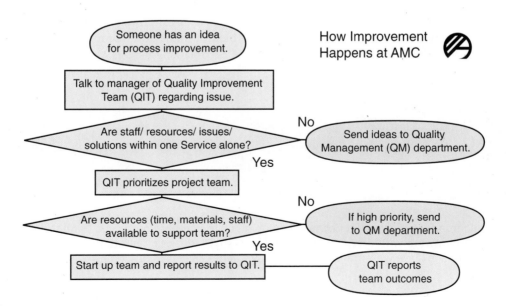

Figure 19-3 Flow Diagram—How Improvement Happens (Courtesy of Albany Medical Center, Albany, NY)

- Multiple paths that show lots of people involved in the activity or delivering the service to the customer. Too many staff involved is wasteful and confusing to the patient.

If the process seems reasonable, with one or two areas needing improvement, then a micro-level analysis of your flow diagram is needed.

- Examine decision symbols (diamonds) that represent quality inspection activities. Can these activities be eliminated? Do some errors go undetected? Is the check redundant? This examination will ensure limited rework and maximum clarity.
- Examine each process in the diagram for redundancy and value. If a step is repeated or does not have any value for the customer, it should be eliminated.
- Examine processes for waiting time areas. The process should be changed to eliminate these wait times.
- Examine all processes for rework loops. A step should not be repeated. Resources are always limited, especially in hospitals today.
- Check that handoffs are smooth and necessary. Handoffs are times when a process is handed from one staff person or department to another. Handoffs always leave room for error. They are also common times for wait areas. During this phase, cause-and-effect diagrams and Pareto charts can be helpful. These tools will be illustrated later.

U: Understand the degree of change needed. In this stage, the team reviews what it knows and enhances its knowledge by reviewing the literature, available data, and competitive benchmarks. How are other health care organizations doing the process?

S: Solution: Select a solution for improvement. The team can brainstorm and then choose the best solution. It can then use the PDCA Cycle to test this solution. An implementation plan should be used to track progress and the steps required. This implementation plan can be in the form of a work plan or Gantt chart. This is a chart in the form of a table that identifies what activity is to be completed, who is responsible for it, and when is it going to be done. (See sample in Figure 19-4.) It outlines the steps needed to implement the change.

Other Improvement Strategies

Improvement strategies identified at the organizational level involve benchmarking, meeting regulatory requirements, identifying opportunities for system changes following sentinel event review, using a balanced scorecard, and using a storyboard.

Benchmarking

Benchmarking is the continual and collaborative discipline of measuring and comparing the results of key work processes with those of the best performers. It is learning how to adapt these best practices to achieve breakthrough process improvement and build healthier communities (Gift & Mosel, 1994). Benchmarking focuses on key services or processes,

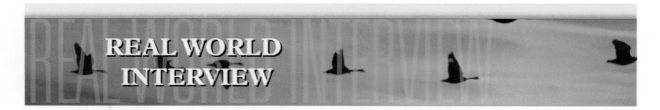

REAL WORLD INTERVIEW

I felt that benchmarking was useful because it allowed us to compare ourselves to other organizations. It allowed us to network with other similar facilities to share ideas and strategies. It allowed us to test our strategies to see if we were making any improvements.

Karen Petronis, RN, MS
Orthopedic Clinical Nurse Specialist

Bed Access Improvement Team
Phase 2 Work Plan: Transition to Daily Management and Evaluation

Activity	Responsible Party	8/98	9/98	10/98	11/98	12/98
1.0 Modify the Team						
1.1 Identify Phase 2 tasks to be completed	Team	■				
1.2 Review & Modify Team Composition/membership	Team	■				
1.3 Develop Work Plan	Planning Team	■				
1.4 Review Work Plan with Team	Myers/Nolan		■			
2.0 Review/Modify Ideal Design						
2.1 Identify Modifications/Opportunities for Additional Change	Team			■		
2.2 Revise Ideal Flow Chart	Team			■		
3.0 Modify Structure & Supports: People/Forms Needed						
3.1 Revise Process Management Structure • Modify job descriptions—triage Manager and Admitting Coordinator	Triage Management Subgroup				■	
3.2 Assess Communication Needed with Nursing Units	Team					
4.0 Draft/Standardize Tasks						
4.1 Draft/Standardize Tasks					■	
5.0 Transition to Daily Operations, Develop Data Collection Process, Evaluate, Monitor						
5.1 Evaluate Bed Access Simulation • Review ED & PACU data • Identify accomplishments and opportunities of structure and ideal process	Team					■
5.2 Develop Plan to Transition Process and Structure to Daily Operations	Planning Team					■
5.3 Develop Data Collection Process	Planning Team					■
5.4 Evaluate Process & Structure (milestone meeting)	Team					■
5.5 Identify Subgroup of Pt Care Delivery System QIT to Monitor Progress	Team					■

Figure 19-4 Gantt Chart/Workplan (Courtesy of Albany Medical Center, Albany, NY)

for example, length of time in the operating room for a total hip replacement or length of stay in hospital postprocedure. A benchmark study will identify gaps in performance and provide options for selection of processes to improve, ideas for redesign of care delivery, and ideas for better ways of meeting customer expectation (Youngberg, 1998).

Regulatory Requirements

The Joint Commission on Accreditation of Healthcare Organizations (JCAHO) has developed standards to guide critical activities performed by health care organizations. Preparation for an accreditation survey and the survey results will provide a wealth of information and data, which can be utilized as ideas for improvement strategies.

Sentinel Event Review

An adverse **sentinel event** is an unexpected occurrence involving death or serious physical or psychological injury to a patient (Joint Commission on Accreditation of Healthcare Organizations, 1998). Events are called sentinel because they require immediate investigation. During analysis of these sentinel events, opportunities for improving the system will arise and should be taken advantage of. Linkage of sentinel event review to the organization's performance improvement system will identify strategies for prevention of future sentinel events. An example of a sentinel event is surgery performed on the wrong side of a patient. Reviewing the surgical process and developing a system to mark the appropriate site is a change in process to prevent future harmful occurrences.

Balanced Scorecard

To ensure value in care, measurement of progress has to be balanced. Generally, four cardinal domains of outcomes are measured; Figure 19-5 illustrates these in the form of a clinical value compass (Caldwell, 1998).

Such an approach allows those reviewing data to examine all aspects of care. For example, patient outcomes are reflected in a patient's functional status and clinical status. Patient satisfaction and cost balance this to ensure value. Data can be arranged to create a balanced scorecard, in an approach that uses the organization's priorities as categories for indicators. For example, three priorities might be customer service, cost-effectiveness, and positive clinical outcomes. These priorities help sort out what should be measured to give a balanced view of whether a strategy is working. Indicators are selected based on what they have in common, so that if a change occurs in the cost-effectiveness category, it will affect the data in another category. For example, if we decrease cost for orthopedic surgery, does that affect the customer's satisfaction positively or negatively? If we decrease the length of stay for these patients, does it increase or decrease complication rates? Once indi-

cators are selected, data are tracked over time at regular intervals (every month or every quarter, for example). Figure 19-6 shows how the balanced scorecard was used on an orthopedic unit. From the control charts, you can see that the total hip pathway length of stay increased and then decreased. The satisfaction scores remained at around 90%, so even though the length of stay decreased, the satisfaction did not deteriorate. The ratio of complications went down; the average number of physical therapy visits varied and then went up. This reporting mechanism offers a balanced view.

Storyboard: How to Share Your Story

Process improvement teams share their work with others using a storyboard. The storyboard usually takes the major steps in the improvement methodology and visually outlines the progress in each step. The storyboard can be displayed in a high-traffic area of the organization to inform other staff of the QI efforts under way. Storyboarding can be done when a process is complete, or used during the process to communicate information.

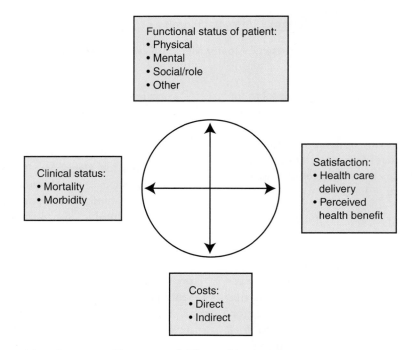

Figure 19-5 Clinical Value Compass (Courtesy of Albany Medical Center, Albany, NY)

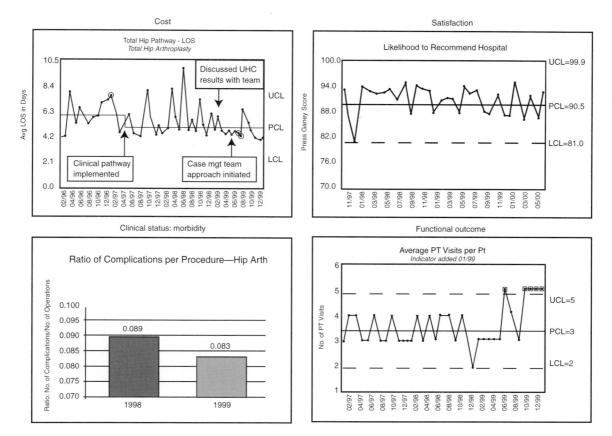

Figure 19-6 Orthopedic Balanced Scorecard (Courtesy of Albany Medical Center, Albany, NY)

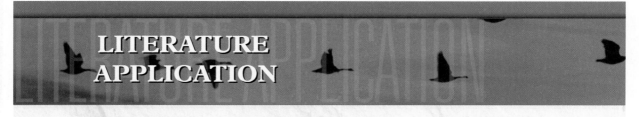

LITERATURE APPLICATION

Citation: Lesar, T., Briceland, L., & Stein, D. (1997). Factors related to errors in medication prescribing. *Journal of the American Medical Association, 277*(4), 312–317.

Discussion: Adverse drug events occur in up to 6.5% of hospitalized patients and account for almost one-fifth of all adverse patient events. Errors in the prescribing and management of drug therapy are common and have been identified as a major cause of adverse drug events. Understanding the many factors contributing to errors should assist in implementation of more effective error prevention strategies. Several easily identified factors are associated with a large proportion of medication prescribing errors.

Implications for Practice: Nurses and doctors can help in identifying ways to improve processes to decrease medication errors. To help focus their efforts, they should review the information available about what factors have the greatest association with errors.

Patient Satisfaction Data

Patient satisfaction data can be obtained in several ways. Most health care facilities get feedback from patients by having them fill out a questionnaire that asks how they felt about their health care encounter. It is most helpful if this data can be compared or benchmarked with other organizations' data. This requires that several organizations use the same data collection tools. All patient responses would be put into a database so the results can be compared. Another method to obtain patient satisfaction information is via a focus group or postcare interview. This means meeting with one or more patients after their discharge and getting feedback on their perceptions of their stay.

Using Data

Several different types of charts are used to examine data in QI efforts. These include time series charts, Pareto charts, histograms, flowcharts, fishbone diagrams, pie charts, and check sheets.

Time Series Data

Time series data (Figure 19-7) allow a QI team to see change in quality over time. A time series chart allows the user to determine whether a process is in control, meaning that the process has normal variation rather than dramatic changes that are not predictable. Although bar charts are useful, there are

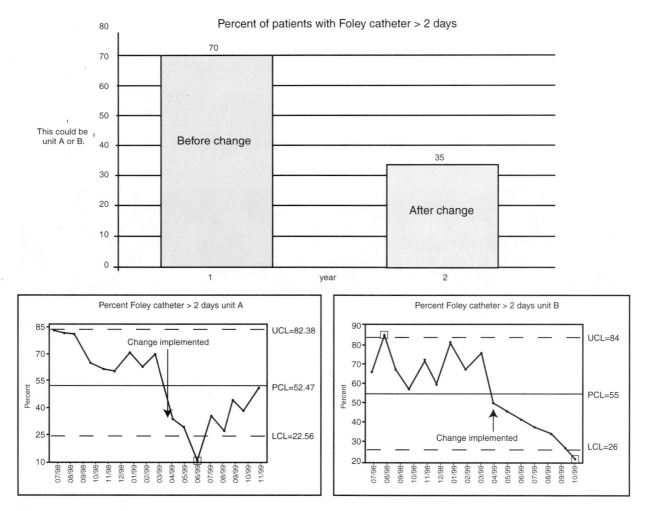

Figure 19-7 Time Series versus Bar Charts (Courtesy of Albany Medical Center, Albany, NY)

times in process improvement efforts when time series data display the process more clearly.

In the bar graph at the top of Figure 19-7 you can see that from year 1 to year 2 the percentage of the time that Foley catheters were in for greater than 2 days decreased dramatically. However, if you look at the time series chart of the same data for two different units, the actual process for each unit is quite different. Unit A had a good initial decrease after the change was implemented. However, it could not hold the gains, and the rate of Foley use has begun to creep back up. Unit B, however, made progress and has continued to decrease its rate over time. Determining next steps for these two units in this process improvement initiative would require very different strategies.

Tracking data over time allows you to see how a process is behaving. A time series graph is used for this. Graphs or charts—rather than tables of numbers—are used to display data because graphs are faster to interpret. As you can see from the graph of the total hip arthroplasty pathway length of stay in Figure 19-6, a time series data graph contains data points at particular intervals, every two months for example. The process centerline (PCL) represents the average and the upper control limit (UCL) and

lower control limit (LCL) represent acceptable boundaries for expected performance (Wheeler, 1993). If the process were changed in some way, you would expect to see the data change at that time. The time series chart is used to look for trends, shifts, and unusual data.

Charts: Pareto, Histogram, Flowcharts, Fishbone Diagrams, Pie Charts, and Check Sheets

In addition to time series data graphs, information can be displayed in several different ways to enhance decision making. These include Pareto diagrams, pie charts, flowcharts, and histograms. Figure 19-8 is an example of a fishbone diagram. (Fishbone diagrams are also referred to as root cause diagrams, cause-and-effect diagrams, or Ishikawa diagrams.) Note that many factors contribute to a problem. Review of a cause-and-effect chart encourages staff to look for all the causes of a problem, not just one cause. Figure 19-9 shows a flowchart, a check sheet, a Pareto chart, and a control chart. A full discussion of these tools is outside the scope of this chapter.

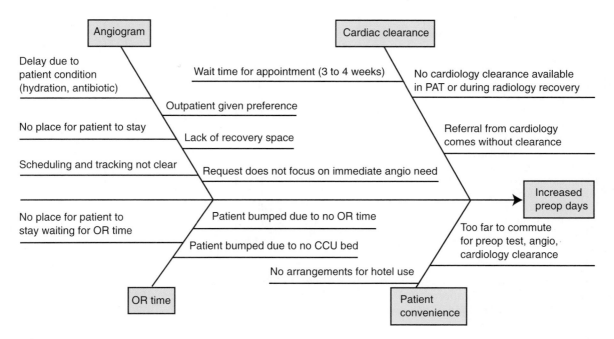

Figure 19-8 Root Cause/Fishbone Diagram

a.

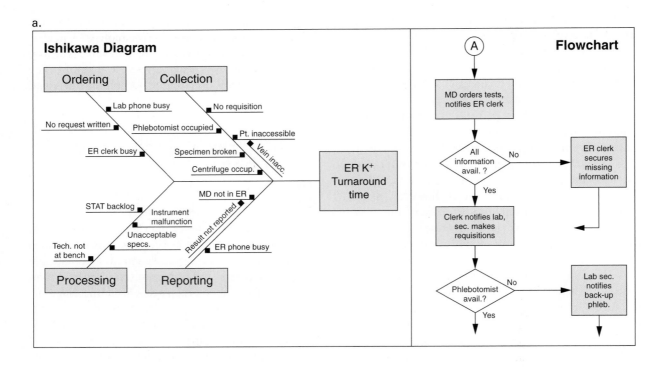

b.

Check Sheet
Delays in production of Se K$^+$ results from 1/1/91 to 1/7/91

Code/Delay Type		Mon	Tue	Wed	Thur	Fri	Sat	Sun	Total
A	Request not written by physician	I	I				I		3
B	Lab phone busy > 2 minutes	I		I		II		I	5
C	Phlebotomists unavailable	III	II	III	III	II	IIII	III	20
D	Requisition not ready	II	I	I	I	I	III	II	11
E	Patient inaccessible	I	I	II	I		II	I	8
F	Vein inaccessible	I		II		I	II		6
G	Centrifuge busy	II		I		I			4
H	Specimen broken	II		I				I	4
I	STAT backlog	III			I		II	I	7
J	Tech. not at bench	II		II		I	II	I	8
K	Unacceptable specimen	I	I		II		I	II	7
L	Lab. sec. unavailable to report	III		I		I			6
M	ER Phone not answered			I			II		3
N	MD not in ER	II	I			II		I	5
O	MD not answer page	I	I	II		II		II	8
P	Results not reported by ER sec.	II	I	II	I	III	II	II	13

(continues)

Figure 19-9 Ishikawa Diagram, Flowchart, Check Sheet, Pareto Chart, and Control Chart (Reprinted with permission from *Clinical Laboratory Management Review*, November/December 1991, 5[6]:448–462. ©Clinical Laboratory Management Association, Inc. All rights reserved)

c.

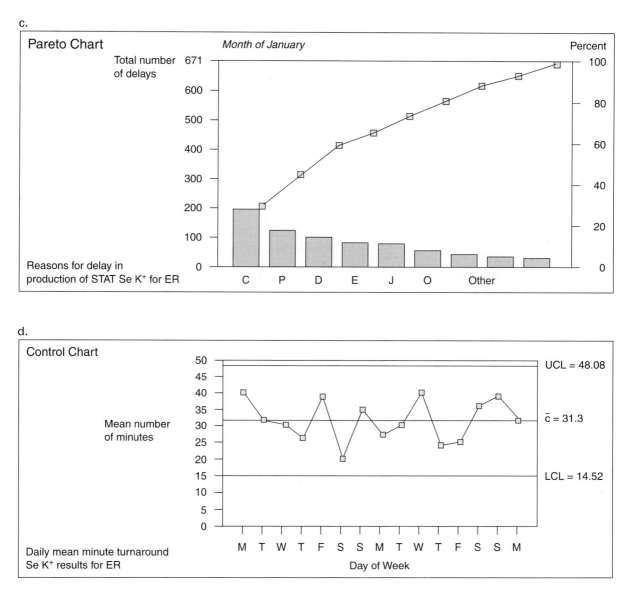

Figure 19-9 *(continued)*

PRINCIPLES IN ACTION IN AN ORGANIZATION

How are these principles and tools of quality management actually used on a day-to-day basis in a health care facility? This is done through setting up a structure for the organization, using a process for quality, and monitoring outcomes.

Organizational Structure

Most organizations today are structured to maximize QI efforts. This allows an organization to be flexible and nimble in a very turbulent health care environment. An organization accomplishes this through an organizational structure that encourages accountability and communication and by focusing all staff on the priorities of the organization.

Figure 19-10 is an organizational chart that shows a structure for quality improvement. Note that it includes staff from the board level to staff on individual quality improvement teams (QITs). Communicating priorities at all levels in the organization is key. Staff members must realize how their day-to-day work influences the accomplishment of strategic goals. Mission, vision, and value statements help

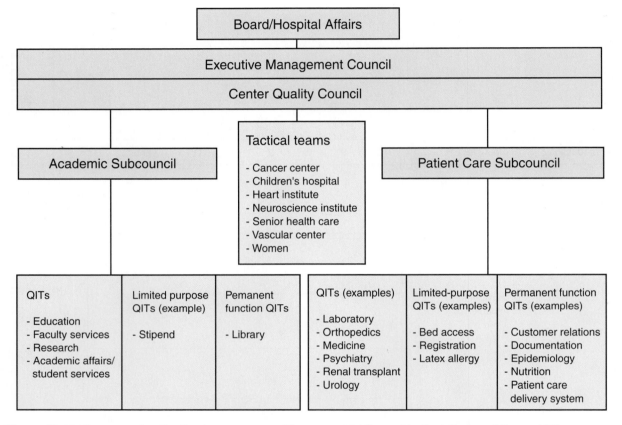

Figure 19-10 Structure for Quality Improvement (Courtesy of Albany Medical Center, Albany, NY)

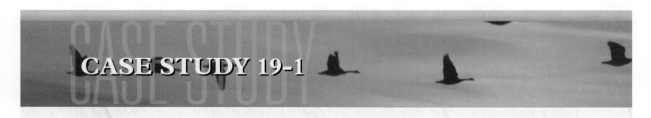

CASE STUDY 19-1

You have been caring for groups of patients post myocardial infarction. You have also developed a good working relationship with the other nursing and medical staff on your unit. You believe that the care delivery on your unit could improve, thus improving patient satisfaction and clinical outcomes and decreasing the length of stay. How would you proceed? Whose support would you enlist first? Who should be involved? What quality indicators could be measured?

CRITICAL THINKING

There are times when some care providers, particularly physicians, see clinical pathways and other standardized guidelines as cookie-cutter medicine. All health care providers like to think they give their patients the best care possible. Standardization and evidence-based clinical guidelines are meant to communicate the latest evidence as to the best practice for a given patient problem. This allows care providers to focus on specific individual patient needs rather than spending energy on determining what the research says is the best evidence-based strategy. In developing a clinical pathway or other standardized guideline, evidence-based practice guidelines should be incorporated. In the absence of evidence-based practices, consensus of the team should be used to develop the clinical pathway. In the absence of consensus, the patient's health care provider should make an independent decision, which is not included in the clinical guideline. A group that was developing a clinical pathway for the care of patients with acute myocardial infarction noted evidence showing that these patients should receive acetylsalicylic acid (ASA) on admission. The research in this area was very clear, and most providers believed this was being done. When a chart audit was performed to determine whether this was, in fact, the practice on the unit, it was discovered that only 48% of the patients were receiving ASA within 8 hours of admission. The team added this to the clinical pathway. After this was implemented, 85% of the patients received ASA within the first 8 hours of admission.

What clinical practices do you see on your clinical unit that are based on an evidence-based clinical pathway? How can you participate in improving the care of more patients using evidence-based clinical pathways?

accomplish this clarity of focus. This is discussed more in Chapter 14.

Outcomes Monitoring

Outcomes are a measurement of the patient response to structure and process. Outcomes measure actual clinical progress. Outcomes can be short term, such as the average length of stay for a patient population, or long term, such as a measure of patients' progress over time (e.g., survival rate for a transplant patient 1, 2, and 3 years after treatment). Outcomes can be studied to identify potential areas of concern. This may lead to an investigation of structure and process to determine any root causes. For example, when a postoperative infection rate was used as an outcome measure, an increase in the number of infections per month was noted. This led the team to review the patient care process being used. It was discovered that, often, preoperative prophylactic antibiotics were not given to the patient because the order was not

written. The team added this order to the initial order set, and all patients received prophylactic antibiotics. The number of postoperative infections decreased.

KEY CONCEPTS

- Quality improvement is a continuous process focused on maintaining regulatory compliance and improving patient care processes and outcomes.
- Patient care needs should drive improvement opportunities.
- Decisions should be driven by data.
- Improvement initiatives should be linked to the organization's mission, vision, and values.
- Organizational goals and objectives should be communicated up and down the organization.
- There should be a balance in improvement goals focused on patient clinical and functional status, cost, and patient satisfaction outcomes.

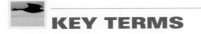

KEY TERMS

benchmarking

diagnosis-related group

performance
  improvement
process

quality assurance

quality improvement

sentinel event

system

REVIEW QUESTIONS

1. Which of the following describes the benchmarking process?
   A. Reviewing your own unit's data for opportunities
   B. Collecting data on an individual patient
   C. Reviewing data in the literature
   D. Comparing your data to that of other organizations to identify opportunities

2. Identifying opportunities in the health care arena is the responsibility of which group?
   A. Administration
   B. Physicians
   C. Patients
   D. Everyone

3. Following a sentinel event, which step would be initiated first?
   A. No action
   B. Corrective action of personnel
   C. Reporting to health department/root cause analysis
   D. Immediate investigation

4. What document defines the purpose of an organization?
   A. Mission
   B. Fishbone diagram
   C. Balanced scorecard
   D. Process flowchart

5. What tool could be used to track a change in a process over time?
   A. Flowchart
   B. Histogram
   C. Time series chart
   D. Pie chart

REVIEW ACTIVITIES

1. Risk management, infection control practitioners, and a benchmark study have revealed that your unit's utilization of Foley catheters is above average. Brainstorm reasons why this may be occurring. Creating a fishbone (root cause) diagram may help.

2. After you have identified the root causes for the overuse of Foley catheters, use the PDCA Cycle to identify improvement strategies.

3. Think about your last clinical rotation experience. Identify one process that you believe could be improved and describe how you would begin improving the process. Using the FOCUS methodology would be helpful.

EXPLORING THE WEB

- Use these sites for potential benchmark data:
  University HealthSystem Consortium (UHC):
  http://www.uhc.org
  Institute for Healthcare Improvement (IHI):
  http://www.ihi.org

- These sites are recommended for a team that is looking for evidence-based guidelines or research studies for a particular diagnosis:
  National Guideline Clearinghouse:
  http://www.guideline.gov/index.asp
  Cochrane Library: *http://www.cochrane.org/cochrane/revabstr/mainindex.htm*
  PubMed's Clinical Queries:
  http://www.ncbi.nlm.nih.gov/entrez/query.fcgi
  Evidence-Based Practice Internet Resources:
  http://www-hsl.mcmaster.ca/ebm/

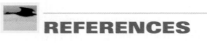

REFERENCES

Al-Assaf, A. F., & Schmele, J. (1997). *Total quality in healthcare.* Boca Raton, FL: St. Lucie Press.

AMC Q series curriculum. (1998). Albany, NY: Albany Medical Center, Quality Management Department.

Berwick, D., & Plsek, P. (1992). *Managing medical quality videotape series.* Woodbridge, NJ: Quality Visions.

Caldwell, C. (1998). *Handbook for managing change in health care.* Milwaukee, WI: ASQ Quality Press.

Crosby, P. B. (1989). *Let's talk quality.* New York: McGraw-Hill.

Deming, W. E. (1986). *Out of the crisis.* Cambridge, MA: Center for Advanced Engineering Study.

Gift, R. G., & Mosel, D. (1994). *Benchmarking in health care: A collaborative approach.* Chicago: American Hospital Publishing.

Joint Commission on Accreditation of Healthcare Organizations. (1998). *Comprehensive accreditation manual for hospitals* (p. AC-5). Oakbrook, IL: Joint Commission on Accreditation of Healthcare Organizations.

Katz, J., & Green, E. (1992). *Managing quality.* St. Louis, MO: Mosby.

Langley, G. J., Nolan, K. M., Norman, C. L., Provost, L. P., & Nolan, T. W. (1996). *The improvement guide.* San Francisco: Jossey-Bass.

Lesar, T., Briceland, I., & Stein, D. (1997). Factors related to errors in medication prescribing. *Journal of the American Medical Association, 277*(4), 312–317.

Plsek, P. E. (1993). Tutorial: Quality improvement project models. *Quality Management in Health Care, 1*(2), 69–81.

Wheeler, D. J. (1993). *Understanding variation: The key to managing chaos.* Knoxville, TN: SPC Press.

Youngberg, B. (1998). *The risk manager's desk reference.* Gaithersburg, MD: Aspen.

SUGGESTED READINGS

Balestracci, Jr., D., & Barlow, J. L. (1994). *Quality improvement: Practical applications for medical group practice.* Englewood, CO: Center for Research in Ambulatory Health Care Administration.

Duffy, J. R. (2000, July-September). Cardiovascular outcomes initiative: Case studies in performance improvement. *Outcomes Management in Nursing Practice, 4*(3), 110–116.

Henry, S. B. (1995, May-June). Informatics: Essential infrastructure for quality assessment and improvement in nursing. *Journal of the American Medical Information Association, 2*(3), 169–182.

Kelly-Heidenthal, P., & Heidenthal, P. R. (1995, March-April). Benchmarking. *Nursing Quality Connections, 4*(5), 4.

King, K. M., & Teo, K. K. (2000, August). Integrating clinical quality improvement strategies with nursing research. *Western Journal of Nursing Research, 22*(5), 596–608.

Kitson, A. (2000, December). Towards evidence-based quality improvement: Perspectives from nursing practice. *International Journal of Quality in Health Care, 12*(6), 459–464.

Koivula, M., Paunonen, M., & Laippala, P. (1998, November). Prerequisites for quality improvement in nursing. *Journal of Nursing Management, 6*(6), 333–342.

Maleyeff, J., Kaminsky, F. C., Jubinville, A., & Fenn, C. (2001, July-August). A guide to using performance measurement systems for continuous improvement. *Journal of Healthcare Quality, 23*(4), 33–37.

Meisenheimer, C. G. (1997). *Improving quality: A guide to effective programs* (2nd ed.). Gaithersburg, MD: Aspen.

Rantz, M. J., Petroski, G. F., Madsen, R. W., Scott, J., Mehr, D. R., Popejoy, L., Hicks, L. L., Porter, R., Zwygart-Stauffacher, M., & Grando, V. (1997, November). Setting thresholds for MDS (Minimum Data Set) quality indicators for nursing home quality improvement reports. *Joint Committee Journal on Quality Improvement, 23*(11), 602–611.

CHAPTER 20

The best outcomes evaluation is likely to come from partnerships of technically proficient analysts and clinicians, each of whom is sensitive to and respectful of the contributions the other can bring
(Robert L. Kane, Professor of Public Health, University of Minnesota)

Strategies to Improve Patient Care Outcomes

Mary Anne Jadlos, MS, ACNP-CS, CWOCN
Glenda Kelman, PhD, ACNP-CS

OBJECTIVES

Upon completion of this chapter, the reader should be able to:

1. Discuss the use of outcomes research in evidence-based practice.
2. Describe selected evidence-based models.
3. Utilize the Model for Improvement to implement evidence-based practice in specific patient care situations.
4. Identify resources available to generate outcomes/benchmarks in clinical practice.

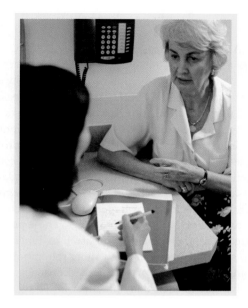

During report, the staff nurse tells you about a 60-year-old woman, Miss Kelly, who was admitted to the unit today with left hip and sciatic pain after a recent fall at home. You immediately begin to think she has a hip fracture. The staff nurse interrupts your thoughts and says, "Wait, there is more. This woman has a new diagnosis of breast cancer and has also developed a pleural effusion, which necessitated the insertion of a chest tube this morning. Her dyspnea has improved since this morning, and her pulse oximetry on 2 liters of oxygen via nasal cannula is 99%."

Miss Kelly has lymphedema of her right hand and arm, and the right breast mass is a very large, open, foul-smelling lesion that bleeds intermittently. She appears anxious and has indicated that she is uncomfortable and afraid to move. She has Tylenol with codeine ordered orally every 4 hours as needed for pain but has been very reluctant to use the medication because she thought it would alter her ability to think and make decisions regarding her care. Results of a bone scan and CT scan of the abdomen and pelvis indicate that she has further metastatic involvement of the left acetabulum. This could be the cause of her left hip pain—tumor replacing the bone. Although the CT scan does not reveal a fracture, Miss Kelly is at high risk for developing a pathological fracture.

Miss Kelly is single, has no children, and lives with her brother and five cats. She does not smoke or drink. She is a retired clerk for the state Department of Labor. She has been followed by a cardiologist for hypertension for several years. She would call for prescription refills and then cancel her appointments because she feared what the doctor would find or say.

What are your thoughts about how you will approach this patient?

What additional data do you need to develop a protocol of care to improve Miss Kelly's outcomes?

What priorities should be addressed to manage Miss Kelly's care?

This chapter will identify strategies used to improve patient care outcomes. Information from nursing theory and an evidence-based practice model for improvement will be applied to a selected patient case study. Some of the terms or the language related to evidence-based practice or evidence-based nursing may be unfamiliar to you, but do not let this intimidate you. By asking the simple question "Why?" you are beginning the journey of gathering data and evidence either to support your current practice or to change how you provide care and interact with patients and families to improve patient care outcomes. The focus is the patient.

EVIDENCE-BASED PRACTICE

Evidence-based practice (EBP) is defined as the conscientious, explicit, and judicious use of current best evidence in making decisions about the care of individual patients (Sackett, Rosenberg, Gray, Haynes, & Richardson, 1996). EBP uses outcomes research and other current research findings to guide the development of appropriate strategies to deliver quality, cost-effective care. Outcomes research provides evidence about benefits, risks, and results of treatments so individuals can make informed decisions and choices to improve their quality of life. Research seeks to understand the end results of particular health care practices and interventions. End results may include changes in a person's ability to function and carry out routine activities of daily living. Outcomes research can also identify potentially effective strategies that can be implemented to improve the quality and value of care.

The Pew Health Professions Commission's *Final Report* (Bellack & O'Neil, 2000) identified 21 competencies for the 21st century to prepare health professionals for the practice environments and organization of the future (also discussed previously in Chapter 1). Four competencies specifically focus on responsibilities related to outcomes and will be addressed in this chapter. They include (1) provide evidence-based, clinically competent care; (2) demonstrate critical thinking, reflection, and problem-solving skills; (3) take responsibility for quality of care and health outcomes at all levels; and (4) contribute to continuous improvement of the health care system.

Historically, health care providers have relied primarily on biomedical parameters or measures such as laboratory and diagnostic tests to determine whether a health intervention is necessary and whether it is successful. However, these measures often do not fully reflect the multidimensional outcomes that matter most to the patients, such as quality of life, family, work, and overall level of functioning. Traditionally, outcome measures have included physical measures, such as blood pressure to assess the effectiveness of antihypertensive medications. They have also sometimes included patient satisfaction measures to assess patient satisfaction with the care or services provided. The Medicare Health Outcomes Survey is used to assess how well health plans improve the functional status of Medicare patients but may not capture how the patient actually feels (Clancy & Eisenberg, 1998).

Role of the ANA

The American Nurses Association (ANA) was an active advocate of outcomes evaluation as early as 1976. Outcomes were emphasized as a measure of quality care. The 1980 ANA *Social Policy Statement* stated that one of the four defining characteristics of nursing is the evaluation of the effects of actions in relation to phenomena. In 1986, the ANA approved policies related to the development of a classification system including outcomes. In 1995, the ANA developed a *Nursing Report Card for Acute Care Settings*, which lists indicators for patient-focused outcomes, structures of care, and care processes. These patient-focused outcome indicators are listed in Table 20-1. Nurses need to recognize and value the importance of using these indicators to achieve safe, quality, cost-effective care in their daily practice

Evolution of EBP

Evidence-based practice has evolved from a nice-to-know perspective to a need-to-know essential strategy in health care. Patients, health care providers, and pay-

TABLE 20-1	ANA Nursing Report Card, Patient-Focused Outcome Indicators
Indicator	**Definition**
Mortality rate	A measure of the number of patients who die following admission to a hospital for care (can be examined over a number of different time periods)
Length of stay	Duration of the inpatient hospital component of a defined episode of illness
Adverse incident rate (total)	Measures the rate at which patients admitted to a hospital for care experience adverse incidents during the course of their stay that are not directly related to the reason for their admission
Medication error rate	Rate at which errors in the administration of medications occur within a given institution
Patient injury rate	Rate at which patients fall or incur physical injuries (unrelated to a surgical or diagnostic procedure) during the course of their hospital stay

(continues)

Table 20-1 *(continued)*

Total complication rate	Rate at which additional diseases or conditions that are related to the patient's original diagnosis are developed in patients receiving care at a hospital
Decubitus ulcer rate	Rate at which patients receiving care at a hospital experience skin breakdown
Nosocomial infection rate (total)	Rate at which patients experience infections (all sites) originating in the hospital
Nosocomial urinary tract infection rate	Rate at which catheterized patients experience urinary tract infection originating in the hospital
Nosocomial pneumonia rate	Rate at which inflammation of the lungs with exudation and consolidation develops in patients during the course of their hospitalization
Nosocomial surgical wound infection rate	Rate at which patients experience surgical wound infections
Patient or family satisfaction with nursing care	A patient's or family's opinion of care received from nursing staff
Patient/family willingness to recommend hospital to others or to use hospital again	Rate at which patients or family would recommend the hospital providing their care to others or agree to return to the hospital for care in the future
Patient adherence to discharge plan	Rate at which patients fully and correctly execute the therapeutic regimen established for the period immediately following discharge
Readmission rate	Rate at which patients return to the hospital within a defined period of time following a hospital stay for unplanned or emergent care related to the same diagnosis addressed during the prior admission
Postdischarge emergency room visits	Number of patient visits to the emergency room, for preventable complaints related to a previous hospital stay, during a defined time period following discharge
Postdischarge unscheduled physician visits	Number of unplanned physician visits, for preventable physician complications related to a previous hospital stay, during a defined time period following discharge
Patient knowledge	The extent to which patients possess the knowledge and skills necessary to care for themselves following discharge, or if the patient is unable to do so, an appropriate member of the patient's social support network is able to provide that care

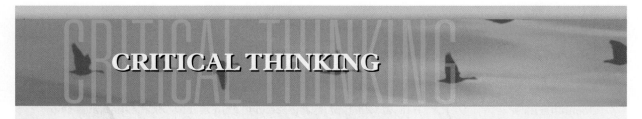

CRITICAL THINKING

You are attending a conference on evidence-based nursing practice. After the conference, you begin to think about your own practices.

Do you need to know about outcome indicators to effectively care for your patients? Why has there been an increase in the number of methicillin-resistant *Staphylococcus aureus* (MRSA) infections in patients on your nursing unit recently? Why are more of your unit's patients being readmitted after being home for only a short period of time?

ers recognize the significance of collecting data and analyzing outcomes to achieve safe, quality, cost-effective care. Outcome strategies used in EBP by nurses and members of the health care team include the creation of clinical protocols, guidelines, pathways, algorithms, and so on, which become the tools for health care interventions. According to the Joint Commission on Accreditation of Healthcare Organizations (JCAHO), a **practice guideline** is defined as a descriptive tool or a standardized specification for care of the typical patient in the typical situation. These guidelines are developed by a formal process that incorporates the best scientific evidence of effectiveness and expert opinions. Synonyms or near synonyms include practice parameter, preferred practice pattern, algorithm, protocol, and clinical standard (1999).

Evidence-based practice is used to guide practice interventions and is most successful when the entire organization and interdisciplinary team buy into EBP and participate and support the process. By linking the care that people receive to the outcomes they experience, EBP or outcomes research has become key to identifying and developing better strategies to monitor and improve the quality of care.

EBP is not a cookbook approach to patient care, however. The nurse and members of the health care team assess each patient and determine whether a guideline is appropriate. Nursing theorists such as Nightingale, Peplau, Benner, and others have identified that the uniqueness of nursing is based upon the relational and integrative nature of healing, involving the person and environments (Bryant, 1998). Nursing is the only discipline that views the whole person within the context of the person's environment. Nurses must not mimic physicians but must focus on the art and science of nursing that comforts, cares, nurtures, heals, and builds on nursing theory to guide practice. There is a difference between evidence-based practice and evidence-based nursing practice. Ingersoll has defined **evidence-based nursing practice** (EBNP) as the conscientious, explicit, and judicious use of theory-derived, research-based information in making decisions about nursing care delivery to individuals or groups of individuals and in consideration of individual needs and preferences (2000). Evidence-based practice has a medical focus, whereas evidence-based nursing practice considers the individual's needs and preferences based on nursing theory and research.

The role of the nurse is to participate in developing a comprehensive, interdisciplinary evidence-based plan of care in conjunction with the patient and members of the health care team. This plan of care integrates the art and science of caring, not merely the medical model of the absence or presence of disease. Nurses need to embrace innovation, creativity, and the use of technology to move beyond the old logic that elevated doing above knowing (Bryant, 1998).

Benner, Hooper-Kyriakidis, Hooper, Stannard, & Eoyang (1998) identify aspects of what they refer to as the skilled know-how of managing a crisis. They state that some of this knowledge is assumed based on training, skill, and experience. Other nursing responsibilities are accepted or imposed based on necessity or a sense of moral obligation. These

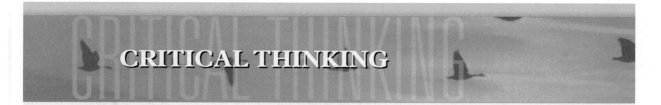

CRITICAL THINKING

Patrick and Carol are having coffee. They are two RNs working in an intensive care unit (ICU) in a community hospital. They are discussing implementation of the congestive heart failure (CHF) pathway. Patrick says, "I don't have enough time to finish my charting. I already stay an hour every day without overtime to finish my charting." Carol responds, "Maybe we could meet with the nurse manager. She may be able to help us."

How can Patrick and Carol be expected to implement this new clinical pathway? How will the use of a clinical pathway improve patient care?

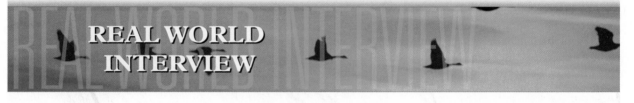

REAL WORLD INTERVIEW

Wow, I just had a very busy night shift. Mr. King is going for a colonoscopy and his colostomy exploded twice overnight. He had so much diarrhea with the colonoscopy preparation. We ran out of supplies, and he has no appliance on right now because I have not had any time to get another one out of the storeroom. I have been so busy. I am taking care of 12 patients and have only one aide to help. It seems like I just keep running from patient to patient. There are so many intravenous meds, mostly every patient is incontinent, and Mr. Ruff is very confused and keeps trying to get out of bed. He almost fell last night. On top of that, the lady in room 21 almost coded. She has congestive heart failure (CHF) and became very short of breath and I had to call the doctor. Her IV infiltrated so we needed to restart that, and then we needed to put a Foley catheter in and give her IV Lasix and morphine. She is much better now, but I called her family because she became very anxious. I am so tired. I wonder if I am making any difference here.

Christina Yerdon, RN

responsibilities might include stocking equipment at the bedside, prioritizing interventions and procedures, organizing the team and orchestrating their actions in a way that enhances their ability to function, recognizing the effect of therapies, and asking for help as appropriate. These skills are all relatively invisible in daily nursing practice. They become more visible in crisis situations. Mastery of and comfort with these skills come only with practice, practice, practice.

Nurses are expected to manage the care of acutely ill patients. Beginning nurses should be encouraged to thoughtfully acknowledge their personal abilities and limitations. There must be a blend between knowing and doing. It is important that the beginning nurse realize that gaining knowledge and skill is a gradual process. As the beginning nurse develops aspects of skilled know-how, she will become aware of her own ability to deliver safe patient care, minimize patient discomfort, decrease

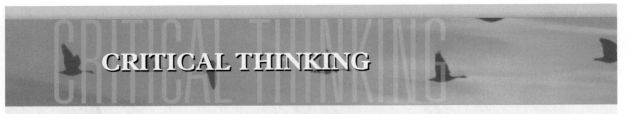

CRITICAL THINKING

An elderly patient is admitted with CHF and venous stasis ulcers on her legs. The doctor orders normal saline gauze dressings to be changed twice a day. The evening staff registered nurse is giving report to the night nurse. She states that the dressings are always wet and they are saturating the bed linens. The registered nurse wonders whether the prescribed dressing regime is the best choice for this patient.

What sources do you currently use to find answers to questions you have about your patients during the course of your shift? What other health care professionals do you talk with about the problems your patients are having? Do you have a preceptor or role model that is available to help you?

stress and anxiety, and assist in optimizing team performance. Guidelines based on EBP can help to direct care but cannot replace learning by hands-on delivery of patient care. As beginning nurses gain clinical experience and learn new theoretical knowledge, they will be able to contribute to the development and revision of EBP guidelines. Remember, EBP guidelines outline practice parameters based on evidence or research, but they do not outline how to deliver individualized patient care.

EVIDENCE-BASED MULTIDISCIPLINARY PRACTICE MODELS

Several models are used in EBP. They include the University of Colorado Hospital model and the Model for Improvement.

The University of Colorado Hospital Model

The University of Colorado Hospital model (Figure 20-1) is an example of an evidence-based multidisciplinary practice model (Goode et al., 2000; Goode & Piedalue, 1999). This model presents a framework for thinking about how you use different sources of information to change or support your practice. The health care team or team member uses valid and cur-

rent research from sources such as journals, conferences, and clinical experts as the basis for clinical decision making. The model depicts nine sources of evidence that are linked to the research core. This model provides a way for the nurse to organize information and data needed not only to care for a patient but also to evaluate the care provided. In other

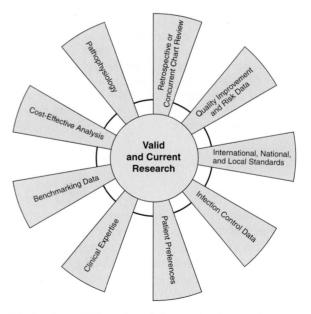

Figure 20-1 University of Colorado Hospital Evidence-Based Multidisciplinary Practice Model (By permission of University of Colorado Hospital Research Council, Denver, CO)

words, did this patient receive the best possible care not only that this institution can offer, but that is available in this world?

The elements of the University of Colorado's practice model can be applied to the case of Miss Kelly in the Opening Scenario of this chapter (Table 20-2). For example, to assess Miss Kelly's progress related to her diagnosis of breast cancer, it would be important to review evidence using institutional and national benchmarks comparing length of stay for Miss Kelly with other breast cancer patients' length of stay. Benchmarking is defined as the continuous process of measuring products, service, and practices against the toughest competitors or those customers recognized as industry leaders (Camp, 1994). The

wound care regime related to nursing time and product use could be analyzed for cost-effectiveness. How much time does it take for a nurse to complete a dressing? How much do the dressings, tape, and other supplies used for the dressing cost?

Pathophysiology would be analyzed by reviewing Miss Kelly's biopsy results, bone scan results, and CT scan results to rule out metastatic disease. These results could be discussed with the physician regarding implications related to the prognosis, treatment, and survival rates for breast cancer. A concurrent or ongoing review could be conducted using the Braden Scale for Predicting Pressure Sore Risk (Bergstrom, Braden, Laguzza, & Holman, 1987) and documenting the assessment score daily.

TABLE 20-2	*Practice Application to Elements of the University of Colorado Hospital Model*
Model Element	**Application**
Benchmarking data	Compare length of stay for Miss Kelly with that of other breast cancer patients in this hospital and other hospitals nationally
Cost-effective analysis	Analyze cost-effectiveness of wound care regimens, including nursing time and use of actual products (e.g., hydrogel vs. normal saline dressings)
Pathophysiology	Review biopsy results/findings of testing for metastatic disease and implications
Retrospective/concurrent chart review	Assess changes in condition related to pressure ulcer development using the Braden Pressure Ulcer Risk Assessment Scale
Quality improvement and risk data	Review and analyze documentation regarding patient progress and risk assessment (e.g., infection, bleeding, pressure ulcer development); outcomes assessment (e.g., pain rating and dosage of narcotic administration)
International, national, and local standards	Assess effectiveness of care related to AHRQ guidelines for cancer pain and pressure ulcers
Infection control data	Review wound culture results and institute appropriate precautions and treatment
Patient preferences	Discuss, document, and implement patient's wishes regarding advance directives
Clinical expertise	Consult acute care nurse practitioner for wound, skin, and pain management

(By permission of University of Colorado Hospital Research Council, Denver, CO)

Data collected for quality improvement purposes could include information on the incidence and management of infection, bleeding, pressure ulcers, and pain. The pain and pressure ulcer guidelines from the Agency for Healthcare Research and Quality (AHRQ; formerly the Agency for Health Care Policy and Research) are examples of national standards that could be used to benchmark and manage cancer pain (AHCPR, 1994a), prevention of pressure ulcers (1992b), and treatment of pressure ulcers (1994b) for Miss Kelly. Infection control data could include a review of wound culture results and the use of appropriate institutional wound precautions. The nurse could discuss with Miss Kelly, document, and then implement Miss Kelly's wishes regarding advance directives. Utilization of clinical expertise could include consulting the acute care nurse practitioners (ACNPs) for input regarding wound, skin, and pain management initially and on an ongoing basis.

The Model for Improvement

Another model for using EBP is the Model for Improvement (Langley, Nolan, Nolan, Norman, & Provost, 1996). Some elements of this model (Figure

20-2) were discussed in chapter 19. The model begins with these questions:

1. What are we trying to accomplish?
2. How will we know that a change is an improvement?
3. What change can we make that will result in improvement?

These three questions provide the foundation for the Model for Improvement and will help focus the use of the Plan, Do, Study, Act (PDSA) Cycle (see Figure 20-3) to complete the Model for Improvement. (Note that the PDSA Cycle was called the Plan-Do-Check-Act (PDCA) Cycle in Chapter 19; different sources may refer to the cycle with either abbreviation.) We will apply the Model for Improvement to the Opening Scenario presented at the beginning of this chapter in relation to pain, pressure ulcers, and wound management.

PAIN MANAGEMENT

Unrelieved pain remains a major health problem, and 50% to 80% of individuals with cancer do not receive adequate pain relief (American Pain Society, 1995; SUPPORT Study Principle Investigators, 1995). In

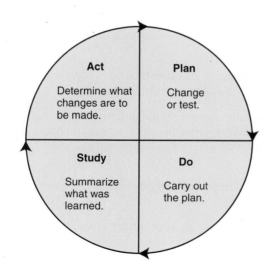

Figure 20-2 The Model for Improvement (From *A Practical Approach to Enhancing Organizational Performance* [p. 7], by G. J. Langley, K. M. Nolan, T. W. Nolan, C. L. Norman, and L. P. Provost, 1996, San Francisco: Jossey-Bass. Reprinted by permission of Jossey-Bass, Inc., a subsidiary of John Wiley & Sons, Inc.)

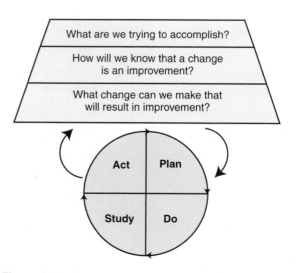

Figure 20-3 The PDSA Cycle (From *A Practical Approach to Enhancing Organizational Performance* [p. 3], by G. J. Langley, K. M. Nolan, T. W. Nolan, C. L. Norman, and L. P. Provost, 1996, San Francisco: Jossey-Bass. Reprinted by permission of Jossey-Bass, Inc., a subsidiary of John Wiley & Sons, Inc.)

August 1997, a collaborative project was initiated with the Robert Wood Johnson Foundation and the Joint Commission on Accreditation of Healthcare Organizations (JCAHO) to integrate pain assessment and management into the standards that JCAHO uses to accredit health care facilities. The pain man-agement standards received approval of the JCAHO board of commissioners in May 1999 and are pub-lished in the accreditation manual for implementa-tion with the 2001 health care organization surveys (Berry & Dahl, 2000). The new pain standard is listed in Table 20-3.

TABLE 20-3	1999–2000 JCAHO Standard for Pain Assessment

Standard

PE.1.4 Pain is assessed in all patients.
(Effective January 1, 2001.)

Intent of PE.1.4

In the initial assessment, the organization identifies patients with pain. When pain is identified, the patient can be treated within the organization or referred for treatment. The scope of treatment is based on the care setting and services provided. A more comprehensive assessment is performed when war-ranted by the patient's condition. This assessment and a measure of pain intensity and quality (e.g., pain character, frequency, location, and duration), appropriate to the patient's age, are recorded in a way that facilitates regular reassessment and follow-up according to criteria developed by the organization.

Examples of Implementation for PE.1.4

1. All patients at admission are asked the following screening or general questions about the pres-ence of pain: Do you have pain now? Have you had pain in the recent past? If the patient responds "yes" to either question, additional assessment data are obtained:

   • Pain intensity (use a pain intensity rating scale appropriate for the patient population; pain intensity is obtained for pain at present, at worst, and at best or least: if at all possible, the pain rating scale is used consistently in the organization and between disciplines);

   • Location (ask the patient to mark on a diagram or point to the site of pain);

   • Quality, patterns of radiation, if any, and character (elicit and record the patient's own words whenever possible);

   • Onset, duration, variations and patterns;

   • Alleviating and aggravating factors;

   • Present pain management regimen and effectiveness;

   • Pain management history (including a medication history, presence of common barriers to reporting pain and using analgesics, past interventions and response, manner of expressing pain);

   • Effects of pain (impact on daily life, function, sleep, appetite, relationships with others, emo-tions, concentration, etc);

   • The patient's pain goal (including pain intensity and goals related to function, activities, quality of life); and

   • Physical exam/observation of the site of pain.

(continues)

Table 20-3 *(continued)*

2. Patients often have more than one site of pain. An assessment system or tools with space to record data on each site is provided on the assessment sheet.

3. A hospital may need to use more than one pain intensity measure, depending on their patient population. For example, a hospital serving both children and adults selects a scale to be used with each of those patient populations. Assessment of cognitively impaired patients may also require assessment of behavioral factors signaling pain or discomfort.

4. Staff are educated about pain assessment and treatment including the barriers to reporting pain and using analgesics. Staff encourage the reporting of pain when a patient and/or family member demonstrates reluctance to discuss pain, denies pain when pain is likely to be present (for example, post-operative, trauma, burns, cardiac emergencies), or does not follow through with prescribed treatments.

5. Pain intensity scales are enlarged and displayed in all areas where assessments are conducted. For organizations using clinical pathways, pain assessment is incorporated in some way, into every appropriate clinical pathway.

   - An organization selects pain intensity measures to insure consistency across departments; for example, the 0-10 scale, Wong Baker FACES Pain Rating Scale (smile-frown), and the Verbal descriptor scale. Adult patients are encouraged to use the 0-10 scale. If they cannot understand or are unwilling to use it, the smile-frown or the verbal scale is used.

   - A unit caring for persons with Alzheimer's disease develops a pain scale for each resident based on their long-standing knowledge of their residents and their knowledge of the common pain syndromes in elderly persons.

   - A pediatric hospital includes, in its introductory information for parents, information about pain and pain assessment, including parents' role in interpreting behavioral changes of their child that may indicate pain or discomfort.

Examples of Evidence of Performance for PE.1.4
(Effective January 1, 2001.)

- Observation of assessment interview
- Interviews with patients and families
- Review of assessment forms or protocols
- Review of clinical records
- Interviews with clinical staff
- Policies and procedures, practice standards, or other processes regarding pain assessment
- Records and content outlines of staff educational offerings
- Educational materials for patients/clients and families

(From *1999–2000 Comprehensive Accreditation Manual for Hospitals: The Official Handbook* (CAMH) [p. PE-8], by Joint Commission on Accreditation of Healthcare Organizations, 1999, Oakbrook Terrace, IL. Reprinted with permission.)

Application of the Model for Improvement to Pain Management

Let's revisit the scenario related to Miss Kelly described at the beginning of this chapter and apply the Model for Improvement.

1. *What are we trying to accomplish?* The overall objective is to reduce or alleviate Miss Kelly's pain, which may be related to a variety of physiological, psychosocial, and spiritual issues. Cancer pain may be related to the breast cancer compression of tissue and nerves, pressure from a pleural effusion, discomfort related to a chest

tube, fear of diagnosis and prognosis, social isolation, and perceived lack of opportunity to participate in spiritual activities.

The nurse can begin by asking Miss Kelly where her pain is and ask her to describe the quality and characteristics of her pain. Miss Kelly may express a range of sensations related to the different sources of her pain. The nurse will ask her to rate her pain on a scale from 0 to 10, with 0 meaning no pain and 10 meaning the highest pain possible. The nurse will then document the pain rating and the degree of relief that medications or other pain relief strategies provide and will also identify any alleviating or aggravating factors. The nurses in conjunction with the other members of the health care team will identify, implement, and document the best strategies that reduce, minimize, or alleviate her pain.

2. *How will we know that a change is an improvement?* Miss Kelly will state that her pain is decreased or relieved. Behaviors that may indicate decreased pain include her verbal or nonverbal expression of pain relief or improved comfort, her ability to reposition herself, and statements such as "I feel more rested," along with an improved mood.

3. *What change can we make that will result in improvement?* To standardize pain management for patients like Miss Kelly, the nursing staff created a protocol that includes a plan to use a trial pain management flow sheet (Figure 20-4). Note that this flow sheet documents the patient's pain status as reported by the patient and pain interventions at various points in time.

Implementation of the PDSA Cycle

The PDSA Cycle can be individual or system focused. It can be used to solve a specific patient problem or to structure strategies to manage groups of patients with common problems. Based on our answers to the three questions, we will apply the PDSA Cycle as follows:

Planning Phase. Once the three Model for Improvement questions have helped staff identify what should be improved, the multidisciplinary staff (RN, MD, pharmacist, and so on) would develop a plan for improvement. The plan would include using

the pain management flow sheet and implementing unit standards for assessing and monitoring patient comfort.

Doing Phase. Nursing staff decided to trial the pain management flow sheet to collect data on Miss Kelly during her hospital stay. All nurses assigned to care for Miss Kelly were asked to complete the documentation tool. Data to be collected would include the patient's pain rating, her nonverbal behaviors, level of consciousness, respiratory rate, side effects, activity, nonpharmacological therapies, pharmacological interventions, and patient teaching.

Studying Phase. Data was collected for a period of 2 weeks. The nurses on the unit met and reviewed the documentation. Several improvements and issues were identified. Documentation of pain assessment and pain parameters had been completed 66% of the time during the 2-week period. Staff nurses reported that they referred to the pain management flow sheet when giving report to the doctor about Miss Kelly's pain status. Pain parameters commonly not documented included assessment and documentation of side effects, activity, and alternate therapy such as nonpharmacological interventions.

Acting Phase. After a meeting with the nurse manager, clinical nurse specialist, doctor, pharmacist, staff nurse, and other health care staff to discuss the findings, the staff agreed to continue to trial the pain management flow sheet for 4 months on all patients admitted to the oncology unit. This next step in the improvement process reflects the use of additional multiple PDSA cycles (Figure 20-5) to improve not only Miss Kelly's individual care but also to improve the total care delivery system.

Multiple Uses of the PDSA Cycle

Multiple PDSA cycles were used to improve care, not just for Miss Kelly but for all patients.

Planning Phase. The inpatient oncology staff agreed to collect data for 4 months using the pain management flow sheet on Miss Kelly and all new patients admitted to the oncology unit. A start date and stop date for the pilot study were identified. The pilot study also included a plan to orient the staff to

PAIN MANAGEMENT FLOW SHEET - DIRECTIONS

1. X PREDOMINANT site of pain on the figures below.
2. Ask patient to rate pain using the Pain Intensity Scale.
3. For VERBAL patients, enter "●" on the flow chart and connect ●----●.
   For NON-VERBAL patients, document in the space provided using the key.
4. Document teaching / analgesia / intervention(s).

	DATE	
	TIME	
	INITIALS	
ASSESSMENT	WORST PAIN 10	
	9	
	8	
	7	
	6	
	5	
	4	
	3	
	2	
	1	
	NO PAIN 0	
	NON-VERBAL BEHAVIOR	
	LOC	
	RESPIRATORY RATE	
	SIDE EFFECTS	
	ACTIVITY	
INTERVENTION	ALTERNATE THERAPY	
	MEDICATION REGIME	
	PCA / EPIDURAL / INTRATHECAL / IV DRIP (Circle) Medication	Concentration /cc
	RATE (cc/hr)	
	BOLUS DOSE (mg)	
	TOTAL cc INFUSED	
	PT / FAMILY TEACHING	

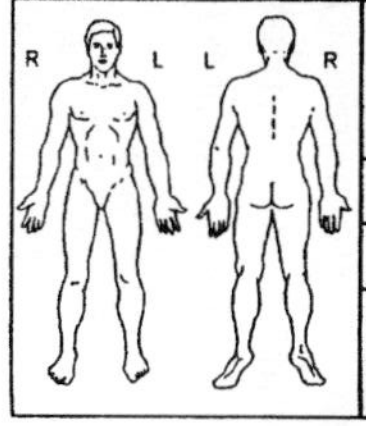

NON-VERBAL BEHAVIORS
G = Grimacing
M = Moaning
R = Restless
— = Not Applicable
Patient-Specific:
1.
2.

LEVEL OF CONSCIOUSNESS (LOC)
0 = Normal Sleep
1 = Awake
2 = Occasionally Drowsy; Easy to arouse
3 = Frequently Drowsy; Easy to arouse
4 = Somnolent; Difficult to arouse

0-10 NUMERIC PAIN INTENSITY SCALE
0 (No Pain) 1 2 3 4 5 6 7 8 9 10 (Pain as bad as you can imagine)

SIDE EFFECTS
N = Nausea
V = Vomiting
CNF = Confusion
C = Constipation
R = Urinary Retention
MSD = Motor / Sensory Deficit
HA = Headache
I = Itching
O = Other
— = Not Applicable

ACTIVITY
B = Bed Rest
C = Chair
A = Ambulation
AA = Anticipated Activity
PT = Physical Therapy

ALTERNATE THERAPY
RP = Reposition
H = Heat
C = Ice Pack
M = Massage
TENS = Tens Unit
D = Distraction
— = Not Applicable

MEDICATION REGIME
(Drug Name/Dose/Route)
1.
2.
3.
4.

PT / FAMILY TEACHING
P = Per Protocol
R = Reinforced
NN = Narrative Note
RSE = Reinforce Side Effects

Figure 20-4 Pain Management Flow Sheet (Copyright 1996 by Oncology Nursing Press, Inc. Reprinted with permission.)

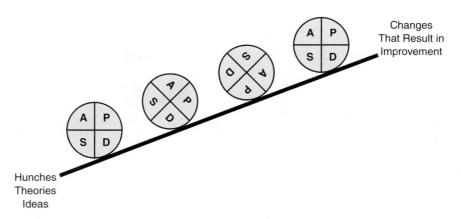

Figure 20-5 Use of Multiple PDSA Cycles (From *A Practical Approach to Enhancing Organizational Performance* [p. 5], by G. J. Langley, K. M. Nolan, T. W. Nolan, C. L. Norman, and L. P. Provost, 1996, San Francisco: Jossey-Bass. Reprinted by permission of Jossey-Bass, Inc., a subsidiary of John Wiley & Sons, Inc.)

the purpose, development, and procedures for using the tool. A plan was also developed to orient the pharmacist and the physicians.

Doing Phase. All nursing staff working on the inpatient oncology unit attended an inservice reviewing the purpose, development, and procedures for using the pain management flow sheet. Once all the staff had completed the orientation, the data collection period was implemented. The pharmacist and physicians were oriented individually by the clinical nurse specialists and provided with an opportunity to ask questions. Data was collected by the nurses for a period of 4 months on all patients admitted to the oncology unit.

Studying Phase. Documentation practices were reviewed after 4 months. Documentation of pain assessment was completed on 78% of all patients' charts on admission to the inpatient unit, 67% were completed 24 hours after admission, and 50% were completed 48 hours after admission. The majority of the unit's nurses agreed that they were using the pain management flow sheet as a basis for their report to the physician regarding the patient's pain status. The pharmacist and the physician reported that they did review the pain management flow sheet approximately 50% of the time, but they most often relied on the staff to verbally share with them the information to improve the patient's pain status.

Acting Phase. A protocol for pain assessment, management, and documentation was developed and integrated with the pain management flow sheet (Figure 20-6). Eventually, this process was published in the oncology literature (Jadlos, Kelman, Marra, & Lanoue, 1996).

This example using the Model for Improvement provides a framework to think about how to apply knowledge and increase the ability to make changes in individual patient care, ultimately resulting in improvement for many patients. The next two applications of the Model for Improvement are still related to the Opening Scenario but focus on other aspects of comfort care, including pressure ulcer and wound management. Benner et al.'s research with critical care nurses provided a description of clinical judgment and thinking-in-action referred to as clinical grasp and clinical forethought. In addition, they identified nine domains of practice common to complex patient care situations. One domain includes providing comfort measures. Benner et al. explain that skin is a point of connection and central or primary to many nursing interventions. Touching a patient; giving a back rub; assessing a wound for erythema, drainage, and odor; changing an ostomy appliance; and caring for an incontinent patient are all points of connection with the patient. One of the most essential aspects of nursing practice is comfort care.

PRESSURE ULCER MANAGEMENT

Pressure ulcers are a significant health concern for all patients with limited mobility and activity levels.

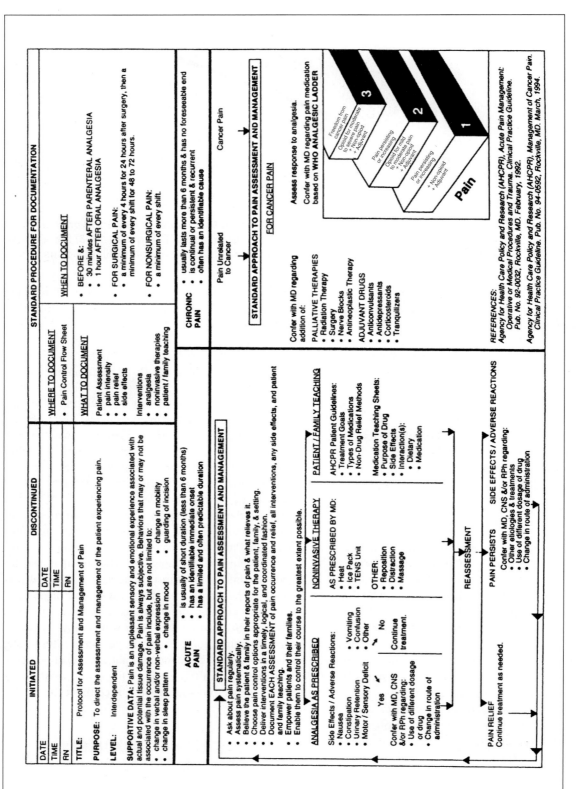
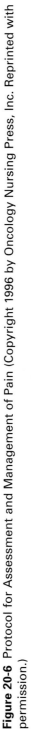

Figure 20-6 Protocol for Assessment and Management of Pain (Copyright 1996 by Oncology Nursing Press, Inc. Reprinted with permission.)

They occur because of a complex interaction among a variety of risk factors in addition to mobility and activity levels. These include environmental factors, such as skin moisture and cutaneous shear forces, as well as intrinsic biological factors, such as a patient's nutritional status and sensory perception. The economic impact of pressure ulcers is significant. The cost in the United States to heal one pressure ulcer has been reported to range from $5,000 to $40,000. Cost analyses reveal that prevention is cost-effective. However, few cost-effectiveness studies measure the cost to achieve measured treatment outcomes (Phillips, 1997).

The Agency for Healthcare Research and Quality (AHRQ) developed national guidelines for dealing with pressure ulcers. *Pressure Ulcers in Adults: Prediction and Prevention* (1992b) is based on research findings and expert multidisciplinary opinion. This guideline first recommends identification of at-risk individuals and identification of the specific factors placing those individuals at risk. The guidelines strongly recommend the use of a validated instrument such as the Braden Scale (Bergstrom, Braden, Laguzza, & Holman, 1987; Bergstrom, Braden, Kemp, Champagne, & Ruby, 1998) (Figure 20-7) to identify patients potentially at risk for the development of pressure ulcers. A protocol should then be initiated for these patients to minimize this risk. The guideline then outlines preventive care to include three categories: skin care and early treatment, mechanical loading and support surfaces, and education.

Prevention of pressure ulcers is imperative when the overall goal is to cure an illness, to rehabilitate the individual, or to help the individual live optimally with a chronic illness. However, when an individual is in the latter stages of a terminal illness and is suffering intractable pain, the primary goal of therapy may be to promote comfort and decrease pain. In this case, frequent repositioning, nutritional support, and other strategies to prevent pressure ulcers may not be consistent with the goal of promoting comfort.

Application of the Model for Improvement to Pressure Ulcer Management

In the scenario presented at the beginning of the chapter, we identified a patient with a need for pain management, and we will now focus on prevention and treatment of pressure ulcers in this same patient. Since admission, Miss Kelly's mobility was limited to bed rest because of multiple factors, including presence of a chest tube, shortness of breath, right arm lymphedema, and metastatic left leg pain from her breast cancer. The Braden Scale for Predicting Pressure Sore Risk demonstrated she was at high risk, with a score of 12 initially and daily for 2 weeks. The preventive interventions from the Skin Care Treatment Plan for Actual Skin Breakdown were implemented upon admission (see Figure 20-8). A dynamic alternating air mattress was placed on Miss Kelly's bed. Miss Kelly's appetite was poor and her serum albumin was low at 1.8 g/dl. When she was repositioned, Miss Kelly continued to complain of a pulling, stretching, sharp pain radiating from the thigh to the lower leg. She rated the pain as an 8 on a scale of 0 to 10. She had started to take oral Tylenol with codeine as needed every 3 to 4 hours. The radiation oncologist initiated a course of radiation therapy to the left leg to help control the leg pain. Her limited mobility necessitated the use of a bedpan for urination and defecation. As a result of her limited mobility and repeated use of the bedpan, Miss Kelly developed a sacral decubitus ulcer and open painful superficial skin breakdown between the buttocks. She tended to lie on her back in bed continuously. When asked why she laid on her back all the time, she stated that her left leg hurt when she moved and that she was afraid her leg would break if she moved the wrong way.

We apply the Model for Improvement and start with the three questions:

1. *What are we trying to accomplish?* The overall goal is to treat and heal the sacral decubitus ulcer, treat and heal the open excoriated skin between the buttocks, and prevent further skin breakdown. The primary risk factors for pressure ulcers are immobility and limited activity levels, so an additional overall goal in managing this patient for pressure ulcer treatment would include improvement in her mobility and activity level.

2. *How will we know that a change is an improvement?* Miss Kelly's sacral decubitus ulcer and the open skin between her buttocks will show signs of healing. Miss Kelly will verbalize less discomfort related to the open skin between her buttocks. Miss Kelly will demonstrate increased

BRADEN SCALE FOR PREDICTING PRESSURE SORE RISK - *Complete* **DAILY**				SCORE
Total Score of 12 or less = high risk for pressure ulcer development				
SENSORY PERCEPTION ability to respond meaningfully to pressure-related discomfort	**1 Completely Limited** Unresponsive (does not moan, flinch, or grasp) to painful stimuli, due to diminished level of consciousness or sedation. **OR** limited ability to feel pain over most of body surface.	**2 Very Limited** Responds only to painful stimuli. Cannot communicate discomfort except by moaning or restlessness. **OR** has a sensory impairment which limits the ability to feel pain or discomfort over 1/2 of body.	**3 Slightly Limited** Responds to verbal commands, but cannot always communicate discomfort or need to be turned. **OR** has some sensory impairment which limits ability to feel pain or discomfort in 1 or 2 extremities.	**4 No Impairment** Responds to verbal commands. Has no sensory deficit which would limit ability to feel or voice pain or discomfort.	
ACTIVITY degree of physical activity	**1 Bedfast** Confined to bed.	**2 Chairfast** Ability to walk severely limited or non-existent. Cannot bear own weight and/or must be assisted into chair or wheelchair.	**3 Walks Occasionally** Walks occasionally during day, but for very short distances with or without assistance. Spends majority of each shift in bed or chair.	**4 Walks Frequently** Walks outside the room at least twice a day and inside room at least once every 2 hours during waking hours.	
MOBILITY ability to change and control body position	**1 Completely Immobile** Does not make even slight changes in body or extremity position without assistance.	**2 Very Limited** Makes occasional slight changes in body or extremity position but unable to make frequent or significant changes independently.	**3 Slightly Limited** Makes frequent though slight changes in body or extremity position independently.	**4 No Limitations** Makes major and frequent changes in position without assistance.	
NUTRITION usual food intake pattern	**1 Very Poor** Never eats a complete meal. Rarely eats more than 1/3 of any food offered. Eats 2 servings or less of protein (meat or dairy products) per day. Takes fluids poorly. Does not take a liquid dietary supplement. **OR** is NPO and/or maintained on clear liquids or IV's for more than 5 days.	**2 Probably Inadequate** Rarely eats a complete meal and generally eats only about 1/2 of any food offered. Protein intake includes only 3 servings of meat or dairy products per day. Occasionally will take a dietary supplement. **OR** receives less than optimum amount of liquid diet or tube feeding.	**3 Adequate** Eats over half of most meals. Eats a total of 4 servings of protein (meat, dairy products) each day. Occasionally will refuse a meal, but will usually take a supplement if offered. **OR** is on a tube feeding or TPN regimen which probably meets most of nutritional needs.	**4 Excellent** Eats most of every meal. Never refuses a meal. Usually eats a total of 4 or more servings of meat and dairy products. Occasionally eats between meals. Does not require supplementation.	
FRICTION & SHEAR	**1 Problem** Requires moderate to maximum assistance in moving. Complete lifting without sliding against sheets is impossible. Frequently slides down in bed or chair, requiring frequent repositioning with maximum assistance. Spasticity, contractures or agitation leads to almost constant friction.	**2 Potential Problem** Moves feebly or requires minimum assistance. During a move skin probably slides to some extent against sheets, chair, restraints, or other devices. Maintains relatively good position in chair or bed most of the time but occasionally slides down.	**3 No Apparent Problem** Moves in bed and in chair independently and has sufficient muscle strength to lift up completely during move. Maintains good position in bed or chair at all times.		
MOISTURE degree to which skin is exposed to moisture	**1 Constantly Moist** Skin is kept moist almost constantly by perspiration, urine, etc. Dampness is detected every time patient is moved or turned.	**2 Very Moist** Skin is often, but not always moist. Linen must be changed at least once a shift.	**3 Occasionally Moist** Skin is occasionally moist, requiring an extra linen change approximately once a day.	**4 Rarely Moist** Skin is usually dry, linen only requires changing at routine intervals.	
Total Score of 12 or less = high risk.				**TOTAL SCORE**	
IMPAIRED TISSUE PERFUSION	Hemoglobin less than 12.6 gm/dl			Problem (/)	
PREDISPOSING MEDICAL CONDITION	Cardiovascular, Respiratory and/or Diabetes			Problem (/)	
DIARRHEA				Problem (/)	

Total Score = 17 or less without skin breakdown initiate Protocol for POTENTIAL Skin Breakdown.
For Stage 1, 2A, 2B, 3, and/or 4 skin breakdown initiate Protocol for ACTUAL Skin Breakdown.

Figure 20-7 Braden Scale for Predicting Pressure Sore Risk (Copyright Barbara Braden and Nancy Bergstrom, 1987. Reprinted with permission.)

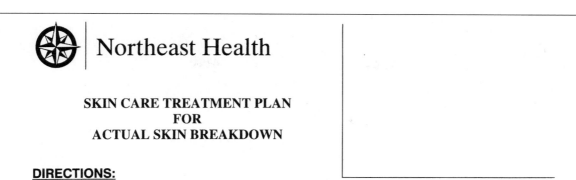

Northeast Health

SKIN CARE TREATMENT PLAN
FOR
ACTUAL SKIN BREAKDOWN

DIRECTIONS:

1. Initiate the Protocol for Treatment of Actual Skin Breakdown.
2. Document the skin care regimen for **Preventive Interventions** as follows:
    a. Enter the start or change date and your initials in the space provided.
    b. In the same column, place a check mark (✔) in the space provided to indicate selected interventions.

		START/ CHANGE DATE				COMMENTS
		INITIAL				
NURSING INTERVENTIONS	INCONTINENCE	Skin Cleanser / Dry Thoroughly				
		Skin Barrier Cream				
	PRESSURE / FRICTION / SHEAR	Air Mattress				
		Elevate heels off bed				
		HOB lower than 30 degrees				
		Assistive devices when transferring				
		If chairfast: Assist back to bed after 2 hours maximum in chair (bid or tid)				
		q2h Turning Schedule				
		Encourage patient to change position or to shift weight frequently.				
		Range of Motion exercises bid				
		Chair Air Cushion				
		Foot Waffle (check) ❑ R ❑ L ❑ Both				
	NUTRITION	Assist with meals				
		Monitor nutritional intake				
		Consult Dietician				
	OTHER	Physical Therapy				

FORM #60601 (6/98)

Figure 20-8 Skin Care Treatment Plan for Actual Skin Breakdown (Courtesy of Northeast Health Samaritan Hospital, Acute Care Division, Troy, NY.)

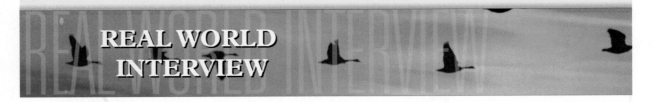

REAL WORLD INTERVIEW

It was very satisfying to care for Miss Kelly. I think she felt cared for and made progress despite the severity of her illness. As it turned out, she had a lot of different worries and concerns that she did not tell us about at first. We were able to see her almost every day, and she grew to trust us. We got to know her and were able to engage her in planning and delivering her care. Miss Kelly said she was afraid about her condition and its treatment. Her physical care was complicated. If her nursing care was not coordinated and monitored closely, she would not have progressed as well as she did and would have developed unnecessary problems. I think that the continuity in care provided by the acute care nurse practitioners helped the entire staff to provide quality care for Miss Kelly, from nursing to physical therapy to medicine to discharge planning. I became a nurse practitioner after being a nurse for 20 years. It has been good for me as a person and as a nurse. I have always thought that there has been a gap between medicine and nursing; that is, that the two have the same goal but very different ways of achieving it. I think that the ACNP working in the hospital fills that gap. My relationship with doctors and nurses has changed. There is more of a team spirit. The patients are so sick, and it is a very hard time for their families. More than ever, they deserve a high level of nursing care. Many families have been caring for patients at home and have an intense interest in them and how they are cared for by us. The nurse practitioners for the Wound, Skin and Ostomy Service spend much of their time coordinating this care. The nurses work hard each day to help our patients. They get very tired and often wonder if what they are doing makes any difference. Their efforts deserve respect and recognition. What better way to do this than to work side by side with them and tell them? Hopefully, they will be inspired to keep going and find new ways to develop their practice.

Mary Anne Jadlos, ACNP
Nurse Practitioner—Wound, Skin, Ostomy Service

mobility in bed and increased activity such as getting out of bed with assistance and sitting in a chair.

3. *What change can we make that will result in improvement?* We will initiate the Protocol for Treatment of Actual Skin Breakdown (Figure 20-9). We will consult the acute care nurse practitioner for additional recommendations regarding treatment of the open skin. We will consult other members of the health care team such as physicians, physical therapists, a nutritionist, and so on. We will conduct a multidisciplinary patient care conference to coordinate strategies for pressure relief, skin care, mobility, and nutrition. Finally, we will involve Miss Kelly and decide on her goals and care recommendations together.

Implementation of the PDSA Cycle

Based on our answers to the three Model for Improvement questions, we will begin the PDSA Cycle as follows:

Planning Phase. A multidisciplinary patient care conference including the patient and her brother, nursing staff, the ACNP, the physician, the physical therapists, the nutritionist, and the clinical resource manager was held. All conference members agreed that a change in Miss Kelly's skin care regimen and activity and mobility was necessary in addition to pain and anxiety relief measures. The nurse practitioner wrote orders for management of the sacral ulcer and the open skin on Miss Kelly's buttocks. A physical therapy consultation was ordered for strengthening exercises

(continues on page 419)

OSHA Category I

TITLE: **PROTOCOL FOR TREATMENT OF ACTUAL SKIN BREAKDOWN**

PURPOSE: **To promote the healing of skin breakdown based on principles of moist wound healing.**

LEVEL: **Independent**

Exception: Use of this protocol for patients with skin breakdown related to medical conditions such as vascular insufficiency or cellulitis must be approved by the physician.

SUPPORTIVE DATA: Wound healing is a complex process including removal of causes of breakdown (pressure, friction, chemical irritation) and the promotion of an environment conducive to tissue healing.

**Infection should be suspected if any of the following are present:

- pus
- increased redness
- change in color of exudate
- peri-wound edema
- elevated WBC count
- uncharacteristic odor
- elevated body temperature

Wound(s) cannot be accurately staged if eschar is present. Wound eschar (scab) is thick, fibrin containing necrotic tissue.

STAGE 1	STAGE 2A	STAGE 2B
Intact skin, erythema, heat, swelling, pain.	Intact skin, erythema, heat, swelling, blister, no drainage.	Skin not intact, scant to moderate bleeding drainage, granulation tissue present. Superficial. Skin tear. Shallow crater.

STANDARD PROCEDURES FOR SKIN BREAKDOWN

1. Complete Braden Scale for Predicting Pressure Sore Risk DAILY

2. Urinary / Fecal Incontinence-related Measures:
   - Wash soiled area and dry thoroughly
   - Consult M.D. regarding condom or indwelling catheter, if necessary
   - Apply barrier ointment to protect skin
   - Apply Fecal Incontinence Collector if Braden Score = 14 or less AND diarrhea

3. Pressure-related Measures:
   - Place air mattress on bed if Braden Score = 14 or less
   - Elevate heels off bed
   - Institute turning schedule
   - Keep HOB lower than 30 degrees, unless higher angle required
   - Utilize assistive devices when transferring or moving patient
   - Encourage maximum mobility as patient condition warrants

   If chairfast:
   - Place chair cushion if patient is unable to shift weight
   - Assist patient back to bed after 2 hours maximum in chair (bid or tid)
   - Assist patient with range of motion exercises at least bid

Impaired Mental Status

No
- Encourage patient to change position or to shift weight frequently and instruct regarding rationale

Yes
- Consult with M.D. regarding Physical Therapy evaluation and/or use of assistive devices

Impaired Nutritional Status
(Braden Nutrition Subscore = 1)

No
- Monitor nutritional intake q shift
- Provide assistance with meals, as necessary

Yes
- Consult Dietician/M.D. regarding nutritional needs
- Monitor nutritional intake q shift
- Provide assistance with meals, as necessary

Impaired Tissue Perfusion
(Hgb less than 12.6 gm/dl)

No
- Consult M.D. regarding routine CBC

Yes
- Consult ET Nurse
- Consult M.D. regarding routine CBC

Rx: ALL STANDARD PROCEDURES FOR SKIN BREAKDOWN

+

**Infected **

No
Rinse with NS
Dry intact skin

Hydrocolloid dressing

Polyurethane Foam dressing

Open to air

Yes
Notify M.D.

Normal Saline Dressing

Dressing Change Parameters:

- leakage of drainage
- interruption in dressing integrity (i.e. loose, wrinkled, or curled edges)

FOR POLYURETHANE FOAM DRESSINGS:
- If intact, change every 5 - 7 days

FOR HYDROCOLLOID DRESSINGS:
- if intact, change:
  every 2 - 3 days

- Expect foul odor and yellow drainage with dressing removal.

Original: 8/8/89

REVIEW: _____

REVISION: 11/11/92
                    6/9/93
                    5/10/95
                    8/9/95
                    1/14/98

(continues)

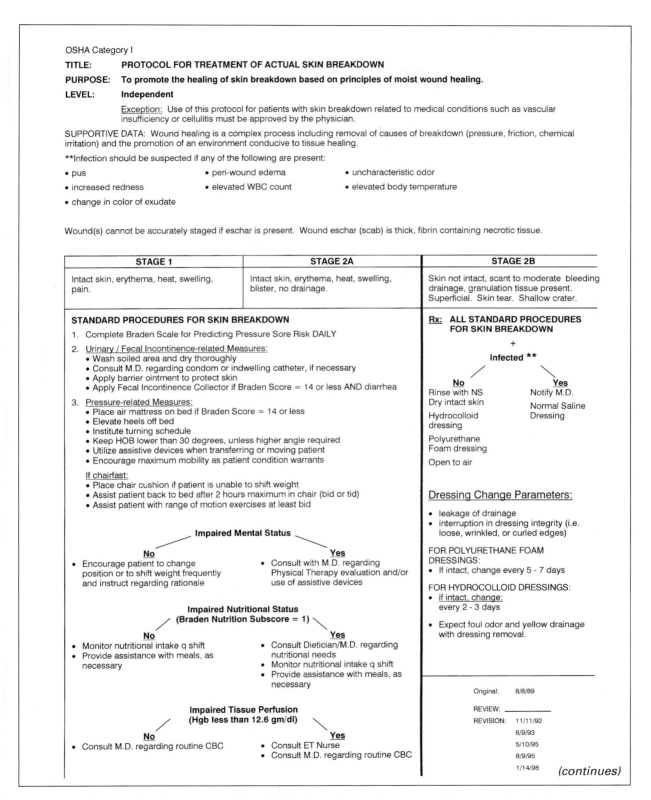

Figure 20-9 Protocol for Treatment of Actual Skin Breakdown (Courtesy of Northeast Health Samaritan Hospital, Acute Care Division, Troy, NY.)

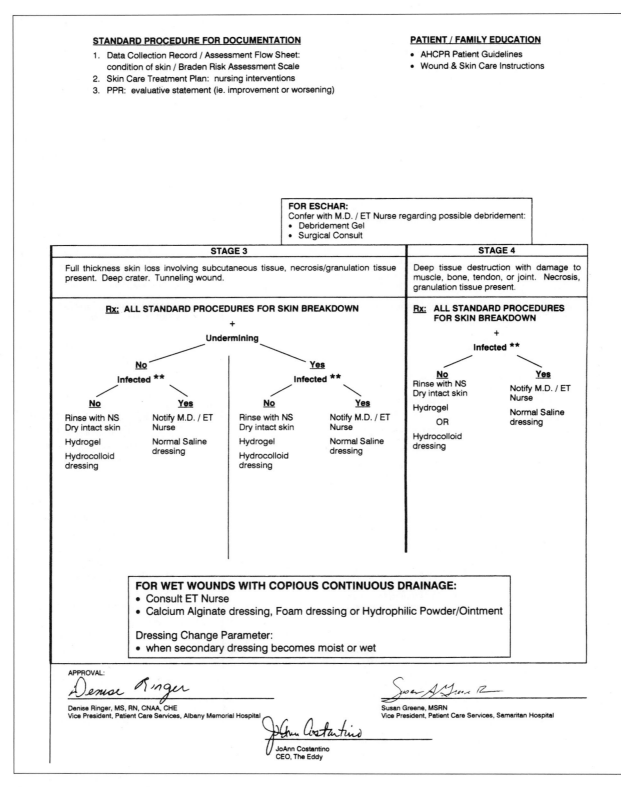

STANDARD PROCEDURE FOR DOCUMENTATION

1. Data Collection Record / Assessment Flow Sheet: condition of skin / Braden Risk Assessment Scale
2. Skin Care Treatment Plan: nursing interventions
3. PPR: evaluative statement (ie. improvement or worsening)

PATIENT / FAMILY EDUCATION

- AHCPR Patient Guidelines
- Wound & Skin Care Instructions

FOR ESCHAR:
Confer with M.D. / ET Nurse regarding possible debridement:
- Debridement Gel
- Surgical Consult

STAGE 3	STAGE 4
Full thickness skin loss involving subcutaneous tissue, necrosis/granulation tissue present. Deep crater. Tunneling wound.	Deep tissue destruction with damage to muscle, bone, tendon, or joint. Necrosis, granulation tissue present.

STAGE 3

Rx: ALL STANDARD PROCEDURES FOR SKIN BREAKDOWN
+
Undermining

No — Infected **
- **No**
  Rinse with NS
  Dry intact skin
  Hydrogel
  Hydrocolloid dressing
- **Yes**
  Notify M.D. / ET Nurse
  Normal Saline dressing

Yes — Infected **
- **No**
  Rinse with NS
  Dry intact skin
  Hydrogel
  Hydrocolloid dressing
- **Yes**
  Notify M.D. / ET Nurse
  Normal Saline dressing

STAGE 4

Rx: ALL STANDARD PROCEDURES FOR SKIN BREAKDOWN
+
Infected **

- **No**
  Rinse with NS
  Dry intact skin
  Hydrogel
  OR
  Hydrocolloid dressing
- **Yes**
  Notify M.D. / ET Nurse
  Normal Saline dressing

FOR WET WOUNDS WITH COPIOUS CONTINUOUS DRAINAGE:
- Consult ET Nurse
- Calcium Alginate dressing, Foam dressing or Hydrophilic Powder/Ointment

Dressing Change Parameter:
- when secondary dressing becomes moist or wet

APPROVAL:

Denise Ringer, MS, RN, CNAA, CHE
Vice President, Patient Care Services, Albany Memorial Hospital

Susan Greene, MSRN
Vice President, Patient Care Services, Samaritan Hospital

JoAnn Costantino
CEO, The Eddy

Figure 20-9 *(continued)*

(continued from page 416)

and non-weight-bearing instruction for the left leg when out of bed. The Protocol for Treatment of Actual Skin Breakdown was continued to guide interventions and the Skin Integrity Flow Chart was used to document the skin care treatment plan for the sacral and buttock ulcers (see Figure 20-10). The Wound and Skin Care Instructions in Figure 20-11 were followed. Hydrogel dressings were initiated twice a day to the open skin of the buttocks and to the sacral ulcer.

A specific schedule of positioning and activities was developed that included the following:

- Less use of pillows to prop Miss Kelly in bed
- Encouragement of the patient to turn herself and shift her weight frequently

- Use of staff assistance to get Miss Kelly out of bed every day for all meals
- Use of staff assistance to help Miss Kelly use the commode instead of the bedpan whenever possible

Doing Phase. The staff nurses implemented the agreed-upon plan of care. They documented the status of Miss Kelly's skin breakdown and worked with the nurse practitioners to assess the progress of the patient's wounds and mobility status. Physical therapists worked with the patient every day on range of motion, transfer techniques, and non-weight-bearing measures. The dietician also was consulted to assess Miss Kelly's nutritional status and made dietary

(continues on page 423)

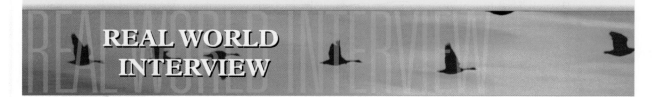

REAL WORLD INTERVIEW

I think every person deserves the kind of care you would want for your own mother and father. This is the attitude I take in caring for my patients. These people are so sick and their families need a lot of support. I do get frustrated because sometimes I don't have enough time to give them everything they need. Miss Kelly is typical of most patients. Her care was very involved and time consuming. The nurse practitioners are a very valuable member of our team. For Miss Kelly, we were able to call them to help us determine how to manage the open tumor on her chest wall. They evaluated not just her draining wound but they also evaluated her overall condition. A specific treatment plan for dressing changes was outlined. This made it possible for us to perform this to give the same care no matter what nurse cared for this patient. Also, the nurse practitioners performed dressing changes themselves frequently. When they did, they also gave Miss Kelly a bath. This was very helpful to us. The nurse practitioners make us feel like we are a part of a team. You can count on them to be there for us. They are easy to talk to and want to know and use our ideas. If we had any concerns or problems about Miss Kelly, we talked to them. For instance, we were having problems with bleeding from the tumor with dressing changes. This made us and the patient nervous. The nurse practitioners listened to us and shared this concern. They tried drenching the old dressing with water before removing it and put more hydrogel on the tumor and used an abdominal pad instead of gauze so that the dressing would not stick to the wound. Once they saw that this worked, they wrote detailed instructions for the nursing staff. The staff really respect the input of the nurse practitioners. They help us with a lot of different problems. In Miss Kelly's case, we found we were not only talking to them about the dressing changes but about her pain control and her poor mobility. Skin care and preventing pressure ulcers was a big concern for us. The nurse practitioners were able to order a special air mattress, and they monitored the condition of Miss Kelly's skin. Having the nurse practitioners involved is helpful because we always knew we could call someone if we needed help. Also, if my assignment changed, I knew Miss Kelly was still being seen almost every day by someone who knew her.

Susan DuPont, LPN
Staff Nurse

SKIN INTEGRITY FLOW CHART

DIRECTIONS:

1. Number wound(s) and circle location on figure(s) below.
2. Document assessment of wound(s) WHEN DRESSING IS CHANGED (at least weekly in home and long-term care settings) using the

Assessment Key:

* i = intact	P = pink	R = red	S = slough	Y = yellow	W = white	E = eschar
** S = superficial (or record in cm.)						
*** S = serosanguinous	B = bloody	Y = yellow	G = green	0 = none		
**** 0 = none	F = foul (possible infection)	C = characteristic				

SKIN CARE TREATMENT PLAN

DIRECTIONS:

1. Document the skin care regimen for **Treatment of Actual Skin Breakdown** as follows:
   a. Enter the start/change date and your initials in the space provided.
   b. Enter the PLANNED FREQUENCY of dressing change in the space provided.

Site # _____
Location _____

		START/ CHANGE DATE			
Wound Type		INITIAL			
DRESSING	Calcium Alginate				
	Foam				
	Hydrocolloid				
	Polyurethane Foam				
	NS Wet-to-Dry				
OINTMENT/POWDER	Debridement Gel				
	Hydrogel				
	Hydrophilic Ointment				
	Hydrophilic Powder				
OTHER	Open to Air				

Date								
Initial								
Stage 1, 2A, 2B, 3, 4 or SW (surgical wound)								
Appearance of wound *								
Appearance of wound margins *								
Size (cm.)								
Depth * *								
Drainage * * *								
Odor * * * *								
Surrounding Skin inflammation (Y / N)								
Surrounding Skin maceration (Y / N)								
Undermining (Y / N)								

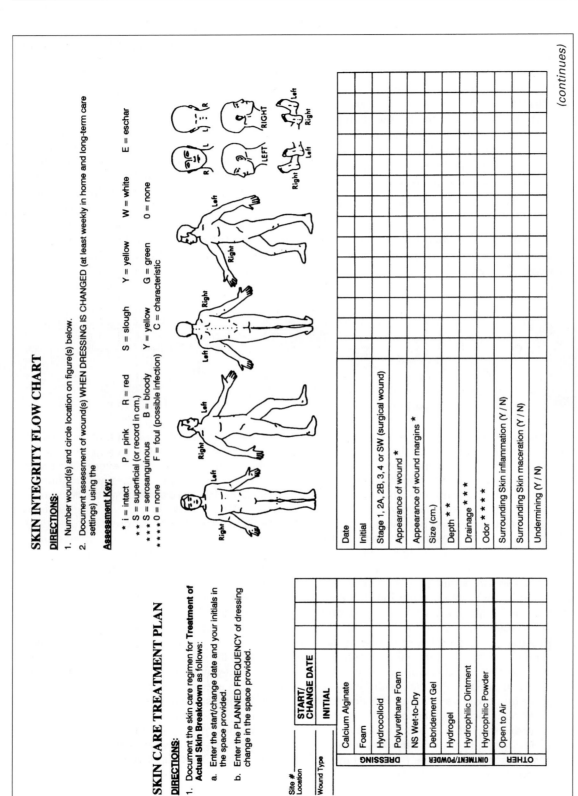

(continues)

Figure 20-10 Skin Integrity Flow Chart (Courtesy of Northeast Health Samaritan Hospital, Acute Care Division, Troy, NY.)

Site # _____
Location _____

		START/		
		CHANGE DATE		
		INITIAL		

Wound Type _____

DRESSING	Calcium Alginate			
	Foam			
	Hydrocolloid			
	Polyurethane Foam			
	NS Wet-to-Dry			
OINTMENT/POWDER	Debridement Gel			
	Hydrogel			
	Hydrophilic Ointment			
	Hydrophilic Powder			
OTHER	Open to Air			

cm 1 2 3 4 5 6 7 8 9 10 11 12

Date
Initial
Stage 1, 2A, 2B, 3, 4 or SW (surgical wound)
Appearance of wound *
Appearance of wound margins *
Size (cm.)
Depth * *
Drainage * * *
Odor * * * *
Surrounding Skin inflammation (Y / N)
Surrounding Skin maceration (Y / N)
Undermining (Y / N)

Assessment Key:
* i = intact   P = pink   R = red   S = slough   Y = yellow   W = white   E = eschar
* * S = superficial (or record in cm.)
* * * S = serosanguinous   B = bloody   Y = yellow   G = green   0 = none
* * * * 0 = none   F = foul (possible infection)   C = characteristic

Site # _____
Location _____

		START/		
		CHANGE DATE		
		INITIAL		

Wound Type _____

DRESSING	Calcium Alginate			
	Foam			
	Hydrocolloid			
	Polyurethane Foam			
	NS Wet-to-Dry			
OINTMENT/POWDER	Debridement Gel			
	Hydrogel			
	Hydrophilic Ointment			
	Hydrophilic Powder			
OTHER	Open to Air			

Date
Initial
Stage 1, 2A, 2B, 3, 4 or SW (surgical wound)
Appearance of wound *
Appearance of wound margins *
Size (cm.)
Depth * *
Drainage * * *
Odor * * * *
Surrounding Skin inflammation (Y / N)
Surrounding Skin maceration (Y / N)
Undermining (Y / N)

Figure 20-10 (continued)

WOUND & SKIN CARE INSTRUCTIONS

LOCATION	PRODUCT	INDICATIONS / GOAL	PROCEDURE
		DRESSINGS	
	CALCIUM ALGINATE **Sorbsan / Calcicare / Tegagen** *Change once a day or if drainage strikes through*	Stage 3/4 ulcer (ie. surgical incision, venous or diabetic ulcer) / copious, continuous drainage/infected or non-infected wound/abdomen, foot, bony prominence **GOAL** *Absorb drainage & promote granulation*	1. Place dressing into wound filling all "dead space". 2. Cover with 4 x 4 gauze dressing. 3. Secure with paper/transparent tape.
	FOAM **Poly-Mem** *Change as directed*	Stage 2/3/4 ulcer (ie. skin tear, stasis ulcer) / moderate to copious, continuous drainage/clean wound bed **GOAL** *Absorb drainage & prevent skin maceration*	1. Place dressing over wound bed. 2. Secure edges with paper/transparent/ Hy-Tape.
	HYDROCOLLOID **Restore / Duoderm / Tegasorb** *Change every 2 to 3 days*	Stage 2/3/4 ulcer (ie. clean, sloughing or necrotic pressure ulcer) / scant to moderate drainage **GOAL** *Debride necrotic tissue & maintain moist wound bed*	1. Remove paper backing, apply dressing. 2. Secure edges with paper/transparent/ Hy-Tape.
	POLYURETHANE FOAM **Flexzan** *Change every 5 to 7 days*	Stage 2B ulcer (ie. skin tear / abrasion) / scant drainage / clean wound bed **GOAL** *Facilitate healing & prevent further damage*	1. Wipe peri-wound skin with "skin prep" or alcohol prep, allow to dry. 2. Remove paper backing, apply dressing. 3. Wipe edges with "skin prep" or tape.
	NORMAL SALINE (NS) WET-TO-DRY *Change (indicate frequency)*	Stage 2/3/4 ulcer (ie. clean, sloughing, necrotic wound bed) / moderate to no drainage **GOAL** *Debride necrotic tissue*	1. Moisten gauze with NS & wring out. 2. Open gauze & place into wound bed, with all surfaces in contact with the gauze. 3. Cover with another gauze & ABD pad. 4. Secure with paper/transparent tape.
		OINTMENTS / POWDERS	
	DEBRIDEMENT GEL **Santyl / Elase / Silvadene** *Change once a day*	Stage 3/4 ulcer (ie. wound with sloughing, necrotic tissue or eschar) / moderate to no drainage **GOAL** *Liquify devitalized tissue*	1. Apply thin coat of barrier ointment to peri-wound skin. 2. Apply debridement ointment to wound bed. 3. Cover with 4 x 4 gauze dressing. 4. Secure with paper/transparent tape.
	HYDROGEL **Restore / Solosite / Tegagel** *Change once a day*	Stage 3 ulcer (ie. abrasion / pressure ulcer) / no drainage / clean wound bed **GOAL** *Maintain moist wound bed*	1. Measure _____ tablespoon(s) gel. 2. Place into wound bed, filling all "dead space". 3. Cover with 4 x 4 gauze dressing. 4. Secure with paper/transparent tape.
	HYDROPHILIC OINTMENT **Dermagran-B** *Change once a day*	Stage 3/4 ulcer (ie. diabetic ulcer) / scant drainage / clean wound bed **GOAL** *Provide topical nutrients (zinc) & maintain moist wound bed*	1. Measure _____ tablespoon(s) gel. 2. Place into wound bed, filling all "dead space". 3. Cover with 4 x 4 gauze dressing. 4. Secure with paper/transparent tape.
	HYDROPHILIC POWDER **Multidex / Chronicure** *Change once a day*	Stage 3/4 ulcer (ie. foot, pressure, or vascular ulcer) / scant to moderate drainage / clean, sloughing wound bed **GOAL** *Absorb drainage, cleanse & maintain moist wound bed*	1. Apply thin layer of powder to wound bed. 2. Cover with a 4 x 4 gauze dressing. 3. Secure with paper/transparent tape.
		DEVICES	
	AIR MATTRESS	Pressure ulcer	Maintain on bed AT ALL TIMES
	CHAIR AIR CUSHION	**GOAL** *Relieve / reduce pressure from bony prominences*	Maintain on chair AT ALL TIMES
	FOOT WAFFLE BOOTS		Maintain on feet/lower legs AT ALL TIMES
		OTHER SKIN CARE DIRECTIONS	

IF QUESTIONS CALL ET NURSE: **Phone:**

Figure 20-11 Wound and Skin Care Instructions (Courtesy of Northeast Health Samaritan Hospital, Acute Care Division, Troy, NY.)

(continued from page 419)

recommendations, which were implemented. Discharge planning was initiated by the clinical resource manager with input from the multidisciplinary team.

Studying Phase. Five days after the proposed plan of care was implemented, the open skin between Miss Kelly's buttocks was completely healed. The sacral ulcer, however, looked the same regarding size, depth, appearance of the wound bed, inflammation, and drainage. The patient had received three cycles of chemotherapy and had completed a course of radiation therapy to the left leg. Miss Kelly's left leg pain was minimal, with the patient giving the pain a score of 3 at its worst level. Miss Kelly was making every effort to get out of bed into the chair. In fact, she tried to get out of bed to the chair on her own at first. She thought the doctor wanted her to do this. After this unsuccessful attempt, the nursing staff and physician reinforced to Miss Kelly that she ask for assistance for all transfers. She did this. She did not change her position much when in bed, however. She stated that she wanted to sit up in bed most of the time and be on her back so she could look out the doorway.

Acting Phase. The nursing staff decided to continue the same care regime for the skin of Miss Kelly's buttocks: The ACNP continued to monitor the sacral ulcer with the staff. A revised local wound care regimen was implemented. The staff agreed to continue the PDSA Cycle until there was evidence of improvement in the condition of the sacral ulcer. Miss Kelly's level of mobility and activity would continue to be monitored and would progress as tolerated.

WOUND MANAGEMENT

Patients with cancer may experience disruptions in skin integrity related to the disease or its treatment. Alteration in skin integrity may be caused by breast cancer with chest wall involvement as in the case of Miss Kelly. Breast tumors are often very vascular and, if superficially eroded, may bleed easily. Chemotherapy-related lowering of the blood counts, particularly white blood cells and platelets, may result in complications such as bleeding or infection.

Tumors also are frequently necrotic and have varying amounts of foul-smelling drainage. Therefore, local wound care needs to incorporate measures to maintain a moist environment, aid debridement, promote epithelialization, and increase comfort. Care must be taken to control exudate and odor, minimize frequency of dressing changes, and remove dressings without trauma.

Application of the Model for Improvement to Wound Management

Miss Kelly, as noted previously, has metastatic breast cancer with a large right breast tumor and right arm lymphedema. The right breast tissue was essentially replaced by tumor and the superficial skin had eroded, producing a draining, bloody, malodorous, necrotic wound. The medical oncologist recommended systemic chemotherapy to decrease the size of the breast tumor and treat the metastatic spread of the disease. Potential side effects of this chemotherapy included lowering of the blood counts with risk of infection and bleeding, hair loss, nausea, vomiting, neuropathy, cardiotoxicity, and muscle and joint aches. These side effects were reviewed with Miss Kelly and her brother. An Infusaport was placed for intravenous access, and the chemotherapy treatments were started. Lowered blood counts related to her chemotherapy did occur and resulted in intermittent bleeding from the breast wound. This complicated Miss Kelly's care.

We start with the three questions:

1. *What are we trying to accomplish?* Our goals are to prevent wound infection and bleeding and control odor and exudate. We will work to facilitate epithelialization, if possible, and promote comfort and preserve Miss Kelly's sense of body image.

2. *How will we know that a change is an improvement?* The size of the wound bed will decrease. There will be minimal or no bleeding from the wound bed. There will be no signs of wound infection.

3. *What change can we make that will result in improvement?* We will consult the acute care nurse practitioner for wound care recommendations. We will conduct a multidisciplinary care conference to coordinate the wound care strategies. Wound care

of Miss Kelly's right breast wound can be coordinated with selected members of the nursing staff who are familiar with the patient. The ACNP may initially change the dressing on a regular basis to ensure consistency, optimize wound healing, and prevent complications.

Implementation of the PDSA Cycle

Based on our answers to the three questions, we will begin the PDSA Cycle as follows.

Planning Phase. The nursing staff and the ACNP examined the right breast wound. Based on this examination, the ACNP recommended a regimen of hydrogel gauze dressing changes twice daily. The ACNP explained to the staff and the patient that the use of a hydrogel dressing would maintain a moist environment, conform easily to the wound, and reduce pain. Removal of the secondary dressing would be easier because of the moist, nonadherent wound surface. Hydrogel also provides some autolytic debridement through softening of necrotic tissue (Bates-Jensen, 1998). If there was a significant amount of loosened necrotic tissue, consideration would be given to removal of the tissue by debridement. Any debridement would be performed by the ACNP or physician. In addition, an antibiotic spray solution for application onto the gauze was prescribed to help decrease the foul odor. The dressing was to be stabilized using mesh netting around the patient's trunk to alleviate the need for taping onto the patient's skin.

Doing Phase. The staff nurses implemented the agreed-upon plan of care. The ACNPs assisted by changing the dressing two to three times a week and communicating with the staff. Miss Kelly's platelet levels were monitored closely and debridement of the wound bed was not performed on the days that the platelet counts were low. If bleeding occurred during the dressing change, the nursing staff was instructed not to apply pressure directly on the wound area but to hold a dry gauze next to the site until the bleeding stopped.

Studying Phase. Eight weeks after the implementation of the proposed plan of care, the patient had received three cycles of chemotherapy. During this time, the patient received antibiotic therapy and colony-stimulating factors (CSFs) to maintain her white blood count and reduce the risk of infection. The topical antibiotic spray was effective in eliminating wound odor. The breast wound had dramatically decreased in size, with 90% of the original wound bed covered by epithelial tissue. The remainder of the wound bed was clean with minimal serous drainage. The patient was much more comfortable as a result.

Acting Phase. As the breast wound continued to heal, the hydrogel was discontinued. The ACNP continued to monitor the breast wound in conjunction with the nursing staff. A revised regimen was implemented using different types of dressings. The staff agreed to continue using the PDSA Cycle until the wound was healed.

KEY CONCEPTS

- Evidence-based practice (EBP) represents an approach to the utilization of current research findings to guide the development of appropriate strategies to deliver quality, cost-effective care.
- Outcomes research provides evidence about benefits, risks, and results of treatment so individuals can make informed decisions and choices to improve their quality of life.
- The American Nurses Association has been an active advocate of outcomes evaluation and has developed a Nursing Report Card for Acute Care Settings that lists indicators for patient-focused outcomes, structures of care, and care processes.
- Guidelines based on evidence-based practice can help the nurse to direct care but cannot replace learning by hands-on delivery of patient care.
- The University of Colorado Hospital model is an example of a multidisciplinary evidence-based practice model for using different sources of information to change or support your practice.
- The Model for Improvement can be applied to a system or an individual.
- Patient care improvement must be based on building and applying knowledge.
- Evidence-based practice is based on knowing why you are doing what you are doing.

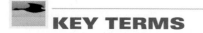

KEY TERMS

benchmarking
evidence-based
   nursing practice
evidence-based practice
practice guideline

REVIEW QUESTIONS

1. To participate effectively in the use of EBNP, nurses must
   A. participate in the development, use, and evaluation of practice guidelines.
   B. read and analyze outcomes of research studies.
   C. involve themselves in everyday patient care and nursing practice.
   D. all of the above

2. Why is it important for nurses to recognize and value patient-focused outcome indicators such as those included on the ANA *Nursing Report Card*?
   A. To achieve safe, quality, cost-effective care for patients in daily practice
   B. To realize that individual nursing practice styles directly affect the rates at which patients recover
   C. To prevent development of unnecessary complications and injury
   D. All of the above

3. Which of the following are examples of national evidence-based practice guidelines?
   A. Hospital policy on how to staff a nursing unit
   B. AHRQ pressure ulcer treatment guidelines
   C. Hospital procedure on how to insert a catheter
   D. JCAHO accreditation standards

REVIEW ACTIVITIES

1. Review the ANA *Nursing Report Card* patient-focused outcome indicators listed in the chapter. Select one of the indicators and review a relevant research study or clinical practice article that discusses the use of evidence-based practice to improve outcomes related to this indicator.

2. The University of Colorado Hospital model is one example of an evidence-based multidisciplinary practice model. This model presents a framework for thinking about how you use different sources of information to change or support your practice. Select a situation from your clinical practice and apply the model. For example, if you were caring for an elderly patient, admitted with a hip fracture sustained during a fall at home, what benchmarking data would you review to compare the patient's length of stay with that of other patient with fractured hips? What standards of care would be used? Are these institutional specific or do they also incorporate any specific outside organizations' guidelines?

3. Another model for achieving improvement is the Model for Improvement. Based on what you have read, consider the three questions:
   a. What are we trying to accomplish?
   b. How will we know that a change is an improvement?
   c. What changers can we make that will result in an improvement?

   Apply the PDSA Cycle to a situation that includes an adolescent's frequent readmissions for exacerbations of asthma.

EXPLORING THE WEB

- The web site for the Agency for Healthcare Research and Quality (AHRQ), formerly the Agency for Health Care Policy and Research (AHCPR), has a clinical information index page that lists evidence reports for topics such as swallowing disorders in stroke patients, evaluation of therapies for stable angina, and access to agency-supported guidelines (e.g., cancer pain, cardiac rehabilitation, pressure ulcers, and so on). *http://www.ahrq.gov*

- If you are interested in reading about evidence-based practice, explore the following web site: *http://www.evidence.org/lpBinCE/lpext.dll?f= template&fn=main-h.htm&2.0*

- The Joint Commission's pain standards are posted at *http://www.jcaho.org/standards_frm. html* (as of March 2, 2002). Questions about the pain standards can be directed to the JCAHO's Standards Interpretation Unit at (630) 792-5000 (e-mail: tmister@jcaho.org).

- Go to *http://www.nursingworld.org/nidsec/index.htm* and find the information about the Nursing Information and Data Set Evaluation Center. Note the ANA Recognized Classification Systems listed.

REFERENCES

Agency for Health Care Policy and Research. (1992a). *Acute pain management: Operative or medical procedures and trauma* (Clinical Practice Guideline, Pub. No. 92-0032). Rockville, MD: Author.

Agency for Health Care Policy and Research. (1992b). *Pressure ulcers in adults: Prediction and prevention* (Clinical Practice Guideline, Pub. No. 92-0047). Rockville, MD: Author.

Agency for Health Care Policy and Research. (1994a). *Management of cancer pain* (Clinical Practice Guideline Pub. No. 94-0592). Rockville, MD: Author.

Agency for Health Care Policy and Research. (1994b). *Treatment of pressure ulcers* (Clinical Practice Guideline, Pub. No. 95-0652). Rockville, MD: Author.

American Nurses Association. (1980*). Social policy statement.* Washington, DC: American Nursing Publishing.

American Nurses Association. (1995). *Nursing report card for acute care settings.* Washington, DC: American Nurses Publishing.

American Pain Society, Quality of Care Committee. (1995). Quality improvement guidelines for the treatment of acute pain and cancer pain. *Journal of the American Medical Association 23,* 1874–1880.

Bates-Jensen, B. M. (1998). Management of necrotic tissue. In C. Sussman & B. M. Bates-Jensen (Eds.), *Wound care: A collaborative practice manual for physical therapists and nurses* (pp. 139–158). Gaithersburg, MD: Aspen.

Bellack, J. P., & O'Neil, E. H. (2000). Recreating nursing practice for a new century: Recommendations and implications of the Pew Health Professions Commission's final report. *Nursing Health Care Perspective, 21*(1), 14–21.

Benner, P. E., Hooper-Kyriakidis, P., Hooper, P. L., Stannard, D., & Eoyang, T., (1998). *Clinical wisdom and interventions in critical care: A thinking-in-action approach.* Philadelphia: Saunders.

Bergstrom, N., Braden, B. J., Kemp, M., Champagne, M., & Ruby, E. (1998). Predicting pressure ulcer risk: A multisite study of the predictive validity of the Braden Scale. *Nursing Research 47,* 261–269.

Bergstrom, N., Braden, B. J., Laguzza, A., & Holman, V. (1987). The Braden Scale for Predicting Pressure Sore Risk. *Nursing Research 36*(4), 205–210.

Berry, P. H., & Dahl, J. L. (2000). The new JCAHO pain standards: Implications for pain management nurses. *Pain Management Nursing, 1,* 3–12.

Bryant, L. (1998). The ontology of the discipline of nursing. *Nursing Science Quarterly, 11,* 145–146.

Camp, R. (1994). Benchmarking applied to healthcare. *The Joint Commission on Quality Improvement 20,* 229–238.

Clancy, C., & Eisenberg, J. (1998). Outcomes research: Measure the end results of health care. *Science, 282,* 245–246.

Goode, C. J., & Piedalue, F. (1999). Evidence-based clinical practice. *Journal of Nursing Administration, 29,* 15–21.

Goode, C. J., Tanaka, D. J., Krugman, M., O'Connor, P. A., Bailey, C., Deutchman, M., & Stolpman, N. M. (2000). Outcomes from use of an evidence-based practice guideline. *Nursing Economic$, 18,* 202–207.

Ingersoll, G. L. (2000). Evidence-based nursing: What it is and what it isn't. *Nursing Outlook, 48,* 151–152.

Jadlos, M. A., Kelman, G. B., Marra, K., & Lanoue, A. (1996). A pain management documentation tool. *Oncology Nursing Forum, 23,* 1451–1454.

Joint Commission on Accreditation of Healthcare Organizations. (1999). *Performance measurement.* Retrieved March 4, 2002, from http://www.jcaho.org/oryx_frm.html

Joint Commission on Accreditation of Healthcare Organizations. (1999). *Comprehensive Accreditation Manual for Hospitals: The Official Handbook (CAMH),* PE-8.

Kane, R. L. (1997). *Understanding health care outcomes research.* (1st ed.). Gaithersburg, MD: Aspen.

Langley, G. J., Nolan, K. M., Nolan, T. W., Norman, C. L., & Provost, L. P. (1996). *The improvement guide: A practical approach to enhancing organizational performance.* San Francisco: Jossey-Bass.

Phillips, T. J. (1997). Cost effectiveness in wound care. In D. Krasner & D. Kane, (Eds.), *Chronic wound care: A clinical source book for healthcare professionals* (pp. 369–372). Wayne, PA: Health Management Publications.

Sackett, D. L., Rosenberg, W. M., Gray, J. A., Haynes, R. B., & Richardson, W. S. (1996). Evidence based medicine: What it is and what it isn't. *British Medical Journal, 312*(7023), 71–72.

SUPPORT Study Principle Investigators. (1995). A controlled trial to improve care for seriously ill hospitalized patients: A study to understand prognoses and preferences for outcomes and risks of treatments (SUPPORT). *Journal of the American Medical Association, 274,* 1591–1598.

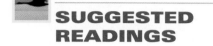

SUGGESTED READINGS

Agency for Health Care Policy and Research. (1999, July 13). *Clinical information: Clinical practice guidelines online.* Retrieved January 30, 2002, from http://www.ahcpr.gov/clinic.

Hess, C. T. (1998). *Nurse's clinical guide: Wound care.* Springhouse, PA: Springhouse.

Krasner, D., & Kane, D. (Eds.). (1997). *Chronic wound care: A clinical source book for healthcare professionals.* Wayne, PA: Health Management Publications.

Morison, M., Moffatt, C., Bridel-Nixon, J., & Bale, S. (1997). *Nursing management of chronic wounds.* London: Mosby.

Sussman, C., & Bates-Jensen, B. M. (Eds.). (1998). *Wound care: A collaborative practice manual for physical therapists and nurses.* Gaithersburg, MD: Aspen.

CHAPTER 21

Decision Making

Sharon Little-Stoetzel, RN, MS

OBJECTIVES

Upon completion of this chapter, the reader should be able to:

1. Apply effective decision making to clinical situations, incorporating critical thinking and problem solving.
2. Facilitate group decision making using various techniques.
3. Apply technology, as appropriate, to decision making.
4. Examine the nurse's role in patient decision making.
5. Examine strategies to improve decision making and build self-confidence.

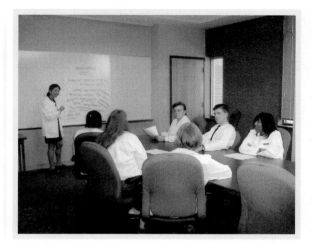

You are a staff nurse in the Emergency Department and have just come from a unit meeting. At the meeting, your nurse manager reported the results of the patient satisfaction survey from the previous year. Patient satisfaction has steadily declined, and for the past 3 months, only 20% of patients were satisfied. The manager selected a task force to investigate potential solutions to this problem and appointed you chairperson. The survey identified some reasons for the dissatisfaction: long waiting periods prior to being seen, not being informed about tests and procedures being performed, and being treated in an impersonal manner.

What should be the first step of the task force?

Can the decision-making process help the group solve the situation?

Rapid changes in the health care environment have expanded the decision-making role of the nurse. Because the health care market is more competitive, decision making by nurses tends to be critical to the agency's survival. Additionally, stringent budgets require that nurse managers and staff alike do more with less. Patient care is more complex as acuity rises. With patients being discharged from acute care institutions earlier, effective decisions regarding treatment must be made in a timely manner.

Critical thinking is essential when making decisions and solving problems. The Pew Health Professions Commission asserted that nurses must "demonstrate critical thinking, reflection, and problem solving skills" to thrive as effective practitioners in the 21st century (Bellack & O'Neil, 2000). This chapter explores the decision-making process and

how it relates to critical thinking and problem solving. Application of decision making models to clinical and management decisions is presented. The chapter examines advantages and limitations to group decision making as well as the use of technology in decision making. Finally, it discusses the nurse's role in patient decision making and strategies for improving the decision-making process.

CRITICAL THINKING

What does it mean to be a critical thinker? Paul (1992) defines critical thinking as "thinking about your thinking while you're thinking in order to make your thinking better" (p.7). Paul is quick to point out that there are many accurate definitions of critical thinking, and most are consistent with each other. A good critical thinker is able to examine decisions from all sides and take into account varying points of view. A good critical thinker does not say, "We've always done it this way," and refuse to consider alternate ways. The critical thinker generates new ideas and alternatives when making decisions. The critical thinker asks "why?" questions about a situation to arrive at the best decision. Four basic skills—critical reading, critical listening, critical writing, and critical speaking—are necessary for the development of critical thinking skills. These skills are part of the process of developing and using thinking for decision making. Ability in these four areas can be measured by the extent to which one achieves the universal intellectual standards illustrated in Table 21-1.

As you begin to apply critical thinking to nursing, use these universal intellectual standards when you are reading material from a textbook, listening to an oral presentation, writing a paper, answering test questions, or presenting ideas in oral form. Ask yourself whether the ideas are clear or unclear, precise or imprecise, specific or vague, accurate or inaccurate, and so forth. You will improve your critical thinking skills over time.

Reflective Thinking

Pesut and Herman (1999) describe **reflective thinking** as watching or observing ourselves as we perform a task or make a decision about a particular situation. We have two selves, the active self and the reflective self. The reflective self watches the active self as it engages in activities. The reflective self acts

TABLE 21-1	The Spectrum of Universal Intellectual Standards

Clear	Unclear
Precise	Imprecise
Specific	Vague
Accurate	Inaccurate
Relevant	Irrelevant
Consistent	Inconsistent
Logical	Illogical
Deep	Superficial
Complete	Incomplete
Significant	Insignificant
Adequate	Inadequate
Fair	Unfair

Adapted from The Foundation for Critical Thinking, Dillon, CA. http://criticalthinking.org/university/unistan.html

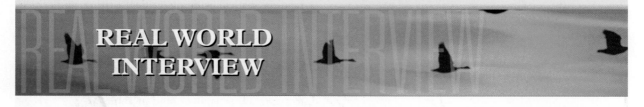

REAL WORLD INTERVIEW

We have found in our organization that if we have to extend a new nursing graduate's orientation, it is usually because we have to help her develop her ability to prioritize and improve her decision-making skills.

Mary A. O'Shea, RN, MN
Nurse Executive

as observer and offers suggestions about the activities. To be a good critical thinker, one must practice reflective thinking. Reflection upon a situation or problem after a decision is made allows the individual to evaluate the decision. Nurse educators assist students to become better reflective thinkers through the use of clinical journals. Using journals helps students reflect on clinical activities and improve their clinical decision-making abilities.

PROBLEM SOLVING

Problem solving is an active process that starts with a problem and ends with a solution. LeStorti et al. (1999) define a problem as the difference between the actual state and the desired state. The problem-solving process consists of the following five steps: identify the problem, gather and analyze data, generate alternatives and select an action, implement the

Methods of Reduction	Cost Savings	Effect on Job Satisfaction	Effect on Patient Satisfaction
Lay off the two most senior full-time employees	$93,500	Significant reduction	Significant reduction
Lay off the two most recently hired full-time employees	$63,200	Significant reduction	Moderate reduction
Reduce by staff attrition	$78,000	Minor reduction	Minor reduction

Figure 21-2 Sample Decision-Making Grid

Elements	Importance Score (out of 10)	Likelihood Score (out of 10)	Risk (multiply scores)
If I work at hospital A			
Learning experience	10	10	100
Good mentor support	8	8	64
Financial reward	6	6	36
Growth potential	8	8	64
Good location	10	10	100
Total			364
If I work at hospital B			
Learning experience	8	8	64
Good mentor support	7	7	49
Financial reward	8	8	64
Growth potential	9	9	81
Good location	6	6	36
Total			294

Figure 21-3 Sample Decision-Making Grid for Weighing Options

depicting the sequence of tasks that must take place to complete a project. Jones and Beck (1996) provide an example of a PERT flow diagram depicting a case management project (see Figure 21-4). The chart shows the amount of time taken to complete the project and the sequence of events to complete the project. An advantage of the PERT diagram is that participants can visualize a complete picture of the project, including the timing of decisions from beginning to end.

14-A.

The vice president for nursing plans to change all units to include case managers. She believes that this can be accomplished within a year and one half. In order for this to be achieved, the following activities and events have to occur:

Activity Symbol	Activity Descriptions	Immediate Predecessor
A.	Form a multidisciplinary advisory group	None
B.	Agree upon definitions	A
C.	Notify members of subcommittees	B
D.	Write job descriptions	C
E.	Advertise for candidates for case manager	D
F.	Review qualifications of candidates	E
G.	Select candidates for case manager	F
H.	Review patient charts	None
I.	Write patient care maps	H
J.	Meet with case managers	None
K.	Orient case managers	J
L.	Orient unit and hospital staff	K
M.	Utilize case management process	L

Events

1.	Project begins
2.	Meeting of multidisciplinary committee
3.	Formation of subcommittees
4.	Subcommittee for job description meets
5.	Subcommittee for patient care maps meets
6.	Candidates for case managers are interviewed
7.	Candidates are hired
8.	Subcommittee for patient care maps meets to finalize maps
9.	Orientation begins
10.	Implementation begins
11.	Project is evaluated

Expected   **Time Calculations**

Activity	Duration
A	0.5 month
B	1 month
C	0.5 month
D	1 month
E	1 month
F	2 months
G	1 month
H	1 month
I	2 months
J	1 month
K&L	1 month
M	3 months

14-B.

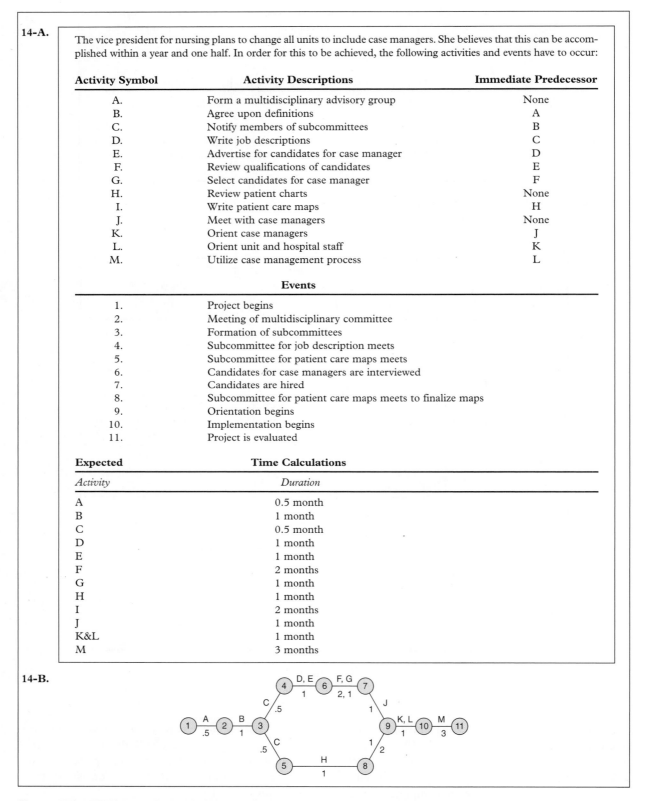

Figure 21-4 PERT Diagram with Critical Path for Implementation of Case Management

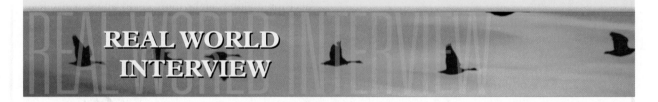

CRITICAL THINKING

You are a new nurse manager and have been in your position for two months. You are working on the holiday schedule, and the unit secretary with the most seniority comes to you and says that she needs both the week of Christmas and the week of New Year's Day off because she will be out of town. You remind her that hospital policy does not allow employees to have both holidays off. The secretary tells you that the previous manager always approved her request and that she has already bought plane tickets. Apply the steps of decision making to this situation.

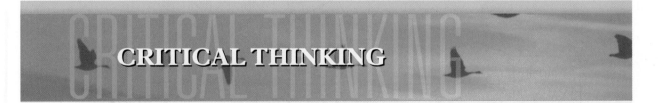

REAL WORLD INTERVIEW

I often find decisions about disciplinary action the most difficult ones to make. But, when I use a decision-making model, it helps me make the best decision. My goal in the decision-making process is often twofold—to help the nurse prevent further disciplinary problems and to help the nurse learn from the situation.

Kathleen Taylor, RN, MS, CCRN
Nurse Manager

CRITICAL THINKING

You are working for a home health agency that employs 17 registered nurses. There have been concerns about staffing and scheduling as the agency's census has increased. The manager has said that until more staff can be hired, there will be an increased need for on-call and overtime scheduling. The manager has given the responsibility to the entire group to figure out the best way to cover the patient assignments.

What would be the best group decision-making strategy to use? What should the group do first?

Decision Tree

A decision tree can be useful in making the alternatives visible. Figure 21-5 is a decision tree for choosing whether to go back to school.

Figure 21-6 identifies a decision analysis tree for a patient who smokes.

Gantt Chart

A Gantt chart can be useful for decision makers to illustrate a project from beginning to end. Figure 21-7 illustrates a Gantt chart used to show the progression of a nursing unit's pilot project.

GROUP DECISION MAKING

Certain situations call for group decision making. Vroom and Yetton (1973) identified certain questions managers should ask themselves before making a decision alone. There are occasions when it is more appropriate for a group to make the decision rather than the individual manager. Each situation is different, and an effective manager adopts the appropriate mode of decision making—group or individual. The eight questions in Table 21-3 may assist the manager in determining which mode to use.

Today's leadership and management styles include people in the decision-making process who will be most affected by the decision. Decisions affecting patient care should be made by those groups implementing the decisions.

The effectiveness of groups depends greatly on the group's members. The size of the group and the personalities of group members are important considerations when choosing participants. More ideas can be generated with groups, thus allowing for more choices. This increases the likelihood of higher-quality outcomes. Another advantage of groups is that when followers participate in the decision-making process, acceptance of the decision is more likely to occur. Additionally, groups may be used as a medium for communication.

A major disadvantage of group decision making is the time involved. Without effective leadership, groups can waste time and be nonproductive. Group decision making can be more costly and can also lead to conflict. Groups can be dominated by one person or become the battleground for a power struggle among assertive members. See Table 21-4 for a listing of the advantages and disadvantages of groups.

Techniques of Group Decision Making

There are various techniques of group decision making. Nominal group technique, Delphi technique, and consensus building are different methods to facilitate group decision making.

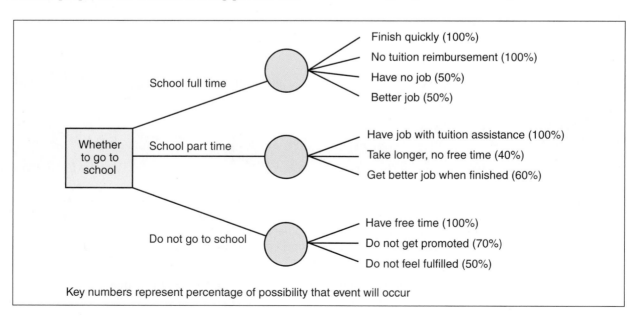

Figure 21-5 Decision Tree for Choosing Whether to Go Back to School

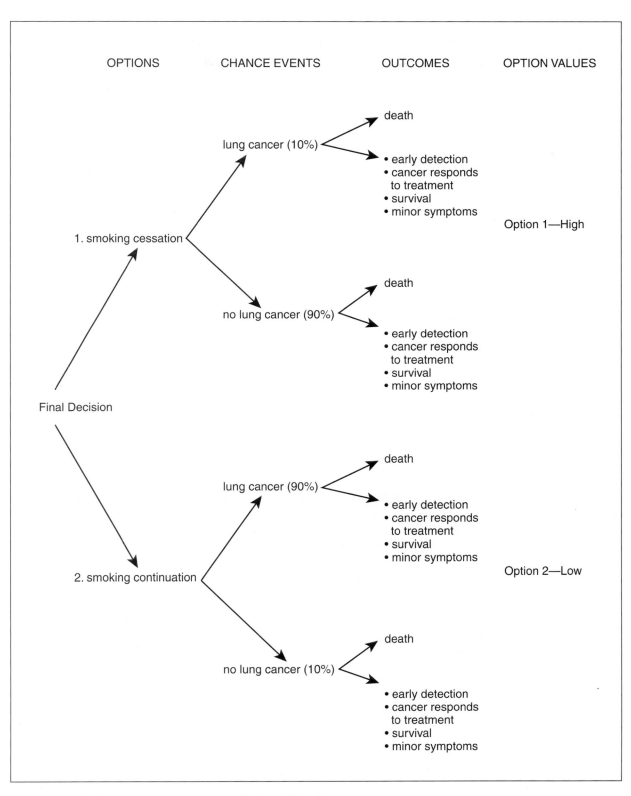

Figure 21-6 Decision Analysis Tree for a Patient Who Smokes

A nurse manager has agreed to have her unit pilot a new care delivery system within six months. The Gantt chart can be used to plan the progression of the project.

Activities	Sept	Oct	Nov	Dec	Jan	Feb	Mar	Apr	May
Discuss project with staff	------ X								
Form an ad hoc planning committee	------	—— X							
Receive report from committee			------ X						
Discuss report with staff			------	—— X					
Educate all staff to the plan					------ —— X				
Implement new system						------	——————		
Evaluate system and make changes							------	——	X

Key
------ Proposed Time
—— Actual Time
X Complete

Figure 21-7 Gantt Chart: Implementation of Care Delivery System

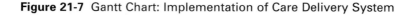

TABLE 21-3   *Individual vs. Group Decision-Making Questions*

1. Does the manager have all the information needed?
2. Do the subordinates have supplementary information needed to make the best decision?
3. Does the manager have all the resources available to obtain sufficient information to make the best decision?
4. Is it absolutely critical that the team accept the decision prior to implementation?
5. Will the team accept the decision I make by myself?
6. Does the course of action chosen make a difference to the organization?
7. Does the team have the best interest of the organization foremost when considering the decision?
8. Will the decision cause undue conflict among the team?

Adapted from *Leadership and Decision-Making* (pp. 21–30), by V. Vroom and P. Yetton, 1973, Pittsburgh, PA: University of Pittsburgh Press.

TABLE 21-4	*Advantages and Disadvantages of Groups*

Advantages

- Easy and inexpensive way to share information
- Opportunities for face-to-face communication
- Opportunity to become connected with a social unit
- Promotion of cohesiveness and loyalty
- Access to a larger resource base
- Forum for constructive problem solving
- Support group
- Facilitation of esprit de corps
- Promotion of ownership of problems and solutions

Disadvantages

- Individual opinions influenced by others
- Individual identity obscured
- Formal and informal role and status positions evolve—hierarchies
- Dependency fostered
- Time consuming
- Inequity of time given to share individual information
- Existence of nonfunctional roles
- Personality conflicts

Nominal Group Technique

The nominal group technique was developed by Delbecq Van de Ven and Gustafson in 1971. The word nominal refers to the nonverbal aspect of this approach (Cawthorpe & Harris, 1999). In the first step, there is no discussion; group members write out their ideas or responses to the identified issue or question posed by the group leader. The second step involves presentation of the ideas of the group members along with the advantages and disadvantages of each. These ideas are presented on a flip board or chart. The third phase may offer an opportunity for discussion to clarify and evaluate the ideas. The fourth phase includes private voting on the ideas. Those ideas receiving the highest rating are the solutions implemented.

Delphi Group Technique

Delphi technique differs from nominal technique in that group members are not meeting face to face. Questionnaires are distributed to group members for their opinions, and these are then summarized and disseminated with the summaries to the group members. This process continues for as many times as necessary for the group members to reach consensus.

An advantage of this technique is that it can involve a large number of participants and thus a greater number of ideas.

Consensus Building

Consensus is defined by *The American Heritage Dictionary* (2000) as "an opinion or position reached by a group as a whole; general agreement or accord" (p. 391). A common misconception is that consensus means everyone agrees with the decision 100%. Contrary to this misunderstanding, consensus means that all group members can live with and fully support the decision regardless of whether they totally agree. This strategy is useful with groups because all group members participate and can realize the contributions each member makes to the decision (Sullivan & Decker, 2001). A disadvantage to the consensus strategy is that decision making requires more time. This strategy should be reserved for important decisions that require strong support from the participants who will implement them. Consensus decision making works well when the decisions are made under the following conditions: all members of the team are affected by the decision; implementation of the solution requires coordination among

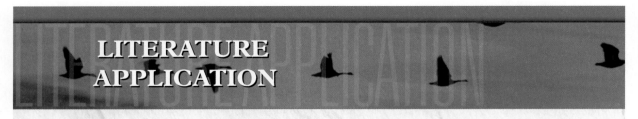

LITERATURE APPLICATION

Citation: Brooks, E. M., & Thomas, S. (1997). The perception and judgment of senior baccalaureate student nurses in clinical decision making. *Advances in Nursing Science, 19*(3), 50–69.

Discussion: One purpose of this study was to identify factors that affect decision making of senior baccalaureate student nurses. The authors used Brooks's Theory of Intrapersonal Awareness (BTIPA), which was based on the nursing theory of King's interacting systems framework. This framework includes perception and judgment as being integral to the nurse-patient relationship. Decisions are influenced by nursing judgment, which in turn, is influenced by values and perceptions. A structured interview and a written, simulated vignette of a clinical situation were given to 18 senior baccalaureate nursing students. The vignette consisted of a man injured in a motor vehicle accident in which his best friend was killed. The family of the injured man did not want him told of his friend's death. The most prominent intrapersonal characteristic affecting how the students made decisions regarding this vignette was experience. Experience was defined as work experience, clinical experience, personal experience, or lack of experience. The second most prominent intrapersonal characteristic was the student's personal values and beliefs. For example, the student would ask herself, "What would I want in this situation?" If someone believes in always telling the truth, then that individual would have a difficult time keeping the patient's death from the other patient.

Implications for Practice: Nurses need to recognize that people make decisions based on their own intrapersonal perceptual awareness. Prior experiences and personal values affect a person's decision making. The authors concluded that students need to be prepared to understand themselves and how their experiences and values will affect the decisions they make.

team members; and the decision is critical, requiring full commitment by team members. Although consensus can be the most time-consuming strategy, it can also be the most gratifying.

Groupthink

Groupthink and consensus building are different. In consensus, the group members work to support the final decision, and individual ideas and opinions are valued. In groupthink, the goal is for everyone to be in 100% agreement. Groupthink discourages questioning and divergent thinking. It hinders creativity and usually leads to inferior decisions (Jarvis, 1997). The potential for groupthink increases as the cohesiveness of the group increases. An important responsibility of the group leader is to recognize symptoms of groupthink. Janis (as cited in Jarvis, 1997) described examples of these symptoms. One symptom is that group members develop an illusion

of invulnerability, believing they can do no wrong. This problem has the greatest potential to develop when the group is powerful and group members view themselves as invincible. The second symptom of groupthink is stereotyping outsiders. This occurs when the group members rely on shared stereotypes—such as, all Democrats are liberal or all Republicans are conservative—to justify their positions. People who challenge or disagree with the decisions are also stereotyped. A third symptom is that group members reassure one another that their interpretation of data and their perspective on matters are correct regardless of the evidence showing otherwise. Old assumptions are never challenged, and members ignore what they do not know or what they do not want to know.

Strategies to avoid groupthink include appointing group members to roles that evaluate how group decision-making occurs. Group leaders should encourage all group members to think independently and verbalize their individual ideas. The leader should allow the group time to gather further data and reflect on data already collected. A primary responsibility of the managers or the group leader is to prevent groupthink from developing.

LIMITATIONS TO EFFECTIVE DECISION MAKING

What are obstacles to effective decision making? Past experiences, values, personal biases, and preconceived ideas affect the way people view problems and situations. Incorporating critical thinking into the decision-making process helps to prevent these factors from distorting the process. Hammond, Keeney, and Raiffa (1998) have identified pitfalls to effective decision-making. Following are pitfalls to avoid:

- Making the decision based upon the first available information
- Being comfortable with the status quo or not wanting to rock the boat
- Making decisions to justify previous decisions even if those decisions are no longer satisfactory
- Pursuing supporting evidence that verifies the decision while ignoring evidence to the contrary
- Presenting the issue in a biased manner or with a leading question
- Assigning inaccurate probabilities to alternatives.

USE OF TECHNOLOGY IN DECISION MAKING

Nurses use technology as a support for decision making. The best source of clinical decision making and judgment is still the professional practitioner. However, computer technology has many uses to support information systems for managers (Tomey, 2000). Patient classification systems, inventory control, scheduling staff, and changes in policies and procedures are but a few examples of how computers can assist managers with tracking the information needed in a management role. Computer software for the clinical practitioner is available for clinical decision making and should be carefully critiqued prior to use.

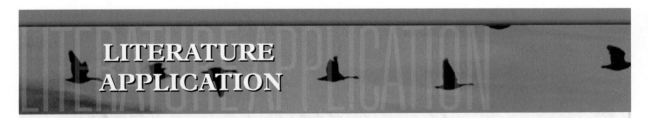

LITERATURE APPLICATION

Citation: Bucknall, T., & Thomas, S. (1997). Nurses' reflections on problems associated with decision-making in critical care settings. *Journal of Advanced Nursing, 25*, 229–237.

Discussion: A questionnaire was sent to 230 practicing critical care nurses to collect data about the problems they experience when making clinical decisions. Lack of time to implement decisions was cited as the most frequent problem. Another problem that frequently was associated with decision making was staying current with the ever-changing treatments and technology. Nurses reported concerns about their abilities to make decisions based on a lack of current knowledge. Other areas in which there were decision-making problems included nurses and physicians having different values about end-of-life treatment. The extent of nurses' autonomy in making decisions was also problematic. Working relationships between nurses and resident physicians were also cited as a frequent problem.

Implications for Practice: Recognizing frequently occurring problems with decision making is an important first step in stopping the problems from recurring. Ways of finding solutions include collaborating with colleagues and researching the nursing literature for information related to identified problems.

NURSES' ROLE IN PATIENT DECISION MAKING

In today's world, patients are taking a more active role in treatment decisions. The consumers of health care are more knowledgeable and cost conscious and have more options than in previous years. Nurses must be aware of patients' rights in making decisions about their treatments, and they must assist patients in their decision making. When patients are active participants, compliance with prescribed treatments is more likely to follow. Empowering the patient in this manner ultimately promotes a more positive outcome.

STRATEGIES TO IMPROVE DECISION MAKING

Comfort with decision making improves with experience. Early in the nurse's career, the nurse is commonly indecisive or uncomfortable with decisions.

Alfaro-LeFevre (1995) has identified several strategies that help to improve critical thinking, which, in turn, will also help to improve decision making. Do you have all the information needed to make a decision? At times, delaying a decision until more information is obtained may be the best approach. Asking "why," "what else," and "what if" questions will help you arrive at the best decision. When more information becomes available, decisions can be revised. Very few decisions are set in stone. Another helpful strategy for improving decision making is to anticipate questions and outcomes. For example, when calling a physician to report a patient's change in condition, the nurse will want to have pertinent information about the patient's vital signs and current medications readily available.

Nurses who practice strategies to promote their own critical thinking will, in turn, be good decision makers. A foundation for good decision making comes with experience and learning from those experiences. Table 21-5 gives the student some additional tips to consider when making decisions. By turning decisions with poor outcomes into learning experiences, nurses will enhance their decision-making ability in the future.

TABLE 21-5	Dos and Don'ts of Decision Making
Do	**Don't**
Make only those decisions that are yours to make.	Make snap decisions.
Write notes and keep ideas visible about decisions to utilize all relevant information.	Waste your time making decisions that do not have to be made.
Write down pros and cons of an issue to help clarify your thinking.	Consider decisions a choice between right and wrong but a choice among alternatives.
Make decisions as you go along rather than letting them accumulate.	Prolong deliberation about decisions.
Consider those affected by your decision.	Regret a decision; it was the right thing to do at the time.
Trust yourself.	Always base decisions on the "way things have always been done."

Adapted from The Small Business Knowledge Base, 1999. Retrieved February 19, 2002, from http://www.bizmove.com.

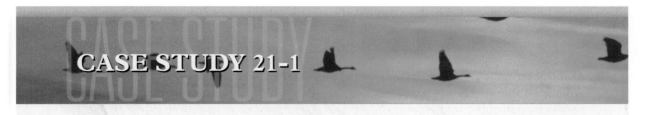

CASE STUDY 21-1

The manager has identified a problem for a group: low patient satisfaction. Patients are dissatisfied with the long waiting periods, lack of information, and impersonal attitude of staff. How will the group solve this problem?

KEY CONCEPTS

- The ever-changing health care system calls for nurses to be effective decision makers. The ability of nurses to make appropriate decisions will affect their employer's ability to survive.
- Critical thinking involves examining situations from every viewpoint when faced with any problem or situation. Use of the universal intellectual standards will improve a nurse's critical thinking.
- Practicing reflective thinking helps individuals become better critical thinkers.
- Problem solving involves five steps: (1) identify the problem, (2) gather and analyze data, (3) generate alternatives and select action, (4) implement the selected action, and (5) evaluate the selected action.
- In the decision-making process, there are five levels: Level 1—identify the need for a decision; Level 2—determine the goal or outcome; Level 3—identify alternatives or actions, along with their benefits and consequences; Level 4—decide on the action and implement; Level 5—evaluate the action.
- Decision-making grids may be helpful when the manager needs to separate multiple factors surrounding a situation during the decision-making process.
- The PERT model is useful for determining timing of decisions.
- There are situations in which the nurse manager makes an individual decision. Other situations call for group decision making.
- Consensus is a strategy utilized when using group decision making.

- To be an effective decision maker, individuals must identify and avoid certain traps during the decision-making process.
- Groupthink occurs when individuals are not allowed to express creativity, question methods, or engage in divergent thinking. Managers must be able to identify the symptoms of groupthink.
- The nurse must recognize the importance of empowering patients in making their own treatment decisions. The nurse needs to provide the patient with information and assist the patient in exploring all possible options.
- There are many strategies to improve your decision making. Obtaining all the information, asking yourself "why" and "what if" questions, and developing good habits of inquiry are a few of the strategies that will help improve your decision making.

KEY TERMS

consensus   problem solving
decision making   reflective thinking
Delphi technique

REVIEW QUESTIONS

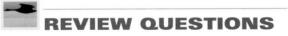

1. Decision making is best described as
   A. the process one uses to solve a problem.
   B. the process one uses to choose between alternatives.
   C. the process one uses to reflect on a certain situation.
   D. the process one uses to generate ideas.

2. Which of the following is the best description of consensus?
   A. Everyone in the group agrees with the decision 100%.
   B. All members of the group vote on the selected action.
   C. Every group member compromises.
   D. Every group member fully supports the decision, once it is made.

3. Which of the following is a symptom of groupthink?
   A. The group members continually disagree with one another.
   B. The group members cannot come to a decision.
   C. The group members stereotype outsiders.
   D. The group members share a common bond.

4. Occasionally, making a decision is difficult because of the multiple factors that surround certain situations. To separate these factors, the nurse manager may utilize a
   A. decision grid.
   B. nominal group technique.
   C. Delphi group technique.
   D. consensus strategy.

REVIEW ACTIVITIES

1. You are the manager of a surgical unit that consists of 12 beds. Your supervisor informs you that 12 more beds will be opened for neurosurgical patients and you are to be the manager. Draw a PERT diagram to depict the sequence of tasks necessary for the completion of the project.

2. The education forms are not being filled out correctly or in a timely manner on new admissions in your medical-surgical unit. Decide on your own the best action to take in this situation. Then, get into a group and attempt to reach consensus on the best action to take. Compare the differences between individual and group decision making. What did you learn about developing consensus?

3. Identify a problem that you have been considering. Using the decision-making grid at the bottom of the page, rate the alternative solutions to the problem that you have been considering on a scale of 1 to 3 on the elements of cost, quality, importance, location, and any other elements that are important to you.

   Did this exercise help you in thinking through your decision?

4. Identify a current problem in health care. Use the problem-solving process in a group to find a solution. Employ the nominal group technique and the Delphi technique.

EXPLORING THE WEB

- Test your critical thinking in critical care with the scenarios on this web site: *http://nursing.umaryland.edu/students/~jkohl/scenario/situatio.htm*
- Note the universal intellectual standards at the Foundation for Critical Thinking: *http://criticalthinking.org/university/unistan.html*
- Visit these critical thinking sites: *http://www.criticalthinking.org http://www.insightassessment.com*
- Note the following site for clinical decision making—this site includes software for clinical decision making: *http://www.apache-msi.com/*
- Review this site on applying artificial intelligence to clinical situations: *http://www.medg.lcs.mit.edu/*

REFERENCES

Alfaro-LeFevre, R. (1995). *Critical thinking in nursing.* Philadelphia: Saunders.
American Heritage Dictionary of the English Language (4th ed.). (2000). Boston, MA: Houghton Mifflin.

	Cost	Quality	Importance	Location	Other
Alternative A					
Alternative B					
Alternative C					

Bellack, J. P., & O'Neil, E. H. (2000). Recreating nursing practice for a new century: Recommendations and implications of the Pew Health Professions Commission's final report. *Nursing and Health Care Perspectives, 21*(1), 14–21.

Brooks, E. M., & Thomas, S. (1997). The perception and judgment of senior baccalaureate student nurses in clinical decision making. *Advances in Nursing Science, 19*(3), 50–69.

Bucknall, T., & Thomas, S. (1997). Nurses' reflections on problems associated with decision-making in critical care settings. *Journal of Advanced Nursing, 25*, 229–237.

Cawthorpe, D., & Harris, D. (1999). Nominal group technique: Assessing staff concerns. *Journal of Nursing Administration, 29*(7/8), 11, 18, 37, 42.

Hammond, J. S., Keeney, R. L., & Raiffa, H. (1998). The hidden traps in decision making. *Harvard Business Review, 76*(5), 47–58.

Huber, D. (2000). *Leadership and nursing care management*. Philadelphia: Saunders.

Huston, C. J., & Marquis, B. L. (1995, May). Seven steps to successful decision-making. *American Journal of Nursing*, 65–68.

Jarvis, C. (1997) *Groupthink*. Retrieved June 2, 1999, from Brunel University web site: http://sol.brunel.ac.uk/~jarvis/bola/communications/groupthink.html

Jones, R. A. P., & Beck, S. E. (1996). *Decision making in nursing*. Clifton Park, NY: Delmar Learning.

LeStorti, A., Cullen, P., Hanzlik, E., Michiels, J. M., Piano, L., Ryan, P. L., & Johnson, W. (1999). Creative thinking in nursing education: Preparing for tomorrow's challenges. *Nursing Outlook, 47*(2), 62–66.

Paul, R. (1992). *Critical thinking: What every person needs to survive in a rapidly changing world*. Santa Rosa, CA: Foundation for Critical Thinking.

Pesut, D. J. & Herman, J. (1999). *Clinical reasoning: The art & science of critical & creative thinking*. Clifton Park, NY: Delmar Learning.

The Small Business Knowledge Base (1999). Retrieved January 19, 2002, from http://www.bizmove.com

Sullivan, E., & Decker, P. (2001). *Effective leadership and management in nursing*. Menlo Park, CA: Addison Wesley Longman.

Tomey, A. (2000). *Guide to nursing management and leadership*. St. Louis, MO: Mosby.

Vroom, V. H., & Yetton, P. W. (1973). *Leadership and decision-making*. Pittsburgh, PA: University of Pittsburgh Press.

SUGGESTED READINGS

Biafore, S. (1999). Predictive solutions bring more power to decision makers. *Health Management Technology, 20*(10), 12–14.

Crandall, S. (1993). How expert clinical educators teach what they know. *Journal of Continuing Education in the Health Professions, 13*, 33–46.

Duchscher, J. (1999). Catching the wave: Understanding the concept of critical thinking. *Journal of Advanced Nursing, 29*(3), 577–583.

Kontryn, V. (1999). Strategic problem solving in the new millennium. *AORN Journal, 70*(6), 1035–1044.

Marquis, B. L., & Huston, C. J. (1998). *Management decision making for nurses: 124 case studies* (3rd ed.). Philadelphia: Lippincott.

Martinez de Castillo, S. L. (1999). *Strategies, techniques, and approaches to thinking: Case studies in clinical nursing*. Philadelphia, PA: Saunders.

Parsons, L. (1999). Building RN confidence for delegation decision-making skills in practice. *Journal for Nurses in Staff Development, 15*(6), 263–269.

Radwin, L. (1995). Conceptualizations of decision making in nursing: Analytic models and "knowing the patient." *Nursing Diagnosis, 6*(1), 16–22.

Recker, D., Bess, C., & Wellens, H. (1996). A decision-making process in shared governance. *Nursing Management, 27*(5), 48A, 48B, 48D.

Schon, D. A. (1987). *Educating the reflective practitioner*. San Francisco: Jossey-Bass.

Schon, D. A. (1989). A symposium on Schon's concept of reflective practice: Critiques, commentaries, illustrations. *Journal of Curriculum and Supervision, 5*(1), 6–9.

Scordo, K. (1997). Reaching consensus through electronic brainstorming. *Computers in Nursing, 15*(2), 33–37.

Simms, L. M., Price, S. A., & Ervin, N. E. (2000). *Professional practice of nursing administration* (3rd ed.). Clifton Park, NY: Delmar Learning.

Swansburg, R. C., & Swansburg, R. J. (2002). *Introductory management and leadership for nurse managers* (3rd ed.). Boston: Jones and Bartlett.

Tabak, N., Bar-tal, Y., & Cohen-Mansfield, J. (1996). Clinical decision making of experienced and novice nurses. *Western Journal of Nursing Research, 18*(5), 534–547.

CHAPTER 22

Every act whatever of man that causes damage to another obliges him whose fault it happened to repair it. . . . (La. Civil Code art. 2315)

Legal Aspects of Patient Care

Judith W. Martin, RN, JD
Sister Kathleen Cain, OSF, JD

OBJECTIVES

Upon completion of this chapter, the reader should be able to:

1. Discuss the effect of public law on nursing practice.
2. Name various federal administrative agencies and their areas of influence.
3. Name the most common areas of nursing practice cited in malpractice actions and list some actions a nurse can take to minimize these risks.
4. Describe the various forms of advanced directives and how these are commonly implemented.
5. Describe risk management and how it is used in the health care setting.
6. Discuss the rights of the nurse as an employee.

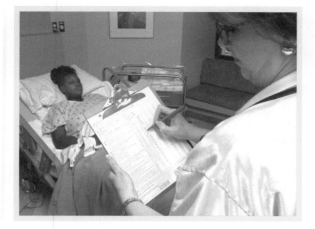

You are working on a geriatric nursing unit when you admit an 82-year-old female, Mrs. Perkins. She has a broken hip and many bruises and skin tears. The family with whom she is living tells you she is confused and falls often. While you are bathing Mrs. Perkins, she begins crying and tells you her grandson pushed her down the stairs and that he often hits her if she does not give him money. She says her daughter does not believe her if she says anything and she is afraid if she complains she will have no one to care for her.

Do you need any additional information to determine the validity of Mrs. Perkins's statement?

If abuse has occurred, what action should you take?

Do patient confidentiality concerns affect any actions you may take?

L aw that affects the relationship between individuals is called civil law. Law that specifies the relationship between citizens and the state is called public law. This chapter reviews how laws are enacted and implemented and how the various types of law affect nursing practice.

SOURCES OF LAW

The authority to make, implement, and interpret laws is generally granted in a constitution. A **constitution** is a set of basic laws that specifies the powers of the various segments of the government and how these segments relate to each other.

Generally, it is the role of a legislative body, both on the federal and state levels, to enact laws. Agencies under the authority of the administrative branch of the government draft the rules that implement the law. Finally, the judicial branch interprets the law as it rules in court cases. Table 22-1 gives examples of these relationships.

Also, a judicial decision may set a precedent that is used by other courts and, over time, has the force of law. This type of law is referred to as common law.

PUBLIC LAW

Public law consists of constitutional law, criminal law, and administrative law and defines a citizen's relationship with government.

Constitutional Law

Several categories of public law affect the practice of nursing. For example, the nurse accommodates patients' constitutional right to practice their religion every time the nurse calls a patient's clergy as requested, follows a specific religious custom for preparation of meals, or prepares a deceased person's remains for burial.

Controversial constitutional rights that may affect the nurse's practice include the recognized constitutional rights of a woman to have an abortion and an individual's right to die (see *Roe v. Wade* [1973] and *Cruzan v. Director* [1990]). Nurses may not believe in either of these rights personally and may refuse to work in areas in which they would have to assist a patient in exercising these rights. Nurses may not, however, interfere with another person's right to have an abortion or to forgo lifesaving measures.

Criminal Law

Criminal law focuses on the actions of individuals that can intentionally do harm to others. Often the victims of such abusive actions are the very young or the very old. These two categories of people generally cannot defend themselves against physical or emotional abuse. The nurse, in caring for patients, may notice that a vulnerable patient has unexplained bruises, fractures, or other injuries. Most states have mandatory statutes that require the nurse to report unexplained or suspicious injuries to the appropriate child or elderly protective agency. Generally, the institution in which the nurse is employed will have clear guidelines to follow in such a situation. Failure

TABLE 22-1	The Three Branches of Government		
	Legislative Branch	**Administrative Branch**	**Judicial Branch**
Example at federal level	Americans with Disabilities Act (ADA) (1990)	The Equal Employment Opportunity Commission (EEOC) publishes rules specifying what employers must do to help a disabled employee.	In 1999, the U.S. Supreme Court interpreted the law to require that to be protected by this law, the individual must have an impairment that limits a major life activity and that is not corrected by medicine or appliances (glasses, blood pressure medicine). *Sutton v. United Airlines* (1999); *Murphy v. United Parcel Service, Inc.* (1999)
Example at state level	Nurse Practice Act	The state board of nursing develops rules specifying the duties of a registered nurse in that state.	Courts and juries determine whether a nurse's actions comply with the law governing the practice of nursing in a state.

to report the problem as required by law can result in the nurse being fined for her inaction.

Another aspect of criminal law affecting nursing practice is the state and federal requirement that criminal background checks be performed on specified categories of prospective employees who will work with the very young or the elderly in institutions such as schools and nursing homes. Again, this is an attempt to protect the most vulnerable citizens from mistreatment or abuse. Failure to conduct the mandated background checks can result in the institution having to defend itself for any harm done by an employee with a past criminal conviction. A recent article related a case in which a hospital was found negligent for failing to conduct a criminal background check or investigate complaints against an employee who later sexually abused a patient (Fiesta, 1999c). However, in another case in which the hospital did investigate such complaints, the appellate court did not find it responsible for the sexual assault on a patient by an employee (Fiesta, 1999c). The rationale for this was that the hospital had done what it was required to do by law in investigating the employee's criminal background and was not liable for these unexpected actions.

The third area in which criminal law concerns affect nursing practice is the prohibition against substance abuse. Both federal and state law requires health care agencies to keep a strict accounting of the use and distribution of regulated drugs. Nurses routinely are expected to keep narcotic records accurate and current.

Nurses' behavior when off duty can also affect their employment status. Abusing alcohol or drugs on one's own time, if discovered, can result in nurses being terminated from employment and their license to practice nursing restricted or revoked (Mantel, 1999). Frequently, boards of nursing have programs for the nurse with a drug problem, and completion of such a program may be required before the nurse can resume practice. Additionally, health care facilities may do random drug screens on their employees to identify those who may be using illegal substances.

Administrative Law

Both the federal government and state governments have administrative laws that affect nursing practice. The laws pertaining to Social Security and, more specifically, Medicare, are interpreted in the *Code of*

CRITICAL THINKING

You work the evening shift in the ICU. You notice that when one particular nurse assigned to the night shift is on duty, all of her patients receive narcotic pain medication at midnight. This is true even when you have observed and documented that some of these patients have diminished responsiveness and no pain complaints when cared for by you or other nurses in the unit. Also, one of your patients complained to his doctor that the pain medication he received from this nurse "didn't work."

Given this scenario what should you do as a nurse? Would you expect to get some guidance from your institution's policy and procedure manual?

Federal Regulations, which contains the administrative rules for the federal government. These rules have specific requirements that hospitals, nursing homes, and other health care providers must adhere to if they are to qualify for payment from federal funds. Likewise, state laws are interpreted in administrative rules that specify licensing requirements for health care providers in the state.

Federal

Administrative law deals with protection of the rights of citizens. It extends some rights and protections beyond those granted in the federal and state constitutions. An example of this type of law, at the federal level, is the Civil Rights Act of 1964, which prohibits many forms of discrimination in the workplace. This law may necessitate that the nurse manager make some scheduling accommodations for such things as an employee's religious practices.

Another federal law that often affects employment in health care facilities is the Age Discrimination in Employment Act of 1967 (ADEA), which protects those 40 years of age and older by prohibiting employers from discriminating on the basis of age in all aspects of employment, including compensation, terms, conditions, and privileges. This law prohibits employers from using age as a factor in limiting or classifying people in any way that would deprive or tend to deprive them of employment opportunities or otherwise adversely affect their status (Nguyen, 2000b).

The Americans with Disabilities Act (ADA), another federal law, protects individuals with disabilities from discrimination-related employment practices. It protects people with a disability who otherwise meet the skill, experience, education, and other job-related requirements for a position of interest. For this law to apply, individuals must have a physical or mental impairment that substantially limits one or more of their major life activities. If the applicant or worker is a qualified individual with a disability who can do the job in question, with or without a reasonable accommodation, then the individual has certain protected rights. These rights include the right to reasonable accommodation to perform the job; to be treated equally by the employer; and to be able to be promoted (Nguyen, 2000a).

Often, nurses must work with older people or people with disabilities who have different capabilities, judgments, and values, and they must be able to recognize and appreciate these differing perspectives and not be biased against the individuals because of these differences (Cofer, 1998).

The Occupational Safety & Health Administration, an administrative agency, works to establish a safe workplace for employees. This includes enacting regulations concerning storage of hazardous substances; protection of employees from infection; and, recently, protection of employees from violence in the workplace. In a recent article, Sheehan noted that a physical attack may come from a coworker, a patient, or a family member and that the nurse must be alert for any warning that such a response is imminent. Some of the questions she suggests the nurse ask in evaluating the potential for violence in a patient include the following:

- Does the individual exhibit anger, irritation, or illogical thought processes?
- Does the patient exhibit confusion and agitation?
- Does the patient lack emotion or have a dull demeanor? (Sheehan, 2000)

These same observations would be valid for assessing the potential for violence in individuals other than patients.

Table 22-2 details some of the federal agencies that are entrusted with enforcement of these laws.

State

An example of a state's administrative law is its nurse practice act. Under nurse practice acts, state boards of nursing are given the authority to define the practice of nursing within certain broad parameters specified by the legislature, mandate the requisite preparation for the practice of nursing, and discipline members of the profession who deviate from the rules governing the practice of nursing. Other professions such as medicine and dentistry have similar practice acts established in state law.

An issue that is currently being discussed and that may affect the practice of nursing in the near future is the debate concerning multistate licensure (Ventura, 1999). This issue has evolved as nurses have crossed state lines in rendering care. It has been suggested that requiring the nurse to obtain a license in each state in which she practices is impractical, inefficient, and costly. Currently, there is discussion about allowing a nurse licensed in one state to practice in another without securing an additional license, a system similar to that used for driver's licenses. The suggested system would also maintain a database containing the licensure and disciplinary history of every nurse in the United States. Concerns raised about such a multistate licensing system include the loss of each state's regulatory control over nurses practicing within its borders, the potential privacy issues associated with such a large database, the cost of maintaining such a system and how this would affect licensing fees for the nurse (Ventura, 1999).

CIVIL LAW

Civil law governs how individuals relate to each other in everyday matters. It encompasses both contract and tort law. Most cases involving nurses fall into the category of civil tort law (Fiesta, 1999a).

Contract Law

Contract law regulates certain transactions between individuals and/or legal entities such as businesses. It also governs transactions between businesses. An agreement between two or more parties must contain

TABLE 22-2	Federal Agencies and Their Areas of Influence in Health Care
Federal Agency	**Area of Influence**
Equal Employment Opportunity Commission (EEOC)	Evaluates complaints of discrimination
Occupational Safety & Health Administration (OSHA)	Establishes a safe working environment
Health and Human Services (HHS)	Regulates hospitals and nursing homes
National Labor Relations Board (NLRB)	Guards the rights of nurses and/or doctors as employees

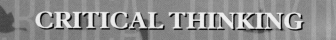

CRITICAL THINKING

You are assigned to a medical-surgical unit, working the night shift. Your supervisor calls and says that one of the registered nurses assigned to the critical care unit has called in sick and you must work that unit instead of your usual assignment. You have never worked in the critical care setting before and have received no orientation to this unit. You are now asked to work there when it is short of staff.

What should you do?

the following elements to be recognized as a legal contract:

- Agreement between two or more legally competent individuals or parties stating what each must or must not do
- Mutual understanding of the terms and obligations that the contract imposes on each party to the contract
- Payment or consideration given for actions taken or not taken pursuant to the agreement

The terms of the contract may be oral or written; however, a written contract may not be legally modified by an oral agreement. Another way this is often expressed is by the phrase "all of the terms of the contract are contained within the four corners of the document," that is, if it is not written, it is not part of the agreement or contract. A contract may be express or implied. In an express contract, the terms of the contract are specified, usually in writing. In an implied contract, a relationship between parties is recognized, although the terms of the agreement are not clearly defined, such as the expectations one has for services from the dry cleaner or the grocer.

The nurse is usually a party to an employment contract. The employed nurse agrees to do the following:

- Adhere to the policies and procedures of the employing entity
- Fulfill the agreed-upon duties of the employer
- Respect the rights and responsibilities of other health care providers in the workplace

In return, the employer agrees to provide the nurse with the following:

- A specified amount of pay for services rendered
- Adequate assistance in providing care
- The supplies and equipment needed to fulfill his responsibilities
- A safe environment in which to work
- Reasonable treatment and behavior from the other health care providers with whom he must interact

This contract may be express or implied, depending on the practices of the employing entity. Sometimes, what is determined to be "reasonable" by the employer is not considered "reasonable" by the nurse. For instance, after 20 years of working as a nurse on the orthopedic unit, a nurse may not view it as reasonable to be pulled to the labor and delivery unit for duty as a nurse there. It would be prudent to express any misgivings to the supervisor and to take assignments that are in keeping with the experience one has on an orthopedic unit.

Tort Law

Black's Law Dictionary (1996) defines **tort** as a private or civil wrong or injury, including action for bad faith breach of contract, for which the court will provide a remedy in the form of an action for damages. A tort can be any of the following:

- The denial of a person's legal right
- The failure to comply with a public duty
- The failure to perform a private duty that results in harm to another

A tort can be unintentional, as occurs in malpractice or neglect, or it can be the intentional infliction of harm such as assault and battery. In a tort suit, the nurse can be named as a defendant because of something she did incorrectly or because she failed to do something that was required. In either case, the suit is usually classified as a tort suit (Fiesta, 1999a). Other tort charges that a nurse may face include assault and battery, false imprisonment, invasion of privacy, defamation, and fraud.

Negligence and Malpractice

If a nurse fails to meet the legal expectations for care, usually defined by the state's nurse practice act, the patient, if harmed by this failure, can initiate an action against the nurse for damages. The term **malpractice** refers to a professional's wrongful conduct in the discharge of his or her professional duties or failure to meet standards of care for the profession, which results in harm to another individual entrusted to the professional's care (Zerwekh & Claborn, 1994). **Negligence** is the failure to provide the care a reasonable person would ordinarily provide in a similar situation.

Simply proving malpractice or negligence is not sufficient to recover damages. Proof of liability or fault requires the proof of the following four elements:

1. A duty or obligation created by law, contract, or standard practice that is owed to the complainant by the professional
2. A breach of this duty, either by omission or commission
3. Harm, which can be physical, emotional, or financial, to the complainant (patient)
4. Proof that the breach of duty caused the complained of harm

A Louisiana appellate court recently described the plaintiff's (patient's) specific burden of proof in a negligence or malpractice case against a nurse as follows:

[T]he three requirements which a plaintiff must satisfy to meet its burden of proving the negligence of a nurse are (1) the nurse must exercise the degree of skill ordinarily employed, under similar circumstances, by the members of the nursing or health care profession in good standing in the same community or locality; (2) the nurse either lacked this degree of knowledge or skill or failed to use reasonable care and diligence, along with her best judgment in the application of that skill; and (3) as a proximate result of this lack of knowledge or skill or the failure to exercise this degree of care, the plaintiff suffered injuries that would not otherwise have occurred. (*Odom v. State Dept. of Health & Hospitals*, [1999])

Once a plaintiff presents his case, the defendant nurse must refute the claims either by showing that if a duty was owed, it was fulfilled or by demonstrating that the breach of that duty was not the cause of the plaintiff's harm.

Proving that a duty was owed is not difficult. The person need only show that the nurse was working on the day in question and was responsible for the plaintiff's care. This can usually be accomplished by producing staffing schedules and assignment sheets.

To demonstrate a breach of duty, the courts employ a *reasonable man* standard by asking what a reasonable nurse would do in a like situation. This is accomplished by reviewing the employing institution's policies and procedures and the state's nurse practice act and hearing testimony from nurses who are accepted as expert witnesses to the standard of nursing practice in the community.

The defendant nurse would employ the same methodology to refute the plaintiff's charges. The nurse would present evidence that the institution's policies and procedures were followed and that the care rendered adhered to accepted nursing standards. To present the nurse's case, the nurse's attorney would also use expert witnesses to document that the care given fulfilled the duty owed, was the kind that would be given by a reasonable nurse in such a circumstance, and that it was not the cause of the plaintiff's harm.

It is not sufficient for a patient plaintiff to show a breach of duty to prevail in a tort suit. He must also show that the breach of the duty caused him harm. Even if it is proved that a nurse made a medication error, if the error was not the cause of the plaintiff's harm, he will not win in recovering damages from the nurse. In a recent malpractice case, a patient with sickle cell anemia died after suffering a cardiopulmonary arrest, attributed to an aspiration that was witnessed by a visitor. The visitor immediately called for and obtained help. Although revived, the patient never regained consciousness and was eventually taken off of life support. At trial, the plaintiff was able to prove that the nurse assigned to this patient did not follow the institution's policy of documenting frequent observations, which were mandated because the patient was receiving a blood transfusion at the time of the cardiac arrest. In reviewing the case on appeal, the appellate court noted the following:

> [T]he record contains no evidence which suggests what could have been done even if the nurse had been seated at his bedside prior to the arrest. Plaintiff has failed to offer any proof that more immediate assistance would have prevented the catastrophic results of his aspiration. Based on the evidence in this record, we conclude that more frequent monitoring would have made no difference. (*Webb v. Tulane Medical Center Hospital*, [1997])

Thus, even though the plaintiff successfully proved a breach of a duty, the breach was not found to be the cause of the patient's death, and the nurse was not found to be guilty of negligence.

Table 22-3 demonstrates the results of a review of appellate decisions in Louisiana from 1995 to 2000.

When a nurse is listed as a party in a medical malpractice lawsuit, the nurse's liability is determined by state laws, such as the nurse practice act, the standards for the practice of nursing, and the institution's policies and procedures. Thus, if Louisiana laws mandate that a nurse must have a doctor's order before doing something, then a doctor's order must be present. Problems arise when the

orders are verbal, and later it is claimed that the nurse misunderstood and acted in error. Another pitfall is illegible writing, which is then misinterpreted and the result causes harm to the patient. Many nurses who have been in practice for a long time have encountered confused doctors who write orders that are contrary to accepted medical practice. In these situations, the nurse must exercise professional judgment and follow the policies and procedures of the institution. Usually these require the nurse to notify the nursing supervisor and the medical director for the area in which the nurse works.

The institution's policies and procedures describe the performance expected of nurses in its employ, and a nurse deviating from them can be liable for negligence or malpractice. Occasionally, such failure to adhere to institutional protocol can result in the employer denying the nurse a defense in a lawsuit.

Practicing nurses must also adhere to the standards of practice for the nursing profession in the community. These standards include such things as checking the five "rights" in medication administration or repositioning the bed-bound patient at regular intervals. It is not uncommon for the nurse to find conflicts between an employer's expectations and the nursing standards of care, resulting in problems such as having insufficient time or staffing to adhere to the standards taught in nursing school or receiving poor evaluations for taking too long to render care. In these situations, the nurse must evaluate what

TABLE 22-3	Louisiana Medical Malpractice Cases in Which Nurses' Actions Were Cited	
Nursing Omission/Commission	**Number of Cases**	**Resolution**
Failure to monitor/assess/communicate findings to appropriate personnel	6	4 decided in patient plaintiff's favor; 2 decided in defendants' favor.
Failure to follow doctor's orders	3	2 decided in patient plaintiff's favor; 1 decided in defendants' favor.
Nursing interventions (such as preventing falls, decubiti, and contractures, and performing sponge counts) were inadequate	7	4 decided in patient plaintiff's favor; 3 decided in defendants' favor

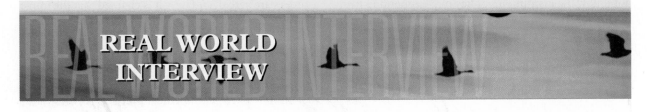

REAL WORLD INTERVIEW

The most common problem areas for a new graduate include the failure to properly document care given, failure to appropriately monitor the patient's condition and document such, and failure to go up the chain of command when physicians are needed and fail to respond. To address these issues, our department provides a risk management orientation for all new nurses during their first week of general orientation. We also meet with individual unit staff at the request of the nurse managers. A program has also been developed and presented to senior nursing students. I tell new graduates they should document, document, and document. If it's not documented, it's not done (as far as the courts are concerned).

Harriet Percy, RN
Risk Manager

standards she must follow to preserve her practice and protect herself from liability, even if this requires a job change.

Assault and Battery

Assault is a threat to touch another in an offensive manner without that person's permission. A **battery** is the touching of another person without that person's consent. In the health care arena, complaints of this nature usually pertain to whether the individual consented to the treatment administered by the health care professional. Most states have laws that require patients to make informed decisions about their treatment.

Fiesta (1999b) explained that informed consent laws protect the patient's right to practice self-determination. The patient has the right to receive sufficient information to make an informed decision about whether to consent or to refuse a procedure. The individual performing the procedure has the responsibility of explaining to the patient the nature of the procedure, benefits, alternatives, and the risks and complications. The signed consent form is used to document that this was done, and it creates a presumption that the patient had been advised of the appropriate risks.

Often the nurse is asked to witness a patient signing a consent form for treatment. When you witness a patient's signature, you are vouching for two

things: that the patient signed the paper and that the patient knows he is signing a consent form (Olsen-Chavarriaga, 2000). For a consent form to be legal, a patient, in most states, must be at least 18 years old; be mentally competent; have the procedures, with their risks and benefits, explained in a manner he can understand; be aware of the available alternatives to the proposed treatment; and consent voluntarily. The nurse must also be familiar with which other people are allowed by state law to consent to medical treatment for another when that person cannot consent for himself. Frequently, these include the person possessing medical power of attorney; a spouse; adult children; or other relatives, if no one is available in one of the other categories listed.

A nurse may also face a charge of battery for failing to honor an advance directive, such as a medical power of attorney, durable power of attorney, or living will. Federal law requires that a hospital ask the patient, upon admission, whether she has a living will; if she does not, the hospital must ask the patient whether she would like to enact one. A **living will** is a written advance directive voluntarily signed by the patient that specifies the type of care she desires if and when she is in a terminal state and cannot sign a consent form or convey this information verbally. It can be a general statement such as "no life sustaining measures" or specific such as "no tube feedings or respirator." Often, the patient's family has difficulty allowing health care personnel to follow the wishes expressed in a living will and conflicts arise. These should be communicated to the hospital ethics committee, pastoral care department, risk management, or whichever hospital department is responsible for handling such issues. If the patient verbalizes her wishes regarding end-of-life care to the family, such difficult situations can sometimes be avoided, and the patient should be encouraged to do this, if possible.

The nurse should be familiar with the requirements for the implementation of a living will in the state where the nurse practices. Figure 22-1 is an example of a living will.

Do Not Resuscitate (DNR) Orders

The attending physician may write a do not resuscitate (DNR) order on an inpatient, which directs the staff not to perform the usual cardiopulmonary resuscitation (CPR) in the event of a sudden cardiopulmonary arrest. The doctor may write such an order without evidence of a living will on the medical record, and the nurse should be familiar with the institution's policies and state law regarding when and how a physician can write such an order in the

---

Sample of a Living Will★

Declaration

Declaration made this _____ day of _____, 2002.

I, _____, being of sound mind, willfully and voluntarily make known my desire that my dying shall not be artificially prolonged under the circumstances set forth below and do hereby declare:

If at any time I should either have a terminal and irreversible incurable injury, disease, or illness or be in a continual profound comatose state with no reasonable chance of recovery, certified by two physicians who have personally examined me, one of whom shall be my attending physician, and the physicians have determined that my death will occur whether or not life-sustaining procedures are utilized and where the application of life-sustaining procedures would serve only to prolong artificially the dying process, I direct that such procedures be withheld or withdrawn and that I be permitted to die naturally with only the administration of medication or the performance of any medical procedure deemed necessary to provide me with comfort care.

In the absence of my ability to give directions regarding the use of such life-sustaining procedures, it is my intention that this declaration shall be honored by my family and physician(s) as the final expression of my legal right to refuse medical or surgical treatment and accept the consequences of such refusal.

I understand the full import of this declaration and I am emotionally and mentally competent to make this declaration.

Signed : _____

City, County, and State of Residence

The declarant has been personally known to me and I believe him/her to be of sound mind.

Witness _____

Witness _____

* See state law requirements.

Figure 22-1 Sample of a Living Will

absence of a living will. Often, a DNR order is considered a medical decision that the doctor can make, preferably in consultation with the family, even without a living will executed by the patient. If the nurse feels such a DNR order is contrary to the patient's or family's wishes, the nurse should consult the policies and procedures of the institution. These may include going up the chain of command until the nurse is satisfied with the course of action. This may entail notifying the nursing supervisor, the medical director, the institution's chief operating officer, state regulators, or the Joint Commission on Accreditation of Healthcare Organizations (JCAHO). Often an institution has an ethics committee that examines such issues and makes a determination of the appropriateness of the order.

False Imprisonment

False imprisonment occurs when individuals are incorrectly led to believe they cannot leave a place. This often occurs because the nurse misinterprets the rights granted to others by legal documents such as powers of attorney and does not allow a patient to leave a facility because the person with the power of attorney (agent) says the patient cannot leave. A **power of attorney** is a legal document executed by an individual (principal) granting another person (agent) the right to perform certain activities in the principal's name. It can be specific, such as "sell my house," or general, such as "make all decisions for me, including health care decisions." In most states, a power of attorney is voluntarily granted by the individual and does not take away the individual's right to exercise his own choices. Thus, if the principal (patient) disagrees with his agent's decisions, the patient's wishes are the ones that prevail. If a situation occurs in which an agent, acting on a power of attorney, disagrees with your patient regarding discharge plans, contact your supervisor for further assistance in deciding an action consistent with your patient's wishes and best interests.

The authority to make medical decisions for another may be granted in a general power of attorney document or in a specific document limited to medical decisions only such as a medical power of attorney. Figure 22-2 is an example of a medical power of attorney. The requirements for a medical power of attorney vary from state to state, as do most legal documents.

A claim of false imprisonment may be based on the inappropriate use of physical or chemical restraints. Federal law mandates that health care institutions employ the least restrictive method of ensuring patient safety. Physical or chemical restraints are to be used only if necessary to protect the patient from harm when all other methods have failed. If the nurse uses restraints on a competent person who is refusing to follow the doctor's orders, the nurse can be charged with false imprisonment or battery. If restraints are used in an emergency situation, the nurse is to contact the doctor immediately after application to secure an order for the restraints. Also, the nurse must check the institution's policies regarding the type and frequency of assessments required for a patient in restraints and how often it is necessary to secure a reorder for the restraints. These policies ensure the patient's safety and must be consistent with state law.

Invasion of Privacy

The nurse is required to respect the privacy of all patients. As a health care practitioner, the nurse may be privy to very personal information and must make every effort to keep it confidential. This often necessitates policing conversations with coworkers that have the potential for being overheard by others so that no patient information is accidentally revealed. Sometimes the protection of a patient's privacy conflicts with the state's mandatory reporting laws for the occurrence of specified infectious diseases such as syphilis or human immunodeficiency virus (HIV). The need to protect an individual's privacy may also conflict with the state's mandatory reporting laws on suspected patient abuse, discussed previously. Other information that state or federal law may require to be revealed include a patient's blood alcohol level, incidences of rape, gunshot wounds, and adverse reactions to certain drugs. Failing to strictly follow reporting laws could lead to criminal, civil, or disciplinary action, termination of employment, or all of these; nurses must consult the institution's policies and confer with its risk management department to ascertain their responsibilities and course of action. The American Nurses Association (ANA) Code for Nurses states that nurses must protect the patient and the public when incompetence or unethical or illegal practice compromise health care and safety. Many states have adopted this concept in their nurse

Sample of Medical Power of Attorney*

By: _____ (Principal)

To: _____ (Agent)

_____ County, _____ (State)

By this instrument of procuration, be it known that on _____ (Date), before me, _____, a notary public, personally came and appeared: _____ (Principal), who is over the age of 18 years, of sound mind, and a resident of _____ County. Principal declared that he/she does grant to the above named agent full power and authority to make health care decisions for principal, in the event he/she is unable to make these decisions for himself/herself for any reason whatsoever. Principal also grants to agent the authority to qualify principal for all government entitlements including, but not limited to, Medicaid, Medicare, and Supplemental Social Security.

This done and passed, at the County and State mentioned above, in the presence of _____ and _____ witnesses, who are both over the age of 18 years and who sign their names along with the principal, _____, and me the notary.

_____ (Principal)

Witness _____

Witness _____

_____
            Notary

I accept the powers granted by this document.

_____ (Agent)

* Check state law requirements.

Figure 22-2 Sample of Medical Power of Attorney

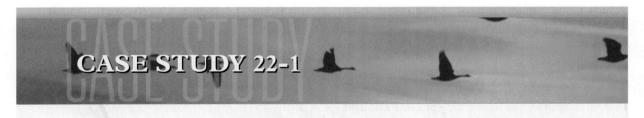

CASE STUDY 22-1

You are working the night shift. One of your patients' physicians has ordered a dose of a medication to be given to a patient that you know is too high for this patient. You are unable to locate the doctor to check the order. What would you do to ensure safe care for your patient?

practice acts, thereby creating a legal obligation to report (Sloan, 1999). If a nurse were to observe unethical behavior in a hospital, he should report this as directed in the institution's policies and procedures manual or by the laws of the state.

Defamation

Defamation is defined as an intentionally false communication/publication (*Black's Law Dictionary*, 1996). Other similar terms used for this tort are *slander*, which is verbal communication. *Libel* is the term for written communication. From its definition, one can see that two essential elements must be proved in a charge of defamation:

1. The information conveyed must be untrue.
2. The false information must be published or communicated to another party.

Note that publication or communication may mean simply telling one other person or writing a friend a letter containing the false information. The nurse may face such an accusation if he communicates inaccurate information to another or if it is claimed that the information charted was untrue. However, several courts have ruled that charting information in a medical record, whether accurate or not, does not constitute publication as required for a charge of defamation.

LEGAL PROTECTIONS IN NURSING PRACTICE

As discussed earlier in this chapter, nursing practice is guided by state nurse practice acts and agency policies and procedures. Other resources for the nurse include Good Samaritan laws, skillful communication, and risk management programs.

Good Samaritan Laws

Good Samaritan laws are laws that have been enacted to protect the health care professional from legal liability. The essential elements of commonly enacted Good Samaritan law are as follows:

- The care is rendered in an emergency situation.
- The health care worker is rendering care without pay.

- The care provided did not recklessly or intentionally cause injury or harm to the injured party.

Note that these laws are intended to protect the volunteer who stops to render care at the scene of an accident. They would not protect an emergency medical technician (EMT) or other health care professionals rendering care at the scene of an accident as part of their assigned duties and for which they receive pay. In doing their duties, these paid emergency personnel would be evaluated according to the standards of their professions.

Skillful Communication

The nurse must communicate accurately and completely both verbally and in writing. In the cases detailed earlier in Table 22-3, more than one-third cited a lack of communication by the nurse. Either the nurse failed to monitor the patient and notify the doctor of a change in the patient's status, or she failed to document the assessments performed. It is essential that the nurse chart accurately and completely. Often a case involving patient care takes several years to come to trial; by that time, the nurse may have no memory of the incident in question and must rely on the written record done at the time of the incident. This record is frequently in the courtroom, blown up to billboard size for all to see. All errors are apparent and omissions stand out by their absence, especially if it is data that should have been recorded per institutional policy. The old adage that "if it isn't written, it wasn't done" will be repeated to the jury numerous times. To protect themselves when charting, nurses should use the FLAT charting acronym: F—factual, L—legible, A—accurate, T—timely

F: Charting should be *factual*—what you see, not what you think happened.
L: Charting should be *legible*, with no erasures. Corrections should be made as you have been taught, with a single line drawn through the error and initialed.
A: Charting should be *accurate* and complete. What color was the drainage and how much was present? How many times, and at what times, was the doctor notified of changes? Was the supervisor notified?

T: Charting should be *timely*, completed as soon after the occurrence as possible. "Late entries" should be avoided or kept to a minimum.

Following Doctors' Orders

In most states, the nurse is required to follow the doctor's orders in giving care to the patient unless doing so would cause the patient harm. To follow this mandate, the nurse must ensure that the orders are clear and accurate. If necessary, the nurse may have to contact the physician for clarification. If the nurse is still uncomfortable following the order, the supervisor should be notified and the institution's policies followed regarding notification. Because of the opportunity for misinterpretation and misunderstanding, verbal orders are not encouraged.

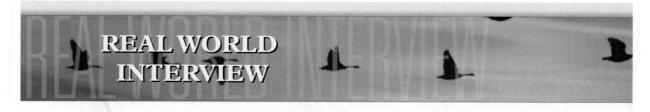

REAL WORLD INTERVIEW

The role of risk management in the health care environment is that of recognition, evaluation, and treatment of risks inherent in the organization. The goal of risk management is improving the quality of care provided by the organization while at the same time protecting its financial integrity. Risk management, while coordinated at a certain level of the organization, is not simply a one-department responsibility, but rather is the responsibility of each employee of the organization.

New graduates in nursing need to understand that in today's competitive health care environment, it is important that each practitioner look for ways to reduce the risks inherent in the delivery of health care. At a time when hospitals are receiving less and less reimbursement, our patients and consumers are demanding higher and higher quality of care.

Health care is at a crossroads, similar to the one that faced private industry during the 1970s. Our customers are demanding that we provide a safe environment and that we consistently strive for continuous quality improvement.

An incident report is a commonly used form that documents a variance from normal protocol or hospital procedures. It is not meant to place blame on an individual practitioner or department. It is used strictly to document the facts surrounding an event so the health care processes can be improved. Thus, the nurse should complete an incident report when any variance from a policy or a procedure is noticed.

When risk management receives the incident reports, they are logged into our database, and monthly reports are forwarded to nurse managers for follow-up and education with their staff.

Incident reports and the subsequent risk management department actions are generally reactive but we also do proactive/preventive interventions in the health care setting. These include the following:

1. Education of students completing their senior year of study in nursing

2. Participation on patient safety, environment of care, pharmacy, nursing, and other hospital committees, which work on proactive programs to reduce risks

3. Facilitation of the slips and falls task force to reduce our patients' fall risk

4. Education of new nurses and physicians on principles of risk management

Harriet Percy, RN
Risk Manager

Risk Management Programs

Risk management programs in health care organizations are designed to identify and correct system problems that contribute to errors in patient care or to employee injury. The emphasis in risk management is on quality improvement and protection of the institution from financial liability. Institutions usually have reporting and tracking forms that record incidents that may lead to financial liability for the institution. Risk management will assist in identifying and correcting the underlying problem that may have led to an incident, such as faulty equipment, staffing concerns, or the need for better orientation for employees. Once a system problem is identified, the risk management department may develop educational programs to address the problem.

The risk management department may also investigate and record information surrounding a patient or employee incident that may result in a lawsuit. This helps personnel remember critical factors if called to testify at a later time. The nurse should notify the risk management department of all reportable incidents and complete all risk management and/or incident report forms as mandated by institutional policies and procedures. Note also that employee complaints of harassment or discrimination can expose the institution to significant liability and should promptly be reported to supervisors and the risk management department, human resources, or whichever department is specified in the institution's policies. See Table 22-4 for a checklist of actions to decrease the risk of nursing liability.

Malpractice/ Professional Liability Insurance

Nurses may need to carry their own malpractice insurance. Nurses often think their actions are adequately covered by the employer's liability insurance, but this is not necessarily so. If, in giving care, the

TABLE 22-4	Actions to Decrease the Risk of Liability

- Communicate with your clients by keeping them informed and listening to what they say.
- Acknowledge unfortunate incidents and express concern about these events without either taking the blame, blaming others, or reacting defensively.
- Chart and time your observations immediately, while facts are still fresh in your mind.
- Take appropriate actions to meet the client's nursing needs.
- Follow the facility's policies and procedures for administering care and reporting incidents.
- Acknowledge and document the reason for any omission or deviation from agency policy, procedure, or standard.
- Maintain clinical competency and acknowledge your limitations. If you do not know how to do something, ask for help.
- Promptly report any concern regarding the quality of care, including the lack of resources with which to provide care, to a nursing administration representative.
- Use appropriate standards of care.
- Document the time of changes in conditions requiring notification of the physician and include the response of the physician.
- Delegate client care based on the documented skills of licensed and unlicensed personnel.
- Treat all clients and their families with kindness and respect.

CRITICAL THINKING

You are the only licensed nurse assigned to give 9 A.M. medications on a 52-bed nursing home unit. To avoid being classified as a drug error according to the institution's policy and usual nursing practice, administration of the medications must occur within 45 minutes of the ordered time. Also, nursing practice mandates you verify the "five rights": the right drug, the right dose, the right patient, the right time, and the right route.

What problems are there with this assignment? What would you do?

nurse fails to comply with the institution's policies and procedures, the institution may deny the nurse a defense, claiming that because of the nurse's failure to follow institutional policy, or because of the nurse working outside his scope of employment, he was not acting as an employee at that time. Also, nurses are being named individually as defendants in malpractice suits more frequently than in the past. Consequently, it is advantageous for the nurse to be assured of a defense independent of that of his employer. Professional liability insurance provides that assurance and pays for an attorney to defend the nurse in a malpractice lawsuit.

Nurse/Attorney Relationship

Despite the nurse's best intentions, a nurse may be named as a defendant in a lawsuit and need to retain the services of an attorney. LaDuke (2000) made the following suggestions for consulting and collaborating with an attorney:

1. Retain a specialist. Generalists are competent to handle many matters, but professional malpractice, professional disciplinary proceedings, and employment disputes are best handled by specialists in those areas.
2. Be attentive. Read the documents the attorney produces and travel to court proceedings to observe the attorney's performance.
3. Notify your insurance carrier as soon as you are aware of any real or potential liability issue. Inform your agent about the status of your case every few months, even if it is unchanged.

4. Keep costs sensible. Your attorney should explain initially how the fee will be computed and how you will be billed. The attorney may require you to pay a retainer fee.
5. Keep informed. The attorney should address your questions and concerns promptly. You are entitled to be kept informed about the status of your case. You are entitled to copies of all correspondence, legal briefs, and other documents.
6. Weed through writing. Your attorney needs to explain all facts and options. Examine all relevant documents and do not hesitate to make corrections in the same way you would correct a medical record by drawing a line through the incorrect or misleading information, writing in the correction, and signing your initials after it.
7. Set your own course. Insist on a collaborative relationship with your attorney for the duration of your case.

KEY CONCEPTS

- Nursing practice is governed by civil, public, and administrative laws.
- Nurses are responsible for providing a safe environment for patients entrusted to their care.
- Nurses need to be familiar with their institution's policies and procedures in giving care and in reporting variances, illegal activities, or unexpected events.
- Nurses must have good oral and written communication skills.

- Common torts include negligence and malpractice, assault and battery, false imprisonment, invasion of privacy, and defamation.
- Nurses need to be familiar with their state nurse practice act.
- Good Samaritan laws exist in many states.
- Risk management programs improve the quality of care and protect the financial integrity of institutions.

KEY TERMS

administrative law	false imprisonment
assault	Good Samaritan laws
battery	living will
civil law	malpractice
common law	negligence
constitution	power of attorney
contract law	public law
defamation	tort

REVIEW QUESTIONS

1. Which of the following is the agency that evaluates complaints of discrimination?
   A. Occupational Safety & Health Administration
   B. Equal Employment Opportunity Commission
   C. Health and Human Services
   D. National Labor Relations Board

2. Which type of law authorizes state boards to enact rules that govern the practice of nursing?
   A. State law
   B. Federal law
   C. Common law
   D. Criminal law

3. An intentionally false communication, either published or spoken, is which of the following?
   A. Assault
   B. Defamation
   C. Malpractice
   D. False imprisonment

4. Invasion of privacy is an example of which of the following?
   A. Tort
   B. Administrative law violation
   C. Good Samaritan law violation
   D. Criminal law violation

5. A body of law that develops through precedents over time and has the force of law is called which of the following?
   A. Contract law
   B. Common law
   C. Public law
   D. Civil law

REVIEW ACTIVITIES

1. Talk to the risk manager at a hospital in which you have your clinical assignments. Ask the risk manager how she handles an incident report. Is it used for improving the hospital's care in the future? How?

2. Review the living will policy at a hospital in which you have your clinical assignments. Notice the forms that patients sign. How do they compare with the living will form in this chapter?

3. Discuss how a nurse's off-duty behavior can affect her practice as a nurse. Can the state board of nursing take action against the nurse's license?

EXPLORING THE WEB

- Go to this site to find malpractice information for your state: *http://www.mcandl.com/states. html*
- Where can you find state and federal laws regulating hospitals? *http://www.findlaw.com*
- You have a patient who is to be transferred to a nursing home for recuperation. Where can you tell the family to look to evaluate the local nursing homes regarding their adherence to the federal regulations for nursing homes? *http://www.medicare.gov/nhcompare/home.asp*
- Where can you find a copy of the ANA Code of Ethics? *http://www.ana.org/ethics/ecode.htm*

REFERENCES

Black's law dictionary (6th ed.). (1996). St. Paul, MN: West.

Cofer, M. J. (1998). How to avoid age bias. *Nursing Management, 29*(11), 34–36.

Court case: Defending against sexual assault charges. (1999). *Nursing99, 29*(6), 71.

Cruzan v. Director, Missouri Department of Health, 110 S. Ct. 2841 (1990).

Fiesta, J. (1999a). Do no harm: When caregivers violate our golden rule, part 1. *Nursing Management, 30*(8), 10–11.

Fiesta, J. (1999b). Informed consent: What health care professionals need to know, part 2. *Nursing Management, 30*(7), 6–7.

Fiesta, J. (1999c). Know your boundaries in sexual assault litigation. *Nursing Management, 30*(10), 10.

LaDuke, S. (2000). What should you expect from your attorney? *Nursing Management, 31*(1), 10.

Mantel, D. L. (1999). Legally speaking: Off-duty doesn't mean off the hook. *RN, 62*(10), 71–74.

Murphy v. United Parcel Service, 527 U.S. 516 (1999).

Nguyen, B. Q. (2000a). ADA coverage: Defining who is a "qualified individual with a disability." *American Journal of Nursing, 100*(1), 87.

Nguyen, B. Q. (2000b). If you're replaced by a younger nurse. *American Journal of Nursing, 100*(3), 82.

Odom v. State Department of Health & Hospitals, 322 So. 2d 91 (La. 1999).

Olsen-Chavarriaga, D. (2000). Informed consent: Do you know your role? *Nursing2000, 30*(5), 60–61.

Roe v. Wade, 410 U.S. 133 (1973).

Sheehan, J. P. (2000). Protect your staff from workplace violence. *Nursing Management, 31*(3), 24–25.

Sloan, A. J. (1999). Legally speaking: Whistleblowing: There are risks! *RN, 62*(7), 65–68.

Sutton v. United Airlines, 527 U.S. 471 (1999).

Ventura, M. J. (1999). The great multistate licensure debate. *RN, 62*(5), 58–62.

Webb v. Tulane Medical Center Hospital, 700 So. 2d 1142 (La. 1997).

Zerwekh, J., & Claborn, J. C. (2000). *Nursing today: Transition and trends* (2nd ed.). Philadelphia: Saunders.

SUGGESTED READINGS

Brown, S. M. (1999). Good Samaritan laws: Protection and limits. *RN, 62*(11), 65–68.

DeLaune, S., & Ladner, P. K. (2002). *Fundamentals of nursing* (2nd ed.). Clifton Park, NY: Delmar Learning.

Fiesta, J. (1999d). Greater need for background checks. *Nursing Management, 30*(11), 26.

Fiesta, J. (1999e). Informed consent: What health care professionals need to know, part 1. *Nursing Management, 30*(6), 8–9.

Fiesta, J. (1999f). When sexual harassment hits home. *Nursing Management, 30*(5), 16–18.

McKee, R. (1999). Clarifying advance directives. *Nursing99, 29*(5), 52–53.

Morris, M. R. (1998). Elder abuse: What the law requires. *RN, 61*(8), 52–53.

Perry, J. (2000). Legislating sharps safety. *Nursing2000, 30*(5), 50–51.

Simpson, R. (1999). Tech talk on multistate licensure. *Nursing Management, 30*(1), 12–13.

Staten, P. A. (1999). How to cover all the bases on informed consent. *Nursing Management, 30*(9), 14.

Sullivan, G. H. (1999). Legally speaking: Minimizing your risk in patient falls. *RN, 62*(4), 69–70.

Sullivan, G. H. (2000). Legally speaking: Keep your charting on course. *RN, 63*(4), 75–79.

Wilkinson, A. P. (1998). Nursing malpractice. *Nursing98, 28*(6), 34–39.

Ventura, M. J. (1999). Legally speaking: When information must be revealed. *RN, 62*(2), 61–62, 64.

CHAPTER 23

Ethical Dimensions of Patient Care

Camille B. Little, MS, RN

OBJECTIVES

Upon completion of this chapter, the reader should be able to:

1. Define ethics.
2. Develop a personal philosophy of professional nursing.
3. Understand and analyze ethical principles and theories as the basis for professional nursing practice.
4. Discuss participation on ethics committees in hospitals.
5. Apply a model for ethical decision making to an ethical dilemma.
6. Examine ethical issues encountered in practice, including cost containment, use of technology, and patients' rights.
7. Incorporate a personal ethic of social responsibility and service into professional practice.
8. Promote an ethical culture within the practice setting.

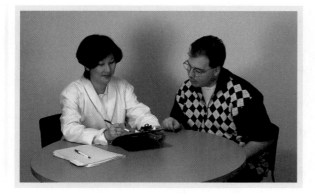

In a large teaching hospital, a patient you are caring for says he does not want to go on living. He has had cancer for several years and states he is tired of being sick. When you ask him whether he has shared these feelings with his family, he says that he does not want them to think he is giving up. You report the patient's statements to the next shift and explain how you encouraged him to talk with his family and his doctor. That evening, the patient suddenly arrests and a code is called. The patient ends up on a ventilator, receives five units of blood, and is comatose.

What are your thoughts about maintaining the patient's life in this situation?

Who should make the decision about the patient's situation since he is comatose?

Nursing has been an ethically principled discipline throughout its history. Nurses are confronted with ethical dilemmas in all types of practice settings. This chapter provides an overview of the nursing profession's ethics and the increased ethical challenges faced by nurses in today's health care environment.

DEFINITION OF ETHICS AND MORALITY

Ethics is the branch of philosophy that concerns the distinction of right from wrong on the basis of a body of knowledge, not just on the basis of opinions. Morality is behavior in accordance with custom or tradition and usually reflects personal or religious beliefs (DeLaune & Ladner, 2002). Ethics governs professional groups and provides a framework for determining the right course of action in a particular situation. For nurses, the actions they take in practice are primarily governed by the ethical principles

of the profession. These principles influence practice, conduct, and relationships that nurses are held accountable for in the delivery of care. Health care ethics, also called bioethics, are ethics specific to health care and serve as a framework to guide behavior in ethical dilemmas. An ethical dilemma occurs when there is a conflict between two or more ethical principles; there is no "correct" decision.

Laws, in contrast, are state and federal government rules that govern all of society. Laws mandate behavior. In some situations in health care, the distinctions between law and ethics are not clear. There may be cases in which ethics and law are congruent; in others, ethics and law may be in conflict (Sullivan & Decker, 2001).

HISTORICAL AND PHILOSOPHICAL INFLUENCES ON NURSING PRACTICE

Nursing practice evolved from the needs of society and has been strongly influenced by religions and women. Society created the profession of nursing for the purpose of meeting specific, perceived health needs (Burkhardt & Nathaniel, 2002). Nursing fulfilled the need to care for people with illnesses. Likewise, a strong instinct for preservation of humanity gave people the motivation to help one another. The concern for health of the community was evident in antiquity and continued as civilizations developed (Donahue, 1985). A complementary relationship evolved as social needs and individual motivation to care for others developed.

Religious Influences

Workers who were engaged in nursing, usually women, were often trained in the doctrines of the church, including unquestioning obedience, humility, and sacrificing one's self for the good of others. An individual nurse did not make independent decisions but followed instructions given by a priest or physician.

Women's Influences

Donahue states that nursing has its origin in the mother-care of helpless infants and must have coexisted with this type of care from earliest times

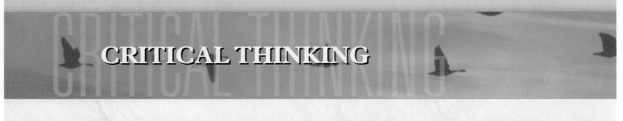

CRITICAL THINKING

Which of the following behaviors is (or are) ethical and illegal? Legal and unethical? Illegal and unethical? Legal and ethical?

- Working in a clinic that performs abortions
- Honoring a terminally ill patient's request to have "no heroic" actions taken
- Discontinuing a comatose patient's life support at the request of the family
- Diverting medications from a patient for your own use

(Donahue, 1985). Mothers cared for family members when they were helpless and sick. During the Christian era, women were selected by Jesus because of the compassion they showed as they ministered to the poor and sick. Thus, Christianity greatly enhanced women's opportunities for useful social service (Donahue, 1985).

Philosophy

Philosophy is the rational investigation of the truths and principles of knowledge, reality, and human conduct. Personal philosophies stem from an individual's beliefs and values. These beliefs and values, in turn, develop based upon a person's experiences in life, cultural influences, and education.

Philosophy of Nursing

A professional nurse's personal philosophy affects her philosophy of nursing. Throughout the nursing educational process, students begin forming their philosophy of nursing. This philosophy is influenced significantly by a student's personal philosophy and experiences. One's personal philosophy should be compatible with the philosophy of the nursing department where she works. This helps the nurse to be an effective leader and practitioner. See Figure 23-1 for a nursing department's philosophy statement. An example of a personal nursing philosophy is:

I believe professional nursing care promotes an optimal level of wellness in body, mind, and spirit to those being served. I believe professional nurses must hold themselves to the highest standards of the profession and honor the profession's code of ethics in all aspects of practice.

ETHICAL THEORIES

The study of ethical behavior has resulted in different theories that may apply to nursing practice and form a framework for ethical decision making. Most familiar among theories in contemporary health care ethics are utilitarianism, a form of teleology, and deontology. Table 23-1 describes these theories.

VIRTUES

Burkhardt and Nathaniel (2002) list four virtues that are more significant than others and that are illustrative of a virtuous person: compassion, discernment, trustworthiness, and integrity. Compassion is a trait nurses have, as perceived by society. It refers to the desire to alleviate suffering. Discernment is possession of acuteness of judgment. Trustworthiness and integrity are traits expected in all people but are especially necessary for professional nurses. These traits form the foundation for an ethically principled discipline and have been endorsed throughout the profession's history (Burkhardt & Nathaniel, 2002).

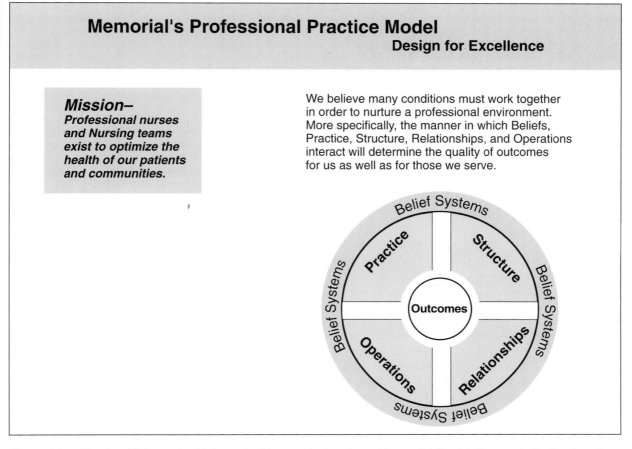

Figure 23-1 Nursing Philosophy (Adapted with permission from Memorial Health System's Professional Practice Philosophy, Springfield, IL)

| TABLE 23-1 | Ethical Theories |

Teleology

Also called *consequentialist theory*. Utilitarianism is one form of teleology.

Theory states that the value of a situation is determined by its consequences. Thus, the outcome of an action—not the action itself—is the criterion for measuring the goodness of that action (e.g., an action is good if it results in a benefit).

Deontology

Also called *formalism*.

Theory states that in determining the ethics of a situation, a person must consider the motives of the actor, not the consequence of the act. This theory was postulated by Immanuel Kant, who established the categorical imperative. The categorical imperative states that one should act only if the action is based on a Universal Principle—that is, everyone would act the same way in a similar situation.

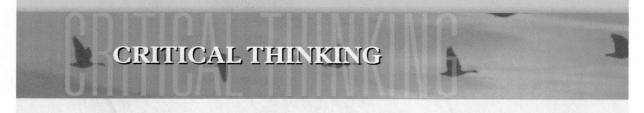

New graduates should formulate a philosophy of nursing based on personal beliefs and values. Reflections on the following questions can assist in the development of a philosophy:

What do you believe about nursing practice? How should professionals conduct themselves? How can you influence patient care based on your nursing philosophy?

CRITICAL THINKING

Mr. Jones smokes three packs of cigarettes a day and is seen in a free clinic for chronic obstructive pulmonary disease. All attempts at getting him to stop smoking have failed. Mr. Jones tells you that smoking is the one pleasure he has in life and he does not want to give it up.

Do you respect Mr. Jones's wishes? Does he still have a right to the free treatment and medications? Are limits to Mr. Jones's treatments justified?

ETHICAL PRINCIPLES AND RULES

In addition to the theories, ethical principles and rules provide a basis for nurses to determine the appropriate action when faced with an ethical dilemma in the practice setting. See Table 23-2 for a summary of the major ethical principles and rules.

Ethics Committees

The complexities found in health care today have presented numerous ethical dilemmas to nurses in patient care, management, and administrative situations. To assist with decision making in these situations, many health care organizations are looking to an organizational ethics committee for assistance. These committees are interdisciplinary in their membership and include representatives from clinical nursing and administration, medicine, clergy, clinical social service, nutritional service, pharmacy, and the legal profession. Additional participants may be invited on an as-needed basis (Figure 23-2).

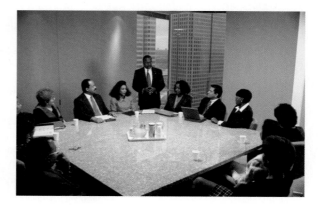

Figure 23-2 Ethics Committee at Work (Photo courtesy of Photodisc)

TABLE 23-2	Ethical Principles and Rules	

Ethical Principle/Rule	Definition	Example
Beneficence	The duty to do good to others and to maintain a balance between benefits and harms.	• Provide all patients, including the terminally ill, with caring attention. • Become familiar with your state laws regarding organ donations. • Treat every patient with respect and courtesy.
Nonmaleficence	The principle of doing no harm.	• Always work within your scope of practice. • Never give information or perform duties you are not qualified to do. • Observe all safety rules and precautions. • Keep areas safe from hazards. • Perform procedures according to facility protocols. Never take shortcuts. • Ask an appropriate person about anything you are unsure of. • Keep your skills up to date.
Justice	The principle of fairness that is served when an individual is given that which he or she is due, owed, deserves, or can legitimately claim.	• Treat all patients equally, regardless of economic or social background. • Learn the state laws and your facility's policies and procedures for handling and reporting suspected abuse.
Autonomy	Respect for an individual's right to self-determination; respect for individual liberty.	• Be sure that patients have consented to all treatments and procedures. • Become familiar with state laws and facility policies dealing with advance directives. • Never release patient information of any kind unless there is a signed release. • Do not discuss patients with anyone who is not professionally involved in their care. • Protect the physical privacy of patients.
Fidelity	The principle of promise keeping; the duty to keep one's promise or word.	• Be sure that necessary contracts have been completed. • Be very careful about what you say to patients. They may only hear the "good news."
Respect for others	The right of people to make their own decision.	• Provide all persons with information for decision making. • Avoid making paternalistic decisions for others.
Veracity	The obligation to tell the truth.	• Admit mistakes promptly. Offer to do whatever is necessary to correct them. • Refuse to participate in any form of fraud. • Give an "honest day's work" every day.

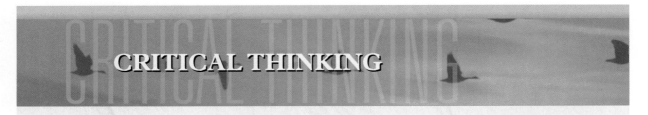

CRITICAL THINKING

You are caring for Mr. Trout, who has been labeled a malingerer. He is in and out of the hospital frequently and always has some type of pain requiring parenteral medications. The order is to give a placebo when he asks for pain medication. When you take the placebo in, Mr. Trout asks you what the medication is.

What principles can guide your actions regarding Mr. Trout? What theories can guide your actions in relation to this patient?

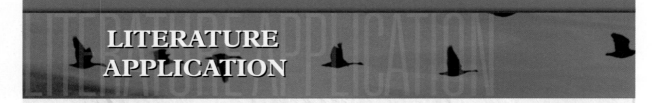

LITERATURE APPLICATION

Citation: Raines, M. L. (2000). Ethical decision making in nurses: Relationships among moral reasoning, coping style, and ethics stress. *JONA's Healthcare Law, Ethics, and Regulation, 2* (1), 29–40.

Discussion: The increasing complexities of health care have led to many ethical dilemmas for nurses. Results from a survey of oncology nurses showed that the nurses experienced an average of 32 different types of ethical dilemmas within the past year. These dilemmas resulted in the nurses experiencing increased stress. The types of ethical issues experienced most frequently were related to pain management, cost containment, decisions in the best interest of the patient, and quality-of-life decisions. The survey also looked at coping strategies that nurses use to deal with stress. Findings indicated nurses used a wide range of positive coping strategies and support resources to help them work through stress. The nurses' primary support consisted of other nurses, but their support resources also included social workers and spouses.

Implications for Practice: Nurses need to develop strategies and have a dependable support system to assist them in coping effectively with the stressful situations encountered in practice.

Anyone on the health care team has the opportunity to refer a situation that has an ethical dilemma associated with it to the ethics committee. Cases, such as the one described in the Opening Scenario, may be referred to the committee for direction. The role of the ethics committee is to provide guidance that assists with decisions involving ethical dilemmas. The ethics committee uses guidelines and criteria developed at the time of its inception to assist with the resolution. In the case in the Opening Scenario,

the ethics committee may invite family members of the patient and other nurses and physicians to assist the ethics committee with the review.

Values

Values are personal beliefs about the truth of ideals, standards, principles, objects, and behaviors that give meaning and direction to life. If you were told that

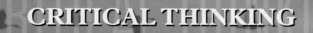

CRITICAL THINKING

Administration announces that the nurse manager must decrease full-time staff by two people. What are the nurse manager's choices? How will the rest of the personnel on the unit view having to work with fewer staff? Will patient care be compromised if staffing is too low? To what extent can the nurse manager compromise personal and unit values?

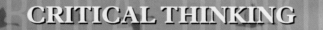

CRITICAL THINKING

A nurse administered the wrong medication to a patient. The patient then had to be transferred to the intensive care unit and required a longer stay in the hospital. The nurse freely admitted the mistake to her nurse manager. The manager recommended that the two of them go talk with the patient and explain what happened. Then the administration heard about the incident and advised the manager against telling the patient immediately about the error. The situation was also referred to the hospital ethics committee. How can the nurse make the right decision? Who is the nurse manager an advocate for? Where does loyalty belong when the patient, the staff nurse, the organization, and self are all involved?

you must pack a bag for a special trip but you may bring only three items from your belongings, what items would you choose? The ones selected are what you value. Suppose the staff, in the Critical Thinking example of a proposed workforce reduction, refused to work under the circumstances they would face if the numbers were reduced as directed? What could be said about the staff's values? What could be said about the administration's values?

Values Clarification

Values clarification is the process of analyzing one's own values to better understand what is truly important. In their classic work *Values and Teaching*, Raths, Harmin, and Simon (1978, p. 47) formulated a theory of values clarification and proposed a three-step process of valuing, as follows:

1. *Choosing*: Beliefs are chosen freely (that is, without coercion) from among alternatives. The choosing step involves analysis of the consequences of various alternatives.
2. *Prizing*: The beliefs that are selected are cherished (that is, prized).
3. *Acting*: The selected beliefs are demonstrated consistently through behavior.

Nurses must understand that values are individual rather than universal; therefore, nurses should not try to impose their own values on clients.

A Guide for Ethical Decision Making

Burkhardt and Nathaniel (2002) developed a guide for decision making, which new nurses may find useful when confronted with an ethical decision. The main points are noted here.

> **Guide for Decision Making**
> - Gather data and identify conflicting moral claims
> - Identify key participants
> - Determine moral perspective and phase of moral development of key participants
> - Determine desired outcomes
> - Identify options
> - Act on the choice
> - Evaluate outcomes of action

ETHICAL ISSUES ENCOUNTERED IN PRACTICE

Numerous events contribute to ethical issues that professional nurses encounter in today's practice. Cost containment and technology and patient rights have all influenced the increased numbers of ethical dilemmas nurses face.

Cost Containment and Issues Related to Technology

Cost containment and the sophisticated technology available in health care today are related. The more technology that is developed and used, the more costly health care becomes. Schroeder (1995) iden-

tifies numerous factors that contribute to the exorbitant costs of receiving treatment in our system. Intensive care units are full of expensive equipment designed to breathe for patients, monitor vital signs automatically, and communicate if the heart is failing in some way. Scores of devices all have the same purpose—to let us know what needs to be done to sustain life.

While the use of technology has brought many benefits, two significant questions arise about its use. When do we refrain from the use of technology? When do we stop using it once we have started? Who is entitled to it in our society?

Patient Rights

The American Hospital Association developed a Patient's Bill of Rights (Table 23-3) with the expectation that when patients and families participate in treatment decisions, the outcome will be more effective care. See the "Exploring the Web" section at the end of this chapter to view this document on-line.

ETHICAL LEADERSHIP AND MANAGEMENT

Nurses have the opportunity to provide leadership in numerous ways and ensure that ethical principles are adhered to throughout all practice settings. Nurse leaders are charged with the responsibility of creating an environment that is ethically principled and accept accountability for upholding the standards of conduct set by the profession. Characteristics of

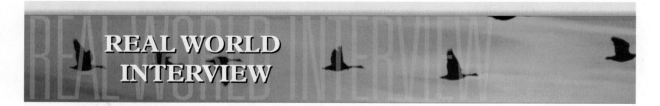

REAL WORLD INTERVIEW

One of my most difficult cases involved a man in his early 40s who was in a coma, ventilator dependent, and declared brain dead. The patient was from a different culture, and when the family arrived 6 weeks later from the country abroad, they refused to allow him to be removed from the ventilator. His parents said they were told by the gods that their son would be well several months in the future. After 2 months in the hospital, the administration began to put pressure on the family to transfer the patient.

Emily Davison, RN
Case Manager

TABLE 23-3	A Patient's Bill of Rights

Introduction

Effective health care requires collaboration between patients and physicians and other health care professionals. Open and honest communication, respect for personal and professional values, and sensitivity to differences are integral to optimal patient care. As the setting for the provision of health services, hospitals must provide a foundation for understanding and respecting the rights and responsibilities of patients, their families, physicians, and other caregivers. Hospitals must ensure a health care ethic that respects the role of patients in decision making about treatment choices and other aspects of their care. Hospitals must be sensitive to cultural, racial, linguistic, religious, age, gender, and other differences as well as the needs of persons with disabilities.

The American Hospital Association presents *A Patient's Bill of Rights* with the expectation that it will contribute to more effective patient care and be supported by the hospital on behalf of the institution, its medical staff, employees, and patients. The American Hospital Association encourages health care institutions to tailor this bill of rights to their patient community by translating and/or simplifying the language of this bill of rights as may be necessary to ensure that patients and their families understand their rights and responsibilities.

Bill of Rights*

1. The patient has the right to considerate and respectful care.

2. The patient has the right to and is encouraged to obtain from physicians and other direct caregivers relevant, current, and understandable information concerning diagnosis, treatment, and prognosis. Except in emergencies when the patient lacks decision-making capacity and the need for treatment is urgent, the patient is entitled to the opportunity to discuss and request information related to the specific procedures and/or treatments, the risks involved, the possible length of recuperation, and the medically reasonable alternatives and their accompanying risks and benefits. Patients have the right to know the identity of physicians, nurses, and others involved in their care, as well as when those involved are students, residents, or other trainees. The patient also has the right to know the immediate and long-term financial implications of treatment choices, insofar as they are known.

3. The patient has the right to make decisions about the plan of care prior to and during the course of treatment and to refuse a recommended treatment or plan of care to the extent permitted by law and hospital policy and to be informed of the medical consequences of this action. In case of such refusal, the patient is entitled to other appropriate care and services that the hospital provides or transfer to another hospital. The hospital should notify patients of any policy that might affect patient choice within the institution.

4. The patient has the right to have an advance directive (such as a living will, health care proxy, or durable power of attorney for health care) concerning treatment or designating a surrogate decision maker with the expectation that the hospital will honor the intent of that directive to the extent permitted by law and hospital policy. Health care institutions must advise patients of their rights under state law and hospital policy to make informed medical choices, ask if the patient has an advance directive, and include that information in patient records. The patient has the right to timely information about hospital policy that may limit its ability to implement fully a legally valid advance directive.

5. The patient has the right to every consideration of privacy. Case discussion, consultation, examination, and treatment should be conducted so as to protect each patient's privacy.

(continues)

Table 23-3 *(continued)*

6. The patient has the right to expect that all communications and records pertaining to his/her care will be treated as confidential by the hospital, except in cases such as suspected abuse and public health hazards when reporting is permitted or required by law. The patient has the right to expect that the hospital will emphasize the confidentiality of this information when it releases it to any other parties entitled to review information in these records.

7. The patient has the right to review the records pertaining to his/her medical care and to have the information explained or interpreted as necessary, except when restricted by law.

8. The patient has the right to expect that, within its capacity and policies, a hospital will make reasonable response to the request of a patient for appropriate and medically indicated care and services. The hospital must provide evaluation, service, and/or referral as indicated by the urgency of the case. When medically appropriate and legally permissible, or when a patient has so requested, a patient may be transferred to another facility. The institution to which the patient is to be transferred must first have accepted the patient for transfer. The patient must also have the benefit of complete information and explanation concerning the need for, risks, benefits, and alternatives to such a transfer.

9. The patient has the right to ask and be informed of the existence of business relationships among the hospital, educational institutions, other health care providers, or payers that may influence the patient's treatment and care.

10. The patient has the right to consent to or decline to participate in proposed research studies or human experimentation affecting care and treatment or requiring direct patient involvement, and to have those studies fully explained prior to consent. A patient who declines to participate in research or experimentation is entitled to the most effective care that the hospital can otherwise provide.

11. The patient has the right to expect reasonable continuity of care when appropriate and to be informed by physicians and other caregivers of available and realistic patient care options when hospital care is no longer appropriate.

12. The patient has the right to be informed of hospital policies and practices that relate to patient care, treatment, and responsibilities. The patient has the right to be informed of available resources for resolving disputes, grievances, and conflicts, such as ethics committees, patient representatives, or other mechanisms available in the institution. The patient has the right to be informed of the hospital's charges for services and available payment methods.

The collaborative nature of health care requires that patients, or their families/surrogates, participate in their care. The effectiveness of care and patient satisfaction with the course of treatment depend, in part, on the patient fulfilling certain responsibilities. Patients are responsible for providing information about past illnesses, hospitalizations, medications, and other matters related to health status. To participate effectively in decision making, patients must be encouraged to take responsibility for requesting additional information or clarification about their health status or treatment when they do not fully understand information and instructions. Patients are also responsible for ensuring that the health care institution has a copy of their written advance directive if they have one. Patients are responsible for informing their physicians and other caregivers if they anticipate problems in following prescribed treatment.

Patients should also be aware of the hospital's obligation to be reasonably efficient and equitable in providing care to other patients and the community. The hospital's rules and regulations are designed to help the hospital meet this obligation. Patients and their families are responsible for making reason-

(continues)

Table 23-3 *(continued)*

able accommodations to the needs of the hospital, other patients, medical staff, and hospital employees. Patients are responsible for providing necessary information for insurance claims and for working with the hospital to make payment arrangements, when necessary.

A person's health depends on much more than health care services. Patients are responsible for recognizing the impact of their life-style on their personal health.

Conclusion

Hospitals have many functions to perform, including the enhancement of health status, health promotion, and the prevention and treatment of injury and disease; the immediate and ongoing care and rehabilitation of patients; the education of health professionals, patients, and the community; and research. All these activities must be conducted with an overriding concern for the values and dignity of patients.

*These rights can be exercised on the patient's behalf by a designated surrogate or proxy decision maker if the patient lacks decision-making capacity, is legally incompetent, or is a minor.

A Patient's Bill of Rights was first adopted by the American Hospital Association in 1973. This revision was approved by the AHA Board of Trustees on October 21, 1992. Copyright 1992 by the American Hospital Association, 840 North Lake Short Drive, Chicago, IL 60611. Printed in the U.S.A. All rights reserved. Reprinted with permission of the American Hospital Association.

ethical leadership identified by Cassidy (1998) are integrity and courage. These are essential attributes for nurse leaders if they are to create an ethical model in the organization. Nurse leaders must also be persistent and committed to bringing about change. Nurse leaders who are dedicated to ethical principles can influence the decisions made by the organization.

Nurse-Physician Relationships

Nurses working in organizations often confront ethical dilemmas in working with patients and their families. To resolve these dilemmas, the nurse must often work closely with the physician. The nurse often finds that physicians hold different beliefs about values, communication, trust and integrity, role responsibilities, and organizational politics and economics. These beliefs affect their ethical beliefs, which, in turn, affect their decisions about treatment, which may lead to nurse-physician conflicts. Strategies to address these ethical conflicts must be identified at the policy and organizational levels. Some policy strategies include the use of multidisciplinary ethical guidelines and ethical administrative guidelines. Some organizational strategies include support for

the development of collaborative ethical teams, an ethical organizational culture, demonstration of the relationship between policy and ethics, and ethical educational approaches and communication (Corley, 1998).

Ethical Codes

One mark of a profession is the determination of ethical behavior for its members. Several nursing organizations have developed codes for ethical behavior. The International Council of Nurses Code for Nurses appears in Table 23-4.

The American Nurses Association has also developed a Code for Nurses. See the "Exploring the Web" section at the end of this chapter for a site to view this document on-line.

The Future

Ethical issues in the future that will challenge nursing practice include the allocation of resources, advanced technologies, an aging population, and an increase in behavior-related health problems. These issues all magnify the importance of professional nurses providing leadership that emphasizes ethical behavior in all practice settings.

TABLE 23-4	*International Council of Nurses Code for Nurses*

The fundamental responsibility of the nurse is fourfold: to promote health, to prevent illness, to restore health, and to alleviate suffering.

The need for nursing is universal. Inherent in nursing is respect for life, dignity, and rights of man. It is unrestricted by considerations of nationality, race, creed, color, age, sex, politics, or social status.

Nurses render health services to the individual, the family, and the community and coordinate their services with those of related groups.

Nurses and People

The nurse's primary responsibility is to those people who require nursing care.

The nurse, in providing care, promotes an environment in which the values, customs, and spiritual beliefs of the individual are respected.

The nurse holds in confidence personal information and uses judgment in sharing this information.

Nurses and Practice

The nurse carries personal responsibility for nursing practice and for maintaining competence by continual learning. The nurse maintains the highest standards of nursing care possible within the reality of a specific situation.

The nurse uses judgment in relation to individual competence when accepting and delegating responsibilities.

The nurse, when acting in a professional capacity, should at all times maintain standards of personal conduct that reflect credit upon the profession.

Nurses and Society

The nurse shares with other citizens the responsibility for initiating and supporting action to meet the health and social needs of the public.

Nurses and Coworkers

The nurse sustains cooperative relationships with coworkers in nursing and other fields. The nurse takes appropriate action to safeguard the individual when his care is endangered by a coworker or any other person.

Nurses and the Profession

The nurse plays the major role in determining and implementing desirable standards of nursing practice and nursing education.

The nurse is active in developing a core of professional knowledge.

The nurse, acting through the professional organization, participates in establishing and maintaining equitable social and economic working conditions in nursing.

From *ICN Code for Nurses: Ethical Concepts Applied to Nursing*, International Council of Nurses, 1973, Geneva: Imprimeries Populaires. Reprinted with permission of International Council of Nurses.

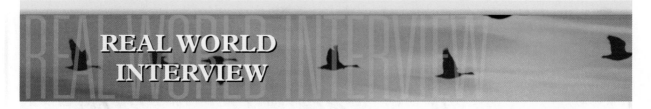

REAL WORLD INTERVIEW

Nurses who work on the maternal-child units in the hospital are faced with dilemmas related to child custody. At times, a newborn is going to be taken into custody by the division of family services. Nurses are informed about this situation, but on occasion the mother is not told until time of discharge to prevent her from fleeing with the infant. This situation creates great stress for the nurses, who are torn between the rights of the mother and what is best for the child. The manager shares the nurses' stress as well as having her own inner struggle about what is ethically right.

Kathi Brinker, RN, BSN
Manager

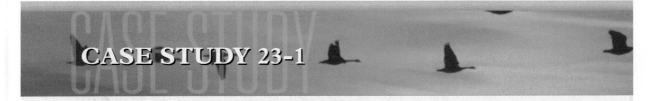

CASE STUDY 23-1

A patient is brought to the hospital in an extremely critical state. The family has supporting documentation that the patient wanted a do not resuscitate (DNR) order at a time such as this. The physician delays writing the order.

How do the nurses caring for the patient deal with this situation if the patient arrests? Who does the nurse advocate for in a situation of this type?

KEY CONCEPTS

- Ethics is the branch of philosophy that concerns the distinction of right from wrong.
- Society created the profession of nursing for the purpose of meeting specific health needs.
- Religious influences helped shape the caring aspect of nursing.
- A personal philosophy stems from an individual's beliefs and values. This personal philosophy will influence an individual's philosophy of nursing.
- Teleology and deontology are two ethical theories.
- Ethical principles and rules include beneficence, nonmaleficence, fidelity, justice, autonomy, respect for others, and veracity.
- Ethics committees provide guidance for decision making about ethical dilemmas that arise in health care settings.
- Values clarification is an important step in the decision-making process.
- The Burkhardt and Nathaniel guide for decision making is a helpful tool.
- Numerous ethical issues face nurses today.
- Patients' rights is an area in which nurses are held accountable.
- Nurses have a contract with society to uphold the trust society places in the nursing profession.
- Nurse leaders who are dedicated to ethical principles can influence organizational ethics.

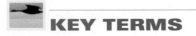
KEY TERMS

autonomy
beneficence
bioethics
deontology
ethical dilemma
ethics
fidelity
justice

morality
nonmaleficence
philosophy
respect for others
teleology
values
veracity

REVIEW QUESTIONS

1. The nurse manager has an ethical responsibility to
   A. the patient.
   B. the organization.
   C. the profession.
   D. the patient, the organization, the profession, and society.

2. The primary role of an ethics committee is to
   A. decide what should be done when ethical dilemmas arise.
   B. prevent the physician from making the wrong decision.
   C. provide guidance for the health care team and family of the patient.
   D. prevent ethical dilemmas from occurring.

3. Ethical dilemmas may be referred to the ethics committee by
   A. physicians only.
   B. nurses, physicians, lawyers, all health care team members, and families of patients.
   C. lawyers only.
   D. hospital administration only.

4. Mrs. Jones rides the elevator to the fifth floor where her husband is a patient. While on the elevator, Mrs. Jones hears two nurses talking about Mr. Jones. They are discussing the potential prognosis and whether he should be told. The nurses are violating which of the following ethical principles?
   A. Autonomy
   B. Confidentiality
   C. Beneficence
   D. Nonmaleficence

REVIEW ACTIVITIES

1. Review the Critical Thinking box in this chapter about Mr. Trout, labeled as a malingerer, who asks what pain medication he is receiving. The nurse knows it is a placebo. Should the nurse tell the patient what the medication is?

   Divide your class into two groups. One group proposes telling the truth and presents the ethical principles that support this position. The other group takes the opposite view and presents the ethical principles that support this position.

2. An elderly woman, age 88, is admitted to the Emergency Department in acute respiratory distress. She does not have a living will, but her daughter has power of attorney (POA) for health care and is a health care professional. The patient has end-stage renal disease, end-stage Alzheimer's disease, and congestive heart failure. Her condition is grave. The doctors want to intubate her and place her on a ventilator. The sons agree. The daughter states that their mother would not want to be on a machine just to prolong her life.

   Divide into groups and discuss the ethical theories that can be applied to this situation. Use the Burkhardt and Nathaniel guide to decision making to help you.

3. As a hospice nurse, you are involved with pain control on a regular basis. Many of the medications prescribed for the management of pain also depress respirations.

   Divide into groups and determine a protocol for the use of these medications, keeping in mind that the purpose of hospice is to promote comfort. Support your decisions with ethical theories and principles.

EXPLORING THE WEB

- See what this web site says about nursing competencies and ethics.
  http://www.ana.org/ojin/ethicol/ethics_2.htm

- What web site could you recommend to nursing managers who need to clarify values of the staff? How else can this web site be used?
  http://www.escape.ca/~rbacal/values.htm

- How is ethics discussed in this web site? Is it congruent with other discussions regarding ethics? *http://www.la.utexas.edu/course-materials/philosophy/bonevac/304/principles.htm*

- Go to the following site to view the American Hospital Association's "Patient's Bill of Rights": *http://www.aha.org/resource/pbillofrights.asp*

- View the American Nurses Association *Code for Nurses with Interpretive Statements* (1985) at: *http://www.ana.org/ethics/1985prov.htm*

- Use the International Council of Nurses web site to find the ICN Code for Nurses: *http://www.icn.ch/icncode.pdf*

REFERENCES

American Hospital Association. (1992). *A patient's bill of rights.* Chicago: Author.

Burkhardt, M. A., & Nathaniel, A. K. (2002). *Ethics & issues in contemporary nursing* (2nd ed.). Clifton Park, NY: Delmar Learning.

Cassidy, V. R. (1998). Ethical leadership in managed care. *Nursing Leadership Forum, 3*(2), 52–57.

Corley, M. (1998). Ethical dimensions of nurse physician relations in critical care. *Nursing Clinics of North America, 33,* 325–337.

DeLaune, S. C., & Ladner, P. K. (2002). *Fundamentals of nursing.* Clifton Park, NY: Delmar Learning.

Donahue, M. P. (1996). *Nursing, the finest art* (2nd ed.). St. Louis, MO: Mosby.

International Council of Nurses. (1973). *Code for nurses.* Geneva: Author.

Raines, M. L. (2000). Ethical decision making in nurses: Relationships among moral reasoning, coping style, and ethics stress. *JONA's Healthcare Law, Ethics, and Regulation, 2*(1), 29–40.

Raths, L., Harmin, M., & Simon, S. (1978). *Values and teaching* (2nd ed.). Columbus, OH: Merrill.

Schroeder, S. A. (1995). Cost containment in U.S. health care. *Academic Medicine, 70*(10), 861–866.

Sullivan, E., & Decker, P. (2001). *Effective leadership and management in nursing* (5th ed.). Upper Saddle River, NJ: Prentice-Hall.

SUGGESTED READINGS

Aiken, T. D., & Catalano, J. T. (1994). *Legal, ethical, and political issues in nursing.* Philadelphia: F. A. Davis.

American Nurses Association. (1985). *Code for nurses with interpretive statements.* Washington, DC: American Nurses Publishing.

American Nurses Association. (1985). *Code of ethics.* Washington, DC: American Nurses Publishing.

Bellack, J. P., & O'Neil, E. H. (2000) Recreating nursing practice for a new century: Recommendations and implications of the Pew Health Professions Commission's final report. *Nursing and Health Care Perspectives, 21*(1), 14–21

Bender, D. (1998). *Biomedical ethics: Opposing viewpoints.* San Diego, CA: Greenhaven.

Bosek, M. (1999). Ethics in practice. *JONA'S Healthcare Law, Ethics, and Regulation, 1*(3), 16–19.

Chambliss, D. (1996). *Beyond caring: Hospitals, nurses, and the social organization of ethics.* Chicago: University of Chicago Press.

Davis, A. J., Aroskar, M. A., Liaschenko, J., & Drought, T. S. (1997). *Ethical dilemmas and nursing practice* (4th ed.). Stamford, CT: Appleton & Lange.

Edge, R. S., & Groves, J. R. (1999). *Ethics of health care: A guide for clinical practice* (2nd ed.). Clifton Park, NY: Delmar Learning.

Ellis, J. R., & Hartley, C. L. (1998). *Nursing in today's world: Challenges, issues, and trends* (6th ed.). Philadelphia: Lippincott.

Hall, J. (1996). *Nursing ethics and law.* Philadelphia: Saunders.

Kindig, D. (1999). Purchasing population health. *Nursing Outlook, 17*(1), 16–22.

Lashley, F. (1997). *The genetics revolution: Implications for nursing.* Washington, DC: American Academy of Nursing.

McDaniel, C. (1998). Enhancing nurses' ethical practice: Development of a clinical ethics program. *Nursing Clinics of North America, 33,* 299–312.

McGee, G. (1999). *Pragmatic bioethics.* Nashville, TN: Vanderbilt University Press.

Schneider, C. E. (1998). *The practice of autonomy: Patients, doctors and medical decisions.* New York: Oxford.

Taylor, C. (1997). Ethical perspectives. In M. Burke & M. Walsh (Eds.), *Gerontologic nursing: Holistic care of the elderly* (pp. 584–600). St. Louis, MO: Mosby.

Woodward, V. (1998). Caring, patient autonomy and the stigma of paternalism. *Journal of Advanced Nursing, 28,* 1046–1052.

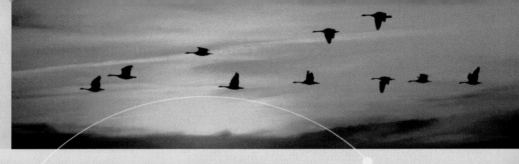

CHAPTER 24

You must be the change you want to see in the world.

(Gandhi)

Cultural Diversity and Spirituality

Karin Polifko-Harris, PhD, RN, CNAA

OBJECTIVES

Upon completion of this chapter, the reader should be able to:

1. Define culture.
2. Discuss the composition of the U.S. population.
3. Identify key cultural nursing theorists.
4. Discuss how culturally competent care can best be delivered.
5. Integrate understanding and respect for spiritual and religious beliefs of different peoples.

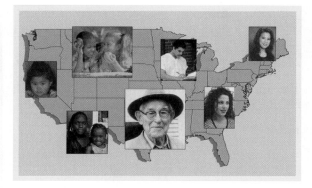

Mr. Wu is brought into the Emergency Department with diaphoresis, nausea, and vomiting, and he is clutching his right shoulder. He is speaking with his wife in Chinese and says he understands only a little English. His wife understands none. Fortunately, Charles Lin, a nurse practitioner, is working this shift and is able to communicate in Chinese with the Wu family. Living in China-town, Mr. Wu often sees a Chinese doctor who prescribes various herbs for his heart problems. While in the Emergency Department, Mr. Wu refuses to take Western medicine and wishes to see an acupuncturist for his pain.

What are your thoughts on how best to provide care for Mr. Wu?

What can you do as a member of the health care team to help Mr. Wu understand what is happening?

Why would Mr. Wu refuse the medication if he entered the hospital?

The United States is a country consisting of many cultures, races, religions, and belief sets. The United States is becoming increasingly diverse and global, with many minority cultures and races developing into majority cultures and races. Newer religions take their place alongside traditional faiths. Both cultural and spiritual differences in people are potential causes for misunderstanding, confusion, and conflict, arising from intolerance and ignorance of these differences. It is imperative that practicing health care providers have an awareness, knowledge, and appreciation for others whose beliefs, values, and practices are different. Culture, religion, and spirituality are closely intertwined and interdependent, especially in the delivery of health care to an ill patient and the patient's family or community. This chapter discusses key points to keep in mind when working and providing care in a culturally diverse environment. Several nursing theorists are

discussed, and trends in diversity are outlined. A section on spirituality includes a discussion on spiritual distress and providing a spiritual assessment to aid in the holistic care of a client. Finally, the beliefs of major world religions are presented.

DEFINING CULTURE, ETHNICITY, ETHNOCENTRISM, VALUES, AND ACCULTURATION

Before one defines a specific culture, one must take into account a person's total environment and that person's relationship to the community. Culture is not defined by the individual; instead, **culture** is defined by the behaviors, norms, belief sets, values, and folkways of a specific group. We grow up with our culture's influences, yet cultural patterns may be altered as we age, or as we move to other communities. As people are exposed to practices within their culture, certain factors are incorporated, shaping one's viewpoints and attitudes (Erlen, 1998). Cultural patterns may be explicit, such as wearing certain clothing, or implicit, such as following religious expectations on certain holidays.

Leininger (1997) states that certain cultural behaviors guide decisions in an expected patterned response, suggesting that practices are learned through direct and indirect observations of others. She believes one's cultural background affects the reactions that are generated by any given situation. A patient's cultural background influences that patient's perceptions of health, wellness, and illness (Spector, 2000; Purnell & Paulanka, 1998). See Table 24-1 for selected characteristics of culture.

Ethnicity is a cultural group's perception of itself (group identity). This self-perception influences how the group's members are perceived by others. Ethnicity involves a sense of belonging and a common social heritage that is passed from one generation to the next. Members of an ethnic group demonstrate their shared sense of identity through common customs and traits. **Ethnocentrism** is the belief that one's own culture or ethnic group is better than all other groups, without considering the merits of the other group.

Race refers to a grouping of people based on biological similarities. Members of a racial group have

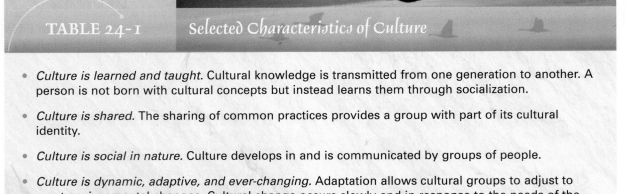

TABLE 24-1 *Selected Characteristics of Culture*

- *Culture is learned and taught.* Cultural knowledge is transmitted from one generation to another. A person is not born with cultural concepts but instead learns them through socialization.

- *Culture is shared.* The sharing of common practices provides a group with part of its cultural identity.

- *Culture is social in nature.* Culture develops in and is communicated by groups of people.

- *Culture is dynamic, adaptive, and ever-changing.* Adaptation allows cultural groups to adjust to meet environmental changes. Cultural change occurs slowly and in response to the needs of the group. It is this dynamic and adaptable nature that allows a culture to survive.

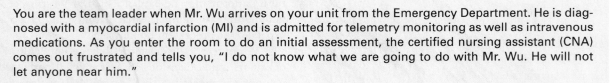

CRITICAL THINKING

You are the team leader when Mr. Wu arrives on your unit from the Emergency Department. He is diagnosed with a myocardial infarction (MI) and is admitted for telemetry monitoring as well as intravenous medications. As you enter the room to do an initial assessment, the certified nursing assistant (CNA) comes out frustrated and tells you, "I do not know what we are going to do with Mr. Wu. He will not let anyone near him."

What is your response to the CNA? What is your first priority regarding care for Mr. Wu? How would you proceed with your assessment? What do you identify as your challenges in caring for Mr. Wu?

similar physical characteristics such as blood group, facial features, and color of skin, hair, and eyes. There is often overlap between racial and ethnic groups because the cultural and biological commonalities support one another (Giger & Davidhizar, 1999). The similarities of people in racial and ethnic groups reinforce a sense of commonality and cohesiveness.

Values are those standards with which a society is maintained. Generally, values are what our families, community, and society teach as right versus wrong, moral or immoral, ethical or unethical (Yukl, 1994). Cultural values have meaning for a particular group and are the desirable behaviors that are reinforced by the culture. Sometimes, a value may be understood and accepted only by the members of a specific cul-

ture, with outside cultures questioning the rationale behind the value. For example, in the American culture, it is generally accepted that the female in a household may hold a job outside the home for a variety of reasons; in other cultures, women are strongly discouraged from working outside the home at all.

The United States once prided itself on its perceived identification as a melting pot, a society in which all cultures would live and take on American cultural values and characteristics. However, in recent years, the emphasis has shifted to maintaining one's cultural identity and acknowledging the differences (Spector, 2000). Members of a minority culture will usually be identified as members of that minority culture; however, they may take on the positive or negative characteristics of the dominant culture. Acculturation is the process by which individuals adjust and adapt either to their host culture or a subculture by altering their own cultural behaviors. Acculturation may be seen in America's Chinatowns: the parents who immigrated may maintain their own native language and customs, such as seeing a Chinese doctor for a physical ailment. The children of the immigrants may speak English as their primary language, with a Chinese dialect as a secondary language, and may seek medical attention from a Western-trained physician for care.

DEFINING U.S. DIVERSITY

The United States has always welcomed, even encouraged, peoples of diverse cultures, races, and ethnicities. According to 1998 census data, 14% of the United States population, or 31.8 million people, speak a primary language in their home other than English. Thiederman (1996) believes, however, that almost 97% of all people living in the United States can speak some English. The states with the highest percentage of those who speak another primary language are: 36% in New Mexico; 31% in California; and 20% in Arizona, Hawaii, New Jersey, New York, and Texas (Stapleton, 1998).

The U.S. ethnic profile is changing quickly. What was once the majority population may no longer be the dominant race, culture, or ethnic group. It is noted by the U.S. Bureau of the Census that immigrant populations are increasing and may be the majority population in some cities and states. Federally defined racial/ethnic groups for census purposes are white, black, Asian/Pacific Islander, Hispanic, and American Indian/Eskimo. An Asian/Pacific Islander is someone from one of 28 Asian countries or the 25 identified Pacific Islander cultures. In the United States, the Chinese, Filipino, and Japanese are the three largest Asian/Pacific Islander groups. The term *Hispanic* identifies anyone with Spanish as a native language or a linkage to Spain or Latin America. Those members comprising the American Indian/Eskimo population are from one of more than 500 tribes and villages within the United States; almost half live outside a reservation (Federal Register, 1996).

According to the 1990 United States Census, by the year 2080 the U.S. cultural mix will be at least 50% minority ethnic groups: Hispanics, 23.4%;

African Americans, 14.7%; Asians and others, 12% (see Figure 24-1 for an illustration of this breakdown). Minority groups are becoming the majority group in many areas of the United States, such as in the urban areas of Miami, San Antonio, Washington, D.C., and Los Angeles.

Racial and Ethnic Diversity of Health Care Providers

Unfortunately, the face of American health care providers does not mirror the population that they care for on a daily basis. Studies have illustrated that the health care industry does not reflect the national trend of racial and ethnic diversity, especially in the physician, nursing, and administrator ranks (Association of American Medical Colleges, 1998). A National Sample Survey completed in 1996 reflects the current demographics of RNs. In 1996, 90% of the total registered nurse workforce was white, non-Hispanic; 4%, black, non-Hispanic; 3%, Asian/Pacific Islander; 2%, Hispanic; and 1%, American Indian/Eskimo (Figure 24-2). Moore (1997) identified that 12% of

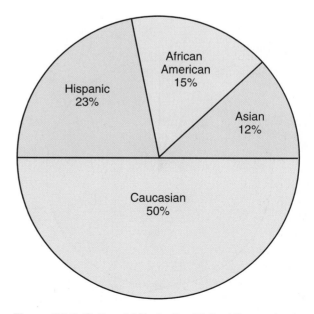

Figure 24-1 Cultural Mix in the United States by the Year 2080 (Data from 1990 U.S. Bureau of the Census)

students entering medical school in 1995 were either black, Indian, Mexican-American, or Puerto Rican. The Association of American Medical Colleges in 1998 identified that only 10% of this minority population became medical students (American Academy of Pediatrics, 2000).

DIVERSITY AWARENESS

The notions of diversity training, diversity awareness, and valuing differences first began appearing in the management, leadership, and social psychology literature in the mid-1980s. Human resource management developed diversity awareness into a focused specialty to meet the demands of an increasingly global workforce, heavily influenced by the Internet. Many organizations began working as direct partners with people of differing cultures, backgrounds, and expectations. As they did, the need for understanding of cultural diversity became both apparent and urgent. Diversity addresses human characteristics that differ from our own and from those of majority

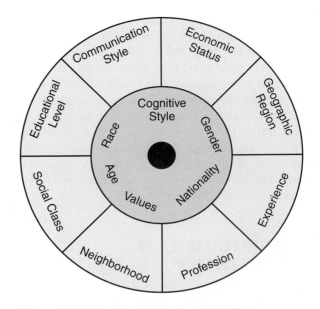

Figure 24-3 Ways in Which People Differ

groups to which we belong. The six primary dimensions of diversity are age, gender, ethnicity/culture, physical abilities, race, and sexual/affectional orientation. It is everyone's responsibility to value difference in people. Figure 24-3 illustrates the many ways in which people differ.

Trends in Health Care Education

Nursing curricula today usually contain components of cultural awareness (Rooda, 1993). Cultural diversity education may also be found in general education requirements. It may be introduced as soon as a student enters the nursing major, perhaps in a separate course or in a thread woven throughout the nursing curricula. Cultural awareness may also be discussed in a leadership course. The importance of cultural education was emphasized by several health care organizations (American Association of Colleges of Nursing, 1998; American Academy of Nursing, 1992; Pew Health Professions Commission, 1995).

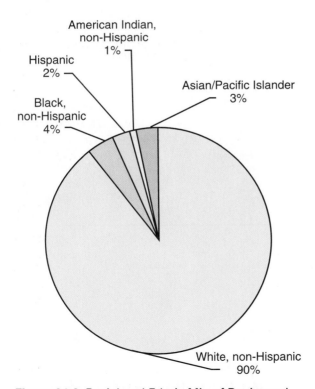

Figure 24-2 Racial and Ethnic Mix of Registered Nurse Population in the United States, 1996

CULTURAL THEORIES

Cultural nursing theories and conceptual models provide a framework for addressing the needs of indi-

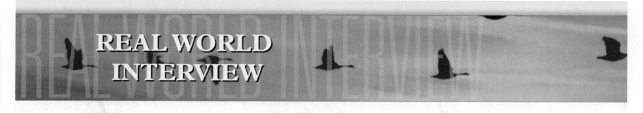

REAL WORLD INTERVIEW

One of the most important things in dealing with a culturally and religiously diverse staff is to value the individual person. Do not expect them to conform to your way of thinking. Everyone has something to contribute, and we need to recognize the differences in people, not just look at them strangely because they may dress in traditional ways or hold beliefs that are not what everyone else holds.

Cathy Robins, RN
Clinical Coordinator

vidual patients and their families while maintaining awareness of cultural differences. Cultural competence is defined by the AAN (1992) as care that is sensitive to issues related to culture, race, gender, and sexual orientation. This care is provided by nurses who use cultural nursing theory, models, and research principles in identifying health care needs. The American Medical Association advocates culturally effective health care, taking into consideration the relationship between the provider and patient. Additionally, the Joint Commission on Accreditation on Healthcare Organizations (2000) has commented on the care of patients regardless of their background or belief sets. In its standards outlining expectations under Patient Rights and Organization Ethics, it is stated that patients have a right to care that is considerate and respectful of their personal values and beliefs (Joint Commission on Accreditation of Healthcare Organizations, 2000).

Transcultural Nursing

Nursing has developed several models of care delivery to help explain relationships between the nurse and culturally diverse clients and their families. Transcultural nursing incorporates concepts found in nursing, sociology, anthropology, and psychiatry. Perhaps the best-known model and theory come from Madeleine Leininger, identified as the founder of transcultural nursing theory, who began her research of transcultural nursing in the 1960s. According to Leininger (1978), **transcultural nursing** is the comparative study and analysis of different cultures and subcultures in the world with respect to their caring

behavior, nursing care and health-illness values, beliefs, and patterns of behavior with the goal of developing a scientific and humanistic body of knowledge to provide culture-specific and culture-universal nursing care practices. Leininger (1997) states that several precepts are inherent in the practice of transcultural nursing. Caring is the first concept: all cultures have expressions of caring and caring behaviors. However, what is defined in one culture may be perceived very differently in another culture. The second concept is that each culture identifies what it considers adequate and necessary care. Most important, application of transcultural nursing to direct patient care requires an acute awareness of each culture's lifestyle patterns; values; beliefs and norms; symbols and rituals; verbal and nonverbal communications; caring behaviors; shared meanings; and rituals of health, wellness, and illness (Leininger, 1997).

Giger and Davidhizar Model

Giger and Davidhizar's Transcultural Assessment Model (1999) offers a method of completing a cultural assessment and evaluating the meanings of cultural variations. Giger and Davidhizar identify five central concepts in their assessment model: transcultural nursing and provision of culturally diverse nursing care; culturally competent care; cultural uniqueness of individuals; culturally sensitive environments; and culturally specific illness and wellness behaviors (Giger & Davidhizar, 1999). The authors further elaborate that transcultural nursing is patient centered and research focused.

Giger and Davidhizar (1999) describe six concepts that are apparent in every cultural group and that need to be kept in mind by nurses when they perform a complete cultural assessment. These six concepts are communication, space, social organization, time, environmental control, and biological variations. The communication concept includes an assessment of both spoken and unspoken language; the space concept includes an assessment of how close people stand to one another, including touch. For example, if we come from a cultural background that encourages touch and closeness, we need to be aware that the members of numerous other cultures require considerably more space and less touch to feel comfortable, especially around strangers. Assessment of social organization reviews cultural identifications such as race, ethnicity, and family patterns.

Every culture has specific ideas about the concept of time and its application in social and personal situations. What may be interpreted as being on time for one culture may be either extremely early or even late for another. Cultural differences are also noted in time orientations of future, present, or past. The concept of environmental control assesses the perceived influence individuals have on their surroundings and their ability to maintain certain cultural health practices. One critical feature of the Giger and Davidhizar model is its inclusion of assessment of biological variations among cultures: Many ethnic and cultural groups are predisposed to certain diseases, have identifying physical characteristics, and have genetic distinctions.

Cultural Competence

Campinha-Bacote (1994) defines cultural competence as a process in which the nurse and patient, family, or community continuously work together to provide optimal care in a culturally diverse environment. Campinha-Bacote identifies four elements necessary to provide culturally competent care. The first element—cultural awareness—builds a sensitivity to another's culture by encouraging self-analysis of one's own prejudices and biases. The goal is for the nurse to move beyond any ethnocentric values to be able to fully appreciate another's culture.

The second element in Campinha-Bacote's model is obtaining cultural knowledge. In this concept, nurses increase their familiarity with various cultures, especially values, practices, and lifestyles. Cultural skill is the third element, which involves a cultural assessment of the patient, including perceptions of health and illness, and identifying possible teaching opportunities. The final element illustrated in this model is the cultural encounter, when the nurse has occasion to experience a culture to refine or modify existing knowledge about a specific cultural group (Campinha-Bacote, Yahle, & Langenkamp, 1996).

Spector's Model

Spector (2000) has expanded on several models to describe the degree to which people's lifestyles reflect their traditional culture, whether European, Asian, African, or Hispanic. In Spector's view, it is assumed that ethnic groups keep their traditional values, beliefs, and norms; this is known as having consistent heritage. The heritage becomes inconsistent when there are acculturation occurrences.

Spector (2000) identifies three categories in her model, the Cultural Heritage Model: culture, religion, and ethnicity. The other six categories in Spector's model are adapted from Giger and Davidhizar's model: space, time, communication, biological variations, social organization, and environmental control.

In completing a cultural assessment of a patient, the nurse would perform an assessment on each of the categories in Table 24-2. She would begin with the six categories from the Giger and Davidhizar model. Of the remaining three categories in the Spector model, all include assessment of primary and extended family members. The cultural category calls for assessment of the language spoken in the culture, any unique folkways, traditions, and practices. The religion category calls for assessment of the historical religious beliefs held by the patient and others in the group, as well as formal religious participation. The final category, ethnicity, involves assessment of the symbolic meanings, values, and traditions of a group and includes migratory status, race, kinship ties, food preferences, and internal and external perceptions of group distinctiveness (Spector, 2000).

PROVIDING CULTURALLY SENSITIVE CARE

Caring for patients requires nurses to take into account the culture of the patient (Erlen, 1998). A cultural assessment can provide insight into health practices, familial relationships, dietary issues, and patient expectations of health care providers. In addition, a cultural assessment can provide insight into a patient's health problems, with potential interventions identified and discussed. Each patient should be identified as an individual belonging to a culture, not merely representing a culture. Health beliefs of the patient are essential to discuss because the patient may have a different interpretation and understanding from what the provider is actually saying or not saying. Effective communication with patients and their families will decrease cultural misunderstandings. See Table 24-3 for a nursing checklist of culturally sensitive care.

MANAGING A CULTURALLY DIVERSE TEAM

Being different in race, culture, gender, age, sexual affections, or abilities is not always seen as positive by many people in an organization. Some may think that being different is a deficit, showing obvious or sometimes not-so-obvious discomfort and displaying prejudices. Others might negate any differences among people, treating everyone the same, regardless of their abilities, values, beliefs, cultural backgrounds,

TABLE 24-2	Spector's Cultural Assessment Categories
Space	Time
Culture	Religion
Social organization	Ethnicity
Communication	Environmental control
	Biological variations

TABLE 24-3	Nursing Checklist for Culturally Sensitive Care

1. Assess and incorporate family history of health care:
   - Fluency in English
   - Extent of family support or disintegration of family
   - Community resources
   - Level of education
   - Change of social status as a result of coming to this country
   - Intimate relationships with people of different backgrounds
   - Level of stress

2. Affirm client strengths and potential for growth.

3. Recognize informal caregivers (family members and significant others) as an integral part of treatment.

4. Demonstrate caring behaviors rather than just tolerating cultural variations in client's behavior.

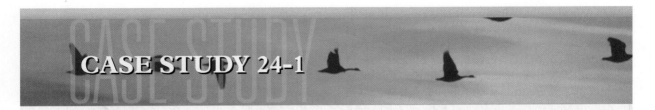

CASE STUDY 24-1

Mrs. Siad is a newly admitted patient. She immigrated from Iraq 4 years ago and has lived in the local community where she is raising a family with her husband. Mrs. Siad, who is Islamic, was admitted for uncontrollable diabetes. She may need to have a great right toe amputation. It becomes clear as you perform the nursing assessment that her husband is clearly in charge of the answers. You, as a male nurse, are feeling quite uncomfortable. Mrs. Siad avoids direct eye contact, and when you ask to assess her feet and move to touch her sheet, her husband gets out of his chair and directs you to stop.

What is your first reaction? How would you handle the situation? What is your plan of care for Mrs. Siad and her family?

REAL WORLD INTERVIEW

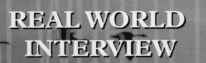

One of the positive things that has happened in my life is that I have been in the military. While in the military, I have worked with many multicultural and multiethnic people. Respect ties everything together. Respect the people you work for and who you work with. Take care of your patients as you would want yourself or your family taken care of. If you work with respect for others, you will conquer prejudices and differences between people.

Janice Couch, RN
Clinical Manager

or potential contributions. There is no one best way to manage a multicultural team. It is critical to remember that each culture has developed its own patterned responses to conflict management, stress, joy, fear, work habits, and communication. The following are a few suggestions for working effectively with a multicultural team:

- When problem solving, be sure to include people who are from different cultural backgrounds, experiences, and abilities. By including a variety of team members, you will obtain a variety of ways to look at an issue, with a variety of ways to solve it.

- Not everyone responds to conflict in the same manner. Some may avoid conflict, while some may want to confront it. Understand how your team works and what the team members' expectations are for the final result. Model respectful behavior.

- Strive to understand what diversity can bring to the group. Focus on the cultural differences and build an appreciation for what everyone can contribute.

- Do not assume that all members of a certain ethnic group, gender, age, or culture act and respond in the same manner. Do not label one culture as preferred over another.

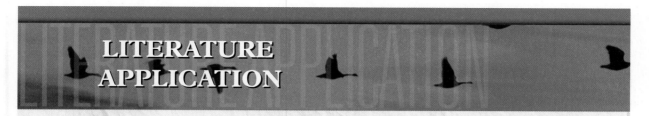

LITERATURE APPLICATION

Citation: Gooden, M. B., Porter, C. P., Gonzalez, R. I., & Mims, B. L. (2001). Rethinking the relationship between nursing and diversity. *American Journal of Nursing, 101*(1), 63–65.

Discussion: The authors believe that—to safeguard human dignity, to circumvent uncertainty and discomfort, and to respect individuality—nursing has embraced the ethic of caring as the sine qua non of the profession, along with concepts of "diversity" and "multiculturalism," as perspectives for interpersonal relations with patients of all races and ethnicities. But regrettably, disabilities, sexual orientation, gender, social class, physical appearance (such as obesity), and ideologies (such as differing political or religious views) have yet to be incorporated into nursing's concept of diversity.

Nurses might begin to initiate discussion among themselves about diversity by defining racial and ethnic minorities as a subset of the population that has a disproportionately high risk of exposure to factors that compromise health (such as environmental toxins, poverty, lack of health care access, and poor housing).

The American Nurses Association (ANA) has written a series of position statements (for example, *Discrimination and Racism in Health Care, Discrimination against Gays and Lesbians in the Military, Decade of Disabled Persons, Cultural Diversity in Nursing Care*); it has created councils and task forces to address issues of diversity in health care; and it has worked diligently for legislation to improve the health of members of racial and ethnic minorities (the Agenda for Health Care Reform and the Nurse Education Act are two examples). Moreover, the ANA's commitment to the incorporation of the concept of diversity into its activities is evidenced by its participation as the only nursing organization on the Steering Committee to Eliminate Racial and Ethnic Disparities in Health, cosponsored by the Department of Health and Human Services and the American Public Health Association.

Implications for Practice: If the nursing profession is to close the health-disparity gap and improve the welfare of the citizens in the United States, it is imperative that nurses rethink the relationship between nursing and diversity.

- Value everyone's differences and recognize their similarities. Seek out experiences with those whose cultural background is different from your own.
- Pay close attention to both verbal and nonverbal communication for cultural cues. Confront, acknowledge, and work with prejudices so that effective communication can occur.
- Ask for clarification. Do not assume.
- Alter your assumptions about others based on their membership in certain groups. For example, do not conclude that all males from a particular culture act a certain way toward females just because they are a member of a certain ethnic group.

- Assist those who are not of the majority cultural group to be successful. As a starting point, include them in informal networking within the organization's culture.

SPIRITUALITY

Religion and spirituality play a large role in many peoples' lives—they influence what people wear, who they can marry, when they seek medical advice, and when they can peacefully die. It is often when people are sick that they seek comfort from religious or spiritual beliefs, seeking strength in their faith or beliefs.

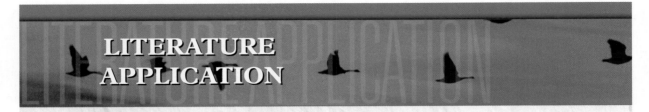

LITERATURE APPLICATION

Citation: Peterson, R., Whitman, H., & Smith, J. (1997). A survey of multicultural awareness among hospital and clinic staff. *Journal of Nursing Care Quality, 11*(6), 52–59.

Discussion: To best meet the needs of its staff of health care providers, an Interdisciplinary Multicultural Patient Care Team was formed at the University of Wisconsin Hospitals and Clinics and UW Children's Hospital in 1994. The article outlines the process the team used as it surveyed its full- and part-time employees regarding their understanding of the system's multicultural issues. Four thousand surveys were distributed, with 21%, or 800, returned. The focus of the tool was to ascertain the level of cultural awareness among employees and to ultimately improve patient outcomes. Among the findings were the need to increase employees' education in the areas of religion, culture, language, and improvement of listening skills.

Implications for Practice: Nurses who develop their cultural awareness can contribute to improved patient outcomes.

Defining Spirituality and Religion

Spirituality and *religion* are two distinct terms, yet they are closely interrelated. Stoll (1989) defines spirituality "as my being: my inner person. It is who I am—unique and alive. My spirituality motivates me to choose meaningful relationships and pursuits. Through my spirituality I give and receive love; I respond to and appreciate God, other people, a sunset, a symphony and spring." Stoll identifies two key dimensions of spirituality in her discussion: the dimension of her relationship with a higher being and the dimension of her relationships with herself and other people, identifying her place in nature. The term **spiritual** refers to a belief in a higher power, an awareness of life and its meaning, the centering of a person with purpose in life. Spiritual does not necessarily mean following an organized religion, but it may mean valuing oneself, one's environment, and those who are part of that surrounding environment. One can be spiritual yet not be a member of a recognized religious group.

Religion is an organized and public belief system of worship and practices that generally has a focus of a god or supernatural power. Religion generally offers an arrangement of symbols and rituals that are meaningful and understood by those who follow and participate in the beliefs and values of the religion. Often, there are rituals that mark significant events and passages in a person's life: birth, adulthood, marriage, and death. However, being a member of a religious group does not make someone spiritual (Long, 1997).

Spiritual Distress

One area of cultural assessment that may produce discomfort for the nurse is the area of spiritual/religious assessment. Many times religion and religious upbringing are topics that are not freely discussed because they are thought to be private information, not to be readily shared. This may be one reason some health care providers may not feel comfortable in assessing their patient's religious beliefs. The North American Nursing Diagnosis Association (NANDA) has identified three nursing diagnoses that address the spiritual care of the patient: spiritual distress (distress of the human spirit), risk for spiritual distress, and readiness for enhanced spiritual well-being (North American Nursing Diagnosis Association, 2001).

Spiritual distress includes questioning the purpose of life and its meaning, refusing to participate in one's usual religious practices, and seeking unusual assistance rather than the usual spiritual or religious support (Tucker, Canobbio, Paquette, & Wells, 1996). Spiritual distress may occur when there is a conflict between what an individual wants or desires to occur and the beliefs of the individual's religion, such as when a Catholic patient uses birth control. Other examples include when an unexpected negative patient outcome occurs, and the patient gets angry at her God, believing that she was being punished or that she was unworthy of getting better.

To provide spiritual care, the nurse does not need focused religious education, just an awareness that a spiritual assessment, much like a cultural assessment, is vital for complete patient care and optimal outcomes. If the nurse becomes aware that the patient is suffering from spiritual distress, then the nurse can decide whether to address it directly with the patient or the patient's family, or whether to bring someone to the patient who may be more helpful, such as the patient's own religious representative.

Spiritual Assessment

Nurses need to ensure that they ask the questions that may lead to better patient outcomes. In a 1998 Duke University study of older adults, it was discovered that those patients who participated in religious activities were 40% less likely to have high blood pressure (Gale Group, 2000). There is more and more interest in the effect that spirituality and reli-

gion play on a person's physical health and well-being (Levin, Larson, & Puchalski, 1997). An integral part of a patient's initial assessment should include data about a patient's spiritual and religious beliefs. This is more than identifying which church a person attends and who their next of kin is. Several spiritual assessment tools are found in the literature (Reed, 1991; Dossey, Keegan, & Guzzetta, 2000; Leininger, 1997; O'Brien, 1999). These tools assist the nurse in asking some of the more abstract questions that may be difficult to define. Questions such as "What in life is important to you?" "What gives your life meaning?" and "Do you pray?" are examples of interview questions that may open up a conversation about spirituality. Asking open-ended questions allows the patient to answer more effectively than a response that requires just a yes or no.

Many nurses do not ask questions about a patient's spirituality or religion because they may have great discomfort in asking the questions, in knowing how to respond, even in identifying what questions to ask. Regardless, it is important to ask these questions, and instead of focusing on the patients' beliefs and practices, it may be better to focus on what patients believe are their needs for health care. A nurse should not assume, much as in a cultural assessment, that just because people are members of one faith that they follow the traditions or rituals of that faith. Spiritual care needs to be individualized, with the patient given the opportunity to participate. It is the nurse's responsibility to call a religious representative if the patient desires this care.

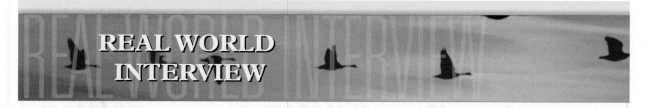

REAL WORLD INTERVIEW

It is sometimes hard for nurses to address completing a spiritual patient assessment if they don't want to look like they are imposing their own beliefs on their patients. Maybe they feel uncomfortable even talking about the topic with patients if they are not even acknowledging their own spirituality. Their comfort level with their own spirituality is going to affect their patient assessments.

Janice Wyatt, RN
Clinical Manager

Religious Beliefs Related to Health Care

The following section offers a brief description of the major religions of the world. A nurse manager should be attentive to the spiritual needs and customs of patients and their families in order to provide holistic nursing care.

Buddhism

Buddhism follows the teaching of Buddha. Buddhist rituals include chanting of last rites at bedside immediately following death. Buddhism discourages drug and alcohol use, and some sects are vegetarian. Illness is seen as a result of negative karma. Cleanliness is viewed as very important. Buddhists are often hesitant to receive treatment such as surgery on holy days.

Christianity

Members of the Christian church profess a belief in Jesus Christ. There are many denominations within the Christian religion, such as Protestant, Catholic, and Episcopalian. These denominations may even have opposite ideas and rituals. A Roman Catholic patient may have beliefs and values that are very different from those of a member of a Protestant church, yet both are professed Christians.

Health care practices vary widely, as do religious activities and even social expectations and traditions. Many Christians use the Bible to guide them in everyday life. A patient may turn to the Bible as a source of encouragement, especially during difficult times. Because of the wide variety of Christian religions, it is imperative that nurses make sure they have an understanding of a patient's belief set when they perform a spiritual assessment. For example, Jehovah's Witnesses will not submit to any blood transfusions, yet other Christian religions have no qualms about accepting this procedure. Seventh-day Adventists have dietary restrictions that include caffeine and alcohol.

Hinduism

Hinduism is believed to be one of the oldest religions in the world. Fasting occurs on specific days of the week, according to which god the Hindu person worships. Most Hindus accept modern medical practices; however, many believe that a person's illness is a result of sins committed in a previous life. Many Hindus are vegetarians. Last rites are carefully prescribed, and family members are often particular about who touches a body after death. A Hindu will most likely be cremated.

Judaism

Judaism is a religion based on the word and laws of God, as written in the book of the Old Testament. There are several different Jewish ideologies. Central to Jewish beliefs is that there is one God. Anyone born of a Jewish mother is considered to be Jewish, as is anyone who formally converts to Judaism. Holy days are many, with the Sabbath beginning on Friday evening at sundown and lasting through sundown on Saturday.

Depending on the ideology followed, some Jewish people have dietary restrictions, known as kosher dietary laws. These laws prohibit the eating of certain meats and eating milk and meat products together during a meal. Upon death, the body is ritually cleansed and buried as soon as possible after death. Autopsy is prohibited in the Jewish faith.

Islam

The religion of Islam comprises many sects of the Islamic faith. Followers perform ritual washing after prayer, which occurs five times a day. Followers of Islam do not eat any pork products, nor do they drink alcoholic beverages. One important ritual is the fasting period in the ninth month of the Muhammadan year, called *Ramadan*; during this period, one fasts during the daytime. Family must be with a dying person. The dying person must confess his sins and ask forgiveness. The family washes the body and only family and friends may touch the body. They usually oppose autopsy. Islamic patients may hold a fatalistic view that interferes with or hinders compliance with the treatment plan.

Agnosticism and Atheism

Two other terms may arise when a nurse cares for a patient and completes a spiritual assessment. If patients state they are **agnostic**, they are not committed to belief in the existence or nonexistence of a god or a supreme being, or perhaps they believe that no one has effectively proven that a god exists. If patients state they are **atheists**, they do not believe in the existence of a god or a supreme being.

KEY CONCEPTS

- As a result of changing demographics in the United States, a majority race or ethnicity today may soon become a minority.
- Health care providers need to more closely mirror the diversity of their patients. Concerted efforts are being made to recruit diverse students to both the medical and nursing professions.
- Culture has a significant influence on the delivery of care for patients, including their interpretations of health and illness and when and how they seek medical attention.
- Diversity characteristics include age, race, ethnicity/culture, sexual/affectional orientation, gender, and physical abilities.
- Transcultural nursing provides a framework for understanding the relationships among the various influences on patient care delivery.
- Understanding a patient's beliefs about health care and illness affects the outcomes of care and leads to culturally competent care.
- Spirituality and religion are two different entities yet are important for the holistic care of a patient.
- Patients often consider spiritual and religious beliefs to be personal information, which may interfere with gathering a spiritual assessment.
- Nurses need to be aware of their own spirituality and beliefs to feel comfortable in discussing spirituality or religious beliefs with a patient.

KEY TERMS

acculturation
agnostic
atheist
culture
ethnicity
ethnocentrism

religion
spiritual
spiritual distress
transcultural nursing
values

REVIEW QUESTIONS

1. Which are important issues to consider when working with a multicultural team?

A. Everyone should be focused on the same goals and objectives.
B. Everyone should be from the same professional background, for example, all nurses.
C. Everyone should have the same values about health care.
D. Everyone should have the same understandings because they all are living in the United States.

2. What would be an appropriate first question when asking patients about their spirituality?
A. "Are you born again?"
B. "You're not Catholic, are you?"
C. "Do you participate in any religious activities?"
D. "When were you baptized?"

REVIEW ACTIVITIES

1. You are a nurse in an HIV clinic that sees a variety of patients from all cultures and ethnicities.

   What type of information is necessary for you to have to effectively take care of your patients? What do you see as some of the challenges in working with your patient population?

2. The hospital where you work is in a predominantly white, non-Hispanic area. Lately, there has been an influx of migrant farm workers from Mexico because local farms cannot find local workers.

   What do you perceive as some of the health needs of the migrant farm workers? What do you see as potential barriers to care for these workers? How would you facilitate the provision of care for these workers and their families?

3. On the unit where you work as a nurse, one particular nurse is adamant about sharing her Christian religious beliefs with patients and their families, regardless of their background, religion, or culture. You have been asked by the evening supervisor to speak with a Jewish family who is upset because the nurse spoke inappropriately to them.

   What do you first do with the family? How can you model the valuing of religious differences with the nurse? What are the potentially positive outcomes of this situation?

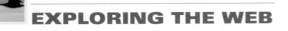

EXPLORING THE WEB

- This web site breaks down the population of the United States: *http://www.census.gov/population/estimates/nation/intfile3-1.txt*

- Language and cultural effects on health care delivery are the focus of this site: *http://www.diversityrx.org*

- Looking for a listing of transcultural nursing references? Try these two sites: *http://www.sunyit.edu/library/culturemed/bib/ transcultural* *http://www.iun.edu/~libemb/trannurs/trannurs. htm*

- The following site has a variety of culture and ethnicity links: *http://www.culturaldiversity.org*

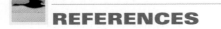

REFERENCES

American Academy of Nursing (1992). AAN expert panel report. *Nursing Outlook, 40*(6), 277–283.

American Academy of Pediatrics (2000). Enhancing the racial and ethnic diversity of the pediatric workforce. *Pediatrics, 105*(1), 129–131.

American Association of Colleges of Nursing. (1998). *Essentials of baccalaureate education for professional nursing practice*. Washington, DC: Author.

Association of American Medical Colleges. (1998). *Minority medical students in medical education: Facts and figures IX*. Washington, DC: Author.

Campinha-Bacote, J. (1994). Cultural competence in psychiatric nursing: A conceptual model. *Nursing Clinics of North America, 29,* 1–8.

Campinha-Bacote, J., Yahle, T., & Langenkamp, M. (1996). The challenge of cultural diversity for nurse educators. *The Journal of Continuing Education in Nursing, 27*(2), 59–64.

Dossey, B. M., & Guzzetta, C. E. (1995). Holistic nursing practice. In B. M. Dossey, L. Keegan, C. E. Guzzetta, & L. G. Kolkmeier (Eds.), *Holistic nursing: A handbook for practice* (pp. 41–52). Gaithersburg, MD: Aspen.

Dossey, B. M., Keegan, L., & Guzzetta, C. E. (2000). *Holistic nursing: A handbook for practice* (3rd ed.). Gaithersburg, MD: Aspen.

Erlen, J. A. (1998). Culture, ethics and respect: The bottom line is understanding. *Orthopaedic Nursing, 17*(6), 79–82.

Federal Register. (1996, November 13). Notice. 61 *Federal Register* 58211–58216.

Gale Group. (2000). Cleveland Medical School programs incorporate spirituality as a prescription for healing. *Jet, 97*(17), 16.

Giger, J. N., & Davidhizar, R. E. (1999). *Transcultural nursing*. Baltimore: Mosby.

Gooden, M. B., Porter, C. P., Gonzales, R. J., & Mims, B. L. (2001). Rethinking the relationship between nursing and diversity. *American Journal of Nursing, 101*(1), 63–65.

Joint Commission on Accreditation of Healthcare Organizations. (2000). *Comprehensive manual for hospitals: The official handbook*. Oakbrook Terrace, IL: Author.

Leininger, M. (1978). *Transcultural nursing: Concepts, theories and practices*. New York: Wiley.

Leininger, M. (1997). Transcultural nursing research to transform nursing education and practice: 40 years. *Image: Journal of Nursing Scholarship, 29,* 341–347.

Levin, J. S., Larson, D. B., & Puchalski, C. M. (1997). Religion and spirituality in medicine: Research and education. *Journal of the American Medical Association, 278*(9), 792–793.

Long, A. (1997). Nursing: A spiritual perspective. *Nursing Ethics, 4,* 496–510.

Moore, J. D. (1997, December 15). The unchanging of healthcare. *Modern Healthcare,* 30–34.

North American Nursing Diagnosis Association. (2001). *NANDA's nursing diagnosis: Definitions and classifications 2001–2002*. Philadelphia: Author.

O'Brien, M. E. (1999). *Spirituality in nursing*. Sudbury, MA: Jones and Bartlett.

Park, H., & Harrison, J. K. (1993). Enhancing managerial cross-cultural awareness and sensitivity: Transactional analysis revisited. *Journal of Management Development, 12*(3), 20–29.

Peterson, R., Whitman, H., & Smith, J. (1997). A survey of multicultural awareness among hospital and clinic staff. *Journal of Nursing Care Quality, 11*(6), 52–59.

Pew Health Professions Commission. (1995). *Critical challenges: Revitalizing the health professions for the twenty-first century*. San Francisco: UCSF Center for the Health Professions.

Purnell, L. D. & Paulanka, B. J. (1998). *Transcultural health care*. Philadelphia: F. A. Davis.

Reed, P. G. (1991). Preferences for spirituality related nursing interventions among terminally ill and nonterminally ill hospitalized adults and well adults. *Applied Nursing Research, 4*(3), 122–128.

Rooda, L. (1993). Knowledge and attitudes toward culturally different patients: Implications for nursing education. *Journal of Nursing Education, 32*(5), 209–213.

Spector, R. (2000). *Cultural diversity in health and illness.* Norwalk, CT: Appleton & Lange.

Stapleton, S. (1998). Emphasis on cultural competence. *American Medical News, 41*(9), 3.

Stoll, R. (1989). The essence of spirituality. In V. Carson (Ed.), *Spiritual dimensions of nursing practice* (pp. 4–23). Philadelphia: Saunders.

Thiederman, S. (1996). Improving communications in a diverse healthcare environment. *Healthcare Financial Management, 50*(11), 72–75.

Tucker, S., Canobbio, M., Paquette, E., & Wells, M. (1996). *Patient care standards: Collaborative planning guides.* St. Louis, MO: Mosby.

Yukl, G. (1994). *Leadership in organizations* (3rd ed.). Englewood Cliffs, NJ: Prentice Hall.

SUGGESTED READINGS

American Association of Colleges of Nursing. (1997). *Statement on diversity and equality of opportunity.* Washington, DC: Author.

Andrews, M. M., & Boyle, J. S. (1995). *Transcultural concepts in nursing care.* Philadelphia: Lippincott.

Block, B. (1983). Assessment guide for ethnic/cultural variations. In M. S. Orque & B. Block (Eds.), *Ethnic nursing care: A multicultural approach* (pp. 49–75). St. Louis, MO: Mosby.

Borkan, J. M., & Neher, J. O. (1991). A development model of ethnosensitivity in family practice training. *Family Medicine, 23*(3), 212–217.

Carpenito, L. J. (1999). *Handbook of nursing diagnosis* (8th ed.). Philadelphia: Lippincott.

Donley, R. (1995). Advanced practice nursing after health care reform. *Nursing Economic$, 13*(2), 84–88.

Elmuti, D. (1993). Managing diversity in the workplace: An immense challenge for both managers and workers. *Industrial Management, 35*(4), 19–22.

Epting, L. A., Glover, S. H., & Boyd, S. D. (1994). Managing diversity. *Health Care Supervisor, 12*(4), 73–83.

Estes, G., & Zitzow, D. (1980). *Heritage consistency as a consideration in counseling Native Americans.* Paper read at the National Indian Education Association Convention, Dallas, TX.

Fine, M. G. (1996). Cultural diversity in the workplace: The state of the field. *Journal of Business Communication, 33*(4), 485–502.

Hofstede, G. (1997). *Cultures and organizations.* New York: McGraw-Hill.

Johnston, W. B., & Packer, A. H. (1987). *Workforce 2000.* Indianapolis, IN: Hudson Institute.

LaFrambose, T., Coleman, L. K., & Gerton, J. (1993). Psychological impact of biculturalism: Evidence and theory. *Psychological Bulletin, 114*(3), 395.

Lauver, D. R. (2000). Commonalities in women's spirituality and women's health. *Advances in Nursing Science, 22*(3), 76–88.

Morrison, T., Conaway, W. A., & Borden, G. A. (1994). *Kiss, bow or shake hands: How to do business in sixty countries.* Holbrook, MA: Adams Media.

Polifko-Harris, K. (1995). *The influence of national culture on work-related values and job satisfaction between American and Filipino registered nurses.* Unpublished doctoral dissertation, Old Dominion University, Norfolk, VA.

Polifko-Harris, K. (2000). Managing a culturally diverse workforce. In L. M. Simms, S. A. Price, & N. E. Ervin (Eds.), *Professional practice of nursing administration* (pp. 567–581). Clifton Park, NY: Delmar Learning.

Praill, D. (1995). Approaches to spiritual care. *Nursing Times, 91*(34), 34–37.

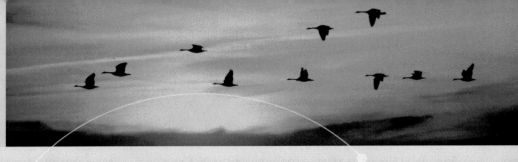

CHAPTER 25

You will have much opposition to encounter. But great works do not prosper without great opposition.

(Florence Nightingale, 1864, cited in Ulrich, 1992)

Collective Bargaining

Janice Tazbir, RN, MS, CCRN

OBJECTIVES

Upon completion of this chapter, the reader should be able to:

1. Review the history of collective bargaining and associated legislation.
2. Discuss collective action models and associated terminology.
3. Identify the American Nurses Association's role and function in collective bargaining.
4. Discuss professionalism in the context of unionization.
5. List pros and cons of collective bargaining.

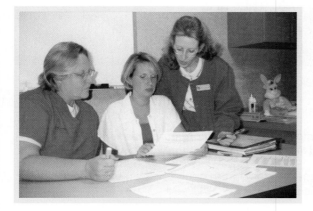

You are a new nurse on an orthopedic unit. When you have lunch, you decide to sit in the conference room because most of the nurses socialize there. You walk into a discussion between two nurses. Jane, a registered nurse with 10 years of experience, states, "I'm tired of low pay and work assignments that are unsafe." Peggy, a registered nurse with 5 years of experience, states, "Have you brought your complaints to management?" Jane replies, "Of course. I point out unsafe situations and the lack of raises, but no one cares." Peggy says, "I bet we would have better success with these issues if we nurses came together as a group."

What are your thoughts about this situation?

What are some of the choices the nurses have?

Historically, nurses have often been perceived as hard-working, submissive women who do what they are told. The scope of nursing has changed so drastically that today nurses cannot afford to have a submissive image and do only what they are told. Patients, their illnesses, and their families are more complex than ever. Nurses are educated to advocate for their patients and themselves. Clinical situations arise in which nurses must voice their opinions and stand up for what is best for patients. To be effective in today's world, nurses must understand the tools available to deal with problems.

Collective action, or simply acting as a group with a single voice, is one method of dealing with problems. **Collective bargaining** is the practice of employees, as a collective group, bargaining with management in reference to wages, work practices, and other benefits. This chapter discusses different types of collective action models and also includes information concerning unionization, as well as professionalism in the context of unionization.

HISTORY OF COLLECTIVE BARGAINING AND COLLECTIVE BARGAINING LEGISLATION IN AMERICA

Collective bargaining and unionization have existed in the United States since the 1790s. Traditionally, people who formed and joined unions were highly skilled craftspeople. People found that by working collectively they could set wages and standards for their trades. The Erdman Act, passed in 1898, was the first federal legislation to deal with collective bargaining. Since then, numerous legislative acts have been passed to ensure the rights of employees (Table 25-1). The rights many workers have today came from the struggles of others with the fortitude to stand up for what they believed was right.

COLLECTIVE ACTION MODELS

One of the main purposes of collective action for nurses is to advance the profession of nursing (Underwood, 1997). Many nurses belong to numerous collectives, including specialty nursing organizations, church organizations, special interest clubs, community groups, and so on. The reason most people belong to these organizations is to better themselves and their communities or to promote and support the special interests of a group. Two types of nursing collective action are discussed in this chapter: workplace advocacy and collective bargaining. Shared governance, another type of collective action, is discussed in another chapter.

Workplace Advocacy

Workplace advocacy refers to activities nurses undertake to address problems in their everyday workplace setting. This type of collective action is probably the most common in nursing. An activity that falls under workplace advocacy is forming a committee to address problems, devise alternatives to achieve optimal care, and invent new ways to implement change.

TABLE 25-1	Summary of Selected Legislation Affecting the Workplace
Year and Title of Legislation	**Summary**
1898: Erdman Act	Outlawed discrimination by employers against union activities
1935: National Labor Relations Act (Wagner Act)	Gave private employees the right to organize unions to demand better wages and safer work environments
1938: Fair Labor Standards Act	Set minimum wage and maximum hours that can be worked before overtime is paid
1947: Taft-Hartley Act	Returned some rights to management; somewhat equalized balance between unions and management
1962: Kennedy Executive Order 10988	Amended National Labor Relations Act to allow public employees to join unions
1964: Civil Rights Act	Set equal employment standards such as equal pay for equal work
1965: Executive Order 11246	Set affirmative action guidelines
1967: Age Discrimination Act	Protects against forced retirement
1973: Rehabilitation Act	Protects rights of disabled people
1973: Vietnam Veterans Act	Provides reemployment rights
1974: Taft-Hartley Amendments to the Wagner Act	Allows nonprofit organizations to join unions

A supportive management will view workplace advocacy as a way to strengthen staff and promote teamwork. If the management is authoritative, however, workplace advocacy may not be encouraged, because it may be perceived as a threat to management and its policies.

Collective Bargaining

In collective bargaining, the group is bargaining with management for what the group desires. If the group cannot achieve its desires through informal collective bargaining with management, the group may decide to use a collective bargaining agent to form a union.

Factors Influencing Nurses to Unionize

In general, nurses who are content in their workplace do not unionize (Hart, 1998). It is when nurses feel powerless that they initiate attempts to unionize.

Other motivations to unionize include the desire to eliminate discrimination and favoritism (Marquis & Huston, 1998). Nurses are also motivated to join unions when they feel the need to communicate concerns and complaints to management without fear of losing their jobs. Many nurses believe that they need a collective voice so that management will hear them and changes will be instituted.

Issues that are commonly the subject of collective bargaining include poor wages, unsafe staffing, health and safety issues, mandatory overtime, poor quality of care, job security, and restructuring issues such as cross-training nurses for areas of specialty other than those in which they were hired to practice (American Nurses Association [ANA], n.d.). Many nurse managers believe that it is best to deal quickly and effectively with issues that arise in order to avoid collective bargaining, because of the increase in costs to the hospital that results from collective bargaining and the limitations it places on managers.

Unions

A **union** is a formal and legal group that works through a collective bargaining agent to present desires to management formally, through the legal context of the National Labor Relations Board.

Table 25-2 lists some collective action terminology. This is useful in understanding the collective bargaining process.

WHISTLE-BLOWING

As patient advocates, nurses protect patients from known harm. Nurses are often aware of health care fraud in the form of people violating laws or endangering public health or safety. However, many nurses who are aware of health care fraud do nothing because of fear of retribution. Fraud costs the federal government and ultimately costs the taxpayer.

Whistle-blowing is the act in which an individual discloses information regarding a violation of a law, rule, or regulation, or a substantial and specific danger to public health or safety. The government recouped more than $135 million during 1995 and 1996 from whistle-blowers exposing fraud (Polston, 1999). Health care fraud can range from filing false claims to performing unnecessary procedures. As patient advocates, nurses have an ethical and moral duty to protect their patients. In 1986, the False Claims Act was modified to encourage whistle-blowers to come forward (Polston, 1999). Whistle-blowing claims are brought in qui tam lawsuits (Polston, 1999), which anyone can file on both the government's behalf and their own behalf. If the government believes an individual has a case of fraud, the government will pay all expenses for the lawsuit and the individual will be entitled to 15% to 25% of the government's recovery (Polston, 1999). The name of

TABLE 25-2	Collective Bargaining Terminology
Term	**Definition**
Agency shop	Synonymous with "open shop." Employees are not required to join the union but may join it.
Arbitration	Last step in a dispute. Indicates a nonpartial third party will be involved and may make the final decision. Arbitration may be voluntary or imposed by the government.
Collective bargaining	The practice of employees, as a collective, bargaining with management in reference to wages, work practices, and other benefits.
Collective bargaining agent	An agent that works with employees to formalize collective bargaining through unionization.
Contract	A set of guidelines and rules voted and agreed upon by union members that guides their work practices, wages, and other benefits.
Dispute	A disagreement between management and the union. A dispute may go through (1) mediation and conciliation, (2) arbitration, and possibly (3) a strike. A dispute may be settled at any stage.
Employee at will	An employee working without a contract. The employee agrees to work under given rules and may be terminated if she breaks any rules imposed by management.

(continues)

Table 25-2 *(continued)*

Fact finding	Fact finding is used in labor management disputes that involve government-owned companies. It is the process in which claims of labor and management are reviewed. In the private sector, fact finding is usually performed by a board of inquiry.
Grievance	A grievance occurs when a union member believes that management has failed to meet the terms of the contract or labor agreement and communicates this to management.
Grievance proceedings	A formal process in which a union member believes that management has failed to meet the terms of the contract. The steps usually include (1) communication of the grievance to management, (2) mediation with a union representative and a member of management, and possibly (3) arbitration. The dispute may be settled at any step.
Lockout	Closing a place of business by management in the course of a labor dispute to attempt to force employees to accept management terms.
Mediation and conciliation	A step in the grievance process in which a nonpartial third party meets with management and the union to assist them in reaching an agreement. In this step, the third party has no actual power in decision making.
National Labor Relations Board	The National Labor Relations Board was formed to implement the Wagner Act. The two major functions of the board include (1) determining and implementing the free democratic choice of employees as to whether they choose to be or choose not to be in a union and (2) preventing and remedying unfair labor practices by employers or unions.
Professional	A person who has knowledge from formal studies and has autonomy.
Self-expression	"The expressing of any views, argument, or opinion, or the dissemination thereof, whether in written, printed, graphic or visual form[,] if such expression contains no threat or reprisal or force or promise of benefit" (National Labor Relations Act, 1994).
Strike	An act in which union members withhold the supply of labor for the purpose of forcing management to accept union terms.
Supervisor	A person with the authority to (1) impart corrective action and (2) delegate to an employee.
Union	A formal and legal group that brings forth desires to management through a collective bargaining agent and within the context of the National Labor Relations Board.
Union dues	Money required of all union employees to support the union and its functions.
Union shop	A place of employment in which all employees are required to join the union and pay dues. *Union shop* is synonymous with the term *closed shop*.
Whistle-blowing	Whistle-blowing is the act in which an individual discloses information regarding a violation of a law, rule, or regulation, or a substantial and specific danger to public health or safety.

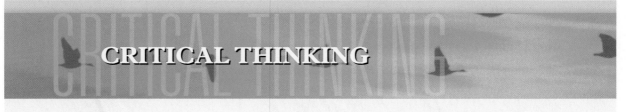

CRITICAL THINKING

You are caring for Mr. Johnson, a 65-year-old man who was admitted for congestive heart failure. He is a retired steelworker from an area steel mill. He states, "I worked in that mill for 30 years, and I am thankful for the union. Because of the union, my medical costs are covered for the rest of my life. The union served me well. Do nurses have unions or groups that help them get what they want?"

How will you respond to Mr. Johnson? Name two collective groups to which you belong. What are these collective groups able to get done as a whole? Are these collective groups more effective and stronger than you are as an individual in these interest areas? What are the downsides of belonging to a collective group?

CRITICAL THINKING

You are a nurse working at an institution in which there is limited flexibility in the scheduling. You want to institute self-scheduling, with the staff nurses responsible for making and maintaining the schedule. Make a plan to present this idea to the manager. How will you elicit the support of other nurses? Now put yourself in the role of the manager. How would you respond to this request?

---

the person filing the suit will not be divulged if the government does not consider the matter to involve health care fraud, thereby protecting the person from any retribution from the employer. The employer will not know who attempted to "blow the whistle." If nurses are aware of fraud in their practice setting, the proper steps for them to take include the following:

- File a qui tam lawsuit in secret with the court.
- Do not let the agency or hospital know you filed a lawsuit.
- Serve a copy of the complaint to the Department of Justice with a written disclosure of all the information you have concerning the fraud.
- If the government decides to go forward with the lawsuit, the government will bear responsibility for litigating the lawsuit, and the government will pay for it.

PROCESS OF UNIONIZATION

The process of choosing a collective bargaining unit and negotiating a contract may take 3 months to 3 years. There are formal steps to follow to legally form a union. A **collective bargaining agent** is an agent that works with employees to formalize collective bargaining through unionization. The American Nurses Association outlines the steps in organizing a collective bargaining unit through a state nurses association in Table 25-3.

Managers' Role

Registered nurses have the legal authority to participate in collective bargaining in the majority of health

TABLE 25-3	Steps in Organizing a Collective Bargaining Unit

Bring together a group of nurses supportive of collective bargaining.

Arrange a meeting with a representative of the state nurses association to discuss organizing.

Assess the feasibility of an organizing campaign at your facility.

Conduct the necessary research, such as what are the needs and/or complaints of the employees, to develop a plan of action.

Establish an organizing committee and subcommittees to facilitate organizing.

Begin the process of obtaining union authorization cards from the National Labor Relations Board to legally vote on a collective bargaining agent.

Schedule an informal meeting for nurses eligible for the collective bargaining unit.

Keep the lines of communication open with nurses.

Seek voluntary recognition from the employer.

Move toward formal organization of the unit.

Seek certification by the National Labor Relations Board as the exclusive bargaining agent of the unit.

Initiate contract negotiations.

(Drawn from "How the Bargaining Process Works," by L. Flanagan, 1991, *American Nurse, 23*(9), 11–12.

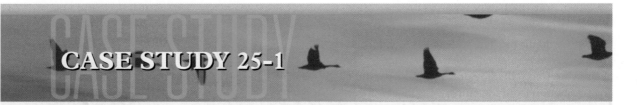

CASE STUDY 25-1

You are a nurse working in a cardiac catheterization unit. You notice that a certain physician routinely performs cardiac catheterizations on patients who are in their early 40s, have no risk factors for cardiac history, and are on Medicaid. The catheterizations are always negative for disease. You love your job but are troubled by this practice. You are fearful that patients will have complications. You ask the physician why these procedures are performed on patients who do not appear to need this testing. His response is, "You don't worry about what I do; these procedures keep us all employed with healthy paychecks." You discuss this with your nursing manager and the chief nursing executive, who both say, "Just do your job and let the doctor decide what is best for your patients."

You decide that whistle-blowing is your next action. What is your first step? Should you notify management of your whistle-blowing? What policies exist in your agency to guide the nurse when the nurse finds unprofessional activities?

care facilities in the country. Over the years, there has been debate over the composition of collective bargaining units in the health care industry. In 1989, the National Labor Relations Board deemed eight collective bargaining units, including one for registered nurses, appropriate in the hospital setting. Some other collective bargaining units in the hospital include licensed practical nurses, secretaries, and housekeepers. Managers who work in a union setting may have up to eight different contracts for various employees. Unionization may result in increased costs for the hospital and may limit the authority of its managers. Table 25-4 lists some ways managers can respond to the threat of collective bargaining (ANA, n.d.).

Employees' Role

Nurses desiring to choose a collective bargaining agent must be sure they carefully follow the laws pertaining to unionization. It is important to carefully choose the collective bargaining agent, such as the American Nurses Association. It is useful to find out about the former success of the agent, details of how nurses will be supported, and where and how the union dues are spent. Spend time talking to other nurses in union settings to see how their contract is structured and if collective bargaining has helped with the issues that led them to unionize in the first place. Table 25-5 lists some suggested activities for the nurse during the process of unionization (ANA, n.d.).

TABLE 25-4	*Manager's Role During Initiation of Unionization*

Know the law; make sure the rights of the nurses as well as the rights of management are clearly understood.

Act clearly within the law, no matter what the organization delegates to you as manager.

Find out the reasons the nurses want collective action.

Discuss and deal with the nurses and the problems directly and effectively.

Distribute lists of cons of unionization such as paying dues.

Distribute examples of unions that did not help with patient care issues.

TABLE 25-5	*Nurse's Role During Initiation of Unionization*

Know your legal rights and the rights of the manager.

Act clearly within the law at all times.

If a manager acts unlawfully, such as firing an employee for organizing, report it to the National Labor Relations Board.

Keep all nurses informed with regular meetings held close to the hospital.

Set meeting times conveniently around shift changes and assist with child care during meetings.

STRIKING

Many nurses are morally opposed to unions because they believe if they are members of a union, they may be forced to strike. In reality, a collective bargaining agent cannot make the decision to strike. The decision to strike is made only if the majority of union members decide to do so. Most nursing collective bargaining agents insert in the contract a no strike clause, stating that striking is not an option for its members. The union members decide upon the no strike clause. Provisions set forth in the 1974 Taft-Hartley Amendments to the Wagner Act guarantee the continuation of adequate patient care by requir-

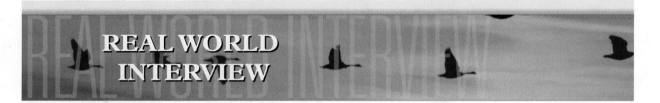

REAL WORLD INTERVIEW

I graduated from a diploma nursing program in 1962. I worked for 5 years and then was home for 15 years raising my children. I wanted to return to nursing and took a refresher course. It was very hard. So much had changed. I made it, though. I think that with the shortage of nurses now, hospitals would be smart to try to make it easier for nurses who have left nursing to return by offering reasonable, supportive refresher courses. I stayed at the hospital I went back to and later retired with just short of 19 years of service. When I retired, I was shocked to find out what my pension was going to be. It was $425 a month—this after almost 19 years of service. If it wasn't for my husband's pension, who, with a high school education, gets almost 10 times what I get, I would never be able to retire. My husband worked through a union. I understand that teachers who work through unions often get 75% of their salary when they retire. Some nurses who are single or divorced would like to retire but simply can't afford to do so. You keep hearing about the poor pay for teachers, and while I agree it should be better, at least they can afford to retire. Who thinks about nurses? It seems to me that more and more of the doctors' work is being given to the nurses and yet a survey I read said that the gap between the doctors' and nurses' pay is greater than what it was at the end of World War II. New nurses should start thinking about retirement benefits when they look for their first job. I know my 40 years as a nurse went fast.

Gerri Kane, RN
Retired Staff Nurse

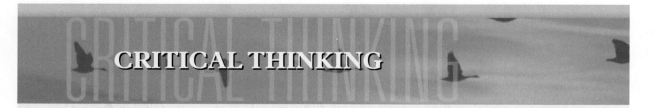

CRITICAL THINKING

You are a nurse working in a hospital that is a union shop. Nurses are concerned about unsafe staffing and floating to units whose patient populations they have not been properly trained to care for. The collective bargaining agent for the union has met with management concerning these issues and nothing has been resolved. There are rumors that a vote to decide whether to strike will take place next week.

What issues make people consider striking? What is the American Nurses Association stance on striking? What steps can be taken to avoid a strike?

ing the union to provide contract expiration notice and advance strike notice, making mediation mandatory, and giving the hospital or agency the option of establishing a board of inquiry prior to work stoppage.

COLLECTIVE BARGAINING AGENTS

Different organizations act as collective bargaining agents for nurses. Some of these are the Teamsters Union, the General Service Employees Union, and the American Nurses Association. The largest collective bargaining agent for nurses is the United American Nurses AFL-CIO. The United American Nurses (UAN) and its constituent member nurse associations, including state nurses associations, are a division of the American Nurses Association (ANA) that serves as a collective bargaining agent. The UAN represents approximately 400,000 nurses. The second largest collective bargaining agent for nurses is the National Union of Hospital and Health Care Employees. It represents 375,000 nurses and health care workers nationally. The third largest collective bargaining agent for nurses is the Service Employees

International Union. It represents 110,000 nurses and health care workers nationally. Other nursing collective bargaining agents are part of the United Autoworkers of America and the United Steelworkers of America (Seltzer, 2001).

American Nurses Association

The **American Nurses Association** (ANA) is a full-service professional organization representing the nation's entire registered nurse population. The ANA represents the 2.6 million registered nurses in the United States through its 54 constituent state and territorial associations. The ANA's mission is to work for the improvement of health standards and availability of health care services for all people, foster high standards for nursing, stimulate and promote the professional development of nurses, and advance their economic and general welfare (ANA, n.d.). The National Labor Relations Board recognizes the ANA as a collective bargaining agent. The fact that the ANA has a dual role of being a professional organization and a collective bargaining agent causes controversy. Some nurses believe that unionization is not professional and that the ANA cannot truly support

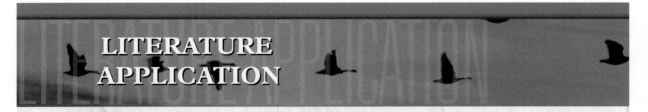

LITERATURE APPLICATION

Citation: Junor, J. (1998). What roles do unions have in preparing nursing leaders to effective change for the future? *Concern, 27*(1), 18–19.

Discussion: Nursing unions do more than serve the needs of their members. Unions empower their members. Examples of what nursing unions can do to empower nurses to prepare them to become nursing leaders include formally teaching them how to be more assertive and introduce political agendas pertinent to nursing issues. By being more assertive and politically active, nurses can realize their individual power and the power nurses have as a collective. Unions also teach nurses the skills of understanding contracts and the importance of documentation.

Implications for Practice: Nurses can grow professionally and personally from active union membership. Union membership provides opportunities for nurses to learn skills such as assertiveness, to understand the political process, and to promote change. Nurses possessing these qualities will have the capacity to lead and the ability to make changes to better the nursing profession.

nursing as a profession if it is also a collective bargaining agent. Because nurse managers are excluded from union membership, many nurse managers believe they have been left outside the organization that is supposed to represent all of nursing. Other nurse managers do not feel this separation ("The Role of Collective Bargaining and Unions," 1998).

The ANA represents the interests of nurses in collective bargaining and in many other areas as well. The ANA advances the nursing profession by fostering high standards for nursing practice and lobbies Congress and regulatory agencies on health care issues affecting nurses and the general public. The ANA initiates many policies involving health care reform. It also publishes its position on issues ranging from whistle-blowing to patients' rights. The ANA recently launched a major campaign to mobilize nurses to address the staffing crisis, to educate and gain support from the public, and to develop and implement initiatives designed to resolve the crisis ("United American Nurses," 2001).

PROFESSIONALISM AND UNIONIZATION

Requirements for a vocation to be considered a profession include (1) a long period of specialized education, (2) a service orientation, and (3) the ability to be autonomous (Jacox, 1980). Jacox (1980) defines autonomy as a characteristic of a profession in which the members of that profession are self-regulating and have control of their functions in the work situation. Nurses agree that specialized education and a service orientation are necessary to become a nurse, but many nurses disagree on the concept of autonomy. This disagreement is the central argument that divides nurses with regard to whether it is professional to be part of a union.

Many nurses believe that for nursing to be considered a profession, nurses must exercise autonomy, and like most professionals, work out issues themselves. Many argue that this cannot be done without unionization. The debate about whether it is professional to be a part of a nurse's union has plagued nursing since the inception of nursing unions.

Definition of Supervisor

Much discussion in nursing unions has revolved around the definition of a supervisor. The National Labor Relations Act (1994), in Title 29 of the United States Code, defines a supervisor as "any individual having authority, in the interest of the employer, to

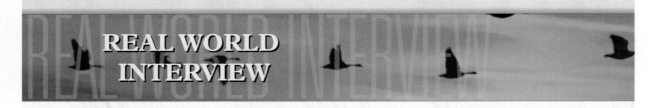

I believe it is professional to be in a union because you have more opportunities to stand up for your patients and your own nursing practice. Having worked in both a union and a nonunion environment, I think being in a union allows you to speak your mind without fear of losing job security. They can't dismiss you for just any reason. There are grievance proceedings. In a nonunion environment, if they don't like you or what you say, they can punish you. But I've also seen the downside of unions. An example is when a contract comes out. The more-senior union nursing staff wants to hold out from agreeing on a contract that does not address all of our concerns while the junior union nursing staff wants to agree on the first contract that is presented. Holding out for what you want is why there is arbitration. The junior nurses don't realize the power of the bargaining unit in nursing. I think most nurses don't realize what we as nurses can accomplish if we stick together.

Susan Zielinski, RN
Staff Nurse

hire, transfer, suspend, lay off, recall, promote, discharge, assign, reward, or discipline other employees, or the responsibility to direct them, or to adjust their grievances, or effectively, to recommend such action, if in connection with the foregoing, the exercise of such authority is not of a merely routine or clerical nature, but requires the use of independent judgment."

Using this definition, conceivably every nurse may be considered a supervisor—if not to another registered nurse, then of licensed practical nurses, nurse's aides, and unlicensed personnel. The larger issue for discussion is, if all nurses are supervisors by definition, can they legally be in a union? Nursing unions do not allow nursing managers or supervisors to unionize. Only nurses defined as employees can unionize. The ambiguity of the terms *employees* and *supervisors* has caused legal disputes (Phan, 1999). Dependent on clarification from the legal system, nurses may not always have the privilege to unionize. This very definition of supervisor has not allowed many other professionals to join unions because, by definition of their roles, they are supervisors.

Physician Unionization

As health maintenance organizations (HMOs) and other health care groups change the face of health care, they are changing the role of physicians. Physicians are considered employees in some settings instead of supervisors and now, like nurses, have the ability to join unions. The recent loss of physician autonomy and lowered wages have prompted many physicians to join unions (Phan, 1999). Similar to what occurred in nursing, physician discontent leads to unionization. Approximately 6% of physicians in the country are already unionized (Charatan, 1999), and the Service Employees International Union has pledged $1 million to recruit salaried physicians, who comprise approximately half of all physicians, to join physician unions (Charatan, 1999). The American Medical Association supports doctors engaging in collective action with employers but does not favor them formally joining unions (Charatan, 1999).

Unionization of University Professors

The unionization of kindergarten through twelfth-grade teachers is established in this country. Now, though, the number of professors at higher education institutions who are choosing to unionize is increasing. Again, wages and work environment have been reasons stimulating university professors to join unions. As the average age of university faculty increases and fewer people show interest in teaching, unions may be able to protect professors from becoming overburdened and financially reward those who enter teaching at the university level.

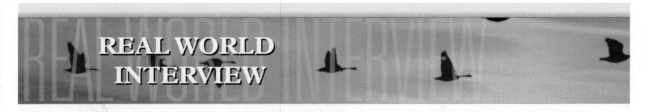

REAL WORLD INTERVIEW

I don't think it's any less professional for a physician to be in a union than any other health care provider. Doctors agree to try to help people. In return, physicians should be able to charge for that service and provide the best care they know how to deliver. Doctors should be able to bargain for better conditions and autonomy like the rest of society. More and more, the governing decision is not so much the patient care as what's cost-effective. Doctors are not making those decisions and that's inherently wrong. As more and more of the medical structure becomes corporate, the workers, which doctors have become, need a means of negotiating with their employers.

Jonathan Fisher, MD
Surgical Resident

MANAGING IN A UNION ENVIRONMENT

Managers must work with the union to manage within the rules and context of contract agreements. In some ways, managing once a union is in place is less difficult because of the explicit language in most union contracts. Corrective actions, rules concerning allowed absences, and so on are agreed upon, voted on, and written in the contract.

Grievance

When a union member believes that management has failed to meet the terms of the contract or labor agreement and communicates this to management, this process is called a **grievance**. All union contracts specify grievance proceedings for union members. Grievance proceedings usually start with an employee who believes there has been wrongdoing on the part of management. Next, the member talks with a union representative, who helps the employee judge whether the act or condition actually justifies a complaint. The union representative uses her knowledge of the contract, knowledge of the National Labor Relations Board, and her judgment to assist the employee. Next, the union member and the union representative meet with the manager to voice the grievance. At this step, the conflict may be resolved. If the conflict is not resolved, the next step may be to appeal management's decision and mediate with a higher-level manager. Grievance proceedings may differ from union to union.

PROS AND CONS OF COLLECTIVE BARGAINING

The decision to support or not to support collective bargaining in the form of a union is a personal one. Table 25-6 summarizes a number of pros and cons of collective bargaining.

TABLE 25-6	*Pros and Cons of Unionization*

Pros	Cons
The contract guides standards.	There is reduced allowance for individuality.
Members are able to be a part of the decision-making process.	Other union members may outvote your decisions.
All union members and management must conform to the terms of the contract without exception.	All union members and management must conform to the terms of the contract without exception.
A process can be instituted to question a manager's authority if a member feels something was done unjustly. More people are involved in the process.	Disputes are not handled with an individual and management only; there is less room for personal judgment.
Union dues are required to make the union work for you.	Union dues must be paid even if individuals do not support unionization.
Unions give a collective voice for employees.	Employee may not agree with the collective voice.
Employees are able to voice concerns to management without fear of job security.	Unions may be perceived by some as not professional.

REAL WORLD INTERVIEW

The union affects my role as manager in many ways. There are so many pros and cons with it. I get frustrated as a manager when I feel like I cannot use my judgment because it may contradict the contract. An example is I had an employee that lost a grandparent that I know was essentially their parent, but I couldn't give them time off because it was not technically their parent. The contract also doesn't allow me to really commend employees that really work hard and do their best every day. The hard-working person's pay and benefits are exactly the same as a mediocre employee. My hands are tied.

If you violate the contract, it becomes a time-consuming project for me as the manager. An example of this is if I chose to give the person time off for the grandparent that died. I would have grievances from other people that I did not give time off for their grandparent's death. I would have to document what I did and why and would ultimately lose the grievance and have to find a way to compensate the other people for not giving them time off. I come from a pro-union family, and I understand how unions can protect employees. In general, it is good for employees to have somebody who is on their side and who treats all as equals. It's hard for me to imagine that there are managers who mistreat their employees in other institutions.

Ann Marie O'Connor, RN
Patient Care Manager

Nurses practicing in the United States have the luxury of many laws to protect individuals in the workplace. If nurses prefer a particular collective action model, they can find that model in action in numerous work settings. Nurses have the ability to choose where they practice and under which model they practice.

KEY CONCEPTS

- Collective bargaining has existed in the United States since 1790.
- The Wagner Act of 1935 gave private employees the legal right to form unions. Since then, numerous legislative acts have been passed to protect employees from unfair work practices.
- Workplace advocacy is a collective action model that is more informal and encompasses the everyday creativity and problem solving that occur in nursing.

- Collective bargaining through unionization is a collective action model that is formal and legally based. It uses a written contract to guide nursing and workplace issues.
- Nurses are often aware of fraud and are fearful to report it. Qui tam lawsuits allow people to discreetly expose health care fraud.
- Nurses who are unhappy in the workplace because of issues such as wages and unsafe staffing often attempt to unionize to rectify workplace problems. Nurses who are not managers have the legal right to unionize. There are specific steps that can be taken to institute a union. Employees and managers must be aware of what steps to take during the initiation of unionization.
- The American Nurses Association is a full-service professional organization that represents the nation's entire registered nurse population. The ANA has a dual role of being a professional organization and a collective bargaining agent for nursing. The ANA is politically active and lobbies on issues affecting nursing and the general public.

- Other professionals who do not have a tradition of unionization are opting to unionize. Physicians and university professors are joining unions for the same reasons that some nurses have chosen to join unions.

KEY TERMS

American Nurses
  Association
collective action
collective bargaining
collective bargaining
  agent

grievance
union
whistle-blowing
workplace advocacy

REVIEW QUESTIONS

1. A manager should do which of the following if nurses are attempting to unionize?
   A. Nothing; most often the union attempt fails.
   B. Do not hire any registered nurses who are pro-union.
   C. Find out the reason nurses want collective action.
   D. Fire the nurse instigating unionization.

2. Workplace advocacy is best defined as
   A. a management-defined solution for the workplace.
   B. holding managers and nurses accountable.
   C. a formal structure that is voted on.
   D. activities nurses undertake to address problems in the workplace.

3. Common reasons nurses unionize include all of the following EXCEPT
   A. patient care issues.
   B. wages.
   C. staffing issues.
   D. being content in the workplace.

4. Which legislation gave unions the right to organize?
   A. National Labor Relations Act (1935)
   B. Fair Labor Standards Act (1938)
   C. Taft-Hartley Act (1947)
   D. Executive Order 11246 (1965)

REVIEW ACTIVITIES

1. You are a new graduate nurse and have begun working on a medical unit. The nurse manager explains to you that the unit uses workplace advocacy. What is workplace advocacy? How will it affect your functioning as a registered nurse on the unit?

2. You are hired in a hospital that is a union shop. How does unionization differ from other collective action models such as workplace advocacy? Give three examples of how unionization differs from workplace advocacy.

3. You are a graduate nurse, and you found out you passed the NCLEX examination. As a registered nurse, you are represented by the American Nurses Association. What is the mission of the ANA? What is meant when it is said that the ANA has a dual role in nursing? Is the ANA active in politics?

EXPLORING THE WEB

- What sites would you recommend to someone inquiring about collective bargaining?
  http://www.www.nursingworld.org
  http://www.www.califnurses.org

- Go to the site for the American Nurses Association and find your state nurses association. What did you learn about your state nurses association? *http://www.nursingworld.org*

- What site would you access to find out the history of collective bargaining?
  http://www.nlrb.gov

- Go to the site for the California Nurses Association and click on some news articles, then on Nursing Practice. What did you learn about nursing and current events?
  http://www.califnurses.org

REFERENCES

American Nurses Association. (n.d.). Mission statement. Retrieved March 2, 2000, from http://www.nursingworld.org

Charatan, F. (1999). American trade union aims to recruit more doctors. *Western Journal of Medicine, 170*(5), 305–306.

Flanagan, L. (1991). How the bargaining process works. *American Nurse, 23*(9), 11–12.

Hart, C. (1998). The state of the unions. *Nursing Times, 94*(15), 36–37.

Jacox, A. (1980). Collective action: The basis for professionalism. *Supervisor Nurse, 11*(9), 22–24.

Junor, J. (1998). What roles do unions have in preparing nursing leaders to effective change for the future? *Concern, 27*(1), 18–19.

Marquis, B., & Huston, C. (1998). *Management decision making for nurses: 124 case studies* (3rd ed.). Philadelphia: Lippincott.

National Labor Relations Act. (1994). Regrieved March 2, 2000, from http://www.nlrb.gov/publicat.html

Phan, C. (1999). Physician unionization: The impact on the medical profession. *Journal of Legal Medicine 20*(1), 114–140.

Polston, M.D. (1999). Whistleblowing: Does the law protect you? *American Journal of Nursing, 99*(1, pt. 1), 26–31.

The role of collective bargaining and unions in advancing the profession of nursing. (1998). *Nursing Trends & Issues, 3*(2), 1–8.

Seltzer, T. M. (2001). Collective bargaining: A wake-up call—part 2. *Nursing Management, 32*(4), 35–37, 48.

Ulrich, B. (1992). *Leadership and management according to Florence Nightingale.* Norwalk, CT: Appleton & Lange.

Underwood, P. (1997). Nurses need collective action to "build" profession. *Michigan Nurse, 70*(10), 3.

United American Nurses (UAN) mobilizes nurses on staffing crisis. (2001). *American Journal of Nursing, 101*(1), 65.

SUGGESTED READINGS

Aging faculty adds to RN shortage. (1999). *Nursing Spectrum* (Greater Chicago/NE Illinois & NW Indiana ed.), *12*(5), 6.

Hellinghausen, A. (1999, August 9). Changes afoot. *NurseWeek,* 27–28.

Jamison, D. T., Frenk, J., Knaul, F. (1998). International collective action in health: Objectives, functions and rationale. *Lancet, 351*(9101), 514–517.

Meir, E. (1999). Politically speaking. *ONS News, 14*(10), 13.

Melville, E. (1995). The history of industrial action in nursing. *Professional Nurse, 11*(2), 84–86.

National Labor Relations Board. (1995). *The First Sixty Years: The Story of the National Labor Relations Board 1935–1995.* Retrieved March 2, 2000, from http://www.nlrb.gov/publicat.html

Nurse staffing law may herald benchmarks. (1999). *Healthcare Benchmarks, 6*(120) 137–138.

Porter-O'Grady, T. (2001). Collective bargaining: The union as partner. *Nursing Management, 32*(6, pt. 1), 30–32.

Reffner, G. (1996). Collectively: Be prepared—each one doing our part. *Hawaii Nurse, 3*(9), 8.

Tone, B. 1999, (August 9). Pulled apart: Does unionizing serve the interests of the profession? *NurseWeek,* 1–5.

Trossman, S. (1998). Doctors increasingly are looking for the union label. *American Nurse, 30*(4), 19.

Walmsley, J. (1996). Collective action brought change. *Kaitiaki: Nursing New Zealand, 9*(1), 28.

Yoder-Wise, P. (Ed.). (1999). *Leading and managing in nursing* (2nd ed.). St. Louis, MO: Mosby.

CHAPTER 26

The future belongs to those who believe in the beauty of their dreams.

(Eleanor Roosevelt)

Career Planning

Karin Polifko-Harris, PhD, RN, CNAA

OBJECTIVES

Upon completion of this chapter, the reader should be able to:

1. Detail the process of a successful nursing job search.
2. Develop a resume and cover letter.
3. Identify appropriate dress for a successful job interview.
4. Discuss potential interview questions and identify acceptable answers.

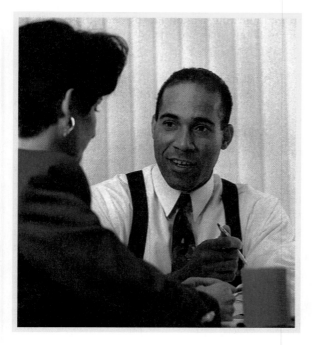

Juliette will be graduating from Great College with her bachelor of science in nursing (BSN) degree in 1 month. She is one of the few students in her class who has not even begun looking for a job. She is beginning to wonder whether she should start now rather than wait until she passes her NCLEX-RN. Everyone else around her excitedly speaks about the job market being wide open, but she is just not motivated to start her job search.

Should Juliette begin her job search now? Should she wait until she takes the NCLEX-RN?

What are some of the positive aspects of waiting to begin her job search until she becomes a registered nurse (RN)? What are some of the negative aspects of waiting?

Where are the opportunities for new graduate nurses?

Starting a new career is an exciting time, but it also may cause a little anxiety, even if you are well prepared. New graduates are no longer under the watchful eyes of their instructors and now must make independent nursing decisions. Experienced registered nurses graduating with a new BSN may find that employers have new expectations. The focus of this chapter on career planning is to give new nursing graduates the tools to seek and obtain a new position. Included in this chapter are tips on resume writing, sample interview questions and answers, and hints on how and where to search for a new job.

BEGINNING A JOB SEARCH

While in school, many new graduates may have had some wonderful experiences during their clinical rotations and after graduation may be interested in staying at the facilities in which they worked. The feeling may be mutual. The staff and nurse manager may be just as interested in having the new graduate as she is in working there. But what if there is no job offer from a clinical agency at which you completed a clinical rotation? Now where do you begin to look for a job as an RN?

The first job out of college is an important one, with availability dependent on the geographical area of the United States. Regardless of the area in which one seeks employment, it takes a focused effort to find and then secure the best opportunity. Finding a job does not happen overnight, and depending on the status of health care economics when the search is begun, it may take as little as a few days or as long as several months. The United States goes through phases of need for professional registered nurses. Some years, new graduates may have difficulty finding full-time employment. This occurred in the mid-1990s. At other times, new graduates may be hired for full-time work before graduation. Depending on the health care environment, new graduates may be hired only for medical-surgical nursing positions. During nursing shortages, new graduates may have more choices and may be able to begin their professional careers in specialty areas such as critical care nursing or home health nursing. Hospitals have always been the largest employers of nurses, but opportunities abound in other sectors of health care, such as home health, insurance companies, managed care companies, and pharmaceutical companies.

The critical first step in your job search is preparation. Know what clinical area you are interested in and what skills you have that may fit that area. Before graduation, ask the nursing faculty members who have worked closely with you during clinical rotations what skills and abilities they perceive you to have, and where they believe you to excel. A trusted mentor, family member, or even classmates may also provide you with some insight as to abilities and strengths. Sometimes it is easier to have someone else see what you do well than for you to see these skills clearly. Do you enjoy a fast-paced environment with multiple tasks? Do you like the unknown, or do you prefer a more routine environment? Do you like psychiatric clients? Young or old clients? Working with a specific specialty such as oncology or cardiac care? What did you like and what did you dislike in your clinical rotations? Did work in a hospital intrigue you, or were you challenged with the community health rotation? New graduates have a generalist background, that is, the ability to deliver care to a variety of patients and their families.

Once a desirable clinical area is identified, then longer-term goals should be reviewed to fully look at lifelong learning and employment opportunities. Essential to career success is understanding yourself—who you are, what challenges you professionally, and what essentially inspires you to work. What is your attitude and initiative? Do you like or shy away from responsibility? What are your abilities? (Hauter, 1997). In completing this phase of self-assessment, the new graduate looks at each job as a career segment. Are there plans to continue schooling? If yes, in what area? What are the long-term (5 years plus) goals? What type of experience would best serve in meeting those goals? For example, if becoming a certified registered nurse anesthetist (CRNA) is a long-term goal, then several steps could be taken to increase the likelihood of achieving that goal (Table 26-1).

By having a long-term goal in mind, you can see where you need to be to stay on target and which job may provide the best opportunities for success. At this point, it is usually helpful to talk with someone who has experience in the field you are interested in pursuing, such as someone actively working in the field. With the long-term goal in mind, the job search can begin.

Newspapers

The first place most people think to begin a job search is the local newspaper. Generally, the Sunday edition has the most thorough job section; local institutions will advertise there and possibly out-of-town institutions as well, depending on the job market. Not all job openings will be listed in the paper, perhaps just the harder-to-fill positions or newer positions. Some employers will run an advertisement specifically for a new graduate, with notice of an internship or preceptorship within the ad. Note the contact name, address, and phone number listed in the ad. It is often helpful to begin a job file. Place clipped ads with the newspaper's name and the date advertised in your file. If you are moving out of the local area, you may want to subscribe ahead of time to the Sunday edition of the paper in the city where you will be moving so that you have a better understanding of available job opportunities.

Bulletin Boards, Employment Telephone Lines

Another place to look for job openings is in health care agencies themselves. Most will have an employment bulletin board located near the human resources

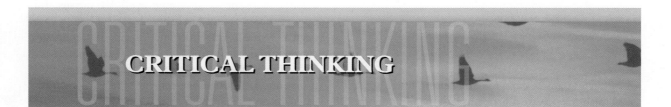

CRITICAL THINKING

Andrea Lightfoot is a new graduate who really enjoyed her clinical rotation in the coronary care unit (CCU). In fact, the staff in the CCU liked her so much, they convinced their nurse manager to offer Andrea a full-time night position after graduation. Andrea has always heard other registered nurses say that a new graduate should work at least a minimum of a year in medical-surgical nursing before transferring to a specialty area of nursing.

What have you heard about working in a specialty area, such as critical care, right after graduation? What are the positives and what are the negatives about taking a first position in a specialty area after graduation? What do you think are the negatives and positives about working on a medical-surgical unit?

TABLE 26-1	*Career Goal*

Goal:	Certified registered nurse anesthetist (CRNA)
Step 1:	Graduate with BSN.
Step 2:	Obtain position in telemetry unit (years 1 to 2).
Step 3:	Obtain position in critical care unit (years 2 to 3).
Step 4:	Apply to CRNA program (years 3 to 4).

department with a listing of RN positions, experience needed, and the contact person. By going directly to the hospital or agency, you will see the available positions and qualifications needed. Also, by going to the agency to view the potential jobs, you can pick up the necessary paperwork to complete an application.

Many health care employers have an employment telephone line or web site that identifies job openings on a weekly basis. Phone numbers may be toll free, especially in those agencies that have multiple openings or attract many people from out of the area. You can find these phone numbers either by directly calling the human resources department, looking up the agency in the Yellow Pages, or perhaps checking the agency's employment web page on the Internet.

Job Fairs

Many employers participate in job fairs, which may be announced on the radio or through the mail or advertised in the paper. A university or college may arrange job fairs for students, asking many employers to come to a designated spot with recruitment materials. Sometimes local, regional, or national educational conferences will also invite agency representatives to recruit, such as the state and national conventions of the National Student Nurses Association. Many employers will send a human resources representative, most likely the nurse recruiter, and possibly a nurse manager. Job fairs are great occasions to see a variety of employers and to compare options and opportunities. These events are to be taken seriously because first impressions are critical in being able to secure an interview after the job fair is over. Job fairs and other recruitment events offer the potential for networking. **Networking** is the con-

tinuous process of initiating and maintaining professional relationships through communication and information sharing (Hadley & Sheldon, 1995). Networking among colleagues is important. It is not always what you know but who you know that may be the key to your next job opportunity.

Electronic Media and the Internet

Perhaps the single largest innovation in the job search is the use of the Internet and the World Wide Web. Where does one begin a job search on the Internet? There are several sources of on-line employment. These sources include search engines; job boards; and agency and company sites such as those for a specific hospital, health care agency, or health care company. Electronic media sites include health care journals. Building a successful job search on the Internet takes some thoughtful preparation.

Search Engines

Search engines are probably the best start to a job search. Identify keywords for the job you are interested in finding, such as *critical care registered nurse* and *Las Vegas*. Following are some examples of search engines:

- Dogpile (allows you to search multiple search engines at one time; this site is known as a metasearch engine): *http://www.dogpile.com*
- Savvy Search (another metasearch engine): *http://savvysearch.com*
- Excite: *http://www.excite.com*
- WebCrawler: *http://www.webcrawler.com*
- Infoseek: *http://www.infoseek.com*

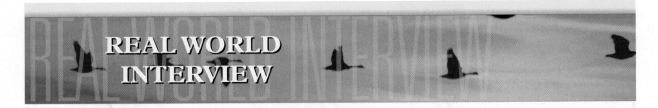

Job Boards

Job boards are another place to look for positions, with some job boards specifically for nursing positions. These sites are maintained by recruiters, employment agencies, and marketing firms that specialize in the industry. Health care organizations may also maintain listings of job opportunities on-line; however, many require membership and passwords to use. Some examples of job boards specific to health care include the following:

- *http://www.healthcareerweb.com*
- *http://www.medjobs.com*
- *http://www.monster.com*: A variety of positions. This site also includes sample interview questions. You will need to narrow your search to health care and nursing opportunities.
- *http://www.aone.org*: This site requires membership to use.

Agency and Corporate Sites

Agency and company sites are specific to a hospital, health system, or other places that employ registered nurses. In fact, many companies that may be indirectly linked to nursing care may have open RN positions. Many hospitals now maintain active web sites with listings of employment opportunities, so this is a great way to begin a job search if you know specifically where you would like to work after graduation. Some examples include the following:

- *http://www.hr.duke.edu*: This site is for work opportunities at Duke University.
- *http://www.amgen.com*: Amgen is a biotechnology company.

Media Sites

Media sites are on-line journals and newspapers. In addition to articles, advertisements, and discussion forums, many on-line journals and media sites maintain job openings. A few examples of these media sites include the following:

- *http://www.rn.com*
- *http://www.careercity.com*

DEVELOPING A RESUME

Resumes are generally the first opportunity a prospective employer has to see who you are and what your qualifications are for a given position. A **resume** is a brief summary of your background, training, and experience as well as your qualifications for a position. It should be viewed as a marketing tool to sell yourself to a prospective employer. Generally, a resume should be no longer than one to two pages, so it needs to contain concise information that clearly identifies your specific skills, strengths, and experiences. A resume should be honest, neat, and easy to read. In companies that are highly desirable to work at, the resume is also often used as a screening tool so that a recruiter's time can best be spent wisely with potential employees who are seen as welcome team members.

There is no one perfect resume style. It is agreed that an effective resume (1) gets the employer's interest; (2) identifies critical areas such as education, work experience, and special qualifications; (3) should be tailored to the employer's needs; (4) creates a favorable first impression about you and your abilities; (5) communicates that you are someone who is a good fit for the position; and (6) is visually appealing. A good resume takes time to prepare; you should ensure that what is presented on paper is truthful and presents you as a capable person who is able to make immediate and sustained contributions to an organization.

A resume contains three basic elements: information about yourself, your education, and your work experience. Although there is no universal format or style, two basic types of resumes—the chronological resume and the functional resume—are generally used, with both types containing the common elements listed in Table 26-2.

TABLE 26-2	*Elements of a Resume*
Identifying information/ Heading	Include your name, address, telephone number, and e-mail address. If you are moving after school, be sure to include a permanent address.
Career objective	Specify your employment target to help recruiters quickly identify your purpose in applying.
Employment data/ Professional experience	Include name of employer, location of employer, dates employed, and job title(s). If you are developing a chronological resume, write about specific job responsibilities, job skills, and any accomplishments while you were employed at each agency or facility. If you are writing a functional resume, include only the name and address of the employer, dates employed, and job title(s). Include relevant clinical experiences, specialty classes, preceptorships, externships, or research projects,
	Keep in mind that prospective employers are interested in your ability to work well with the public and other employees, your positive communication skills, and your ability to maintain a strong work ethic.
Military experience	Include rank, service, assignment, dates, and significant experiences.
Formal education and specialized training	Note where you attended school, the school's address, the degree you received (for example, BSN), the date you completed your studies, and any special achievements, such as grade point average (especially if it was 3.0 or better), any leadership positions held, any membership in student or professional organizations, and any specialized training.
Professional organizations and memberships	Identify memberships and any offices held.
Awards and honors (optional)	If you are a new graduate without a significant work history, you could include high school and college honors and awards.
References	The statement "References available upon request" can be placed on the last line of a resume. You can either provide a listing of references on the application, or bring a separate reference list to a job interview. Include at least 3 professional references, with names, titles, addresses, and phone numbers—but only after receiving permission from these persons to use them as references. Do not use family, friends, or neighbors as references. Notify your references when you interview to let them know they may be contacted.

The Chronological Resume

The chronological resume is the more common type of resume. Jobs are listed in reverse chronological order; that is, the most recent job held is listed first, the job before that is listed next, and so on.

A chronological resume is good for those with a steady work history, or new graduates without a significant employment history. It is easier to write than other resume formats. However, there are some potential problems with a chronological resume. It can highlight gaps in employment; and special qualifications, skills, and talents are more difficult to spot quickly. For those who may be in their second or third careers, a chronological resume may not easily illustrate the fit among careers. For someone returning to work after many years of absence, it does not readily show how that person's experiences apply to the position sought. Figure 26-1 illustrates a chronological resume for a new graduate.

The Functional Resume

A functional resume is a good tool for people who have had multiple careers or who want to dramatically change their career focus. Skills and abilities are emphasized rather than progressive job responsibilities. Disadvantages to the functional resume include its unfamiliarity to employers—most are familiar with the chronological resume—and the fact that it is more difficult to write this resume. Figure 26-2 is an example of a functional resume for an experienced RN.

Resume Writing Using Action Verbs, Phrases with Meaning

The most difficult task in writing a resume is describing what you have accomplished using action verbs and phrases with meaning. Weigh your choice of words. Remember, you have the attention of recruiters for an average of only 30 seconds as they review your resume. Every word is critical. Every descriptive phrase should have significant meaning. Use meaningful phrases such as *desire to achieve, organizational ability, results oriented,* and *attention to detail.* Use meaningful phrases when one word does not fully express the complete thought. When writing a resume, keep in mind it is not boasting to write about what you do well. If you do not write about your strengths, no one else will and you may not have an opportunity to even obtain an interview. Table 26-3 is a summary of action verbs for resume preparation.

TABLE 26-3	List of Action Verbs for Resume			
accomplished	delivered	identified	operated	reorganized
achieved	demonstrated	increased	organized	revamped
administered	designed	initiated	oversaw	revised
analyzed	developed	innovated	performed	simplified
approved	directed	instituted	planned	solved
built	earned	launched	proposed	streamlined
communicated	eliminated	listed	provided	supervised
completed	established	maintained	purchased	taught
conceived	evaluated	managed	redesigned	terminated
conducted	expanded	mastered	reduced	trained
coordinated	explored	motivated	reengineered	transformed
created	generated	negotiated	reinforced	utilized

Caitlin O'Malley
2424 Sailing Avenue
Cherry Hill, NJ 08080
(609) 444-2212 (home)
cat24@excite.net

OBJECTIVE: An entry-level position as a pediatric registered nurse

EDUCATION: Bachelor of Science in Nursing, May 2002
                  University of Pennsylvania, Philadelphia, PA

                  Highlights: *   Maintained 3.66 GPA, Dean's list
                                *   Senior class president, junior class advocate
                                *   220-hour preceptorship on the Oncology Unit at the
                                    Children's Hospital of Philadelphia

EXPERIENCE: Patient Care Assistant, Labor and Delivery
                  St. Mary's Medical Center, Philadelphia, PA
                  (August 2000–present)

                  Duties: *   Assist in the preparation of the operating room
                                *   Provide basic patient care monitoring, including
                                    vital signs, phlebotomy, glucose screening
                                *   Prepare and stock patient rooms

                  Life Guard and Camp Counselor
                  Camp Perry, Point Pleasant, NJ
                  (Summers 1996–1999)

                  Duties: *   Supervise waterfront for 150 campers along with three
                                    additional lifeguards
                                *   Perform basic camp counselor duties, including direct
                                    supervision of campers ages 9 to 14

CERTIFICATION: Certified as a Basic Life Support Provider, 1996–present

PROFESSIONAL
ORGANIZATIONS: Nursing Student Association, University of Pennsylvania Chapter
                  National Student Nurses Association
                  American Red Cross, Blood Drive Volunteer
                  Philadelphia Free Clinic, Registration Volunteer

Figure 26-1 Resume—Chronological

Chung Tao, BSN, RN
48 Windmere Drive
Virginia Beach, VA 23456
(757) 436-2880
chungtao@aol.com

OBJECTIVE: A department-level nursing management position within an ambulatory care center

HIGHLIGHTS OF QUALIFICATIONS

- Highly organized with ability to coordinate multiple tasks and projects
- Administer an annual $1.2 million budget
- Supervise 24 professional and paraprofessional employees

RELEVANT EXPERIENCE

Management

- Planned, designed, and implemented a 12-bed, in-hospital, short-stay unit
- Developed and managed $1.2 million operational and capital budget
- Interviewed and hired new personnel, both professional and paraprofessional
- Implemented self-scheduling in the short-stay operating room
- Coordinated JCAHO site visit for the Surgical Operating Center

Clinical

- Maintain clinical competency in both inpatient and outpatient surgical nursing
- Act as code team coordinator for the Surgical Operating Center
- Established clinical competency expectations for staff members

Community Service

- Hospital representative for the bimonthly community blood drive
- President, Parent Teacher Association

ACADEMIC PREPARATION

May 2002	Bachelor of Science in Nursing
	University of North Carolina at Charlotte, Charlotte, NC
May 1990	Associate of Science in Nursing
	Los Angeles Community College, Los Angeles, CA

EMPLOYMENT HISTORY

2001–present	Nurse Manager, Short Stay Unit
	Mercy Hospital, Charlotte, NC
1999–2001	Nurse Manager, Operating Room
	University Hospital, Charlotte, NC
1996–1999	Assistant Nurse Manager, Operating Room
	Charlotte Memorial Hospital, Charlotte, NC
1993–1996	Staff Nurse, Recovery Room
	San Francisco General Hospital, San Francisco, CA
1990–1993	Staff Nurse, General Surgical Care Unit
	Inner City Medical Center, Los Angeles, CA

PROFESSIONAL CERTIFICATIONS

2000–present	Advanced Cardiac Life Support instructor
1999–present	Advanced Cardiac Life Support provider
1994–1999	Certified Medical-Surgical Nurse, Generalist,
	American Nurses Association Credentialing Center

PROFESSIONAL MEMBERSHIPS

- American Nurses Association, North Carolina Nurses Association
- American Organization of Nurse Executives, North Carolina Organization of Nurse Executives

Figure 26-2 Resume—Functional

Try to eliminate as much extraneous wording as possible from your resume, and be cautious of using abbreviations. Use a spell checker and then have someone else review your resume for errors. Word processing programs are not perfect and may not pick up all misspelled words. It also is helpful, once the resume is written, to apply Grammatik, which is a program built into both Corel WordPerfect and Microsoft Word that reviews the spelling, punctuation, and grammar of your copy.

In printing a resume for a nursing position, it is best to use white, ivory, or pale gray paper of good quality. All office supply stores have resume-grade paper, often with matching envelopes. Again, you may have only one opportunity to make a good impression. Use a printer that prints clearly and darkly. Choose a legible, professional font such as Times New Roman or Arial. If your resume runs more than one page, place your name and the number 2 at the top left-hand corner of the second page.

Writing a Cover Letter

A resume should always have a letter of introduction, known as the cover letter. It is a one-page letter designed to entice the prospective employer to become interested enough to read the resume. It does not reiterate the entire resume but presents highlights and a summary of the essential points found on the resume. Figure 26-3 is an example of a cover letter.

Developing an Electronic Resume

With the growth of the Internet and the expansion of the World Wide Web, many sites offer not only job openings but also the option of e-mailing a cover letter and resume directly to an address. Sending a resume via e-mail requires special considerations, especially if the desired result is a clean, neat appearance. You need to be able to send your resume via e-mail so that the recipient will be able to read the resume, regardless of the software the recipient is using.

There are several ways to create an electronic resume, including writing the resume using standard word processing software such as Microsoft Word or WordPerfect. Type the resume using the word processing software and then save it in one of three formats: ASCII plain text (.txt), rich-text (.rtf), or as hypertext (.html). ASCII text files are the most common types of data files found on the Internet. This

type allows for simplicity in reading the text but does not allow any type of text formatting such as boldface characters, bullets, underlining, or italics. The recipient receives plain, clear text without any identifying marks, tabs, or visually appealing formatting. If you want to highlight a specific area, then use a character like an asterisk (*).

It is important to use keywords in sending an electronic resume. Keywords are what are picked up by a recruiter's computer program. When recruiters are looking for someone with specific skills, they perform a search using keywords such as *pediatric nurse practitioner* or *oncology registered nurse*. Recruiters' reliance on keywords reinforces the recommendation that resumes should not be written in complete sentences and paragraphs but in cogent thoughts and phrases. Be sure to use correct grammar, spelling, and punctuation. Do not use all capital letters to type messages because doing so makes it appear as though the writer is shouting.

Table 26-4 identifies the steps to follow in creating an electronic resume.

Tracking Job Leads

When you begin to develop a sense of what positions are available, it is helpful to organize the job search. Figure 26-4 is one example of a method to track progress on job leads.

DRESSING FOR A SUCCESSFUL INTERVIEW

A registered nurse is considered a professional, with professional dress expected for the interview. Casual clothing, such as khakis and polo shirts, gives the impression that you do not take this interview seriously. A good rule of thumb is to wear what you would consider business attire (Figure 26-5). Interview clothing may not be worn on a daily basis, but perhaps it is worn to special functions or events. For women, a suit with skirt, a tailored pantsuit, or a neat dress is appropriate. For men, a neatly tailored shirt with tie, pants, and perhaps a sport coat would be appropriate to wear to an interview for a staff nurse position. It is best to dress conservatively rather than in a trendy manner. Makeup, perfume, and jewelry should be minimal. Be sure to turn off all cell phones and pagers so that all your attention can be directed at the interviewer.

Caitlin O'Malley
2424 Sailing Avenue
Cherry Hill, NJ 08080
(609) 444-2212

April 10, 2002

Ms. Vanetha Raj, BSN, RN
Nurse Recruiter
Shore Memorial Hospital
100 Seashore Drive
Point Pleasant, NJ 07726

Dear Ms. Raj:

This letter is in response to your advertisement in the April 10, 2002 issue of the Philadelphia Inquirer for a registered nurse in the pediatrics ward. I completed my pediatric clinical rotation at Children's Hospital of Philadelphia and since that time I have had a strong interest in developing a career in pediatric nursing.

I am currently enrolled in the Bachelor of Science in Nursing program at the University of Pennsylvania and plan to graduate in May 2002. My GPA in nursing is currently a 3.66, and I am active in professional activities such as the Nursing Student Association, Omicron Delta, and as a senior mentor to undergraduate nursing majors. I am highly motivated and enjoy working with children and their families. I look forward to learning as much as I can about the nursing profession in my new position.

Thank you for your time and consideration of my resume. I look forward to speaking with you in the near future to discuss the potential of employment as a registered nurse at Shore Memorial Hospital. I will be calling within the next week to check on the status of my application. I may be reached at home at (609) 444-2212.

Sincerely,

Caitlin O'Malley

Figure 26-3 Cover Letter

TABLE 26-4 — *Creating an Electronic Resume*

Step 1: In the word processing program, set margins so that 6.5 inches of text are displayed. This is seen easily by the majority of e-mail programs.

Step 2: Write the resume using a font in 12-point type, such as Courier 12 or Times New Roman 12.

Step 3: Save the resume as a text-only file with line breaks. Do not use the Tab key. Use the space bar instead. Use the left justification format.

Step 4: Open this new file in a text editor such as Microsoft Notepad.

Step 5: Review the resume. This is how the recipient will see the resume once it is transmitted via e-mail. Pay careful attention to unsupported formats or those formats that your word processing program may not be able to read. You may have to add ASCII-supported characters such as asterisks to make the resume easier to view. Proofread!

Step 6: Copy and paste the resume in the body of a test e-mail message. Maybe send it back to yourself or a friend who uses a different e-mail program to see how the recipient views your resume.

Step 7: When sending a resume electronically, a cover letter should also accompany the resume. Rather than sending both the cover letter and the resume in the text area, or as separate attachments, the preferred approach is to send the cover letter in the text portion of the e-mail, and attach the resume.

Adapted from *Electronic resumes and online networking* (p. 72), by R. Smith, 1999, Franklin Lakes, NJ: Career Press.

Company	Telephone Number	Contact Name	Resume Sent/Date	Interview Date	Thank You Letter	Follow-Up

Figure 26-4 Tracker for Job Leads

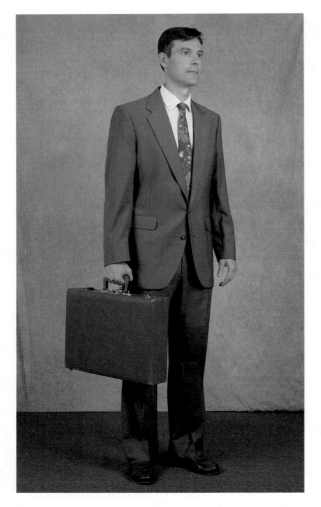

Figure 26-5 Interview attire should be neat and professional.

PLANNING FOR THE INTERVIEW

Successful preparation for a job interview begins before you enter the building. It begins at home. The first step in putting your best foot forward is to do a self-assessment. A self-assessment is sometimes difficult to do, as many of us do not really like to talk about ourselves and perceive it to be boastful. In an interview situation, however, you are expected to highlight your strengths and abilities and discuss how you would be a good fit within the organization. Know what clinical areas you want to work in.

The second step in planning for an interview is to find out about the organization. How is the organization viewed by the community? The patients and their families? The health care providers? What are the mission and values of the organization, and do they agree with your values?

Interview Questions

When preparing for an interview, it is often helpful to rehearse questions and answers with another person—a friend, professional colleague, or family member—who will be honest with you and let you know what impression you make during your responses. Table 26-5 contains 10 common interview questions with suggested guidelines for responding. They may provide you with a beginning point to successfully answer the question. You need to answer all questions honestly, and you need to be positive about your experiences and skills in a nonboastful manner.

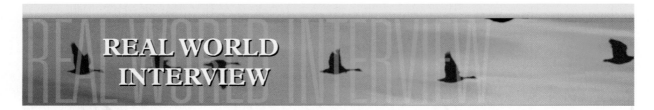

REAL WORLD INTERVIEW

As a clinical coordinator, I need to see that seasoned nurses nurture and develop new graduates to the best of their potential. In choosing a preceptor, I look for someone who has patience, enjoys teaching, and is confident in their own abilities as a professional. I also look to match people with similar personalities because not everyone works well with every personality. I need to know sooner rather than later if a match between a preceptor and a new graduate isn't working.

Christine Vera, RN
Clinical Coordinator

TABLE 26-5	*Interview Questions*

Question	Potential Response
Tell me about yourself.	Do not go into a long list, but have two to three traits that are solid (e.g., "I am a positive person and look for new learning experiences").
Why do you want to work here?	Describe several attributes of the work environment, the staff, or the patients (e.g., "I enjoyed my rotation on 5 West—the staff worked as a team and I am looking for that type of support in my first position").
What do you want to be doing in 5 years?	Identify a long-term goal and figure out how to achieve it with progressive responsibilities and achievements.
What are your qualifications?	Discuss experiences that you have had that qualify you for the new position.
What are your strengths?	This is a favorite question. Look at the job description. What qualities do you have that are required? Are you able to work under stress, are you organized, are you eager to learn new skills, do you enjoy new challenges?
What would your references say?	You may want to ask your references this question. Would they say you are easily distracted or focused? A team player or solo player? A problem solver or one who ignores problems?
Are you interested in more schooling?	Most who have just graduated may want to say no, but an employer wants someone who is interested in lifelong learning, especially in the nursing profession.
What has been your biggest success?	Think of a success ahead of time that may fit with the organization. It does not have to be in nursing.
What has been your greatest failure?	Again, think ahead, but this time, make sure you can state what you learned from the negative experience. After all, to fail is to learn, so state what you would do differently next time and why.
Why do you want to leave your current job?	For an RN, you can say that you are seeking new responsibilities, experiences, and challenges. Give an example of a new experience you are looking for.

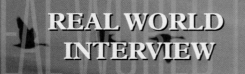

REAL WORLD INTERVIEW

Being a new graduate can bring a high anxiety level, so one of the most supportive things we as experienced nurses can do is take a new graduate under our wing. A new graduate has been in a highly structured environment while in school, and sometimes, as seasoned nurses, we tend to forget the amount of independence that we have in our decision making.

Lori Mattingly, RN

You will also be offered the opportunity to ask questions of the interviewer, so be prepared with several that clearly illustrate your interest in the organization and your willingness to become a valued team member. It is best to have your questions written down so that if you are under a little stress, you do not forget to ask specific questions. See Table 26-6 for some sample questions that you might want to investigate.

Showing more interest in personal gain than in contributing to the employer is one sure way to lose employment opportunities. However, you need the information in these questions before making a deci-

sion on whether to accept the job. Nevertheless, you must first concentrate on convincing the employer that you are the person for the job.

WRITING A THANK YOU LETTER

After your interview, you should send a thank you letter to the interviewer for his time and interest in you as a prospective employee. Many people do not take the time to write a personal note, and this will set you

---

TABLE 26-6   *Sample Questions to Ask During an Interview*

- How can I prepare myself to work on this unit and do a good job?

- What shift will I be scheduled to work? Will I rotate shifts?

- Who is my preceptor?

- What type of orientation will I receive? How long is it?

- What holidays am I scheduled to work?

- What type of benefits are offered with this position? (Health, dental, retirement, holiday time, sick time, continuing education opportunities, educational reimbursement)

- May I have a copy of the job description and performance appraisal form? When will I be evaluated?

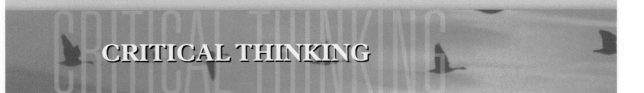

CRITICAL THINKING

Robert Mondiani is interviewing for a night staff nurse position, and the manager notices that he has held three jobs as a staff nurse in 7 years. She asks him why he left his jobs. Robert does not always agree with his managers' rotating schedules because they assume he can work the rotations since he is single and does not have any children. They frequently assign him to more than his share of rotating shifts because the majority of Robert's coworkers are married and have children. Robert has other obligations that he needs time for, including taking care of an ailing father.

How should Robert respond to the nurse manager when she asks about his job turnover? Is this critical information for the manager? Should Robert say anything about his sick father? What should he say?

apart from other potential employees as someone who is professional and sincerely interested in joining the organization. Include in the letter your availability either for an additional future interview or employment. Figure 26-6 illustrates a thank you letter as a follow-up to an interview.

Caitlin O'Malley
2424 Sailing Avenue
Cherry Hill, NJ 08080
(609) 444-2212

April 26, 2002

Ms. Vanetha Raj, BSN, RN
Nurse Recruiter
Shore Memorial Hospital
100 Seashore Drive
Point Pleasant, NJ 07726

Dear Ms. Raj:

    Thank you for the time you spent with me as I interviewed for a position as a registered nurse at Shore Memorial Hospital. I enjoyed meeting the pediatric nurse manager and several of the staff nurses yesterday and was especially impressed with the sense of professionalism among the staff.

    I have requested that my transcripts be sent directly to your office and I will have three of my instructors complete the reference forms you gave me. I look forward to hearing from you soon about my second interview and will contact you in two weeks as directed.

                                      Sincerely,

                                        Caitlin O'Malley

Figure 26-6 Follow-Up to Interview Letter

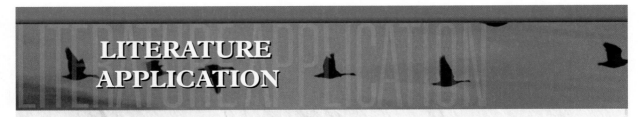

LITERATURE APPLICATION

Citation: Happell, B. (2000). Student interest in perioperative nursing as a career. *AORN Journal, 71,* 600–605.

Discussion: Perioperative nursing is a field in which students receive little or no clinical experience while enrolled in school because of curricula that are loaded with other subjects; the result is that students do not have exposure to perioperative nursing. It is hypothesized that many students choose a first job opportunity based on experiences while in school, with many nursing students not choosing the perioperative specialty as a first or second career because of nonexposure. Happell's article discusses students' career preferences both prior to and after school. With the decline of available perioperative nurses, the author suggests that including a perioperative clinical experience during school may increase the number of new graduates choosing to work in this field.

Implications for Practice: Selection of clinical experience sites often affects new graduates' choice of work experience. Faculty should choose clinical experience sites carefully.

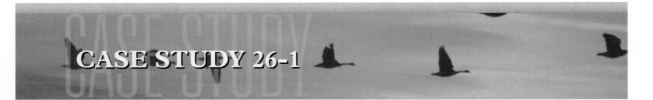

CASE STUDY 26-1

Maria Diaz is a senior nursing student working as a patient care assistant on an oncology floor in a small community hospital. Maria is well liked by the staff of the floor and is offered a full-time registered nurse position upon graduation. While Maria is flattered and relieved that she has an offer, she feels that she should at least interview at another local hospital for comparison. She thinks she may know someone who is employed at another facility in town.

How would Maria begin her job search? What are the key elements to securing an interview at the other hospital? Once Maria has an interview, what type of questions should she be prepared to answer from the interviewer? What type of questions should Maria be prepared to ask?

RESIGNING FROM A CURRENT POSITION

If you are currently employed, you may have to offer your resignation once you have secured a position in a new agency. Regardless of your feelings about your current position, a resignation letter should never leave a bad impression on the reader. After all, you may need a reference from your employer in the future and you should always keep that fact in mind when tendering a resignation. Figure 26-7 is an example of a resignation letter.

Michael Dodson, BSN, RN
1268 Starboard Drive
Williamsburg, VA 22306

October 15, 2002

Abigail Hess, MSN, RN
Administrator, 6 West Surgical
University Medical Center
1 University Avenue
Williamsburg, VA 22306

Dear Ms. Hess:

It is with regret that I offer my resignation as a staff nurse on 6 West Surgical, effective November 15, 2002. I have taken a new position as the nurse manager of the Telemetry Unit at the Veteran's Hospital.

I have very much enjoyed my three years as a staff nurse on 6 West Surgical. I feel that there were numerous opportunities to learn and expand my nursing knowledge as well as to work with supportive physicians and staff members.

Thank you very much for the privilege of working with you and a truly dedicated nursing staff.

Sincerely,

Michael Dodson, BSN, RN
Staff Nurse

Figure 26-7 Letter of Resignation

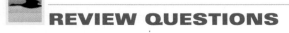

KEY CONCEPTS

- The critical first step in a successful job search is determining what clinical area you are interested in and what skills you have that may fit with that particular area.
- Newspapers, electronic media and the Internet, job fairs, employment hot lines, human resources departments, and networking are all possible avenues for job opportunities.
- An effective resume will (1) get the employer's interest; (2) identify critical areas such as education, work experience, and special qualifications; (3) be tailored to the employer's needs; (4) create a favorable first impression about you and your abilities; (5) communicate that you are someone who is a good fit for the position; and (6) be visually appealing.
- The purpose of a cover letter is to entice the prospective employer to become interested enough to read the resume.
- In dressing for an interview, it is best to dress professionally and conservatively rather than in a trendy or casual manner.
- When preparing for an interview, practice answering potential interview questions with a colleague, friend, or family member before the actual interview so that you have practiced answers to difficult questions.
- In addition to asking questions about shifts and rotation schedules, it is important to ask questions about other aspects of your prospective job, such as the benefit package, educational opportunities, orientation and preceptorship, and evaluation practices.

KEY TERMS

networking   resume

REVIEW QUESTIONS

1. Which of the following is the best response to the interview question "What are your strengths?"

A. "I have many. Where do you want me to begin?"
B. "I have strong communication skills, both written and verbal, and I am someone who values completing a task."
C. "I think I am well liked and get along with everyone."
D. "Well, I am just a new nurse without many strengths right now, but I will be learning with this new job."

2. Which of the following components are absolutely necessary to include in a resume?
A. Identifying information, career objective, employment experiences, education, and professional organizations
B. Identifying information, employment experiences, education, professional organizations, and awards and honors
C. Identifying information, employment experiences, education, professional organizations, and references
D. Identifying information, employment experiences, education, and professional organizations.

3. When creating an electronic resume, which of the following is essential?
A. Setting margins so that 7 inches of text are displayed in a word processing program
B. Using a type font in 12 point, such as Courier 12 or Times New Roman 12
C. Saving the resume using the right justification format
D. Using the bold and underline function in the resume as a way of highlighting information

4. What is the primary function of a cover letter?
A. To entice the prospective employer to become interested enough to read the resume
B. To have a letter to include with your resume
C. To include references that are not listed on a resume
D. To reiterate all that is on your resume

REVIEW ACTIVITIES

1. You are graduating in 2 months from a BSN program. Develop a resume using the chronological format found in Figure 26-1. Develop a resume using the functional format found in Figure 26-2.

2. While looking on a web site for a hospital out of state, you notice that you can submit a resume electronically for a job position that you are interested in applying for. What are the differences between an electronic resume and a traditional paper resume? Develop an electronic resume using the suggestions found in Table 26-4.

3. You are a nurse who has been asked to interview for a new position as team leader of the orthopedic floor. Develop a cover letter expressing interest in the position. Develop a listing of appropriate interview questions for the nurse manager of the floor.

4. Review the *AJN Career Guide, January 2001,* How to Interview on Your Terms, pp. 16–18 (Russo, 2001). How can this guide help prepare you for interviewing for a nursing position?

EXPLORING THE WEB

- Review this reference from the U.S. Department of Labor, which maintains occupational statistics: *http://stats.hls.gov/oco/ocos083.htm*
- Review these generalized web sites for nursing issues:
  http://www.nursingworld.org
  http://www.nursingcenter.com
  http://nursing.net
  http://www.nurseweek.com
  http://www.medzilla.com
  http://www.medsearch.com
- Review these good examples of letters of application in a variety of situations: *http://www.career.vt.edu/JOBSEARC/coversamples.htm*

REFERENCES

Hadley, J., & Sheldon, B. (1995). *The smart woman's guide to networking.* Philadelphia: Chelsea House.

Happell, B. (2000). Student interest in perioperative nursing as a career. *AORN Journal, 71,* 600–605.

Hauter, J. (1997). *The smart woman's guide to career success.* Philadelphia: Chelsea House.

Russo, E. (2001). *How to interview on your own terms.* AJN career guide, 2001 (pp. 16–18). Philadelphia: Lippincott.

Smith, R. (1999). *Electronic resumes and online networking.* Franklin Lakes, NJ: Career Press.

SUGGESTED READINGS

Bozell, J. (1999*). Anatomy of a job search—a nurse's guide to finding and landing the job you want.* Philadelphia: Springhouse.

DeLuca, M. J., & DeLuca, N. F. (1997). *Wow! Resumes for creative careers.* New York: McGraw-Hill.

Kennedy, J. L. (1999). *Resumes for dummies.* Foster City, CA: IDG Books Worldwide.

Lore, N. (1998). *The Pathfinder.* New York: Simon & Schuster.

Potter, R. (1998). *100 best resumes for today's hottest jobs.* New York: Macmillan.

Sussman, D. (2000). Roads less traveled. Retrieved February 2, 2002, from http://www.nurseweek.com/news/features/00-07/path.html

Weinberg, J. (1996). Your references: Important allies in your job campaign. *South Carolina Nurse, 3*(2), 15.

Weinberg, J. (1997). Mail vs. telephone—How should you initiate contact with your targeted employers? *South Carolina Nurse, 4*(1), 9–10.

Welton, R. H., & Morton, P. G. (1995). Strategies for writing an effective resume. *Critical Care Nurse, 15*(3), 118–126.

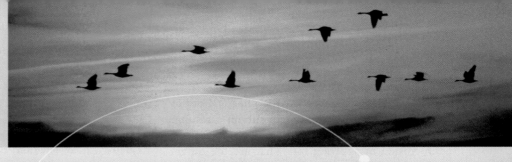

CHAPTER 27

Emerging Opportunities

Stephen Jones, MS, RNC, PNP, ET

OBJECTIVES

Upon completion of this chapter, the reader should be able to:

1. Discuss the many nursing opportunities available upon graduation.
2. Discuss advanced nursing practice and other nontraditional nursing roles.
3. Identify various opportunities for certification.
4. Review hospital- and nonhospital-based nursing practice.
5. Identify directions for the future of nursing.

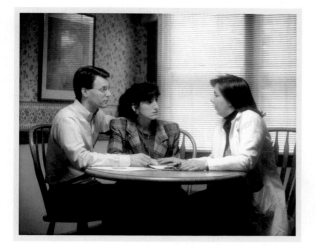

You are within 4 months of graduation. Your thoughts are focused on moving to a nice city and getting a good job in a health care setting that will stimulate and educate you. You also know individuals who have been nurses for a while. They are doing seemingly incredible activities and interventions. Many are able to write prescriptions, and some even have flexible hours. There are numerous questions the graduating nurse needs to consider:

Where do you see yourself 1 year, 5 years, and 10 years from now?

What are your real life situations and circumstances regarding family, ability to relocate, hours to work?

Do you have financial constraints?

What are your strengths and weaknesses?

Health care facilities have been experiencing nursing shortages since the mid-1980s. In the early 1990s, there was a temporary ease in the nursing shortage. This easing, however, was short-lived; at the turn of the 21st century, the nursing demand far exceeded the supply of registered professional nurses. Nurses, who comprise the largest group of health care professionals in America, determine the quality of health care (Chiara, 1993). Nurses apply their holistic knowledge to help individuals manage the changes brought on by illness or disease, educate them about preventive health care, and, in general, attempt to improve the quality of health care. Many factors have caused the nursing shortages over the past 25 years, especially since the mid-1980s. In particular, the number of chronically ill and frail elderly patients has increased, and the demand for nurses who can care for them far exceeds

the supply. In addition, the various restructuring efforts in our nation's health care system have made nursing jobs less attractive. The nursing shortage that started in the mid-1990s and carried over to the new millennium is expected to not only continue but worsen by the year 2020. This shortage is different from those of the past in several ways. Factors contributing to the most recent shortage include an aging nursing population, a declining number of nursing students in the academic pipeline, and the need for more accommodating working conditions for nurses. Statistical data show the following (National League for Nursing, 2001):

- Average age of nurses: 43.4 years
- Average associate professor's age: 52.0 years
- Steady decline in enrollment in nursing education programs from 1995 to 1999 and a 13.6% decline in graduates
- 32% of nursing graduates were BS prepared and 10% were MS prepared in 1999
- Steady decline in the number of NCLEX-RN exams taken from 1994 to 1999

Throughout its history, nursing has always responded to changes in society's health care needs. From the days of Florence Nightingale and her service in the mid-1800s to Lillian Wald and public health nursing in the early 1900s, to Martha Rogers in the 1930s and 1940s suggesting that nurses prepare themselves to handle the health issues that arise from space travel, nursing has met society's changing health care needs by expanding the roles of nurses. For decades, nurses in acute care settings have been taking on advanced and expanded roles on evening, night, and weekend shifts.

Many of the changes in nursing have evolved naturally and logically. Positions such as staff nurse, nurse manager, director of nursing, and case manager and organizations such as visiting nurse associations and public health organizations are a direct reflection of these evolutions. Nursing has established itself in hospitals, ambulatory clinics, physicians' offices, and community and school settings. An issue confronting nurses, however, has been identifying what a nurse really is, because many levels of educational preparation exist. In December 1965, the American Nurses Association (ANA) House of Delegates (HOD) adopted a motion that the ANA continue to work toward baccalaureate education as the educational foundation for professional nursing practice. By 1985, the ANA House of Delegates agreed to urge state nursing associations to establish the BS degree with a major in nursing as the minimum educational requirement for licensure and to retain the title of registered nurse (American Nurses Association [ANA], 2000). To date, there are still a variety of paths an individual can take to become a registered nurse. These include a 2-year associate degree, a 3-year diploma, and a 4-year baccalaureate degree. In deciding which education option to pursue, students should consider their future, that is, where they want to be in 5 to 10 years. If advanced

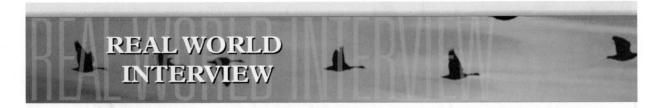

REAL WORLD INTERVIEW

What a difference a year makes! It is hard to believe a year has gone by since I graduated, but it also seems like an eternity. I remember the anxiety of taking the NCLEX, applying for jobs, and starting orientation as a new grad. Since that time, I have grown tremendously as a nurse. I remember feeling nervous about my newfound independence, but facing and overcoming the challenges has helped me gain confidence. Juggling a full assignment as a staff nurse, I am learning to prioritize and organize like never before. Through this transition process from student nurse to RN, I continue to grow each day. There are so many different opportunities as I look to the future. I do not know where my career will be in 5 or 10 years, but I am excited to explore the possibilities.

Danielle Shippey, RN, BSN

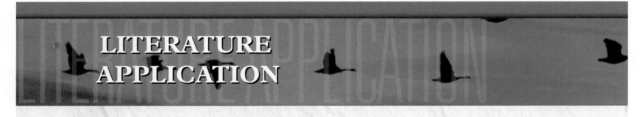

LITERATURE APPLICATION

Citation: Maurer, M. C. (1994). *An identification of factors influencing pre-professional socialization of aspirants to the nursing profession.* Unpublished doctoral thesis, Loyola University of Chicago.

Discussion: Health care facilities have been in the throes of a nursing shortage since the mid-1980s. There are many studies that examine nurse retention but few that address specifically what motivates individuals to choose nursing as a career. This study sought to understand why women and men were choosing to enter nursing. Using a qualitative methodology of in-depth, nonstructured interviews, 22 prenursing students were interviewed. Their responses were categorized under two primary themes: career attractors and career facilitators. The study showed that in nursing, altruism and self-fulfillment were the key career attractors and motivators.

Implications for Practice: Individuals are attracted to a career in nursing because of their altruism and desire for self-fulfillment. A secondary finding was identification of the importance of role models (career facilitators) and the importance of observing practicing nurses in action as major influences to enter the profession.

practice is a desired goal, then a baccalaureate education is the required first step toward that goal.

A major advancement within nursing has been the emergence of several areas of advanced nursing practice: the certified registered nurse anesthetist (CRNA), the clinical nurse specialist (CNS), the nurse practitioner (NP), and the certified nurse-midwife (CNM). Nurses within these roles assume expanded functions and additional responsibilities, often crossing over into what had been viewed as the role of medicine. The 20th century was a unique time in nursing's history; the profession struggled to assume its rightful role in the health care arena with its members performing traditional nursing roles, yet it significantly upgraded its educational, clinical, research, and managerial focus. This chapter will examine emerging opportunities for both new graduates who would prefer not to assume advanced or expanded nursing roles and those who are contemplating advanced or expanded roles.

EMERGING OPPORTUNITIES

Within the traditional hospital setting, the levels of nursing hierarchy are established: vice president/director of nursing, managers, and staff nurses. This hierarchy allows for promotion and advancement. Since the mid-1980s, the trend has been to flatten the levels of nursing management, that is, have fewer managers and additional clinical bedside nurses.

Certification

A process of certification through various organizations and agencies exists for nurses. Certification is the process by which a nongovernmental agency or association certifies that an individual licensed to practice a profession has met certain predetermined standards specified by that profession for practice (Table 27-1). The process of certification allows nurses to demonstrate a specific educational or clinical expertise for their patient population. Many certifications last up to 5 years and the nurse may recertify by either retesting or completing the needed number of continuing education contact hours. Many different organizations issue certification credentials for nursing. See the *American Journal of Nursing Career Guide 2001* for a listing of more than 80 certifications available to nurses ("Your Guide to Certification," 2001).

Traveling Nurse

As the demand for nursing has increased, the supply has often been very low, and hospitals are frequently understaffed. One option to fill the nursing shortage is the traveling nurse. These nurses usually work in 3-month assignments on the same unit. They travel to various locations throughout the United States. The financial charge by the traveling nurse company to the employing hospital for a traveler is usually very high, often greater than $50 per hour. The traveling nurse's salary may be similar to that of her fellow employees or higher.

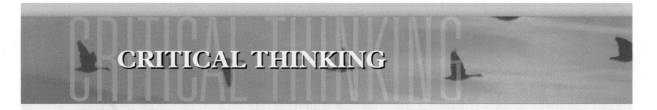

CRITICAL THINKING

Many nurses are certified in their area of specialty. You are thinking about taking the certification examination but are not sure you really want to spend the time required to prepare for it. Some reflections on what certification might do for you are useful:

What is the reason you want to take this examination? Will becoming certified make a difference in your job? Will becoming certified allow you to further progress in your position? Is certification required for licensure?

TABLE 27-1	*Nursing Certification*	
Certification examples	ACLS	advanced cardiac life support
	BLS	basic life support
	CEN	certified emergency nurse
	CCRN	critical care registered nurse
	NRP	neonatal resuscitation program
	PALS	pediatric advanced life support
Selected certifying organizations	AANA	American Association of Nurse Anesthetists
	ACCN	Association of Critical Care Nurses
	ANCC	American Nurses Credentialing Center
	AWHONN	Association of Women's Health, Obstetric, and Neonatal Nurses
	NANN	National Association of Neonatal Nurses
	NAPNAP	National Association of Pediatric Nurse Associates and Practitioners
	WOCN	Wound, Ostomy, and Continence Nurses Society
Examples of specializations	Community health nurse	
	Informatics nurse	
	Inpatient obstetric nurse	
	Medical-surgical nurse	
	Nursing administration	
	Nursing case management	
	Pediatric nurse	
	Perinatal nurse	
	Psychiatric and mental health nurse	

The benefits to the health care institution of using traveling nurses include having a nurse with a variety of experiences providing continuity of care for a 3-month period. These traveling nurses often need only the basic hospital and unit orientation because they come with skills applicable to their area of practice ("Travel Nursing Spotlight," 1999). Traveling nurses need to be aware of differing nursing methodologies and licensure requirements from state to state and will require a license for each state in which they practice. Traveling nurses should also ensure that

their contract stipulates clearly what their assignment is and what the institution and agency expect of them. Most travelers exhibit flexibility, adaptability, assertiveness, strong organizational and interpersonal skills, confidence, independence, and the ability to learn new skills and techniques (Penny, 1997).

If traveling is in your blood, adventure also lies outside of the United States, as many foreign countries actively recruit American nurses, especially Middle East countries such as Saudi Arabia and Kuwait. This is an opportunity to see other areas of the world, work with different cultures, and learn other interventions. Many of the traveling nurse companies advertise in nursing journals as well as over the Internet. The *American Journal of Nursing Career Guide 2001* discusses international nursing and includes international nursing employment contacts.

Medical Sales/ Pharmaceutical Representatives

Some nurses have left clinical staff nursing and have become representatives for companies that work in conjunction with traditional health care institutions. These include companies involved in pharmaceutical sales, durable medical equipment, home care, and insurance coverage, as well as health maintenance organizations (HMOs). These opportunities afford the nurse a perspective into corporate America and the workings of the world of business. There are frequently many salary enhancements, or perks, given with these positions, including having a company car, going on business trips and attending meetings, participating in profit-sharing and stock option plans, and meeting a variety of health care personnel. It can

be difficult, however, especially with pharmaceutical sales, to meet sales quotas, provide for your customers, and survive the ups and downs of the business world.

Registered nurses are usually seen as desirable employees for these types of positions because of their knowledge of pharmacology, technology, and health care systems. They understand how items are supposed to work yet are excellent problem solvers when events are not going well.

Case Manager

Aliotta defined case management as a "collaborative process which assesses, plans, implements and evaluates options and services to meet individual health needs along the continuum of care through communication and the use of available resources to promote quality cost effective outcomes" (Dickerson, Peters, Walkowiak, & Brewer, 1999, p. 52). The case manager position was created to help hospitals meet demands to deliver care at lower costs (Nolan, Harris, Kufta, Opfer, & Turner, 1998). The nurse case manager should have expert clinical skills and knowledge of the health care system, health care finances,

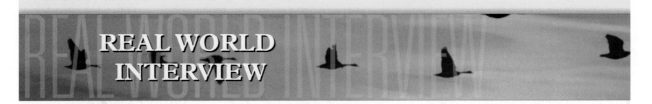

REAL WORLD INTERVIEW

After receiving my BSN in nursing and passing the NCLEX, I entered the field of nursing in 1998. My career started on a busy pediatric unit filled with an assortment of medical and surgical patients. As my clinical nursing skills greatly improved, I became interested in participating in many of the unit's committees, such as the quality improvement team. This introduced me to the field of case management. As a pediatric case manager, I work with the quality improvement teams to increase patient care quality. Through collaborating with health care teams, we hope to improve care across the continuum. As a case manager, I advocate for the patient to ensure that appropriate nursing and medical interventions are implemented in a timely manner. A case manager also functions as a resource to families, patients, and staff in facilitating education and assisting with the utilization of community resources. Finally, I screen all pediatric patients for appropriateness of admission and length of stay. By doing so, I identify cases that potentially may not be covered by insurance and work to utilize resources to promote the patient's best outcome.

Jennifer Rivera, BSN, RN
Case Manager

and legal issues, as well as be an effective communicator (Strassner, 1996). Within the case management model, the nurse case manager will utilize various tools, such as practice guidelines, critical pathways, variance analysis, protocols, and outcome measurement tools, to achieve quality and cost-effective outcomes. Nurse case managers must provide care that focuses on outcome achievement and assist in arranging, coordinating, and monitoring patient care services. The goals are essentially twofold: patient-oriented care and system-oriented care (Stahl, 1996). Patient-oriented goals include improving access to health care services, providing services that meet the patient's needs, and facilitating support for informal caregivers. The system-oriented goals include coordinating the service delivery systems so that services are accessed more easily, preventing unnecessary use of services, and containing costs.

Nurse Entrepreneur

Many nurses are leaving the bedside for the world of entrepreneurship in a variety of consultative, educational, or technical areas (Manthey, 1999). With this risk-taking move, these individuals quickly learn that success is based on high-quality work, patient satisfaction, and establishing and building effective relationships.

The concept of entrepreneurship is not a new one. The term is an interpretation of a French word that means "to undertake" (Simpson, 1998). At the start of the 20th century, nurses functioned independently and contracted directly with the patient or family to provide care (Dickerson & Nash, 1999). It was not until the 1930s that nurses moved into the hospital setting and became employees. Following are characteristics of today's nurse entrepreneur (Wilson, 1998; Simpson, 1998):

- Having creativity and independence
- Being responsive to a perceived need or stepping into a void
- Assuming accountability and being your own boss
- Being market focused
- Having good financial foresight
- Having common sense
- Facing the possibility of success or failure
- Taking an opportunity brought about by change

As with any job, there are benefits and drawbacks to becoming a nurse entrepreneur. The benefits include job satisfaction, flexibility in choosing opportunities, and being able to do exactly what you want to do. Some of the downsides of entrepreneurship include tough competition; riding the highs and lows of the market; finding the right product or service to sell; and providing for your own health insurance. It is important to decide what nursing service you want to provide and develop a solid business plan. Expect to use your personal savings to cover initial start-up expenses, and plan to develop marketing strategies to spread the word about your business. Table 27-2 and Table 27-3 provide additional information about establishing a business plan. As Manthey indicated in 1999, "The process of deciding how to package my experience in such a way as to sell it was one of my most important learning experiences as a consultant" (p. 82).

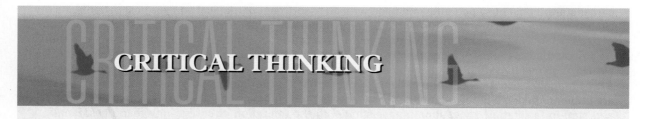

CRITICAL THINKING

You know several individuals who are working as nurse entrepreneurs in some nursing niche in the health care system.

Do you think this is where you want to be in 1 year? In 5 years? In 10 years? Consider what basic nursing experience you should develop now if you want to accomplish this.

TABLE 27-2 Process of Establishing a Business Plan

Nursing Process	Business Process
Assess	• Develop an idea/concept: short term versus long term • Perform a market survey and feasibility study: determine consumer, clientele, location, and business forecast • Identify resources available: financial, technology, and business support
Plan	• Develop market strategies and financial plan based on market survey and feasibility studies • Develop product information: literature, brochures, pamphlets • Develop advertising/public relation methods and material • Schedule appropriate time to deliver product information and services
Implement	• Implement business concepts: direct and indirect methods with follow-up (mailings, telephone, Internet) • Perform services/deliver products or service
Evaluate	• Perform periodic assessment of business plan: monthly, biannually and annually • Identify strengths and weaknesses, and implement changes

TABLE 27-3 Elements of a Business Plan

Resources	• Financial: required capital, personal savings, loans, investors • Technology: computer with encryption capabilities, phone, fax, cell phone, beeper, car, credit card provider • Business Support Services: Better Business Bureau, Chamber of Commerce, personal contacts, accountant/financial planner
Expenses	• Labor: self, employees, benefits, wages • Supplies: office supplies (paper, envelopes, stamps, business cards, and so on), technology (computer, phone, fax, car, telephone, and so on) • Fees: professional services, equipment repair/maintenance, purchased services • General and administrative: utilities, leases/rentals/mortgages, phone services, depreciation, continuing education/tuition, travel, health insurance, post office box
Revenue	• Direct result of services and/or products provided and sold

ADVANCED PRACTICE NURSING

The concept of advanced practice nursing originated in the mid to late 19th century, with the creation of the role of nurse anesthetist. The concept further developed in the 20th century with nurse-midwifery (1925 with the Frontier Nursing Service in rural Kentucky), clinical nurse specialists (1955 at Rutgers University), and finally, nurse practitioners (1965 at University of Colorado with Loretta Ford).

Why is there a need for advanced practice nurses (APNs)? The last quarter of the 20th century taught that detection, prevention, promotion, early intervention, and education are not only cost-effective but also rational. APNs are ideally suited to deliver this type of health care. Many Americans have been disenfranchised from advances in the health sciences, namely the poor, minority groups, the uninsured or underinsured, and individuals suffering from chronic poor health. This segment of our society is especially vulnerable and one that APNs can certainly assist.

According to the American Association of Colleges of Nursing (AACN) task force, "Advanced practice nurses must be master's or doctorally prepared. Critical reflective thinking, self-directed learning, and leadership skills are mandated expectations for health-care providers in the 21st century" (O'Flynn, 1996, p. 432). Advanced practice nursing, therefore, builds on the foundation of professional nursing practice and responds to the health care needs of the country. The future for APNs will be built on their ability to be politically astute and savvy and take an active role in their own destiny, giving evidence of and demonstrating their worth.

This evidence can be provided through research studies as well as through the APN's day-to-day contributions. Are the APN's contributions unique and valuable, and can this be shown to others? Mezey and McGivern (1993, p. 57) provide some examples regarding outcome evaluation:

- Clinical nurse specialist (CNS): In a hospital setting, the CNS must be able to identify how performance contributes to the patient-focused mission and goals of the organization. Does the CNS's practice reduce length of stay, improve patient outcomes, or enhance the efficiency of staff nurses?

- Certified nurse midwife (CNM): The CNM's ability to better meet patient needs, or to provide services to groups of patients at a lower cost than services provided by physicians, should be measureable.
- Nurse practitioner (NP): In an outpatient setting, the NP would need to document both the quantity and quality of services provided to patients and the NP's ability to reduce hospitalization rates.
- Certified registered nurse anesthetist (CRNA): In evaluating anesthesia services in a chronic low back pain clinic, the CRNA would want to clearly document quality of service and patient outcomes.

The remainder of this chapter will examine the current types of expanded roles and advanced practice nursing, looking first at two opportunities that do not require a master's degree: enterostomal therapy and flight nursing.

Wound, Ostomy, Continence Nurse Specialist

The field of enterostomal therapy was initiated in 1958 at the Cleveland Clinic, with the first enterostomal therapists (ETs) being nonnurses. The first nursing training program was started in 1961, and in 1972 new standards for the schools of enterostomal therapy were established. The year 1976 marked a significant change when the governing body of the International Association of Enterostomal Therapists determined that only registered nurses would be admitted to enterostomal therapy educational programs. After this the scope of practice was expanded beyond just caring for ostomies to include skin care, management of draining wounds and fistulas, pressure sores, and incontinence. At this point, the entry requirements into an enterostomal therapy nursing education program (ETNEP) changed to be a bachelor's degree with a major in nursing.

Nurses with this training and education practice both in hospitals and community-based settings such as visiting nurse associations, public health, nursing homes, and long-term care facilities. Over the past 20 years, these specialists have truly become the clinical experts in managing patients with ostomies, alterations in skin integrity, and wounds.

Flight Nursing

In numerous tertiary care centers, nurses are functioning in the role of flight nurse for both helicopter and fixed-wing transports. Over the years, numerous television shows and movies have portrayed these nurses, in their jumpsuits and helmets, landing on the helipad on the top of the hospital. Flight nursing actually started in 1933 with the emergency Flight Corps of the Armed Services and was prevalent in both the Korean and Vietnam wars. The concept of an air ambulance was initiated in Denver in 1972, and today there are more than 230 air programs in the United States (Semonin-Holleran, 1996). One needs numerous advanced technical skills to practice flight nursing, such as patient intubation, EKG interpretation, intravenous (IV) and chest tube insertion, medication administration, sedation, and central line placement. In addition, numerous certifications are required, including pediatric advanced life support (PALS), neonatal resuscitation program (NRP), and advanced cardiac life support (ACLS).

The vast majority of flight teams consist of a registered nurse and a respiratory therapist. While team members follow established health care protocols, they still make many independent decisions regarding crisis intervention. These nurses are truly functioning in an expanded role, providing care to infants, children, and adult patients while performing a variety of therapeutic interventions. Flight nurses also provide education to outlying communities and volunteer in emergency situations.

At this time, there are no true national standards for becoming a flight nurse. Many flight nurses, however, have a baccalaureate degree (BS) and many of the certifications listed previously. Some flight nurses may have additional critical care certifications such as critical care registered nurse (CCRN) or certified emergency nurse (CEN). In addition to the advanced certifications, education, and clinical skills, nurses qualifying for flight nursing need a strong critical care/Emergency Room background, with demonstrated clinical skills in a variety of areas. An extensive training program is also provided. This includes clinical rotations, ambulance and flight observation/ride time, and classroom training. Upon becoming a flight nurse, it is essential that nurses maintain continuing education and certification credits and attend courses offered by agencies such as the U.S. Department of Transportation, the National Flight Nurses Association, and the Emergency Nurses Association.

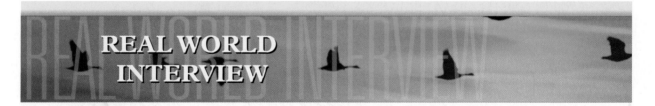

REAL WORLD INTERVIEW

This field of practice has grown tremendously over the past 20 years and provides the individual with a myriad of clinical challenges on a daily basis. The Wound, Ostomy, Continence (WOC) nurse functions in the role of an independent advanced nurse clinician and is uniquely prepared to assume the role of a specialist in three scopes of practice: wounds, ostomy, and continence. In caring for patients with these alterations, the WOC nurse's practice component may include clinical practice, consultation, education, research, and administration. In addition, the WOC nurse can function effectively in a variety of health care settings and is skilled in collaborative practice with the interdisciplinary team that is required for comprehensive patient care management.

Jane Carmel, MA, RN, CWOCN
ETNEP Director

Certified Registered Nurse Anesthetist (CRNA)

The first recorded nurse administering anesthesia was Sister Mary Bernard, a Catholic nun, in 1877. Alice Magaw, however, is considered the mother of anesthesia for her outstanding contributions to the field (Garde, 1996). She was also the first nurse anesthetist to publish articles and perform research on the practice of anesthesia. Between 1909 and 1914, four formal educational programs for nurse anesthetists were established. Currently, there are more than 90 approved programs.

The **certified registered nurse anesthetist** (CRNA) is an advanced practice nurse specialty requiring the graduate to obtain a master's degree. This individual takes care of the patient's anesthesia needs before, during, and after surgery or other procedures alone or in conjunction with other health care professionals. In fact, CRNAs are the sole anesthesia providers for approximately 50% of all hospitals and more than 65% of rural hospitals. CRNAs also provide about 65% of the 26 million anesthetics given yearly (American Association of Nurse Anes-

thetists [AANA], 2000). CRNA programs require a bachelor's of science in nursing as well as at least 1 year of acute care nursing.

Certified Nurse-Midwife (CNM)

Midwifery has existed from the beginning of humankind, and throughout history has played a vital and integral role in a community's growth. In the 1920s, Mary Breckenridge (a British midwife), along with other British midwives, worked with the Frontier Nursing Services in Kentucky to provide services for the rural population. The first American midwifery program was established in 1932, with the curriculum adapted and modified from the British model. In 1955, the American College of Nurse-Midwives (ACNM) was formed, with its main goals focused on setting standards for practice and education.

Currently, there are more than 40 basic nurse-midwifery educational programs, with most offering the master's degree, while some provide a certificate. Since 1980, CNMs have been allowed to practice in

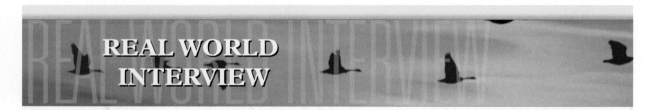

REAL WORLD INTERVIEW

Becoming a flight nurse after being a pediatric intensive care nurse for 7 1/2 years was a huge role change, especially because of the autonomy I now have. I am responsible for performing an assessment on a patient, and then delivering care based on my findings. The care a flight nurse delivers is based on diagnosis-specific standards of care. Many times the patient diagnosis is known, such as when a patient is being transferred from a hospital, but it is the flight nurse's responsibility to ensure that the previous care initiated is still appropriate for this patient. The physical environment is also very different from my previous role. Many of the patients I encounter are located in a very small community hospital with limited resources. When I have a flight mission at an accident scene, the patient may be in an ambulance, trapped in a vehicle, on the ground, or in their house. Once the patient is initially assessed and stabilized, they are moved to the confined and noisy environment of the helicopter. I think that the biggest change from being a staff nurse to a flight nurse is the limited resources available while on a call. Although physician consult is only a radio or phone call away, I am expected to make autonomous clinical decisions in order to save the patient valuable time in receiving lifesaving therapies. At times, I must rely solely on my own experience and that of my partner.

Allison Goodell, BSN, RN, NREMT-P
Flight Nurse

a variety of settings, including hospitals, homes, and birthing centers, providing care for women throughout the childbearing cycle as well as postpartum (Mezey & McGivern, 1993). Nurse-midwives and collaborating physicians agree upon the protocols and procedures. Health education, as well as delivering newborns, comprises a large part of the clinical activities, including the teaching of self-care skills and preparation for childbirth and child rearing. The ANA asserts that the CNM can "provide well woman gynecological and low risk obstetrical care, including prenatal, labor and delivery, and post partum care" (ANA, n.d.).

Clinical Nurse Specialist (CNS)

By the turn of the 20th century, the greatest percentage of APNs were the clinical nurse specialists, whose origins can be traced back to 1938 (Mezey & McGivern, 1993). Reiter first coined the term *nurse clinician* in 1943 to designate a nurse with advanced clinical competence and recommended that such clinicians get their preparation in graduate nursing education programs. Educators first developed the clinical nurse specialist (CNS) role because of their concern for improving nursing care. They believed that improvement was dependent upon increasing expertise at the bedside, giving both direct and indirect care, and incorporating role modeling and consultation (Pinelli, 1997). The CNS role has evolved to include many specialties; the first CNS master's program in psychiatry was started by Peplau in 1955 at Rutgers University.

The impressive development of the psychiatric CNS role helped to initiate the other CNS specialty programs. Following the passage and enactment of the Nurse Training Act in 1965, clinical specialization in graduate education increased tremendously. Graduates would provide a high level of specialized nursing care, as well as serve as change agents in hospital settings.

The CNS is primarily hospital based, practicing in secondary and tertiary care inpatient settings and serving as a consultant in addressing issues in patient care and health care systems (Sperhac & Strodtbeck, 1997). The ANA states that CNSs are registered nurses with advanced nursing degrees, master's degree or doctorate, who are experts in a specialized area of clinical practice" (ANA, 2001A).

A good portion of time is spent in the hospital, in both staff and patient/family education, as well as developing protocols, standards, and pathways that will guide nursing practice. Within the role, the CNS serves as a direct care provider, educator/consultant, researcher, and leader. Their focus can be broad, encompassing adult, pediatric, and obstetric patients, or narrow, including areas such as oncology, the cardiopulmonary system, the pulmonary system, and so on. A study by Wyers, Grove, and Pastorino in 1985 listed essential CNS competencies:

- Developing an in-depth knowledge base
- Demonstrating clinical expertise in a selected area of clinical practice
- Serving as a role model
- Serving as a practitioner/teacher, consultant, researcher

Nurse Practitioner (NP)

The last decade of the 20th century witnessed a large increase in the number of nurse practitioner programs and graduates (Ford, 1997). This was driven in part, perhaps, by the changing health care system, hospital downsizing, an increase in ambulatory care, and constraints on managed care. In addition, the American Medical Association called for a decrease in admissions to medical school. Simultaneously, the federal government practically eliminated the graduate medical education (GME) funds given to hospitals with residency programs. Many of these circumstances are not unlike those that existed when Loretta Ford, a doctorally prepared registered nurse, and Henry Silver, a physician, started the first nurse practitioner training program at the University of Colorado in 1965 (Hoekelman, 1998). A nurse practitioner (NP) is an advanced practice nurse who has education beyond the bachelor's degree in a clinical specialty area strongly focused on primary care, though some subspecialties are hospital based. NPs have received specialized training (most often at the master's level) in diagnosing and treating illnesses and providing health care maintenance. Some of the reasons behind the success of this program included a shortage of health care providers, maldistribution of physicians, and concern over the quality of foreign-trained medical graduates (Wilson, 1994). Within 10 years of Dr. Ford's first NP program, 65 other NP programs were created. The second NP program was started at Duke in 1966, the birthplace of the first physician's assistant program. By 1999, NPs in all

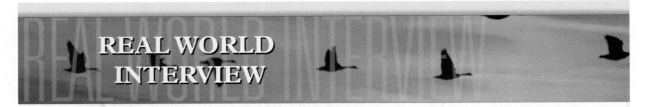

REAL WORLD INTERVIEW

As NPs face the new millennium, it is advisable to listen to the wisdom of the famous author on China, Pearl Buck, who said, "To understand today, you have to search yesterday." Further, to envision the future, think "outside the box" creatively, constructively, and globally. Unfortunately, most people hate change; so do professionals. By their very nature, professionals can become myopic, territorial, and conservative. Some that are so resistant to change become arrogant, self-important, and greedy. Nursing must face the future differently. Tomorrow's practitioners will face globalization, not only of economics but of every field of human endeavor. Demographics, technological advances, transportation, and communication will expand beyond imagination and at lightning speed. Health information will no longer belong exclusively to the health professions. The Internet will see to that. The challenge for NPs is to be proactive rather than reactive in creating a social, cultural, political, and physical environment in which to successfully live, work, and thrive as a responsible member of the new society and as an advocate for our patients and their families. So, thoroughly examine the past, keep the enduring human values of caring, compassion, and courage in nursing, listen to your best teachers—the patients—and create your own future accordingly.

Loretta Ford, EdD, RN, FAAN
Founder, Nurse Practitioner Program

states could be directly reimbursed by Medicare and could write prescriptions (Ventura & Grandinetti, 1999).

Although NPs have become fully integrated into the clinical delivery system, they have often been legally and financially dependent on physicians for their jobs. While some NPs work independently, most states allow NPs to work collaboratively with a physician. This differs from the physician assistant, who works under the direct supervision of the physician. Research data confirm that NPs are competent in delivering primary care that is satisfactory, acceptable to patients, and cost-effective. The keys to the success of the NP role have been the autonomous yet collaborative nature of the practice; accountability as a direct provider of health care services; emphasis on clinical decision making as a foundational clinical skill; the focus on health and healthy lifestyles as a foundation of practice; and the cost-effective, accessible nature of the practice. These basic attributes of NP practice hold true regardless of setting or specialty focus (Ford, 1997).

While many NPs have practiced in primary nonhospital, non-acute care settings, the neonatal nurse practitioner (NNP) has been hospital based for many years. Recently, a new role, the acute care nurse practitioner (ACNP), has been created. These positions also have a collaborative rather than subordinate relationship with physicians (Geier, 1999). As with all NPs, the ACNP is blending nursing and medicine by taking a holistic patient management approach while using collaborative treatment protocols frequently involving procedures previously done only by physicians, such as lumbar punctures, chest tube insertion, writing medication prescriptions, and so on.

While the performance of such roles bodes well for nursing in general and NPs specifically, there is also some discussion about NPs taking on too much within the health care system; the concern is that "if nurses take on an increasing amount of technical and medical work, then characteristics highly valued in the profession may be threatened, . . . for example, skill in caring and communication and in providing a holistic approach to patients treatments" (Dowling, Barrett, & West, 1995, p. 311). It is clear that while NPs provide autonomous practice and competent patient management, they also must protect their holistic, caring nursing role (Geier, 1999).

Clinical Nurse Specialist/Nurse Practitioner (CNS/NP): A Combined Role

Since the mid-1980s, there has been frequent discussion about merging the CNS and NP roles. There are many studies supporting this change as well as opposing it (Cronenwett, 1995; Pinelli, 1997; Sperhac & Strodtbeck, 1997). In 1990, the ANA Council of Clinical Nurse Specialists and the Council of Primary Health Care Nurse Practitioners merged, which sent a powerful message regarding these two national professional's organizations' position on the

issue. Despite this, at the end of the 20th century, while there are some dual-role educational programs and individuals functioning as both a CNS and NP, many education programs and clinical practice areas are separate. Following are some factors to consider when examining these two roles (Pinelli, 1997):

- Different patient populations covered by CNS and NP
- Possible future role for CNS and NP
- Narrower perspective and focus for the NP
- "Horizontal violence" within nursing—nurses fighting among themselves

There are both advantages and disadvantages to merging the roles (Table 27-4). Some predict that

TABLE 27-4	CNS/NP Merger: Advantages and Disadvantages

Advantages	Disadvantages
• Many similarities: education, clinical settings	• Different scopes of practice: CNS is primarily in tertiary care, NP primarily in ambulatory and primary care
• Expanding and overlapping practice settings	
• Increased power in numbers	• Legal issue of trying to include CNS in existing advanced practice legislation
• Cost savings to universities and education programs	
• Increased marketability	• Increased length of graduate education program
	• Continued blurring and role confusion

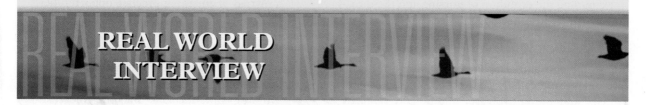

REAL WORLD INTERVIEW

Currently, I am functioning as a CNS/NP. When I made the decision to go on to graduate school in order to become an advanced practice nurse, I carefully examined many different schools of nursing and came to the decision that if I wanted to be a nurse practitioner, then I should go to the school where it all started. For me, that was the University of Rochester, where Dr. Loretta Ford had moved in the mid-1970s. The knowledge and skills I obtained throughout my graduate education, including clinical rotations, course work, and finally master's thesis, were supportive of where I wanted to be in a few years, as I combined the two roles both educationally and clinically. I have also had the wonderful opportunity to practice what I preach in the pediatric clinical setting where I have been working since the early 1980s.

Stephen Jones, MS, RNC, PNP, ET

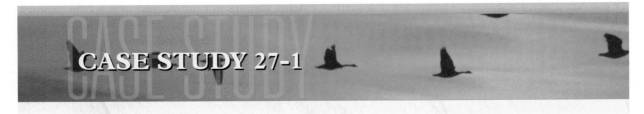

CASE STUDY

CASE STUDY 27-1

It is March of your senior year at college. You have been offered a position as a staff nurse at a hospital where you really wanted to work. For the past several weeks during your last clinical rotation, however, you have had the opportunity to work with an advanced practice nurse. You start to think that perhaps this is what you would like to do, and you know of a few colleges that will take graduates right into their master's program.

Is this something you could do? Should do?

In coming to an answer, consider the following:

- Have the clinical rotations you had as a student prepared you for an advanced practice role?
- What resources are available to you that would provide information in guiding your decision?
- Would spending time working as a staff nurse better prepare you to be an advanced practice nurse?

eventually the two roles will merge as a result of supply and marketplace demands. Additional educational programs for each, however, could still be available for clinical nurse specialists not desiring to spend the majority of their time in clinical practice, such as CNS/consultant, CNS/educator.

DIRECTION FOR THE FUTURE

In examining the evolution of nursing and the direction in which it is heading, the ANA believes that more effective utilization of registered nurses to provide primary health care services is part of the solution to the cost and accessibility problems in health care today. Studies have shown that 60% to 80% of primary and preventive care, traditionally done by doctors, can be done by a nurse for less money (Mezey & McGivern, 1993, p. 604).

The 21st century holds a great deal of promise, but there are many questions to be answered regarding the cost, accessibility, and quality of the health care system in the United States. Nursing has a wonderful opportunity to be a leader in the changing health care delivery system. Few other professions provide as many options. There is a world of emerging opportunities as you prepare to enter the workforce. Take your time, research the possibilities, organize your plan, and live your dream. As Sophia Palmer said in 1897 at the first convention of the American Society of Superintendents of Training Schools for Nursing, "Organization is the power of the day. Without it, nothing great is accomplished" (ANA, 2001B).

KEY CONCEPTS

- Nursing is one of the few professions possessing a myriad of emerging practice opportunities.
- Certification is a process readily available to any registered nurse.
- Case management is a growing subspecialty within the hospital setting, with case managers increasingly in demand.
- Nursing practice has become increasingly specialized.
- There are numerous types of advanced practice nurses (APNs), within both the hospital and community settings. Some examples of these roles include the CNS, NP, CNS/NP, CRNA, and CNM.
- Expanded role opportunities include the WOC nurse and the flight nurse.
- While the CNS is primarily hospital based, NPs practice both in hospitals and community-based settings.

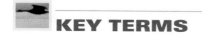

KEY TERMS

certification
certified registered
  nurse anesthetist

clinical nurse specialist
nurse practitioner

REVIEW QUESTIONS

1. The process of certification allows the registered nurse to
   A. demonstrate clinical expertise.
   B. demonstrate educational expertise.
   C. demonstrate clinical and/or educational expertise.
   D. demonstrate advanced nursing degrees.

2. The hospital-based case manager's primary focus is
   A. providing care and services that focus on outcome.
   B. making sure all the patient's expenses are taken care of.
   C. guiding medical and nursing protocols.
   D. ensuring that each patient has a primary nurse.

3. To be a successful nurse entrepreneur, it is imperative that the individual
   A. be able to attain a sizable loan from a bank to help with start-up costs.
   B. attain credit card approval.
   C. understand how the stock market functions.
   D. develop a solid business plan.

4. Which of the following is the best method of determining the effectiveness of an APN's practice?
   A. Patient satisfaction guide.
   B. Fewer hospital admissions
   C. Improved patient outcomes
   D. Number of research studies

5. APNs provide both nursing and health care services. APNs can best fulfill this mission by
   A. performing and then publishing research.
   B. building on the foundation of professional nursing and responding to patients' health care needs.
   C. maintaining as many certifications as possible.
   D. managing patients in both the hospital and outpatient settings.

REVIEW ACTIVITIES

1. Finally, you have graduated and moved to the city of your choice and are working at the health care facility of your choice. You are starting to apply all the knowledge and skills that you gained at school. You are around all levels and types of mentors and role models and are witnessing firsthand the activities of new and experienced staff nurses, as well as those of advanced practice nurses.

   What are some of your initial thoughts on where you will be in 1, 3, 5, or 10 years from now? Discuss how you will determine your progress.

2. Review the salary survey in the March 2001 issue of *Nursing 2001*, pp. 44–47. How will the information help you plan your future goals?

3. Review the salary survey in the July 30, 2001, issue of *Modern Healthcare*, p. 27. Notice how various health care executives are compensated. How will this information help you plan your future goals?

4. Review the Guide to Certification in the *American Journal of Nursing Career Guide 2001*, p. 40. How will this information help you plan your future goals?

5. Review the article on international nursing in the *American Journal of Nursing Career Guide 2001*, p. 12. How will this information help you plan your future goals?

EXPLORING THE WEB

Which sites should you visit regularly, both for your own personal and professional growth?

General Interest and Nursing Issues:

- Centers for Disease Control
  http://www.cdc.gov
- National Institutes of Health
  http://www.nih.gov
- National League for Nursing
  http://www.nln.org
- American Nurses Association (ANA)
  http://www.nursingworld.org
- ANA certification listing
  http://www.nursingworld.org/ANCC/certify/cert/catalogs/index.htm#general

- Center for Nursing
  http://www.nursingcenter.com
- National Council of State Boards of Nursing
  http://www.ncsbn.org
- General nursing interest site
  http://www.allnurses.com
- Health care information
  http://www.medscape.com
  http://www.docguide.com

Specialty Issues:

- American Association of Nurse Anesthetists
  http://www.aana.com/about
- Flight nursing *http://www.flightweb.com*
- Small Business Administration
  http://www.sbaonline.sba.gov
- Service Corps of Retired Executives
  http://www.score.org
- Traveling nurses
  http://www.springnet.com
  http://www.healthcareers-online.com

REFERENCES

American Association of Nurse Anesthetists. (2000). Retrieved March 6, 2000, from www.aana.com/about

American Nurses Association [ANA]. (2000). Press release. Retrieved February 25, 2000, from www.ana.org

American Nurses Association [ANA]. (2001A). Retrieved February 25, 2000, from www.ana.org/readroom/position/index.htm.

American Nurses Association [ANA]. (2001B). Where we come from. Retrieved February 28, 2002, from http://www.nursingworld.org/centenn/index.htm

American Nurses Association [ANA]. (n.d.). Press release. Retrieved February 25, 2000, from www.ana.org/pressrelease

Chiara, M. (1993). *Making a difference: An ethnography of women's career motivations, values and work satisfaction in nursing.* Unpublished doctoral dissertation, Northwestern University, Evanston, IL.

Cronenwett, L. R. (1995). Molding the future of advanced practice nursing. *Nursing Outlook, 43*(3), 112–118.

Dickerson, P. S., & Nash, B. A. (1999). Hospital extra. Nurse entrepreneurs as educators. *American Journal of Nursing, 99*(6), 24A, 24D.

Dickerson, S. S., Peters, D., Walkowiak, J. A., & Brewer, C. (1999). Active learning strategies to teach case management. *Nurse Educator, 24*(5), 52–57.

Dowling, S., Barrett, S., & West, R. (1995). With nurse practitioners, who needs house officers? *British Medical Journal, 311*, 309–313.

Ford, L. C. (1997). Advanced practice nursing. A deviant comes of age . . . the NP in acute care. *Heart & Lung: Journal of Acute & Critical Care, 26*(2), 87–91.

Garde, J. F. (1996). The nurse anesthesia profession: a past, present and future perspective. *Nursing Clinics of North America, 31,* 567–580.

Geier, W. (1999). Caring side-by-side with acute care nurse practitioners. *Nursing Management, 30*(9), 32–34.

Hoeckelman, C. R. (1998). A program to increase health care for children: The pediatric nurse practitioner program by Henry K. Silver, MD, Loretta C. Ford, EdD, and Susan G. Stearly, MS, Pediatrics, 1967, 39: 756–760. *Pediatrics, 102*(1 Pt. 2), 245–247.

Manthey, M. (1999). Financial management for entrepreneurs. *Nursing Administration Quarterly, 23*(4), 81–85.

Maurer, M. C. (1994). *An identification of factors influencing pre-professional socialization of aspirants to the nursing profession.* Unpublished doctoral thesis, Loyola University of Chicago.

Mee, C. L., & Carey, K. W. (2001). Nursing 2001 salary survey. *Nursing2001, 31*(3), 44–47.

Mezey, M., & McGivern, D. (Eds.). (1993). *Nurses, nurse practitioners.* New York: Springer.

National League for Nursing [NLN]. (2001). Press release. Retrieved January 31, 2001, from www.nln.org

Nolan, M. T., Harris, A., Kufta, A., Opfer, N., & Turner, H. (1998). Preparing nurses for the acute care case manager role: Educational needs identified by existing case managers. *Journal of Continuing Education in Nursing, 29*(3), 130–134, 142–143.

O'Flynn, A. (1996). The preparation of advanced practice nurses. *Nursing Clinics of North America, 31*, 429–448.

Penny, J. T. (1997). What a travel nurse company seeks in you . . . Nursing 97 travel nursing guide. *Nursing 1997. 27*(6), 69.

Pinelli, J. M. (1997). The clinical nurse specialist/nurse practitioner: Oxymoron or match made in heaven? *Canadian Journal of Nursing Administration, 10*(1), 85–110.

Semonin-Holleran, R. (1996). Career options. These nurses take flight. *RN, 59*(9), 57, 59–60, 70–71.

Simpson, R. L. (1998). Nursing informatics. From nurse to nursing informatics consultant: A lesson in entrepreneurship. *Nursing Administration Quarterly, 22*(2), 87–90.

Sperhac, A., & Strodtbeck, F. (1997). Advanced practice nursing: New opportunities for blended roles. *American Journal of Maternity and Child Nursing, 22*(6), 287–293.

Stahl, D. (1996). Case management in subacute care. *Nursing Management, 27*(8), 20–22.

Steinhauer, R. G. (2001). International nursing. In *AJN Career Guide 2001—Part 2*, pp. 12–15.

Strassner, L. F. (1996). The ABC's of case management: A review of the basics. *Nursing Case Management, 1*(1), 22–30.

Travel nursing spotlight: Agency alternative. *Nursing99, 29*(6), 78–79.

Ventura, M., & Grandinetti, D. (1999). NP progress report: A survey. *RN, 62*(7), 33–35.

Wilson, C. K. (1998). Mentoring the entrepreneur. *Nursing Administration Quarterly, 22*(2), 1–12.

Wilson, D. (1994). Nurse practitioners: The early years (1965–1974). *Nurse Practitioner, 19*(12), 26, 28, 31.

Wyers, M. E., Grove, S. K., & Pastorino, C. (1985). Clinical nurse specialist: In search of the right role. *Nursing Health Care, 6*(4), 202–207.

Your guide to certification. (2001, January). *American Journal of Nursing Career Guide 2001—Part 2*, 40–49.

SUGGESTED READINGS

Ackerman, M. H. (1997). The acute care nurse practitioner: Evolution of the clinical nurse specialist? *Heart & Lung, 26*(2), 85–86.

Andrews, M., & Wallis, M. (1999). Mentorship in nursing: A literature review. *Journal of Advanced Nursing, 29*(1), 210–217.

Bankert, M. (1989). *Watchful care: A history of America's nurse anesthetists*. New York: The Continuum Publishing Company.

Barmford, O., & Gibson, F. (1999). The clinical nurse specialist role: Criteria for the post, valuing clinical experience and educational preparation. *Advancing Clinical Nursing, 3*(1), 21–26.

Bryan, S. (1996). Flight nursing. *Journal of Emergency Nursing, 22*(6), 491–493.

Carlisle, D. (1996, June 5–11). Crossing the line. Nurse anesthetists. *NursingTimes, 92*(23), 26–27, 29.

Elder, R., & Bullough, B. (1990). Nurse practitioners and clinical nurse specialists: Are the roles merging? *Clinical Nurse Specialist, 4*(2), 78–84.

Ford, L. C. (1995). Nurse practitioners: Myths and misconceptions. *The Pulse, 32*(4), 9–10.

Kersbergen, A. L. (1996). Case management: A rich history of coordinating care to control costs. *Nursing Outlook, 44*(4), 169–172.

Kirchheimer, B. (2001, July 30). Reaping the rewards. *Modern Healthcare*, 27–38.

Knaus, V., Felten, S., Burton, S., Fobes, P., & Davis, K. (1997). The use of nurse practitioners in the acute care setting. *Journal of Nursing Administration, 27*(2), 20–27.

Llewellyn, A. (1995). Case management. *Nursing Spectrum* (Florida ed.), *5*(6), 5.

Manthey, M. (1999). I never saw myself as a change agent. *Reflections, 25*(2), 19–21.

Marion, J. (1999). Change from within. *Reflections, 25*(20), 10–12.

Naughton, M., & Nolan, M. (1998). Developing nursing's future role: A challenge for the millennium. *British Journal of Nursing, 7*, 983–986.

Newell, M. (1998). Transitioning the critical care nurse from ICU to high-tech homecare. *Critical Care Nursing Clinics of North America, 10*, 259–266.

Pearson, L.J. (1999). Annual update of how each state stands on legislative issues affecting advanced practice. *The Nurse Practitioner, 24*(1), 16–82.

Porter-O'Grady, T. (1998). The making of a nurse entrepreneur. *Seminars for Nurse Managers, 6*(1), 34–40.

Schaffner, J. W., Ludwig-Beymer, P., & Wiggins, J. (1995). Utilization of advanced practice nurses in healthcare systems and multispecialty group practice. *Journal of Nursing Administration, 25*(12), 37–43.

Schulmeister, L. (1999). Starting a nursing consultation practice. *Clinical Nurse Specialist, 13*(2), 94–100.

Simms, L., Price, S., & Ervin, N. (2000). *Professional practice of nursing administration* (3rd ed.). Clifton Park, NY: Delmar Learning.

Tahan, H. A. (1998). Case management: A heritage more than a century old. *Nursing Case Management, 3*(2), 55–62.

Taylor, M. A. (1999). The clinic of last resort. *Reflections, 25*(2), 25–30.

Travel nurse spotlight: Travel nurse web sites. (1999). *Nursing99, 29*(6), 80–81.

Trinosky-Lind, P., & Olson, S. (1998). Clinical options. Students in flight nursing. *Nurse Educator, 23*(1), 9–11.

Van Slyck, A. (1999). The stamina to succeed. *Reflections, 25*(2), 13–15.

Young, S. W., & Sowell, R. L. (1997). A case management curricular model: The challenge for nursing education. *Nurse Educator, 22*(5), 13–18.

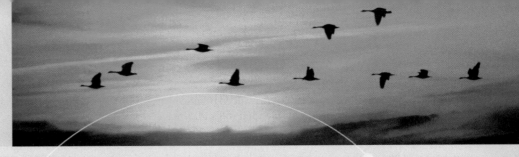

CHAPTER 28

Your First Job

Lyn LaBarre, MS, RN, CEN

Don't try to be popular. Concentrate instead on competence, honesty, and fairness.

(Sharon LaDuke, 2000)

OBJECTIVES

Upon completion of this chapter, the reader should be able to:

1. Identify key elements to consider in choosing a nursing position.
2. Describe typical components of health care orientation.
3. Discuss types of performance feedback.
4. Compare and contrast organizational responses to performance.
5. Discuss specific strategies to enhance the beginning nursing manager role.
6. Identify mechanisms to enhance professional growth.

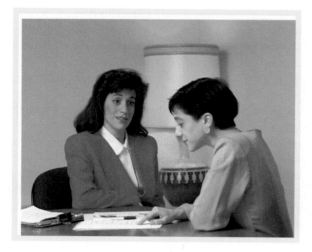

Congratulations! You have just completed your nursing educational requirements, and graduation is 1 week away. You have decided to stay in this geographic area and have received three job offers: a 12-hour night position in the surgical intensive care unit of a regional teaching hospital, a rotating shift 8-hour position on a community hospital's medical-surgical floor, and a public health nursing position with your county's health department.

Which position should you accept?

What factors will help you decide which is the best fit for you?

G raduation brings the transition from the role of student to that of registered nurse. A nurse's first job is an opportunity to solidify skills learned in school. It is also the time to establish relationships with mentors and to set down a foundation for future professional growth. This chapter will discuss important considerations regarding your first job.

CHOOSING A POSITION

In the current job market, new nurses are in the enviable position of having broad choices for their first job. Hospitals now recruit new nurses to specialty areas such as obstetrics, psychiatry, and critical care, as well as to the traditional medical-surgical units. Community health organizations are also anxious to hire recent graduates. The federal government proj-

ects that between the years 2000 and 2006, the need for RNs will grow by 21% ("Staffing Models," 2000). How does a new nurse select the best job?

Patient Types

One of the most important considerations in selecting a job is choosing the best fit for you in a patient care environment. New nurses who start their career on a general medical or surgical unit typically manage patients with a variety of diagnoses. They learn diverse technical and assessment skills. These nurses develop a working knowledge of many common medications and patient teaching scenarios. In contrast, nurses who choose an entry position on a specialty unit focus on patients with specific diseases, body system disorders, or age groups, such as a cardiology, obstetrics, or neonatology patient. Community health nursing positions can be broad spectrum, sharing the characteristics of a medical or surgical nursing role, or being more specialized, for example, a community neonatal nurse.

Work Environment

Another facet to consider in choosing a first position is the opportunity to develop organizational skills. In a critical care or specialty area, nurses need to develop the ability to prioritize and plan care for limited numbers of patients, who need highly specialized assessments and technical care. In contrast, the nurse whose first job is on a general floor must organize care for a diverse and much larger group of patients. A new nurse in the community may work alone for most of the day, seeing patients one at a time. Even though each area requires specific skills, the organizational skills for all these nurses include effective time management.

Another consideration in weighing possible positions is the available schedule. Flexible scheduling is a primary concern for Generation X employees (Cox, 1997). Many health care organizations now offer a variety of schedules. Twelve-hour shifts are particularly popular because a full-time nurse can work as few as three shifts per week. For the patient, this means fewer changes in nursing personnel within a day but less continuity throughout the hospital stay. For the new nurse, a 12-hour shift can be a long work day, but it allows increased flexibility in personal time. Some organizations offer rotations between daytime and other shifts. Others award the more popular day shifts by seniority. When choosing a position, it is important to find out about the process for changing to a different schedule after hiring. Some hospitals restrict new nurses from changing positions for a set period of time. Following are some other questions to ask about your schedule: What will my weekend commitment be? How many holidays will I be expected to work each year? Does the health care organization use a self-scheduling system, in which nurses select their own schedule according to unit guidelines, or is time assigned? If time is assigned, how much notice will be required to have a certain day off?

Pay is an obvious element in choosing your first job, but the best-paying job offer is not necessarily the wisest choice, even from a financial point of view. Health care organizations in the same geographic area tend to offer competitive salaries at the start of employment. It is important to ask about an employer's salary policy. Does the hospital you are considering give a raise once you have passed your NCLEX, or would any potential raise be held until your first-year anniversary? Are nurses paid extra for having a BSN degree? What are the differentials, if any, for weekend work or working off shifts? Be sure that nurses are paid for orientation shifts and required courses. When comparing offers between two health care organizations, ask how many hours are paid for a typical workweek. Some employers pay for a full 8- or 12-hour shift by allowing for a 30-minute overlap at change of shifts. Other organizations do not expect staff nurses to overlap, resulting in a shorter shift. Thus at some facilities, a typical pay week includes 40 hours, while at others nurses routinely work 37.5 hours per week.

Finally, work environments in health care organizations can vary tremendously. Are you more comfortable in a smaller hospital setting in which it is relatively easy to find your way around and everyone knows each other? Or do you prefer the more complex, perhaps less personal setting of a large teaching facility? Do you enjoy working with resident physicians in a teaching hospital, or will you be more satisfied interacting with community-based, private attending physicians?

Orientation Considerations

Different health care organizations also can have very different approaches to new employee orientation and education. Because orientation is a key component of the transition between being a student nurse and becoming a first-time manager of patients, it is important to establish what the organization offers during orientation. Consider the following questions:

- How long should I expect to be in orientation?
- Is it tailored to my learning needs, or is it the same for all incoming nurses?
- Does it all occur at the beginning of my new position, or will it be offered in stages?

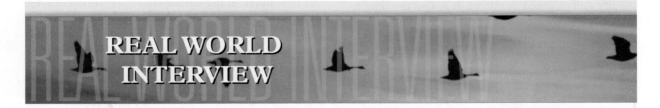

REAL WORLD INTERVIEW

When I graduated from nursing school, I had several choices. The community hospital I had worked in as an LPN while I was in nursing school offered to hire me as an RN. I considered taking that position because I was comfortable at that hospital, and it was close to home. I also interviewed at a large academic teaching hospital 40 miles from my home. I decided to take the position at the large teaching hospital as I felt I would learn more at the academic center, and at this stage in my career, the opportunities made the commute worthwhile.

Ken Simek, RN
Recent Graduate

- What ongoing education will be available to me?
- Will I be paid for time in education programs?
- In case of short staffing, will I be pulled from orientation?

Many new nurses feel pressured to find just the right setting for their first job, particularly if they have a long-term goal of working in a subspecialty. The focus in the first job needs to be on refining assessment and technical skills and learning to be organized in the delivery of nursing care. These skills, coupled with a positive work record regarding attendance, flexibility, and attitude, will ensure the new nurse of many future opportunities.

ORIENTATION TO YOUR NEW JOB

Orientation fosters a smooth transition from graduate to practicing nurse. At its completion, a new nurse should be able to demonstrate competency in the basic skills needed for safe patient care.

General Orientation

Many health care organizations divide nursing orientation into general and unit-specific sections. General orientation includes information and skills measurement, which all nurses new to the facility need, regardless of their eventual unit assignment. Two examples of information discussed at orientation are validation of cardiopulmonary resuscitation competency and an introduction to policies regarding medication administration. General orientation also typically includes explanations of human resource policies and opportunities to hear from representatives of various departments within the organization. Organizational safety skills and procedures are also part of general orientation (Burke, 2000).

Some organizations offer sections of general orientation as written materials or on videotape. This allows a more flexible orientation schedule. It is particularly beneficial for new employees who are available to attend orientation only outside daytime hours. Figure 28-1 is a sample schedule for the first week of general orientation at one medical center.

Most facilities offer general orientation first, followed by unit-specific orientation. In this case, new nurses may not actually spend a shift on their unit for 2 weeks after starting work. Other nurse edu-

cators plan orientation so that nurses go to their home unit very early, reserving some of the general content for later in the orientation schedule. The challenge is to get information to the new employees in an order that makes sense, while still giving them the context provided by spending time in their new work area (Meinecke, 2000).

General orientations are outcome based, requiring the orientee to demonstrate competency, perhaps by written tests or skills measurement (Burke, 2000). Some organizations tailor their general orientation to the individual learners. In this case, an experienced nurse may opt to challenge particular orientation classes by successfully completing the demonstration or written test.

Unit-Specific Orientation

Unit-based orientation, whether it follows the general orientation or is interspersed throughout, focuses on the specific competencies a new nurse needs to care for the diagnoses and ages of patients typical to the assigned unit. These competencies include technical skills as well as beginning mastery of unit-specific processes. Some of the content covered may include topics such as what paperwork is necessary for new admissions and how to get an IV pump for medications.

Most organizations have developed unit-specific competency tools that list those skills orientees need to demonstrate. These lists provide a useful road map with which to plan a learner-specific orientation. Figure 28-2 is an excerpt from an Emergency Department's unit-based orientation tool.

Identifying Your Own Learning Needs

New graduates begin orientation with varied clinical experiences and competencies. Often, beginning nurses are asked to self-rate their level of knowledge or experience with various patient care skills. It is important for new nurses to identify their own learning needs as they become more familiar with their work environment. Orientation is the ideal time for the new nurse to observe coworkers and establish learning priorities. One way to do this is to ask questions of the preceptor or nurse educator. This provides feedback and molds the orientation to the learner's needs.

**RN Orientation Template
Week One**

Monday Perdiems/Weekend Staff attend May 21	Tuesday Perdiems/Weekend attend May 22 **0745 meet in main lobby**	Wednesday Perdiems/Weekend attend May 23	Thursday Perdiems/Weekend attend May 24	Friday May 25
Human Resource/ Safety Education *Remember to sign in on your unit if you want to get paid for the days you attend orientation.	8:00-11:30 Intro/Tour Nursing at AMC Education Opportunities 11:30-12:00 Tina Raggio-Project Learn 12:00-1:00 Lunch 1:00-2:00 Delegation/Assigning *Donna Harat* 2:00-4:30 Modules **some orientees may need to attend the SMS Computer class in the P building from 11:30-2:30-check with Educator**	08:00-11:00 Documentation Standards of Care, protocols, I/O, graphic, Clinical Pathways Unit Day Prep *(ED exempt: modules)* 11:00-11:30 Restraints 11:30-12:00 Back Video Nurse Scheduling 12:00-1:00 Lunch 1:00-4:30 Skills Lab Afternoon Emergency Care and Mock Code (ACLS or PALS exempt and does not apply to NICU), IV/Phlebotomy Skills, Accucheck, PCA Pump	08:00-09:30 Modules 09:30-11:00 Epidemiology *Carolyn Scott* 11:00-11:30 Lunch 11:30-2:30 SMS Computer Class 3:00-4:00 Math Calculation Class (**optional-check with Educator**) 4:00-4:30 Planning for next week/core orientation/orientee assessment forms	07:30-10:30 SMS Computer/P Building-If needed 10:30-12:00 **Independent Activities on Unit of Hire or Modules** 12:00-1:00 Meet with Director **Main 4 Office** **Lunch Provided** 1:00-2:00 Pastoral Care **Room U477** 2:00-4:00 Modules

Required Modules:

Age Specific ☐	IV Therapy ☐	Blood and Blood Products ☐	RN Medication ☐☐	Patient Rights ☐
Peds or Adult Emergency Care☐	Latex Allergy☐	Patient Classification ☐	
Order Transcription (not for ED, PACU)☐	Pain Management☐	Documentation ☐	CPR: (see handout)

Dept of Education- #262-3705

Figure 28-1 Registered Professional Nurse General Orientation Schedule Template—Week One (Courtesy of Albany Medical Center, Albany, NY)

Name	Preceptor	Unit/Dept. Emergency Dept Date:		
At the completion of orientation the RPN will perform technical nursing skills specific to the age and characteristics of the patients served consistent with the Standards of Nursing Practice.				
Self Evaluation Scale 1 2 3	RPN Technical Skill Checklist		Method of Validation/ Code	Date Met/ Initials

	1. Cardiovascular
	  A. Initiate IV therapy
	   1. Adult, non-trauma
	   2. Trauma patient
	   3. Pediatric
	   4. Newborn
	   5. Phlebotomy percutaneous approach
	  B. Blood sampling:
	   1. arterial line,
	   2. blood sampling: port-a-cath
	   3. Triple lumen/ trauma cath/ central line
	  C. Central venous line management: securing/ dressing/ caps/ tubing
	   1. Trauma catheter/ triple lumen
	   2. Implanted device external access (i.e., Hickman)
	   3. PICC line
	   4. Port-a-cath
	  D. Infusion pumps
	   1. IV pumps
	   2. Syringe pumps
	   3. Programmable pediatric pump
	   4. Patient Controlled Analgesia
	  E. Spacelab bedside and Central monitors
	   1. Cardiac rhythm interpretation
	  F. Defibrillator operation
	   1. Zoll
	   2. Physiocontrol 10 and 9
	  G. External transcutaneous pacer–Zoll
	  H. Transvenous pacer pack: Emergent
	  I. Transvenous pacer pack: Urgent
	   1. Pulse generator
	   2. Ushkow's lead
	  J. Blood Products administration
	  K. Level I blood warmer and rapid infuser
	  L. Spun Hct
	  M. Utilization of doppler for vascular assessment			

	2. Gastro-intestinal
	  A. Tubes & Drains
	   1. Salem sump/ Nasogastric tube (age appropriate size)
	    a. Measuring
	    b. cetacaine administration
	    c. securing
	   2. Gastric decontamination/ lavage (Code Blue)			

Figure 28-2 Emergency Department Competency-Based Orientation Tool Sample Page, Excerpt (Courtesy of Albany Medical Center, Albany, NY)

Socialization

Socialization to the new workplace is another important part of orientation. Preceptors can play a key role in introducing the new nurse to coworkers and other members of the health team. The orientee needs to be introduced to the specific functions and roles of those people who interact daily with the nurses on the unit (Marrelli, 1997). This helps the new nurse identify relationships within the unit and between the unit and the larger health care organization. In practice areas where staff are infrequently together, such as a home health agency, socialization can be difficult. Some nurse managers may arrange a luncheon or coffee hour to introduce new staff members to the work group.

Working with Patients

When you begin to work with patients during your orientation, you soon begin to realize that you are a nurse now. Patients expect you to have the answer. This can be a little intimidating at first. The first time you experience an emergency by yourself, it can be unnerving to realize that you are the nurse in charge of your patient. Hopefully your nursing education and hospital orientation have prepared you for this moment. You can instill confidence by keeping your knowledge base up to date and by looking and acting professional. The more experience you have, the easier this will become.

Work to put your patients at ease and demonstrate a sense of caring to them. Work to become a nursing expert in your patient's eyes and relay to the patient that you possess a body of nursing care knowledge. Demonstrate to your patients that they can trust you, and they will want to continue their relationship with you.

Working with Doctors

Sometimes new graduates are intimidated by the doctors they work with. Cardillo (2001) gives several tips on working with doctors. She suggests that it is useful to establish rapport and introduce yourself to the doctors you work with. Do not be intimidated. You and the doctor are both on the health care team to meet the patient's goals. At least one study has indicated that when nurses and doctors work together, patient death rates or readmission rates decrease (Baggs & Ryan, 1990). Both you and the doctor are important to your patient's welfare.

Cardillo (2001) also suggests that nurses be assertive. Do not call a doctor and say, "I'm sorry to bother you." You are not bothering her. That is her job and you are doing your job by calling her. If you do not understand something, ask questions. Many doctors love to teach. Be honest and up front. Tell the doctor if something is new to you.

Show respect and consideration for the doctors you work with but do not be a doormat. Give due respect and expect the same from them. If the doctor is out of line, you might say, "I don't appreciate being spoken to in that way," or "I would appreciate being spoken to in a civil tone of voice and I promise to do the same with you," or something similar.

Finally, Cardillo (2001) suggests that nurses seek clarification from the doctor if an order is unclear. If an order is inappropriate or incorrect, rather than saying, "This order does not seem appropriate for this patient," which would likely put the doctor on the defensive, try, "Teach me something, Dr. Jones; I've never seen a dose of Lopressor that high. Can you explain the therapeutic dynamics to me?" or "Dr. Smith, I can't figure out why you ordered a brain scan on this patient. Can you help me out here?" This approach usually results in the doctor either reevaluating an order or changing it. If the doctor does not change an order that you think is inappropriate, let your supervisor know and follow the guidelines of the agency that you work for regarding what to do when an inappropriate order is given. Remember, diplomacy works wonders, and it is your license on the line.

Learning Styles

Educators have long realized that people learn in different ways, based in part on their previous experiences. At each stage of the learning process, individuals have different learning styles and need different interventions from their preceptors or leaders. There are over 20 different learning styles in the literature. New graduates orienting to the clinical area need a preceptor who gives specific directions. They need details and demonstrations of skills. New nurses benefit if the preceptor or educator breaks tasks down into components so that they can readily see the proper order or priority of items. As nurses become more experienced, they do well with a teaching style that emphasizes collaboration and relates the new material to the learner's frame of reference. Taking a learning style inventory can help bring awareness to the orientation process. It can be difficult to match a teaching style to a learning style.

Preceptors

Ideally, the nurse manager assigns each new orientee to a preceptor who understands the need to match his teaching style to the new nurse's learning needs. In many organizations, the learner follows the preceptor's schedule so that orientation is consistent. A successful preceptor is clinically experienced, enjoys teaching, and is committed to the role. Good preceptors need to be familiar with the organization's policies and procedures and willing to share knowledge with their orientees (Meinecke, 2000). The best preceptors are active and purposeful with their charges (Marquis & Huston, 2000). They model

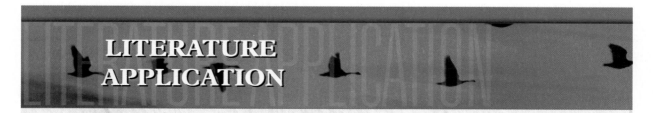

LITERATURE APPLICATION

Citation: McNeese-Smith, D. K. (2000). Job stages of entry, mastery, and disengagement among nurses. *Journal of Nursing Administration, 30*(3), 140–147.

Discussion: Career stages have been conceptualized by a number of researchers. McNeese-Smith surveyed practicing nurses to identify characteristics common to nurses in each stage. The author found that nurses in the entry stage seek to identify with the expectations of their new job. If they receive support from their supervisor and develop realistic goals, they move into the mastery stage. In the mastery level, the focus is on accomplishment and professional growth. At some point while in this stage, nurses begin to perceive themselves as experts.

The third stage, disengagement, begins only if nurses believe their current position no longer offers challenges or growth. The high esteem of the nurse in the mastery phase is replaced by boredom and declining performance. At this point, the nurse usually leaves the position.

Implications for Practice: Nurses move through stages in their professional development. Those who remain actively involved and seek professional growth avoid disengagement.

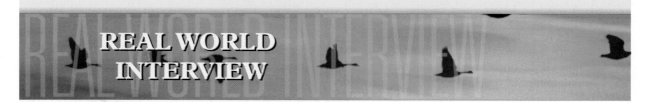

REAL WORLD INTERVIEW

I just finished my unit-based orientation a few weeks ago. Because I'm working in a critical care area, my general orientation included a critical care course, so I wasn't on my unit too much at first. I had two preceptors most of the time—one while I was on the day shift so I could attend classes some days, and the second when I moved to my regular night hours. My preceptors were great—they supported me, taught me new technical skills, and helped me figure out the order to do things. The idea of coming off orientation was scary at first, but I was able to work my schedule so I was on duty the same shifts as my preceptor the first few nights. This gave me the security of knowing I would have a resource available when I needed it.

Jennifer Holscher, RN

behaviors and think out loud in the hearing range of their orientees (Fey & Miltner, 2000).

In some larger organizations, one preceptor is assigned to a group of new nurses. Together, the several orientees work with the preceptor to master core competencies before being assigned to their home unit. For example, several new graduates hired for medical or surgical floors may all be assigned temporarily to one unit, with one preceptor. This has the advantage of providing peer supports to the new nurses and may be more efficient and less expensive than a traditional one-on-one relationship.

In 1974, Kramer described "reality shock" and discussed the difficulties some new graduates have in adjusting to the work environment. Kramer identified a conflict between new graduates' expectations and the reality of their first nursing position. A skilled preceptor can assist new nurses through this transition by offering them opportunities to validate their impressions. The support of other new nurses in a similar situation, such as those participating in the same core orientation, is particularly helpful (Marquis & Huston, 2000).

PERFORMANCE FEEDBACK

"So, how am I doing?" Everyone wants feedback about their performance, particularly when they are in a new position. Some preceptors and managers recognize new employees for their progress, but in many cases, the new nurse needs to solicit their feedback. A concrete mechanism to measure one's own performance is through the objective learning materials provided by nurse educators. New nurses must successfully pass the written and technical portions of orientation. If the organization has a competency-based orientation tool, the new nurse must meet its performance criteria.

Preceptor Assessment

While in orientation, new graduates should meet at regular intervals with their preceptor and manager to review progress (Fey & Miltner, 2000). This evaluation time is important to make certain that new nurses are being assigned to clinical experiences that match their learning needs. It also provides a chance to ensure a smooth interpersonal relationship between orientee and preceptor. At these meetings, the preceptor, manager, and learner should set goals for the next interval. For example, by the end of next week, the orientee will have progressed to an independent patient assessment, completed a patient admission, and increased his workload to a four-patient assignment.

At each of these sessions, it is important for the new nurse to solicit feedback. Ask, "How do you think I'm doing? Am I at the level you would expect? What should I focus on next?" Answers to questions such as these allow the orientee to measure progress.

Formal Performance Evaluation

To maintain accreditation, health care organizations are required to administer performance evaluations for each employee at regular intervals. Individual facilities set their own policies identifying the process and time frames. For many, annual evaluations are the norm.

What should nurses expect from their first formal evaluation? The individual and the nurse manager meet to review progress since either the last evaluation or date of hiring. The evaluation should be objective, based on the nurse's performance as measured against the job description. See Figure 28-3 for an example of a job description.

Most performance evaluations use some sort of checklist, reflecting whether the individual being evaluated meets standards, exceeds standards, or falls below the organization's standards.

Formal performance evaluation between the manager and staff member serves several purposes. The evaluation is used to ensure competence in the skills required for safe patient care. It is also an opportunity to recognize the nurse's accomplishments in the evaluation period, which can be a real morale boost (Marriner-Tomey, 2000). This is the ideal time for the manager to enhance future performance by coaching, setting goals, and identifying learning needs (Lachman, 2000). At the end of the performance evaluation, both the manager and the staff member should have a clear understanding of what needs to happen in the next year for that nurse to grow and continue to be successful.

360-Degree Feedback

Some health care organizations have moved to an evaluation program known as **360-degree feedback**.

ALBANY MEDICAL CENTER HOSPITAL PATIENT CARE SERVICES
Job Description

JOB TITLE: REGISTERED PROFESSIONAL NURSE

Exempt (Y/N): No	JOB CODE:
SALARY LEVEL: N25.1-4	DOT CODE:
SHIFT:	DIVISION: PATIENT CARE SVC
LOCATION: NURSING UNITS	DEPARTMENT:
EMPLOYEE NAME:	SUPERVISOR: NURSE MANAGER
PREPARED BY: AMY BALUCH	DATE: 03/22/95
APPROVED BY:	DATE:

SUMMARY: The Registered Professional Nurse utilizes the nursing process to diagnose and treat human responses to actual or potential health problems. The New York State Nurse Practice Act and A.N.A. Code for Nurses with Interpretive Statements guide the practice of the Registered Professional Nurse. The primary responsibilities of the Registered Professional Nurse as leader of the Patient Care Team is coordination of patient care through the continuum, education, and advocacy.

ESSENTIAL DUTIES AND RESPONSIBILITIES include the following. Other duties may be assigned.

- Performs an ongoing and systematic assessment, focusing on physiologic, psychologic, and cognitive status.

- Develops a goal directed plan of care which is standards based. Involves patient and/or significant other (S.O.) and health care team members in patient care planning.

- Implements care through utilization and adherence to established standards which define the structure, process and desired patient outcomes of nursing process.

- Evaluates effectiveness of care in progressing patients toward desired outcomes. Revises plan of care based on evaluation of outcomes.

- Demonstrates competency in knowledge base, skill level and psychomotor skills.

- Demonstrates applied knowledge base in areas of structure standards, standards of care, protocols and patient care resources/references. Practices in compliance with state and federal regulations.

- Demonstrates knowledge of Patient Bill of Rights by incorporating it into their practice.

- Demonstrates ability to identify, plan, implement and evaluate patient/S.O. education needs.

- Participates in development and attainment of unit and service patient care goals.

- Organizes and coordinates delivery of patient care in an efficient and cost effective manner.

- Documents the nursing process in a timely, accurate and complete manner, following established guidelines.

- Utilizes standards in applying the nursing process for the delivery of patient care.

- Participates in unit and service quality management activities.

- Demonstrates self-directed learning and participation in continuing education to meet own professional development.

- Participates in team development activities for unit and service.

(continues)

Figure 28-3 Albany Medical Center, Hospital Patient Care Services Job Description for Registered Professional Nurses (Courtesy of Albany Medical Center, Albany, NY)

- Demonstrates responsibility and accountability for professional standards and for own professional practice.

- Supports research and its implications for practice.

- Adheres to unit and human resource policies.

- Establishes and maintains direct, honest and open professional relationships with all health care team members, patients, and significant others.

- Seeks guidance and direction for successful performance of self and team, to meet patient care outcomes.

- Incorporates into practice an awareness of legal and risk management issues and their implications.

QUALIFICATION REQUIREMENTS: To perform this job successfully, an individual must be able to perform each essential duty satisfactorily. The requirements listed below are representative of the knowledge, skill, and/or ability required. Reasonable accommodations may be made to enable individuals with disabilities to perform the essential functions.

EDUCATION and/or EXPERIENCE: Graduate of an approved program in professional nursing. Must hold current New York State registration or possess a limited permit to practice in the State of New York.

LANGUAGE SKILLS: Ability to read and interpret documents such as safety rules and procedure manuals. Ability to document patient care on established forms. Ability to speak effectively to patients, family members, and other employees of organization.

MATHEMATICAL SKILLS: Ability to add, subtract, multiply, and divide in all units of measure, using whole numbers, common fractions, and decimals. Ability to compute rate, ratio, and percent.

REASONING ABILITY: Ability to identify problems, collect data, establish facts, and draw valid conclusions.

PHYSICAL DEMANDS: The physical demands described here are representative of those that must be met by an employee to successfully perform the essential functions of this job. Reasonable accommodations may be made to enable individuals with disabilities to perform the essential functions.

While performing the duties of this job, the employee is regularly required to stand; walk; use hands to probe, handle, or feel objects, tools, or controls; reach with hands and arms; and speak or hear. The employee is occasionally required to sit or stoop, kneel, or crouch.

The employee must regularly lift and/or move up to 100 pounds and frequently lift and/or move more than 100 pounds. Specific vision abilities required by this job include close vision, distance vision, peripheral vision, depth perception, and the ability to adjust focus.

WORK ENVIRONMENT: The work environment characteristics described here are representative of those an employee encounters while performing the essential functions of this job. Reasonable accommodations may be made to enable individuals with disabilities to perform the essential functions.

While performing the duties of this job, the employee is regularly exposed to bloodborne pathogens.

The noise level in the work environment is usually moderate.

rev. 9/95
rev. 6/96

Figure 28-3 *(continued)*

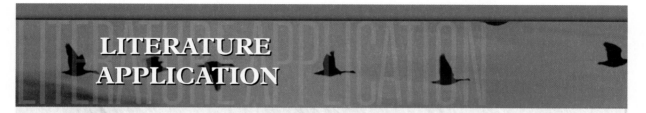

LITERATURE APPLICATION

Citation: Snodgrass, S. G. (2001, June 10). Wish you were a star? Become one! *Chicago Tribune*, D1.

Discussion: The most logical way to predict your future is to create it, so if you want to be a star, start by becoming a top performer now. Companies are drawn to those who use up-to-date skills and leadership to produce measurable results. Organizations seek such people out. Surprisingly, few people understand this. You can begin to position yourself now with exceptional performance.

Start by delivering more than you promise and consistently outperform yourself. Exceed expectations on a regular basis, seek more responsibility, value teamwork and diversity, provide leadership, and always go beyond the call of duty. Communicate effectively and know how to network with others. Be resourceful, comfortable with ambiguity, and open to saying, "I don't know, but I'll find out." In addition, take initiative and persevere until you reach quantifiable results. Finally, assume some personal risk by thinking outside the box and exploring bold, new solutions to challenges. Provide yourself with a margin of confidence through lifelong learning. Be open, flexible, and adapt to new ideas. Spend time with those who challenge your thinking.

You should also be creative, seek innovative solutions, and supplement your past experience with a fresh perspective. Learn how to put your ideas into action and be persistent because achieving results takes time. In addition, do your homework. Understand the business agenda and close any gaps between what you are and what you could be. In other words, define your goals, then create and implement a personal development plan. Finally, demonstrate respect for others, and apply the golden rule. Achieving great results with great behavior enables your star to rise. You can begin the process right now with these specific steps:

- See the big picture. Know why your job was created, how it relates to your organization, and what opportunities it contains. You can positively influence outcomes through performance and achievement.
- Invest in your organization; make decisions as if you owned the company. Determine which actions promise the most significant impact, and then pursue them with zeal.
- Push your comfort zone by seeking challenges, finding the positive in negative situations, taking action, and learning from the past.
- Make time for people; understand the culture, values, and beliefs of the organization; keep things in perspective; and have fun.
- Inspire those around you to exceed expectations; also, convey a sense of urgency, and consistently drive issues to closure.

After you do all this, how do you ensure that you will be noticed? Ask how your company identifies and rewards top performers. Inquire as to whether there is a high-potential category. You should pursue an environment in which the best are recognized and valued. It should be an organization that provides career growth, lifelong learning, and development opportunities.

You also want meaningful work, an opportunity to contribute, and an environment that prizes new ideas and fresh perspectives. In addition, you deserve honest feedback and the opportunity to provide the same in return. Finally, seek an organization that energizes and empowers you, encourages your good health, respects your point of view, and honors your performance. Many such organizations abound.

Implications for Practice: Though a business professional wrote this article, the advice rings true for nurses as well.

In this system, an individual is assessed by a variety of people in order to provide a broader perspective (Marriner-Tomey, 2000). For example, a nurse may complete a self-assessment and submit a packet detailing the year's progress. This may include documentation of inservices completed in the assessment period, samples of charting, and details related to committee work. The appraisal process also includes peer reviews, evaluation by the nurse's immediate supervisor, and patient interviews (Edwards & Ewen, 1996).

With 360-degree feedback, the individual can potentially receive a broader, more balanced assessment. To be consistent and objective, nurses who are asked to evaluate their peers need orientation to the process and the specific tool being used (Marriner-Tomey, 2000). Overall, 360-degree feedback can be time consuming to complete, yet provides valuable information.

Setting Goals

A key component of any performance appraisal is the opportunity to set goals for the coming year. Goals that are measurable and clearly articulated are more likely to be met (Lachman, 2000). These should be developed jointly by the nurse being evaluated and the nurse's manager.

A sample performance goals outline might look like the following:

By the next scheduled performance assessment, nurse Joanne Johnson will do the following:

- Successfully complete the advanced pediatric assessment course
- Assume the primary nurse role for patients with an anticipated length of stay of greater than 3 days
- Become an active participant on a unit-based or hospitalwide committee.

ORGANIZATIONAL RESPONSES TO PERFORMANCE

Many health care organizations have a merit-based compensation structure that is tied to performance evaluations. Employees' pay raises are matched to their performance. But most health care organizations are looking for other ways—in addition to

money—to create job satisfaction. Studies have demonstrated that recognition is one of the most important ways health care organizations have to motivate employee performance (Nelson, 1994).

Employee Recognition Programs

Many health care organizations have developed formal recognition activities. These may take the form of surprising an Employee of the Month with balloons and a plaque, bringing in a national speaker for a celebration of Nurses Day, or presenting recognition pins for years of service. One popular recognition involves selecting an employee from each unit to attend a quarterly luncheon with the organization's administrator. At the luncheon, employees are recognized individually for their contributions to patient care, based on the narratives submitted by the nominating individuals. Figure 28-4 and Figure 28-5 are sample forms used in such a program.

Corrective Action Programs

Sometimes, appraisal feedback indicates the need for significant performance improvement. Most health care organizations have a prescribed corrective action program. One of the first steps in helping employees improve their performance is identifying whether the poor performance is developmental or related to a failure to follow policies or procedures. For example, a nurse may be having difficulty completing assignments in an appropriate time frame. It is unlikely that the nurse's problem is related to a lack of understanding of the rules. Instead, the manager needs to coach the employee, assisting the nurse with whatever support will help him improve (Grensing-Pophal, 2000). It may be that the nurse needs remedial work in some particular technical skill or feedback specifically directed to organizing a patient assignment, either of which can affect the nurse's ability to complete the shift on time.

Another category of corrective action is disciplinary corrective action. In this case, an employee receives feedback for failing to follow the organization's policies. Excessive absenteeism is an example. As with the previous example, the goal is to assist the nurse to improve performance. Most organizations have a series of progressive steps for corrective action

Success Stories Nomination Form

Name: _____

Position: _____ Unit/Dept: _____

Reason for Selection:

_____

_____

_____

_____

_____

_____

_____

_____

_____

_____

Submitted by: Name: _____

Unit/ Ext: _____

Please return complete form to:
Marketing and Retention Committee
M4 Mailbox / MC 73

Figure 28-4 Success Stories Nomination Form (Courtesy of Albany Medical Center, Albany, NY)

ALBANY MEDICAL CENTER

43 New Scotland Avenue, Albany, New York 12208-3478

October 8, 2002

Dear Managers,

The Marketing and Retention Committee, along with Mary Nolan, has been sponsoring Success Stories luncheons to recognize staff. This December 14, 2002, we will extend this luncheon to include a new staff member, of less than a year on your unit, to accompany the staff member who has been chosen by yourself, another staff member, or the previous Success Story candidate.

Please take this opportunity to submit the name of a staff member who you feel has a positive impact on your department and helps make it a successful one. The individual chosen will receive an invitation to a luncheon with Mary Nolan.

Submissions must be returned to Carole West, Marketing and Retention mailbox on M4, MC73, by November 16, 2002.

Thank you, and we look forward to honoring your "Success Story". If you have any questions, please feel free to call me in the Emergency Department, 262-3131. Your staff member will be honored from noon to 2 PM on December 14, 2002.

Sincerely,

Carole West, RN
Success Luncheon Chairman

Figure 28-5 Invitation to Success Stories Luncheon (Courtesy of Albany Medical Center, Albany, NY)

in cases in which employee performance does not improve. For example, a manager may begin by providing a verbal warning to an employee whose attendance is minimally acceptable. If the nurse's attendance problem continues, the nurse may receive a written warning. Without improvement, this could proceed to a suspension, final warning, and eventually termination.

In **progressive discipline**, the manager and employee's mutual goal is to take steps to correct performance to bring it back to an acceptable level. In a union environment, the employee may have the right to union representation after a verbal reprimand. It offers a stepwise process with opportunities for continued feedback and clarification of expectations. In any event, the corrective action applied by the manager must be fair. Employees should be forewarned of the consequences of violating an institution's policies so that there are no surprises (Marquis & Huston, 2000). The corrective action should be consistent and impartial—each person is treated the same each time the rule is broken. Figure 28-6 is a sample corrective action documentation tool.

THE NURSE AS A FIRST-TIME MANAGER OF A SMALL PATIENT GROUP

The registered nurse responsible for direct care of a small group of patients is functioning as a first-line nurse manager. This nurse is responsible for linking each patient to the resources that the patient needs. This often involves supervising other licensed and unlicensed assistive personnel (UAP) involved in direct patient care.

Relating to Other Disciplines

As Burke points out, given the complexity of health care organizations in our country, the successful interconnection among departments is a potential source of tremendous strength (2000). The registered nurse who understands the functions of the respiratory therapists, case managers, and vendors for durable medical equipment will be able to efficiently incorporate their contributions in planning for effec-

tive patient care (Marrelli, 1997). In many settings, diagnosis-specific care plans articulate the anticipated relationships among disciplines. For example, a nursing care plan for a patient admitted for a CVA may include consultation with physical therapy on day 2 and an evaluation for home care needs on day 3. It is important for nurses to develop strong relationships with representatives of the many other disciplines whose practices interface with the nursing role.

Delegation to Team Members

In the current health care environment, lengths of stay are shorter despite increased patient acuity and complexity. The nurse who is responsible for a group of patients also needs to work with other nurses and unlicensed personnel to provide safe patient care. This usually involves delegating specific responsibilities to others. A nurse who delegates effectively assigns routine tasks to a coworker, freeing the RN for more-complex planning or care. The RN needs to match the coworkers' skills with the delegated task. One way to do this is through open-ended questions (Keeling, Adair, Seider, & Kirksey, 2000). The RN may ask the LPN what materials she usually uses for a particular wound dressing. At the same time, the RN needs to ensure that the LPN knows what must be reported back, for example, in this case, a saturated dressing. Despite delegating the task, the RN should continue to evaluate the ongoing needs of the patient (Calloway, 1999).

It is easy to fall into the trap of overdelegating or underdelegating, particularly for new nurses. Some nurses are hesitant to delegate activities to others because they are afraid their teammates will resent being asked to do a specific task. They worry they will be seen as lazy or lacking ability. Or they may hesitate to delegate out of a belief that they can do the task better or faster themselves (Marquis & Huston, 2000).

Other nurses delegate more care than is appropriate or safe. Nurses who overdelegate may do so because they are poor time managers or because they personally lack the skill required. It may be that they failed to first assess their patients or are unfamiliar with their coworkers' competencies (Calloway, 1999).

Performance feedback is a crucial element of delegation. It is important to openly recognize team members' contributions to safe patient care (Keeling

ALBANY MEDICAL CENTER
Corrective Action Notice

Employee's Name: _____ Job Title: _____

Division: ( ) Center ( ) College ( ) Hospital Department: _____

PART I: CORRECTIVE ACTION HISTORY

Date of Corrective Action	Reason For Corrective Action	Level of Corrective Action Applied
1. / /	_____	_____
2. / /	_____	_____
3. / /	_____	_____
4. / /	_____	_____
5. / /	_____	_____
( )	Check here if no previous corrective action issued	

PART II: CURRENT OFFENSE REQUIRING CORRECTIVE ACTION

Date of Offense: _____/_____/_____
Level of Corrective Action Being Applied: ( ) Written Warning ( ) Final Warning
Category of Offense: ( ) Job Performance ( ) Absenteeism/Tardiness ( ) Misconduct ( ) Other

Description of Offense: _____
_____
_____
_____
_____

Expected Improvement And Plan For Correction: _____
_____
_____
_____
_____

Suspension Without Pay (Pending Investigation)
Description of Incident: _____
_____

_____   _____/_____/_____   Follow-Up Date: _____/_____/_____
Manager's Signature   Date

The offense(s) described above is in violation of Albany Medical Center's policies governing the conduct and/or performance standards of it's employees. The reason for and level of Corrective Action being issued has been fully explained to me, and I understand that I must correct my job performance and/or conduct immediately. My job performance and/or conduct must remain at an acceptable level following improvement or further action up to and including discharge will be taken.

_____   _____/_____/_____
Employee's Signature   Date

Original Copy: Human Resources (Hospital Paid Staff) College Personnel Services (College Paid Staff)   Department Copy: Manager   Employee Copy
H-170 (Rev. 11/91)

Figure 28-6 Corrective Action Notice Documentation Tool (Courtesy of Albany Medical Center, Albany, NY)

et al., 2000). In an instance in which the nurse is not satisfied with the outcome of a delegated task, it is equally important to discuss the assignment with the coworker individually. Perhaps the nurse's directions were unclear, or misunderstood, or failed to include an important time frame. Taking the time to provide feedback demonstrates the respect and value a nurse places on her teammates' contributions.

Levels of Authority

Sometimes, when one delegates an assignment to a team member, that person questions the parameters of the assignment. If, for example, the RN in charge of a group of patients delegates a patient's ostomy teaching to another RN on the team, that RN may hear that assignment several ways. For example, the RN may think, "I need to do the ostomy appliance change while the patient's wife is here." Or, "I need

to assess what the patient has learned already and report back to the RN." Or, finally, "I need to develop a teaching plan with the patient and begin to implement it today."

These three possibilities demonstrate the importance of delegating clearly and specifically and defining the level of authority being delegated. Sharon Cox, a nursing leadership consultant, describes four possible levels of authority to be used when delegating a task to a coworker (1997):

1. Collect data, find out the facts, assess the situation, and report back to the team leader.
2. Collect data and make a recommendation back to the team leader.
3. Assess the situation, make a recommendation, report back, and then implement that recommendation.
4. Assess the situation and carry out the task as the coworker believes is appropriate.

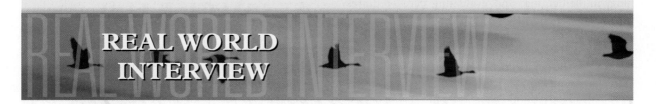

REAL WORLD INTERVIEW

I remember my first job in nursing about 40 years ago. It was as a staff nurse on a general medical-surgical unit. I had a wonderful preceptor, Ed Fuss, RN. He worked with me and helped me until gradually I could assume my full role as a staff nurse on the unit. It took a while. It was very stressful to care for the 42 patients on that unit. After my orientation period, I would sometimes be the only RN, though I would have several licensed practical nurses and nurse aids working with me. I had to quickly learn appropriate delegation techniques.

Nursing has been a great career for me. I have worked as a nurse in Indiana, Illinois, New York, Oklahoma, and Wisconsin. Besides other nursing positions that I have held, I often work as a per diem agency nurse in various Emergency Departments. I find I can move quickly into the culture of a new unit by being friendly, helping others on the unit, and keeping my nursing skills up to date. I notice that people in other professions often complain about being concerned that they will lose their job. In nursing, I have not had to worry about job layoffs. I always have been able to get an interesting nursing job doing something I like.

I have had nurse friends who have worked as nurse practitioners, nurse chaplains, traveling nurses, seminar teachers, missionary nurses, nurse lawyers, nurse managers, informatics nurses, nurses in a homeless shelter, nurses on a cruise boat, etc. There are all kinds of nursing opportunities. I also like stopping at the scene of an accident and knowing I can help. It has been my privilege to be a nurse. How many other professions can say they save lives for a living!

Patricia Kelly-Heidenthal, RN, MSN

An agreement as to the level of authority at the time the task is delegated prevents each party from making inaccurate assumptions about the other's accountability for the delegated assignment. See Chapter 13 for more discussion of delegation.

The Charge Role

Many hospital-based nurses, especially those who work evening or night shifts, rapidly progress from being assigned responsibility for a small group of patients to being assigned to the charge role for the shift. Particularly on medical and surgical floors, the charge nurse continues to care for a group of patients but also may coordinate care for the rest of the unit. He may be responsible for assigning the workload of the nursing staff for the shift.

The nurse as first-time charge nurse often has high expectations for his own performance and can easily become stressed in the new role. It is helpful to recognize that the nursing process—assessing, planning, implementing, and evaluating care—requires organizational and priority-setting skills that directly apply to the charge nurse role (Marrelli, 1997). It is a matter of perceiving and delegating patient care needs from the perspective of the unit as a whole. The new charge nurse must let go of the need to be perfect. Instead, he should concentrate on staying organized and focused on what is best for the patients. It is also important to recognize and utilize the available resources for problem solving, such as coworkers or the facility supervisor.

Articulating Expectations. As a first-time charge nurse, it is important to build relationships with other staff members as well as coworkers from other disciplines. One way to develop these relationships is by sharing expectations (Cox, 1997). This may be as simple as sitting down over coffee and agreeing to certain behaviors, such as "We will maintain a patient focus, as evidenced by answering call lights quickly." Some performance expectations may be more generic, applying to relationships more than specific patient care items, but they still need to be clearly spelled out ("Seven Tips," 2000). For example, "If you disagree with me, you will talk to me about it before you discuss our disagreement with others." These specific expectations help establish a level of trust and prevent the need for mind reading. They open the doorway for clear communication so that when a problem develops, it is easier to approach the individual involved.

STRATEGIES FOR PROFESSIONAL GROWTH

New nurses are more likely to stay in their positions if they are challenged and have opportunities for professional growth ("Getting X-ers to Stay," 2000). Some health care facilities have a wealth of available educational opportunities. Others, particularly smaller organizations, may require the nurse looking for experiences to be more creative. The best place to

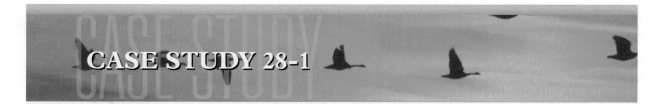

CASE STUDY 28-1

You are the charge nurse for the evening shift on a general surgical floor. A patient care associate (PCA) working on your shift brings you a complaint. He says that the nurse he is assigned to work with this evening is not doing her share. She is sitting at the desk visiting with the unit secretary while he answers all the call lights. She has also assigned him the task of setting up a traction bed, which he has done only once in orientation 2 months ago. As the charge nurse, how would you respond to the PCA? Would you talk to the nurse he is working with? What is the priority issue in this situation?

start is with the experts on and around the nursing unit. Suppose you have developed an interest in learning more about cardiac arrhythmias. If your hospital offers an EKG interpretation course, great! Sign up! If not, there are lots of other ways to grow in this area. Talk to your nurse manager and educator about your interest. Ask them about classes, or ask them to refer you to experts in your geographic area. Speak to the cardiologist when she is making rounds on your unit. Ask her for the name of an interventional cardiologist so you can observe a cardiac catheterization. Ask to spend a day shadowing in a coronary care unit. Do not limit your search to nurses and physicians. Often other health disciplines overlap with nursing's interests, and you may be able to tap into opportunities with another discipline.

Not all nurses have the motivation or time for a lot of formal professional growth activities. What is important is to stay challenged. Find a particular skill or interest in your position, and expand it. What do you like best of all the things you did today? Working with the patient's family? Teaching the new diabetic? Starting that IV? Whatever it is, look for opportunities to become your unit's expert at it.

Cross Training

Given today's shortage of nurses, the national trend is toward increased floating and offering nurses cross training to new areas (Benefield et al., 2000). Cross training is another opportunity for individual growth. While some organizations have strict guidelines to limit the practice of floating nurses, other health care facilities expect nurses to routinely float to either a related unit or an area particularly in need of assistance.

It is important for nurses in their first job to be articulate about their competencies for a new patient population if they are asked to float. They need to be sure the manager assigning them is aware of their experience level. Nurses should not accept total responsibility for an area or population in which they have not achieved competency. It may be more appropriate to assign an inexperienced nurse to specific tasks to help on the unit rather than asking that nurse to take a typical patient assignment on an unfamiliar unit.

One way to minimize the stress of being asked to float to a different unit is to volunteer ahead of time to cross train to the new area. This has many advantages. It allows the nurse the opportunity to experience working with different ages or types of patients. Besides learning new skills, it gives a nurse the chance to see how the other half lives. For example, a nurse who has worked only on a medical floor may regard accepting an admission from the Emergency Department (ED) as something to be worked into the shift, based on other patient care needs. After cross training to the ED, and seeing admitted patients waiting on stretchers in the hall, that nurse may have a new appreciation of the need to negotiate for timely acceptance of ED admissions to the floor.

Cross training has some long-term benefits as well. If a new nurse is considering a career in a specialty, spending some time cross training to that population can help the nurse decide whether she wants to pursue that field. Cross training also is beneficial to the nurse seeking a new position. When a nurse is applying for a new job, experience in more than one clinical area enhances a resume and makes the individual a stronger candidate.

Some health care organizations reward nurses who volunteer to cross train so they can safely float to different areas. These rewards may be monetary. Other institutions offer nonmonetary incentives, such as reduced weekend or holiday commitments, as rewards for cross training or floating.

Identifying a Mentor

Developing a mentoring relationship with a more experienced, successful nurse is another mechanism for professional growth. A mentor coaches a novice nurse and helps the novice develop skills and career direction (Shaffer, Tallarica, & Walsh, 2000). A mentor may introduce the younger nurse to professional networking opportunities. A good person to assist the new nurse in a workplace ethical dilemma may well be his mentor.

How does a new nurse find a mentor? First, the new nurse needs to communicate a willingness to learn and grow. A newer nurse usually needs to seek out a prospective mentor rather than wait to be approached by one. An ideal mentor is an experienced nurse who is willing to support and counsel other nurses when asked (Shaffer et al., 2000). This may lead to a formal structured relationship or a more informal role-modeling association.

Nurses who have been successful preceptors are often potential mentors because they are com-

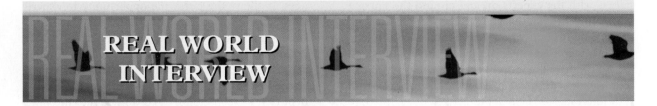

There is a national nursing shortage, most acutely realized in nursing specialty areas such as critical care, operating room, and pediatrics. Staffing and scheduling practices directly affect nursing personnel costs, patient care outcomes, and recruitment and retention of nurses. At a Midwest university hospital, a specialty cluster-nursing program was implemented to respond to the nursing shortage. The specialty cluster-nursing program consisted of grouping several inpatient units and related specialty clinics with similar patient care requirements together. Nurses hired into the cardiac, oncology, pediatrics, and trauma clusters are offered a special fellowship orientation program.

Nurses working the cardiac cluster can work on the cardiac medical intensive care unit, cardiac medical step-down unit, cardiac surgery intensive care unit, and cardiac surgery step-down unit. Nurses working the medical cluster can work on pulmonary, geriatric, psychiatry, and general medicine inpatient units. Nurses working the neuroscience cluster can work on orthopedics, rehabilitation, and neurology inpatient units. Nurses working the oncology cluster can work on the pediatric oncology clinic, adult oncology unit, or the adult hematology/oncology clinic or adult surgical unit. Nurses working the pediatric cluster can work on the infant/toddler, adolescent, hematology, and pediatric intensive care inpatient units. Nurses working the surgical cluster can work on general surgery, plastics and otolaryngology, transplant, peripheral vascular, and security inpatient units. Finally, nurses working the trauma cluster can work on the trauma life support intensive care unit, Emergency Department, burn unit, and general surgery inpatient unit.

This program creates opportunities for nurses to develop expertise and specialty knowledge in patient populations that cross multiple units. Nurses skilled in the specialty cluster are preassigned to one or more settings within the cluster based on projected staffing requirements. Staffing adjustments are made for each scheduling period for patient acuity changes, changes in patient volume, extended leaves, and sick leaves. Scheduling specialty cluster staff prior to the beginning of a work schedule minimizes floating of unit-based staff on a shift-by-shift basis. The cluster program with the fellowship orientation has become an effective nurse retention strategy.

Patricia Dianne Padjen, RN, MBA, MS, EdD
Manager, EMS Program

mitted to helping another nurse learn and grow. Even though the preceptor role is more narrow and defined, the role can easily be expanded to a more informal mentoring relationship.

The Internet is a newer mentoring resource. Nurses can develop relationships through special-interest chat rooms or by e-mailing experts in other geographic areas. There are forums for questions and answers, often on specific patient populations, disease processes, or operational issues. Want to get some expert advice on a particular patient problem? Spend some time on the Internet.

Developing Professional Goals

Once a new nurse has mastered the skills for day-to-day nursing care in her place of work, what is next? How does a nurse measure professional growth? For many nurses, the answer to these questions is a clinical ladder.

Clinical Ladder

A **clinical ladder** is a program established by some health care organizations to encourage nurses to

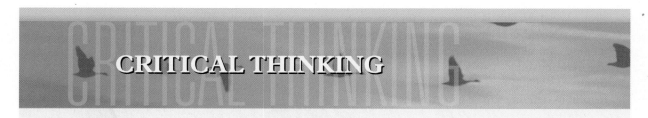

CRITICAL THINKING

You have just begun interviewing for your first nursing job.

What type of nursing recognition programs would appeal to you? What opportunities are available in your community to network with nurses from other institutions? For you, would monetary or scheduling rewards be more of an incentive to cross train on another unit? What are some measurable professional goals for your first year as a registered nurse?

earn promotions and gain recognition and increased pay by meeting specific requirements. Although the criteria may vary, most programs have three or four distinct levels. Some also offer the nurse the opportunity to seek promotion in a specific track, within a clinical, educational, or managerial focus. Thus, it is possible for a new nurse to choose a clinical nursing track and move through the organization's promotional levels by meeting those requirements. For example, to be promoted from a new graduate level to a Level II RN, the nurse may be required to complete a specialty course such as Advanced Cardiac Life Support (ACLS) or EKG interpretation, join a unit- or hospital-based committee, and finish the preceptor course. Besides offering opportunity for promotion, these programs offer an objective way to measure a nurse's achievements. Clinical ladders can be time-consuming to complete yet they provide valuable information.

Specialty Certifications

Many health care organizations encourage their staff to become certified. Nearly all nursing specialties now offer board certification exams to validate expert knowledge of that particular discipline. Emergency nurses may sit for the Certified Emergency Exam and the Advanced Cardiac Life Support Exam. Nurses who specialize in critical care may take the critical care certifying exam to earn their CCRN. Successfully passing a certification exam is another measure of professional growth and offers the benefit of national recognition of one's credentials.

KEY CONCEPTS

- When choosing a first nursing position, it is important to contemplate the differences in developmental opportunities between specialty and general medical-surgical units. Environmental, scheduling, and orientation options are also important considerations.
- Organizational orientation is both general and unit based. Orientation is a time for developing strong relationships with preceptors and members of other disciplines, as well as for mastering competencies needed for safe patient care.
- Nurses receive performance feedback both informally and as part of periodic evaluations. This input is valuable in developing personal goals.
- Health care organizations have mechanisms to recognize employee contributions. Many of these programs reward success, both monetarily and through recognition programs. Corrective action programs can be used to coach an employee who is having performance problems and to foster change in an employee who is failing to follow policies.
- Given the increasing complexity of health care today, it is crucial for the first-time nurse to develop strong relationships with team members and representatives of other health care disciplines. The new nurse needs to delegate appropriately and specify defining levels of authority with her coworkers. Relationships with coworkers are enhanced when staff members mutually agree to performance expectations.

- Professional growth is important for job satisfaction. Organizational opportunities for growth include clinical ladders and developing mentoring relationships. Cross training is another means to expand one's experiences and can be helpful in defining future career plans.

KEY TERMS

clinical ladder   self-scheduling
progressive discipline   360-degree feedback

REVIEW QUESTIONS

1. General orientation includes which of the following?
   A. Information all nurses new to a facility need
   B. Mastery of unit-specific processes
   C. Patient care for a specific diagnostic group of patients
   D. Patient care for a specific age group of patients

2. Which of the following is usually NOT necessary to do in your first job in nursing?
   A. Learning to be organized
   B. Developing a good attendance record
   C. Refining your assessment skills
   D. Completing written performance evaluations of the UAP that report to you

3. Preceptors who work with new nursing graduates should have all of the following characteristics EXCEPT
   A. be clinically experienced.
   B. enjoy teaching.
   C. committment to the preceptor role.
   D. ability to float to specialty units.

4. All of the following are career stages of nurses, as conceptualized by McNeese-Smith, EXCEPT
   A. entry.
   B. mastery.
   C. accomplishment.
   D. disengagement.

5. The corrective action process usually contains all of the following EXCEPT

A. verbal warning.
B. written warning.
C. final warning.
D. transfer to another unit.

REVIEW ACTIVITIES

1. You will be graduating from your nursing program in 3 months. Identify several possible employment opportunities in your desired locale. Prepare examples of questions you will ask as part of choosing a position. What factors are most important to you in choosing a position?

2. You have been working as a new graduate for a year and have done well. Your nurse manager asks you to be the relief charge nurse on your unit for the 3 P.M. to 11 P.M. shift. What type of orientation will you need for this position? How can you work with a mentor to do well in this position?

3. You are interested in the concept of 360-degree feedback. Who could you ask to give you feedback on your clinical performance to achieve 360-degree feedback?

4. Review a recent nurse salary survey—for example, see Charles, Piper, Mailey, Davis, and Baigis (2000) in the References section. How do nursing salaries in your area compare?

EXPLORING THE WEB

- There are many web sites specific to nursing employment opportunities. Try some of these:
  http://www.rnwanted.com
  http://www.healthopps.com
  http://www.healthcareers-online.com

- If you have a specialty area in mind, it is worth the time to explore the Web for more details. How will this help you as you prepare for interviews?

- Look up the Association of Pediatric Oncology Nurses: *http://www.apon.org*

  Association of Rehabilitation Nurses:
  http://www.rehabnurse.org

  Association of Women's Health, Obstetric and Neonatal Nurses: *http://www.awhonn.org*

- If you are interested in trauma nursing, try *http://www.emergency.com*

REFERENCES

Baggs, J. G., & Ryan, S. A. (1990). ICU nurse-physician collaboration and nursing satisfaction. *Nursing Economic$, 8*(6), 386–392.

Benefield, L. E., Clifford, J., Cox, S., Hagenow, N. R., Hastings, C., Kobs, A. E., Mayer, G. G., Porter-O'Grady, T., Stahl, D. A., Valentine, N. M., & Wolgin, E. (2000). Nursing leaders predict top trends for 2000. *Nursing Management, 31*(1), 21–23.

Burke, A. (2000). Organization-wide competency and education. *Nursing Management, 31*(2), 20–25.

Calloway, S. D. (1999). Delegating tasks: Know the legal risks. *ED Nursing, 3*(2), 22–23.

Cardillo, D. W. (2001). *Your first year as a nurse.* Roseville, CA: Prima.

Charles, J. P., Piper, S., Mailey, S. K., David, P., & Baigis, J. (2000). Nurse salaries in Washington D.C. and nationally. *Nursing Economic$, 18*(5), 243–249

Cox, S. H. (1997, November). *Motivation and morale: Coin of the realm.* Symposium conducted at Nursing Management Congress, Chicago, IL.

Edwards, M. R., & Ewen, A. J. (1996). *360 feedback.* New York: American Management Association.

Fey, M. K., & Miltner, R. S. (2000). A competency-based orientation program for new graduate nurses. *Journal of Nursing Administration, 30,* 126–132.

Getting X-ers to stay. (2000). *Management Briefings for Nurse Leaders, 1*(5), 3.

Grensing-Pophal, L. (2000). Give-and-take feedback. *Nursing Management, 31*(2), 27– 28.

Keeling, B., Adair, J., Seider, D., & Kirksey, G. (2000). Appropriate delegation. *American Journal of Nursing, 100*(12), 24A–24D.

Kramer, M. (1974). *Reality shock: Why nurses leave nursing.* St. Louis, MO: Mosby.

Lachman, V. D. (2000). Coaching techniques. *Nursing Management, 31*(1), 15–19.

LaDuke, S. (2000). Putting you to the test. *Nursing Management, 31*(5), 20–21.

Marquis, B. L., & Huston, C. J. (2000). *Leadership roles and management: Functions in nursing* (3rd ed.). Philadelphia: Lippincott.

Marrelli, T. M. (1997). *The nurse manager's survival guide* (2nd ed.). St. Louis, MO: Mosby.

Marriner-Tomey, A. (2000). *Guide to nursing management and leadership* (6th ed.). St. Louis, MO: Mosby.

McNeese-Smith, D. K. (2000). Job stages of entry, mastery, and disengagement among nurses. *Journal of Nursing Administration, 30*(3), 140–147.

Meinecke, J. (2000). Orientation: Six ways to avoid throwing new nurses to the wolves. *Nursing Management, 31*(2), 30.

Nelson, B. (1994). *1001 ways to reward employees.* New York: Workman.

Seven tips to improve nurse performance. (2000). *Management Briefings for Nurse Leaders, 1*(5), 7.

Shaffer, B., Tallarica, B., & Walsh, J. (2000). Win-win mentoring. *Nursing Management, 31*(1), 32–34.

Snodgrass, S. G. (2001, June 10). Wish you were a star? Become one! *Chicago Tribune,* D1.

Staffing models: Nurse shortage spurs hunt for perfect ratios. (2000). *Healthcare Benchmarks, 7*(2), 13–17.

SUGGESTED READINGS

Belkin, L. (1997, June 15). How can we save the next victim? *The New York Times Magazine,* pp. 29–33.

Blanchard, K., Carlos, J. P., & Randolph, A. (1999). *The three keys to empowerment.* San Francisco: Berrett-Koehler.

Connelly, L. M., Yoder, L. H., & Miner-Williams, D. (2000). Hidden charges: Top competencies to develop in a charge nurse. *Nursing Management, 31*(5), 27–29.

Diehl-Oplinger, L., & Kaminski, M. F. (2000). Need critical care nurses? Inquire within. *Nursing Management, 31*(3), 44–46.

Fletcher, C. E. (1997). Failure mode and effects analysis: An interdisciplinary way to analyze and reduce medication errors. *Journal of Nursing Administration, 27*(12), 19–26.

Friedman, P. (1994). *How to deal with difficult people* (2nd ed.). Mission, KS: SkillPath.

Johnson, C. (2000). We made a mistake. *Nursing Management, 31*(4), 22–24.

Lee, L. A. (2000). Buzzwords with a basis: Motivation, mentoring, empowerment. *Nursing Management, 31*(10), 24–27.

Ringerman, E. S., & Ventura, S. (2000). An outcomes approach to skill mix change in critical care. *Nursing Management, 31*(10), 42–46.

Spann, K. (2000). How do you rate your team's teamwork? *Nursing Management, 31*(1), 45.

Urden, L. D., & Rogers, S. (2000). Out in front. *Nursing Management, 31*(7), 27–30.

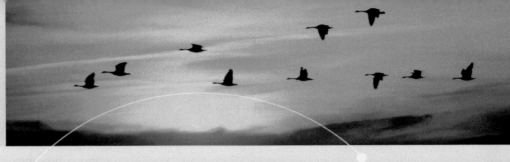

CHAPTER 29

Healthy Living: Personal and Professional Needs

Mary Elaine Koren, RN, DNSc

OBJECTIVES

Upon completion of this chapter, the reader should be able to:

1. Define health.
2. Identify the six concepts of physical, intellectual, emotional, professional, social, and spiritual health.
3. Describe strategies to maintain physical, intellectual, emotional, professional, social, and spiritual health.
4. Discuss occupational health hazards for nurses.
5. Describe methods of personal financial planning.

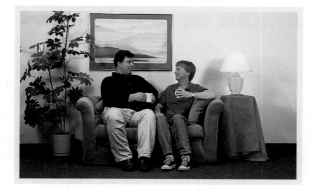

You get up early to work the day shift. On your drive to work, you grab a cup of coffee and a doughnut to sustain you through the morning. It is one of those busy days. The phone is ringing off the hook, patients are not stable, family members are demanding, physicians are slow to answer your page, the laboratory delivers misinformation. It is now noon, and there is no time for lunch. You run down to the vending machines for a Coke and peanut butter crackers to keep you going until the end of your shift. Five o'clock rolls around and you have worked 2 hours overtime and are exhausted. You are already late for your community meeting this evening. You race through a fast-food restaurant for a hamburger, fries, and a milkshake. When you finally arrive home late in the evening, you reward yourself with cookies and a bowl of ice cream and fall into bed. You have given so much throughout the day. There has been little time for good nutrition.

What factors contributed to your poor eating habits in this scenario?

What recommendations would you have to improve your nutrition in this scenario?

Can eating become a crutch for your daily stress?

How can you model the behaviors you teach your patients?

Nursing is a caring profession. Nurses spend their days helping others, many times at the expense of themselves. But who is there to care for the nurse at the end of the shift? If there is nothing left for them, they will not be able to give to their patients. Those that they care for also look to them to model healthy living. If they do not try to live by the standards set for their patients, they will lose a certain amount of credibility in their patients' eyes. How then can they balance the demands of work with their personal needs? The first step is to gather

information. This chapter provides an overview of good health. Many strategies for healthy living are discussed based on six organizing concepts. This chapter also discusses financial planning and occupational health hazards for nurses.

DEFINITION OF HEALTH

Patients and nurses alike strive to maintain good health. But what does health mean? There are various ways of defining health. *Random House Webster's Unabridged Dictionary* (1998) defines health as the "general condition of the body or mind with reference to soundness and vigor." Health as a concept has been in the literature since the inception of modern nursing. Florence Nightingale described health as "being well and using every power the individual possesses to the fullest extent" (Nightingale, 1969 [1860], p. 334). The World Health Organization (1998) describes health as a "state of complete physical, social, and mental well-being, and not merely the absence of disease or infirmity. Health is a resource for everyday life, not the object of living. It is a positive concept emphasizing social and personal resources as well as physical capabilities."

Pender (1996) views health as multidimensional and consisting of biophysical, spiritual, environmental, and cultural aspects. Pender (1996) also states that health, as a concept, is difficult to define because of its complexity. But she does define health as "the actualization of inherent and acquired human potential through goal directed behavior, competent self-care, and satisfying relationships with others while adjustments are made as needed to maintain structural integrity and harmony with relevant environments" (p. 22). Roy and Andrews (1999) define health as "a state or a process of being and becoming an integrated and whole person" (p. 31). Not only is health a complex concept, but it is also dynamic and in a constant state of change.

Health is holistic and multidimensional. All the parts of the whole must be in balance and work together to produce the end result of good health.

Goals for Healthy People 2010

In January 2000, more than 1,500 individuals, health professionals, and organizations convened in

Washington, D.C. to discuss health promotion and disease prevention for the United States population (U.S. Department of Health and Human Services, 2001). The task was to outline specific goals that would enable Americans to maintain their health and avoid disease.

Healthy People 2010 has developed two overall goals for the nation: (1) to encourage those of all ages to increase their life expectancy as well as improve their overall quality of life and (2) to eliminate disparities among various pockets of the population. Ten leading health indicators will be used to measure the overall goals for the nation. Each of these leading indicators reflects a major health concern for the 21st century (Table 29-1).

AREAS OF HEALTH

Health is a complex and dynamic state of being. A healthy person must balance various aspects in life to achieve and maintain good health. When one area of life is affected, general health is also affected. There is overlap among each area, but for purposes of discussion in this chapter, health has been divided into the following elements: physical health, intellectual health, emotional health, professional health, social health, and spiritual health (Figure 29-1).

Our bodies are dynamic and ever changing. Each element of health is constantly adjusting to outside stimuli and attempting to bring balance in life. For example, if one is tired, that fatigue can slow mental acuity. It is easy to become short tempered, which in turn can affect our relationships with oth-

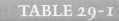

TABLE 29-1	*Healthy People 2010 Indicators*

Physical activity	Responsible sexual behavior	Environmental quality
Overweight and obesity	Mental health	Immunization
Tobacco use	Injury and violence	Access to health care
Substance abuse		

CRITICAL THINKING

What does health mean? McWilliam, Spence Laschinger, and Weston (1999) interviewed 23 nursing and medical students and preceptors to obtain their definition of good health. Participants defined health in a broad sense as not only the absence of disease but also general overall well-being. A student in the study stated that "the way you live your life is going to play a role in how you practice" (p. 101). Maintaining good health is not only important to a nurse's overall well-being, but it will also affect the quality of care provided to patients. Only when you feel good are you able to deliver optimal patient care. Nurses also serve as role models for patients.

How then can nurses, when under tremendous stress on a daily basis, strive toward good health? As you think about your own health, how would you define health? What inhibits you from engaging in healthy behaviors?

ers. By making a conscious decision to sleep longer, we can potentially influence not only our physical well-being but also our ability to think clearly, our emotional state, and how we relate to others. The remainder of this chapter will explore in more depth each of the various elements of health.

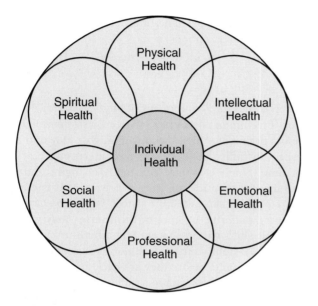

Figure 29-1 Elements of Health

PHYSICAL HEALTH

Physical health, the first element of health, encompasses nutrition as well as exercise coupled with a balanced amount of sleep. Physical health also includes health preventive behaviors such as avoiding smoking and having annual Pap smears and other screening procedures that detect health problems early.

The first step in maintaining good physical health is to do an assessment. Table 29-2 provides a self-assessment of physical health. This tool is designed to assess trends only.

Nutrition

Maintaining good nutrition—one aspect of physical health—is often a difficult task. Finding the time and motivation to eat a nutritious diet in our fast-paced world is not easy. When we eat properly, we feel better and perform tasks at a higher level.

Calculation of Body Mass Index

The newest and most accurate method for assessing body weight in relation to height is to calculate the body mass index (BMI). You can calculate this at

TABLE 29-2	Physical Health Assessment		
Question		**Yes**	**No**
1. I eat three balanced meals a day.			
2. I exercise 30 minutes 3 times a week.			
3. I enjoy exercising.			
4. I exercise with a friend.			
5. I rarely eat between meals.			
6. I sleep 8 hours a night.			
7. I wake up refreshed most mornings.			
8. I sleep soundly without waking up during the night.			

http://www.nhlbi.nih.gov/guidelines/obesity/bmi_tbl.htm. The National Institute of Health (n.d.) has established the following guidelines for interpretation of the BMI:

- 18.5 to 24.9 is optimal health
- 25 to 29.9 is overweight
- 30 and above is obese
- Below 18.5 is considered underweight

Benefits of Exercise

Following nutritional guidelines is not enough to maintain physical health. Daily exercise is another essential ingredient for healthy living. Exercise provides many benefits. It can improve cardiovascular function by lowering cholesterol and blood pressure and strengthening heart muscle. Exercise can boost the immune response to disease. Weight-bearing exercises are especially helpful for calcium uptake in bones. Exercise also improves flexibility and endurance and decreases fat deposition. Exercise can also make you feel better mentally. With exercise usually comes fewer depressive thoughts, less anxiety, an increase in self-confidence, and increased mental acuity (Maraldo, 1999).

Practical Exercise Suggestions

There are many different types of exercise from which to choose. Find one that you are passionate about and one that you truly enjoy. Finding friends who participate in the same activity can help you keep the commitment. When you decide, try to engage in the activity a minimum of three times a week for 30 minutes at a time. Start slowly and gradually build.

There are many ways to get exercise. You can set up an exercise program using videotapes or reference books; for example, Nelson (1997) outlines an entire exercise program for you. Following is a list of some suggestions:

- Walking
- Jogging
- Cycling
- Swimming
- Rowing
- Yoga and tai chi
- Golf and tennis
- Skiing
- Team sports, such as volleyball or basketball
- Dancing

If you are having trouble getting started, you can spend time at a health spa. There are many spas throughout the country, tailored to various budgets. Miller (1998) has published an entire book filled with listings of health spas. The Internet may also provide other health spa options.

Sleep

Sleep is the third component of physical health. It is not uncommon for nurses to sleep less than eight hours per night. Nurses who work nights may find it especially difficult to sleep for an uninterrupted block of time. Nurses who are constantly changing shifts are more susceptible to sleep deprivation. It is estimated that it can take from 4 to 6 weeks to change sleeping patterns. In spite of this, nurses may work multiple shifts within a week. Still other nurses work 10- and 12-hour shifts and do not have a lot of time in between shifts before they are back at work again. If it is necessary to swing to a different shift, it is best to rotate from days to evenings to nights. People generally adapt better if shift rotation is done clockwise (Rogers, 1997). Physicians, family members, and critically ill patients place heavy demands on nurses. Many nurses find it a challenge to leave thoughts of patients and the day's activities at work. This also contributes to insomnia (Davidhizar, Poole, & Giger, 1996).

Assessment of Sleep Deprivation

How do you know if you are sleep deprived? If you answer yes to any of the following questions, you might well be suffering from lack of sleep (Wilson, 2000).

- Do you ever fall asleep at work?
- Is it difficult to get out of bed in the morning?
- Are you tired or irritable at work?
- Do you have trouble concentrating or remembering things at work?
- Do you ever doze off to sleep on your drive home from work?

Deleterious Effects of Sleep Deprivation

Current research indicates that there are many negative effects of sleep deprivation. Sleep-deprived individuals become petulant and find it difficult to remember or concentrate on the simplest tasks. If sleep deprivation occurs for a very long period of time, paranoia and hallucinations can occur. Other effects include overeating, hypersexuality, and increased susceptibility to viral infections (Davidhizar, Poole, & Giger, 1996; Turek & Zee, 1999). A period of 24 hours of wakefulness is equivalent to a blood alcohol level of 0.10% (Dawson & Reid, 1997) in terms of impaired cognitive and psychomotor skills. Even more frightening are the potential negative effects for patients. Taffinder, McManus, Russell, and Darzi (1998) found that surgeons who were sleep deprived committed 20% more errors and took approximately 14% longer to perform simulated surgery than when well rested.

There is no magic formula to guarantee a good night's sleep, but the following suggestions may improve the quality of your sleep life:

- Make sleep a priority. Make a conscious decision to obtain adequate sleep every night.
- Do not use caffeine as a stimulant to stay awake or alcohol as a tool to fall asleep.
- Try drinking warm milk or decaffeinated tea at bedtime. Establish a routine before bed that is repeated nightly.
- Reserve your bed only for sleeping. Watching television or doing paperwork in bed can cause sleepiness early and interfere with sleep patterns.
- If you are constantly thinking about work when in bed, keep a set of index cards near your bed. Write down any thoughts you have while in bed

CRITICAL THINKING

Keep a diary for 1 week of all that you eat, the type and amount of exercise you do and how many hours of sleep you get each night. See Figure 29-2 for a sample activity diary. At the end of the week, assess to see how well you have taken care of yourself. Is this a typical week? Do you need to make any changes? Were there any surprises? You can also record for several weeks and compare the outcomes.

	Breakfast	Lunch	Dinner	Snacks	Exercise Type/ Duration	Hours of Sleep
Monday						
Tuesday						
Wednesday						
Thursday						
Friday						
Saturday						
Sunday						

Figure 29-2 Sample Activity Diary

and then think about these ideas when you wake up, not while trying to fall asleep. (Davidhizar, Poole, & Giger, 1996; Ehrman, 1998)

Adequate sleep, good nutrition, and proper exercise all go hand in hand. When individuals are tired, they may eat more to compensate for the lack of sleep. Overeating can lead to unnecessary weight gain. And the weight gain, and fatigue can lead to a lack of exercise. Proper balance among the three is critical.

INTELLECTUAL HEALTH

Intellectual health is the second element of health and encompasses those activities that maintain intellectual curiosity. Intellectual health consists of the knowledge we accumulate and the ability to think. Intellectually healthy people are able to clearly process information and make sound decisions. They learn from experience and are flexible and remain open to new ideas. For purposes of this chapter, the term *intellectual health* also includes doing personal financial planning.

The first step in maintaining intellectual health is assessment. Table 29-3 contains an assessment tool for intellectual health; this tool is designed to assess trends only.

Intellectual Acuity

Just as it is important to find a type of exercise you are passionate about, so it is important to find some activity outside nursing that is of interest. The list is endless—antique shopping, reading, painting, sewing, photography, and so on. Develop a new hobby. Keep your mind sharp by staying abreast of developments within your interest area. Another way to maintain intellectual acuity is to establish and maintain a financial portfolio.

Personal Financial Planning

The first step in personal financial planning is to identify your annual salary. Mee and Carey (2000)

TABLE 29-3	Intellectual Health Assessment		
Question		**Yes**	**No**
1. I read at least one book a month.			
2. I have a hobby I enjoy.			
3. I belong to a club or organization.			
4. I have a 401K or 403b savings plan for retirement.			
5. I have invested in a mutual bond fund.			
6. I have invested in a mutual stock fund.			
7. I know how much money I have invested in Social Security.			
8. I have a money market account.			

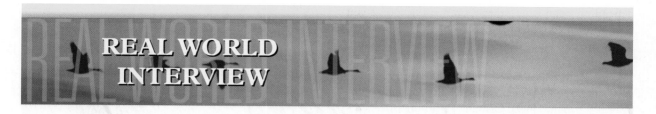

REAL WORLD INTERVIEW

The first savings option to consider as a new investor is either a 401K or the 403b. Your employer may contribute matching funds. Invest the maximum amount in this fund. Find a good high-growth fund and invest at least half of your savings here initially. If you don't have a 401K or 403b, invest in a Roth individual retirement account (Roth IRA). Other savings you may invest your money in are mutual funds and municipal bonds. I suggest investing in individual stocks only if you have some extra money. Investing in individual stocks can be risky.

Ron Rotondo
Investment Representative

surveyed 2,784 nurses throughout the country and found that the average salary for nurses with 5 or fewer years of experience was $33,054.00, and the mean starting wage was $15.41 per hour.

Next, begin to think about the percentage of your salary you want to save; most experts recommend 10% to 15%. There is no better time than now to invest in your future. Now is the time to begin saving for such things as a home, your children's education, and even retirement no matter what your age.

Savings for retirement are three-pronged: (1) Social Security funds, (2) employee retirement funds, and (3) additional personal savings.

Social Security

Social Security is automatically taken out of every paycheck by the federal government. The benefits from Social Security will not cover retirement expenses with today's projected life span. You will need other retirement money. You should annually check the accuracy of your Social Security account by reviewing the information sent to you by the Social Security Administration.

Employee Retirement Funds

The most common retirement funds are the 401K or 403b plans. The only difference between the two is that the 403b is a plan offered by a nonprofit organization and the 401K is offered by a for-profit organization. Otherwise, the two plans are exactly alike.

For purposes of this discussion, the term *401K* will be used.

Both the employee and employer contribute money to a 401K. This is a great way to save because many health care institutions will match the funds that you contribute. Once your money is put into the fund, it is tax sheltered, meaning you do not pay any taxes on the amount contributed until it is withdrawn. For example, if you earn $35,000 per year and contribute $3,500 to the 401K, you will be taxed on only $31,500 of income. If the money is withdrawn before you reach the age of $59^{1}/_{2}$, you will pay a 10% federal penalty. This is an incentive to keep the money in the account until retirement; the plan should be considered a long-term investment.

Once the money is in the fund, you must decide how the company administering the plan will invest it for you. You have two basic choices: bond mutual funds or stock mutual funds. Each of these investment opportunities has risks and benefits (Orman, 1997). Several reliable information sources rank these funds for quality. These include the annual ratings by *Consumer Reports* and the Morningstar ratings available through the Internet. (See "Exploring the Web" at the end of this chapter.)

Individual Retirement Account (IRA). Another type of retirement fund is the individual retirement account (IRA). This account is an option for anyone with sufficient employment income. Contributions cannot exceed $3,000 per year (for 2002). This fund may or may not be tax deductible, depending upon what other retirement accounts you hold and which type of IRA you open (Tyson, 2000). There are two kinds of IRAs: the traditional IRA and the Roth. The Roth IRA was first introduced in 1998. A Roth IRA is taxed prior to the investment but grows tax free and there is no penalty for early withdrawal (Orman, 1999). Orman (1999) highly recommends the Roth IRA and the 401K for investments.

Personal Savings Vehicles

After investing in retirement funds, you also have a few more options for investment. You can open a money market account. This is similar to a bank checking account, though it often requires a larger minimum amount of money to open the account. The interest rate is higher than that of a passbook savings account or a traditional bank checking account, and you have check-writing privileges. This is a place for money that you do not want to diminish in value (Tyson, 2000).

You also have the option to invest in stock mutual funds or bond mutual funds or individual stocks or individual bonds outside of your retirement account. You have the option of investing in individual stocks and bonds, but such an investment requires more research. You can start by reviewing Valueline at your local library (see "Exploring the Web" at the end of this chapter for Valueline). The key to successful investment is to diversify, meaning to spread your money around in many different types of investment options, stocks, bonds, mutual funds, and so on.

How to Educate Yourself

There are many ways to learn more about investments. Brokerage firms offer classes periodically. Try taking a course on personal finance at your junior college. You can also go to the Internet for advice (see "Exploring the Web" at the end of this chapter).

Another option is to hire a financial planner, but that can become expensive (Barker, 2000). The last suggestion is to read. Many of the books on the best-sellers list discuss personal finance. Suze Orman (1997) is an author that many find easy to understand and very relevant.

EMOTIONAL HEALTH

Emotional health is the third element of health. Our emotions express how we are feeling about an event. Emotions can be intense, and each emotion evokes a strong response. Our challenge as human beings is to acknowledge the emotion and then respond appropriately. It is important to have balance between our thought processes and the emotion we are feeling; otherwise, disharmony occurs. Emotions are what make us human. Truly, emotions are one of our greatest gifts and add spice to our lives (Dossey & Keegan, 2000).

Take a minute to assess your emotional state (Table 29-4); this tool is designed to assess trends only. The first step toward emotional health is acknowledgment of feelings.

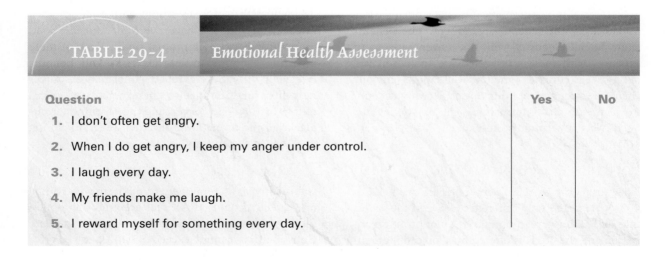

| TABLE 29-4 | Emotional Health Assessment |

Question	Yes	No
1. I don't often get angry.		
2. When I do get angry, I keep my anger under control.		
3. I laugh every day.		
4. My friends make me laugh.		
5. I reward myself for something every day.		

Anger

Anger is a common emotion that we all may feel. As a matter of fact, anger is pervasive in our society today. Peterson (2000) talks about road rage, airplane rage, outraged customers, and rage at youth sporting events. The causes for the anger are numerous and include rapid change in society, primarily the result of high technology; a lack of privacy, because we are accessible to work at all hours through cell phones and beepers; a sense of entitlement; a lack of family connection; and perhaps overcrowding.

There seems to be a spillover of anger into the nursing profession. Thomas (1998) has interviewed numerous staff nurses about anger at work. There are many causes for the nurses' anger: inadequate staffing and unreasonable workload, mismanagement of patients, lack of administrative support, demeaning treatment by other health care providers, feeling like scapegoats for mistakes within the system, and feeling powerless to influence difficult situations.

Ways to Cope with Anger

When confronted with an angry person, it is wise to think the problem through rationally and then respond in a calm manner. Grensing-Pophal (1998) recommends three steps in resolving conflict. First, listen attentively to the other person. Choose a quiet, private room where you will not be interrupted. Listen without bias and without mentally preparing your next response. Second, think about what the speaker has said as if you were a third party. Try to be objective and work out a solution that is agreeable to both parties. Third, respond without anger and work toward a resolution.

Sometimes anger and frustration are caused by sensory overload or overcommitment. It is important to have time for yourself. If nurses are to be effective caretakers, they first must care for themselves. Saying no, be it to a supervisor, friend, or family member, may at times be necessary. Learn to say no.

Humor

Laughter is the best medicine. Laughter has many benefits: it's free; it's a natural tranquilizer that is nonfattening and sodium free; and, best of all, it's contagious (Grensing-Pophal, 1998). Humor can also affect you physiologically. It can enhance the immune system and boost the cardiovascular and respiratory systems (Lannon, 2000). Laughter is a critical stress reliever (Figure 29-3).

Ways to Make You Laugh

Set a goal for yourself—not to let a day go by without a hearty laugh. Surround yourself with people who can joke about life. Read a humorous book; watch a funny television program or movie. See how many people you can get to smile in a day. Treat others at work to a little laughter. It is a great way to engender trust and teamwork. Laughter is not incongruent with dignity and respect. Appropriate humor with all coworkers, no matter what their position, can work wonders (Grensing-Pophal, 1999).

Stress Management

Many things can be done to relieve the emotional stress of life. See Table 29-5 for a few suggestions (Lannon, 2000; DeLaune, 1993).

If these suggestions do not help, there are other options. You can seek out professional counseling. And yes, sometimes nurses need a little extra help. You would be the first to call a counselor for a patient, so

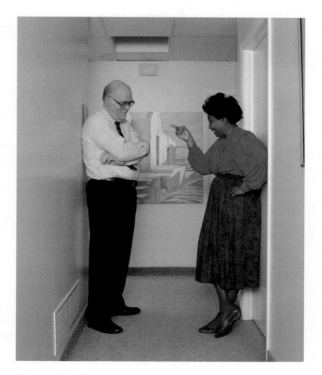

Figure 29-3 Laughter is an effective stress reliever.

TABLE 29-5 *Stress Relief Suggestions*

Meditate.	Do relaxation exercises.	Be polite to all.
Think peaceful thoughts.	Do something different for lunch.	Take a walk.
See things as others might.	Give yourself a pat on the back.	Read.
Forgive your mistakes.	Join a support group.	Join a club.
Do not procrastinate.	Talk about your worries.	Sing a song.
Set realistic goals.	Be affectionate.	Forgive and forget.
Do a good deed.	View problems as a challenge.	Listen to music.
Vary your routine.	Get/give a massage.	Take a hot bath.
Appreciate what you have.	Say a prayer.	Call an old friend.
Focus on the positive.	Expect to be successful.	Let go of the need to be perfect.

LITERATURE APPLICATION

Citation: Healy, C., & McKay, M. (1999). Identifying sources of stress and job satisfaction in the nursing environment. *Australian Journal of Advanced Nursing, 17*(2), 30–35.

Discussion: One hundred twenty-nine nurses from a large private hospital filled out questionnaires related to job stress and job satisfaction. The findings from the questions indicated that a burdensome workload was the nurses' primary concern followed by unclear treatment protocols, conflict with doctors, and dealing with dying patients. Sixty-six of the 129 who completed questionnaires also submitted written descriptions of stressful work situations. This subgroup of 66 nurses elaborated on situations not covered in the initial questionnaire. Conflict among the nursing staff was identified as the most stressful occurrence. The conflict among the staff was caused by the inexperience of some nurses, criticism from other nurses, concern regarding other nurses' practice, and lack of support. The second most commonly cited stressful circumstance was the enormous workload.

Implications for Practice: Nursing administration needs to be aware of the stress and workload of nurses. Providing nursing leaders with quantifiable data concerning nursing responsibilities is most helpful. Nurses are at risk for job burnout as a result of the intensity and duration of the stressors at work. A high level of stress may also affect the quality of patient care. Nurses need to address the staffing issues and continue to care for themselves.

why not help yourself? There are also employee assistance programs that can help. Ask your human resource department at work.

Avoiding Thought Distortions

Research on thinking processes has shown that people sometimes make mistakes in the way they perceive information and think about the world around them. When people are depressed, their automatic thoughts are loaded with distorted thinking. If one can recognize this distorted thinking (Table 29-6), one can begin to turn life in a more positive direction.

PROFESSIONAL HEALTH

Professional health is the fourth element of health. A person is professionally healthy when he is satisfied

with his career choice and thinks that there is continual opportunity for growth. The professionally healthy individual is goal directed and seeks every opportunity to obtain knowledge and new learning experiences. You can assess your professional health by using Table 29-7; this tool is designed to assess trends only.

Ways to Maintain Professional Health

There are numerous ways to continue to advance your career. Ask yourself where you want to be 5, 10, and 15 years from now. If you do not have an overall plan, work can become very monotonous.

It is important to seek out others within the health care field. Find a more experienced nurse you can relate to or who can act as a mentor. This nurse can provide guidance and support when problems arise. Network with other nurses and health care professionals. You can learn an enormous amount from

---

TABLE 29-6   *Thought Distortions*

Thought distortion	Example
All-or-nothing thinking: seeing things only in absolutes	If I leave this job, no one will respect me.
Overgeneralization: interpreting every small setback as a never-ending pattern of defeat	Everyone here is so smart; I'm a real loser.
Dwelling on negatives: ignoring multiple positive experiences	I made a mistake. I'm not good enough to be a nurse.
Jumping to conclusions: assuming that others are reacting negatively without definite evidence	I don't know why I study. Everyone thinks I'm going to fail the NCLEX anyway.
Pessimism: automatically predicting that things will turn out badly	It's only a matter of time before everything falls apart for me.
Reasoning from feeling: thinking that if one feels bad, one must be bad.	My head hurts because I'm a bad person.
Obligations: living life around a succession of too many "shoulds," "shouldn'ts," "musts," "oughts," and "have-tos."	I should marry Joe. Everyone likes him.

TABLE 29-7	*Professional Health Assessment*		
Question		**Yes**	**No**
1. I have professional goals.			
2. I have a mentor.			
3. I have attended at least three workshops in the past year.			
4. I subscribe to three nursing journals.			
5. I belong to at least one professional organization.			
6. I use appropriate personal protective equipment.			
7. I never recap a needle.			
8. I use good body mechanics when transferring patients.			
9. I follow standards of care when handling gaseous waste, disinfectants, and chemotherapy.			
10. I follow standards of care in dealing with radiation equipment.			

others. Keep in touch with some of your favorite faculty members. They will enjoy hearing from you and can also offer useful advice. Join at least one professional organization. Attend as many workshops and professional meetings as possible. Many of these presentations may be paid for by your employer. After attending professional conferences, do not forget to apply for continuing education units (CEUs).

Read as often as possible. If questions arise at work, come home and look up the information in your books or on the Internet, or go to the medical library. Subscribe to at least three professional journals related to your specialty area (Kimmel, 1998).

Occupational Hazards Common among Nurses

An important aspect of professional health is avoidance of occupational hazards. The U.S. Bureau of Labor Statistics (1999) states that the incidence of nonfatal occupational injuries and illnesses for 1999 was 7.5 per 100 full-time workers for those employed in health care facilities. This is the second highest rate of occupational injury among workers employed in the service industry. Nurses are at risk for injury on the job.

There are numerous suggestions for safeguarding against various hazards in the workplace. For purposes of discussion, occupational hazards can be divided into four major categories: (1) infectious agents, (2) environmental agents, (3) physical agents, and (4) chemical agents.

Infectious Agents

Infectious agents are transmitted either through direct contact with an infected patient or by contamination with body fluids or secretions (Rogers, 1997). The major infectious agents are HIV, herpes, tuberculosis, and hepatitis. Needle-stick injuries account for about 80% to 90% of the transmissions of infectious diseases among health care workers. The chance of a seroconversion (a serological test in which antibodies change from a negative reading to a positive one) to HIV is about 1 in every 278 contaminated needles. There is a 0.3% risk for infection after exposure to the HIV virus. The risk for hepatitis B is as high as 30% after one needle-stick exposure, whereas hepatitis C carries only a 1% to 10% risk of transmission after a needle injury (Davis, August, & Salome, 1999).

Although the majority of infectious agents are transmitted through blood, herpes simplex virus can be transmitted by direct contact with an infected lesion. Varicella-zoster, commonly called shingles, is transmitted through respiratory droplets. Hepatitis A is transmitted primarily via diarrhea as a result of poor hygienic practices among health care workers. The incidence of tuberculosis has been decreasing, especially since 1983. The Centers for Disease Control and Prevention (2000) reported an 8.1% decline in reported cases between 1997 and 1998 and a 5.9% decline between 1998 and 1999. See Table 29-8 for safeguards for occupational hazards.

Environmental Agents

Another group of occupational hazards is environmental agents. These include all those agents within the hospital that may lead to injury. The most prevalent include violence, shift work, air quality, and mold and fungus. Nurses are at risk for workplace violence. Carroll (1999) surveyed 586 nurses from seven states and found that 32% of the respondents had been victims of violence at work. Of the 32% of the nurses attacked, 72% were staff nurses.

Poor air quality in the workplace is yet another environmental risk that may lead to symptoms such as shortness of breath, eye and nose irritation, headaches, contact dermatitis, joint pain, memory problems, and reproductive difficulties. Two common contributors to poor air quality are glutaraldehyde, a

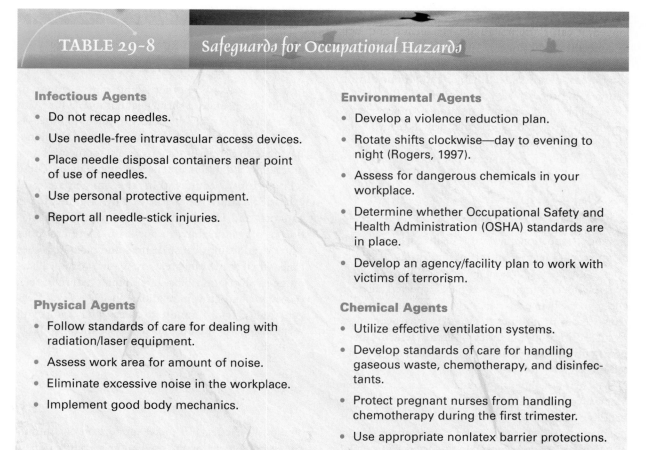

TABLE 29-8 *Safeguards for Occupational Hazards*

Infectious Agents

- Do not recap needles.
- Use needle-free intravascular access devices.
- Place needle disposal containers near point of use of needles.
- Use personal protective equipment.
- Report all needle-stick injuries.

Physical Agents

- Follow standards of care for dealing with radiation/laser equipment.
- Assess work area for amount of noise.
- Eliminate excessive noise in the workplace.
- Implement good body mechanics.

Environmental Agents

- Develop a violence reduction plan.
- Rotate shifts clockwise—day to evening to night (Rogers, 1997).
- Assess for dangerous chemicals in your workplace.
- Determine whether Occupational Safety and Health Administration (OSHA) standards are in place.
- Develop an agency/facility plan to work with victims of terrorism.

Chemical Agents

- Utilize effective ventilation systems.
- Develop standards of care for handling gaseous waste, chemotherapy, and disinfectants.
- Protect pregnant nurses from handling chemotherapy during the first trimester.
- Use appropriate nonlatex barrier protections.
- Develop policies and procedures to ensure safety from latex allergies.

chemical used to disinfect many commonly used instruments, and laser plume smoke, which is emitted after laser treatment (Wilburn, 1999). Air quality can also be influenced by mold and fungus, which are often found in carpeting and in ceiling tiles. The presence of mold and fungus can lead to asthma and other respiratory problems.

Physical Agents

Physical agents are another occupational hazard and include radiation, noise, and back strain. Radiation exposure is common among health care workers. Radiation is used for both diagnostic and treatment interventions. Overexposure has been linked to cancer and reproductive disorders (Rogers, 1997). Laser treatment carries the risk of eye and skin injury if the instruments are not handled properly. Noise is another physical hazard that can lead to hearing loss. Further, if exposure to noise is excessive and prolonged, it can cause irritability, headaches, and lack of concentration (Rogers, 1997). Special care units are especially noisy with alarms, ventilators, suction equipment, monitors, call lights, and so on. Lifting patients improperly is yet another risk factor for nurses. The most common method of transfer is to grip the patient under the axilla, which places force on the lifter's lumbar-sacral area (Owen, 1999). Lifting a load too large or using poor body mechanics may exacerbate the situation.

Chemical Agents

Another occupational hazard is chemical agents such as anesthetic agents, antineoplastic drugs, disinfectants, and latex gloves. Those health care workers exposed to anesthetic gases have reported adverse effects to the hepatic, renal, nervous, and immune systems. Exposure to anesthetic gases may occur as a result of improperly inflated endotracheal tubes, poorly fitting oxygen masks, or gas lines that are fitted incorrectly (Rogers, 1997).

Chemotherapeutic agents also raise concerns. Valanis, Vollmer, and Steele (1999) found that nurses handling antineoplastics during their first trimester of pregnancy were at greater risk for spontaneous abortion than nurses not exposed to the drugs. Partners of male nurses handling these same drugs had a similar pattern of miscarriage; however, it was not statistically significant. Nurses exposed to chemotherapy have cited the following symptoms: light-headedness, nasal sores, alopecia, flushing, decreased white blood cells, and rashes (Rogers, 1997).

Disinfectants are chemical agents that are of concern to nurses. Besides the gaseous effects of glutaraldehyde, which were discussed earlier, glutaraldehyde can also cause skin problems. Ethylene oxide, a chemical commonly used to sterilize surgical equipment, has been reported to have carcinogenic effects.

Latex glove exposure is the last type of chemical concern for nurses. It has been reported that approximately 8% to 12% of health care workers are allergic to latex (Worthington, 1999). Reactions to latex range from a simple contact dermatitis to a more systemic reaction to an anaphylactic crisis. This reaction is caused by an increased sensitivity to the proteins found in the natural rubber of latex gloves (Rogers, 1997).

SOCIAL HEALTH

Social health is another significant element of health. The essence of social health is interacting with other people. Having the ability to relate to others is essential for life. Few can survive completely alone. We relate to people at various levels—some we know intimately and others are mere acquaintances. These relationships occur within the immediate and extended family; at work; and within the local, national, and international community. These relationships give meaning to our lives. There are times when relationships cause distress and pain and other times when they bring great joy. We strive toward harmony in all relationships. It is human nature to seek out others and grow in relationships (Dossey & Keegan, 2000). Take a minute to assess your status with relationships by taking the self-assessment in Table 29-9; this tool is designed to assess trends only.

Impact of Social Relationships

The positive effects of social support on health outcomes have been documented in the literature (Chesney & Darbes, 1998). If these interactions are frequent, that only adds to good health. In other words, the more you see your friends, the healthier

TABLE 29-9	Social Health Assessment	Yes	No
Question			
1. I go out with my friends at least once a week.			
2. I see my family at least twice a month.			
3. I have one friend I can confide in.			
4. I have some friends who are very different from me.			
5. Not all of my friends are nurses.			
6. I do volunteer work.			

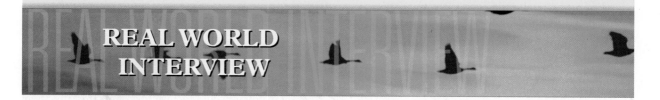

REAL WORLD INTERVIEW

I try to integrate my personal and professional life by organizing and prioritizing at the beginning of each day. Each night I outline with my family who needs to be where and how my husband and I will get the children to their various activities. In this way, I know my family will be taken care of during the day while I am at work. My family is my first priority. I view my social life in much the same manner. What needs to be accomplished today and how will I go about achieving this?

I organize my professional life every morning before I officially begin my day. I ask myself what are the issues that most need my attention today. Each Friday is "turnaround time." I assess the events of the week and determine all the good things that I did and those things that I could improve upon. I make sure I reward myself for the positives. I encourage all my managers to implement this weekly method of evaluation.

I have also developed a competency-based checklist for my managers. This is a tool that I use to continually assess and guide improvement of the managers. The tool outlines communication, leadership, decision making, interpersonal skills, just to name a few. I may begin by going over the assessment areas weekly and gradually taper the time needed to teach and assess the managers. Once the manager has mastered an area, there is no longer a need to use the tool. It is my goal for the managers to exhibit competency in all areas.

Another way that I try to keep balance in my life is to work hard and play hard. I make sure that I have fun on my weekends. It is important that I have humor in my life on a daily basis. My staff can laugh at me and I at them. This is healthy and a great stress reliever. Family and friends are very important to me. I try to incorporate family and friends into my daily life.

Corinne Haviley, RN, MS
Director, Ambulatory Care Services

you become. The variety of those relationships may also keep you healthy. The greater the diversity of the relationships, such as professional, family, neighborhood, or church relationships, the more likely you are to remain healthy.

Try to interact with friends in person as often as possible. Cell phones and e-mail are helpful forms of communication, but nothing is more effective than face-to-face conversation. Be careful, though, to stay away from negative relationships and people who do not treat you well. Sometimes it is difficult to end a friendship, but if the relationship is destructive, it may be in your best interest to end it.

Another way to build relationships is through rituals. For example, celebrate Christmas with friends by seeing *The Nutcracker* or play tennis with a friend once a week. But do not forget about your friends of the past. Phone a friend from the past or contact a family member you have argued with (Hallowell, 2000).

Finally, another way to establish friendships is through volunteerism. For example, join the American Red Cross as a disaster volunteer or pursue another activity that you find rewarding. It is also a good way to be aware of community issues.

SPIRITUAL HEALTH

Spiritual health, the last element of health, is the ability to find strength from within. This strength results from a connection with a higher being or power (Chilton, 1998). It is through our spirituality that we find meaning in life. It is the essence behind how we live our lives. It also is a piece of our lives that needs attention and development. You can determine what your spiritual needs are by answering the questions in Table 29-10; this tool is designed to assess trends only.

Religion and Health

Koenig (1999) has extensively researched religion and health. His findings lend some scientific support to the positive effects of prayer and religious involvement. Koenig (1999) found that older adults who are religiously active (based on attendance at religious services) are more physically fit and live longer than those who are less religious. It appears that prayer does have a positive impact on health outcomes. See the "Suggested Readings" for other resources on spirituality.

DECISION MAKING

Every day we make decisions. There are some days when we may decide to care for others and put their needs before our own. But there are still other days when we need to care for and nurture ourselves. The decision is always up to us. These decisions are often complicated and difficult to make. The goal of this chapter has been to provide you with some thoughts that will guide your decisions concerning your health.

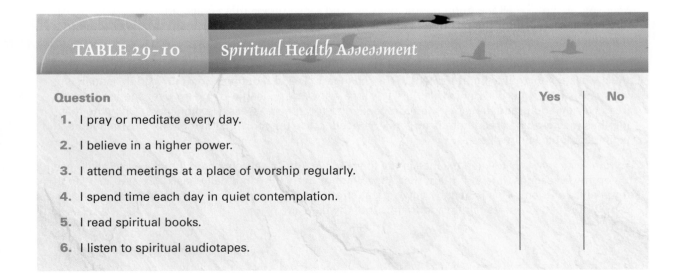

TABLE 29-10 *Spiritual Health Assessment*

Question	Yes	No
1. I pray or meditate every day.		
2. I believe in a higher power.		
3. I attend meetings at a place of worship regularly.		
4. I spend time each day in quiet contemplation.		
5. I read spiritual books.		
6. I listen to spiritual audiotapes.		

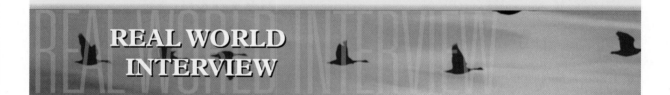

CRITICAL THINKING

Take a minimum of 10 minutes to sit and think about the day's activities. Make sure you are comfortable and will not be interrupted by any outside stimuli. Ask yourself what was good about the day and what might have been improved. What can you learn from today's events? If you choose the early morning as a time of reflection, you can also use this time to plan your day. It is a time for relaxation just for you. Try reading some inspirational passages (see the Suggested Readings for some ideas). Or you might find soaking in the bathtub to be the best alternative. No matter how busy you become, do not forget to save time for yourself. The busier you become, the more important it is to take time to reflect and relax. Be good to you!

REAL WORLD INTERVIEW

I have learned a lot in the 9 months that I have practiced nursing. I used to say yes to overtime each time when asked. I thought I needed the experience and that I owed it to the staff. I have since learned to say no. I have also learned that I need to take care of me. I used to come home and eat a lot and fall into bed. I gained weight and felt awful. Now I either go for a walk or to the health club after work. I volunteer at my church youth organization part time whenever I can. I have also developed my own routine in delivering patient care. I am better organized and leave on time. I have gained more confidence in my clinical decisions. For example, I had a patient who I thought should not be extubated from the ventilator. I tried to voice my opinion to the resident on call but was overridden by the attending physician. The charge nurse was also supportive of keeping the patient intubated. As it turned out, the patient was extubated for a half-hour and then reintubated. I felt bad for the unnecessary procedure for the patient, but it did boost my confidence. I know now that in the future, I will be even more assertive with physicians concerning the welfare of my patients.

When I am scared in a clinical situation, I try not to let fear paralyze me. I try to think everything through logically. I have found that the better I understand what I am doing, the better nurse I become. I'm always trying to learn new things. I've been to about five seminars this year and I subscribe to three nursing journals. I want to learn as much as I can.

Nayiri M. Birazian, RN
New Staff Nurse

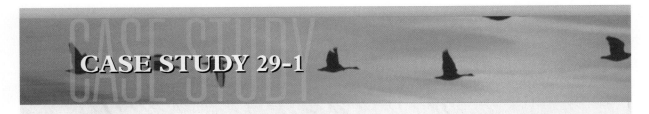

CASE STUDY 29-1

You have been working for a home health agency for about 1 year now. One of your best friends at work, another nurse, asks your advice about how to maintain a healthier lifestyle. She states she is 10 pounds overweight and does not really exercise much. She says she feels like all she does is work and come home and go to sleep. She says she does not have fun in life anymore. She states that college life is great compared to all the stress at work.

What advice would you give your friend about how to stay healthy? What would your first priority be in offering advice? What other major areas of consideration would you explore with your friend?

KEY CONCEPTS

- To provide quality patient care, nurses need to first take care of themselves and maintain a healthy lifestyle.
- Health is not just the absence of disease, it is the state of complete balance of physical, intellectual, emotional, professional, social, and spiritual well-being.
- The ability to care for yourself consists of multiple dimensions that overlap and interact constantly. If one dimension is affected, all dimensions are affected.
- Nurses' physical health encompasses good nutrition, proper exercise, and adequate sleep.
- Intellectual health is the ability to maintain mental acuity. It is important to keep current in both professional and personal arenas.
- An important piece of intellectual health is adequate financial planning. Now is the time to begin saving.
- Emotional health includes laughter, an essential ingredient of healthy living.
- Maintaining many different types of relationships helps to keep you healthy.
- Spiritual well-being—the ability to relate to a higher being—is another essential element of good health. Spirituality needs to be continually nurtured, as do our friendships.
- To stay healthy, you must make a conscious decision to maintain each area of health. The choice is yours.

KEY TERMS

emotional health
401K
403b
health
intellectual health
money market account

physical health
professional health
Roth IRA
social health
spiritual health
traditional IRA

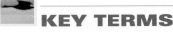

REVIEW QUESTIONS

1. Nurses who sustain a needle-stick injury are at greatest risk for which of the following infections?
   A. Hepatitis A
   B. HIV
   C. Hepatitis B
   D. Hepatitis C

2. Glutaraldehyde, a common disinfectant used to clean instruments, can cause all of the following symptoms EXCEPT
   A. contact dermatitis.
   B. difficulty breathing.
   C. anorexia.
   D. eye and nose irritation.

3. You have $1,000 that you would like to deposit into an account. Which of the following would offer the highest interest rate with the greatest flexibility in accessing the money?
   A. Money market account
   B. Passbook savings account

C. Traditional bank checking account
D. Traditional IRA

4. The optimal method for rotating shifts to decrease fatigue is
A. rotate clockwise.
B. rotate counterclockwise.
C. rotate nights to days only.
D. rotate evenings to days only.

REVIEW ACTIVITIES

1. Try doing a short relaxation exercise. Take a deep breath in and let it out. Take slow, deep breaths that originate from the diaphragm. Tighten the muscles in your right arm for 30 seconds and release. Your arm should feel totally limp and relaxed. Do the same with your left arm. Tighten the muscles in your right leg for 30 seconds and release. Repeat with the left leg. Pull in your stomach muscles for 30 seconds and release. Tighten the muscles in your buttocks and release. Continue to breathe in and out deeply. You can practice this brief exercise anytime or anywhere. If you are having a particularly hectic day, take a minute to do a relaxation exercise. You can vary the exercise by flexing any group of muscles you want.

2. Your best friend is getting married next month, and you are the maid of honor. You have been invited to a shower to be held out of town in honor of your friend this next weekend. You have already purchased a nonrefundable airline ticket to attend the shower. You work in a very small intensive care unit. You have been working 10- and 12-hour shifts and are near exhaustion. Your head nurse calls you 2 days before you are to leave for the shower and asks you to work the weekend. One of the staff has been involved in a serious car accident, and there is no one else to work. What would you do?

    If you work this weekend, you would disappoint your best friend and lose the money for your ticket. You are already exhausted and you do not know how effective you would be at work. You know you need the break.

    If you do not work, you would be letting the rest of the staff down. They have been there for you, and now it is your turn to help them. You find it very hard to say no. You are a young nurse and you should "pay your dues." How could you relax when you know that you are needed elsewhere?

3. You were recently hired to help set up a nurse-managed clinic in the community. You need to order all the supplies and equipment.

    What equipment and supplies do you need to keep in mind to protect you and your staff from contracting any infectious diseases?

EXPLORING THE WEB

- Calculate your BMI and determine your life expectancy and health risks at *http://www.healthstatus.com*.

- Try one of the following sites to retrieve information on dietary supplements, nutrition, and alternative medicine:
  http://www.nutritionsite.com
  http://www.alternativemedicine.com
  http://www.homeopathic.net

- Go to *http://www.mpowercafe.com* for information on a 401K.

- Dugas (1999) recommends two web sites for retirement information: Quicken.com (*http://www.quicken.com/retirement/planner*) and Charles Schwab (*http://www.schwab.com* and click on *Retirement Planning*). Various investment firms also have retirement information at their web sites.

- Fidelity Investments: *http://www300.fidelity.com*. Click on *Retirement Center* and follow the different retirement options.

- Vanguard: *http://www.vanguard.com*. Click on *Personal Investors* and then click on the *Planning & Advice* tab, where you will find basic retirement planning information.

- Valueline: *http://www.valueline.com*. Click on *What's New? Retirement Planners*.

- Morningstar: *http://www.morningstar.com*. Click on *Retirement*.

Resources for Violence Prevention:

- The ANA's Workplace Violence: Can You Close the Door? Call (800) 274-4ANA *http://www.nursingworld.org/dlwa/osh/violence.htm*

- Guidelines for Preventing Workplace Violence for Healthcare and Social Service Workers. U.S. Department of Labor, OSHA 3148-1996, available on-line: *http://www.osha-slc.gov/SLTC/ workplaceviolence/guideline.html*

- Violence Potential Assessment Tool. Contact Victoria Carroll at (970) 416-6811.

Resources for Needle Sticks

General resource links: *http://www.medamicus. com/resources.asp*

- Safer Needle Devices: Protecting Health Care Workers
  http://www.osha-slc.gov/SLTC/needlestick/ saferneedledevices/saferneedledevices.html
- American Nurses Association *http://www. nursingworld.org/needlestick/nshome.htm*
- Centers for Disease Control and Prevention *http://www.cdc.gov/health/needlesticks.htm*

Resources for Latex Allergy

- ANA's position paper on Latex Allergy
  http://www.nursingworld.org/readroom/ position/workplac/wklatex.htm
  or call (800) 274-4ANA
- OSHA *http://www.osha-slc.gov/SLTC/ latexallergy/*

Resource for Back Strain

- Occupational Safety and Health Administration's ergonomics information
  http://www.osha-slc.gov/SLTC/ergonomics Call (202) 693-1999.

REFERENCES

Barker, R. (2000, January 24). A small price to pay for retirement. *Business Week,* 183–184.

Carroll, V. (1999). Workplace violence. *American Journal of Nursing, 99*(3), 60.

Centers for Disease Control and Prevention. (2000). *Reported tuberculosis in the United States, 1999.* Retrieved January 20, 2002, from http://www.cdc. gov/nchstp/tb/surv/surv99/surv99.htm

Chesney, M., & Darbes, L. (1998). Social support and heart disease in women: Implications for intervention. In K. Orth-Gomer, M. Chesnye, & N. K. Wenger (Eds.), *Women, stress and heart disease* (pp. 165–182). Mahwah, NJ: Erlbaum.

Chilton, B. (1998). Recognizing spirituality. *Image: Journal of Nursing Scholarship, 30*(4), 400–401.

Davidhizar, R., Poole, V. L., & Giger, J. N. (1996). Power nap rejuvenates body, mind. *Pennsylvania Nurse, 51*(3), 6–7.

Davis, G., August, S., & Salome, R. (1999). Nurses at risk call to mobilize. *American Journal of Nursing, 99*(5), 44–46.

Dawson, D., & Reid, K. (1997). Fatigue, alcohol and performance impairment. *Nature, 338*(6639), 235.

DeLaune, S. C. (1993). Learned optimism. *Aspen's Advisor for the Nurse Executive, 8*(11), 8.

Dossey, B. M., & Keegan, L. (2000). Self-assessments: Facilitating healing in self and others. In B. M. Dossey, L. Keegan, C. E. Guzzetta, & L. G. Kolkmeier (Eds.), *Holistic nursing: A handbook for practice* (pp. 361–374). Gaithersburg, MD: Aspen.

Dugas, C. (1999, December 3). Retirement calculators figure it out. *USA Today,* 3B.

Ehrman, J. (1998, June). A good night's sleep? Merely a dream for millions. *The NIH Word on Health.* Retrieved January 20, 2002, from www.nih.gov/ news/WordonHealth/jun98/story02.htm#TOP

Grensing-Pophal, L. (1998). Resolving conflicts: It's as easy as 1-2-3. *Nursing98, 28*(9), 63.

Grensing-Pophal, L. (1999). Multi-tasking made easy. *Nursing99, 29*(2), 55–56.

Hallowell, E. (2000). Strong relationships really do help ensure good health. *Bottom Line Health, 14*(2), 3–4.

Healy, C., & McKay, M. (1999). Identifying sources of stress and job satisfaction in the nursing environment. *Australian Journal of Advanced Nursing, 17*(2), 30–35.

Kimmel, L. (1998). Just got your pin? *Nursing98, 28*(5), 63.

Koenig, H. G. (1999). The healing power of faith. *Annals of Long-Term Care, 7*(10), 381–384.

Lannon, P. (2000, April 27). Laughter, fun is key to combating stress. *The Doings Newspapers,* 63.

Maraldo, P. (1999). *Women's health for dummies.* Chicago: IDG Books Worldwide.

McWilliam, C. L., Spence Laschinger, H. K., & Weston, W. (1999). Health promotion amongst nurses and physicians: What is the human experience? *American Journal of Health Behavior, 23*(2), 95–103.

Mee, C. L., & Carey, K. (2000). Salary survey. *Nursing2000, 30*(4), 58–61.

Miller, J. (1998). *Healing centers and retreats.* Santa Fe, NM: John Muir Publications.

National Institute of Health (n.d.). *Body mass index calculator.* Retrieved February 2, 2002, from http:// www.nhlbi.nih.gov/guidelines/obesity/bmi_tbl.htm

Nelson, M. (1997). *Strong women stay young.* New York: Bantam Books.

Nightingale, F. (1969). *Notes on nursing.* New York: Dover. (Original work published 1860.)

Orman. S. (1997). *The 9 steps to financial freedom.* New York: Crown.

Orman, S. (1999). *The courage to be rich: Creating a life of material and spiritual abundance.* New York: Riverhead Books.

Owen, B. D. (1999). Preventing back injuries. *American Journal of Nursing, 99*(5), 76.

Pender, N. (1996). *Health promotion in nursing practice.* Norwalk, CT: Appleton & Lange.

Peterson, K. (2000, July 18). Why is everyone so short-tempered. *USA Today,* 1A.

Random House Webster's unabridged dictionary. (1998). New York: Random House.

Rogers, B. (1997). Health hazards in nursing and health care: An overview. *American Journal of Infection Control, 25*(3), 248–261.

Roy, C., & Andrews, H. A. (1999). *The Roy adaptation model.* Stamford, CT: Appleton & Lange.

Taffinder, H. J., McManus, I. C., Russell, R. C. G., & Darzi, A. (1998). Effect of sleep deprivation on surgeons' dexterity on laparoscopy simulator. *The Lancet, 352,* 1191.

Thomas, S. P. (1998). *Transforming nurses' anger and pain: Steps toward healing.* New York: Springer.

Turek, F. W., & Zee, P. C. (1999). *Regulation of sleep and circadian rhythms.* New York: Marcel Dekker.

Tyson, E. (2000). *Personal finance for dummies.* Chicago: IDG Books Worldwide.

U.S. Bureau of Labor Statistics. (1999, December). *Workplace injury and illness summary.* Retrieved April 30, 2002, from www.bls.gov/iif/

U.S. Department of Health and Human Services. (2001). *Healthy People 2010: Goals.* Retrieved January 2, 2002, from http://www.health.gov/healthypeople/LHI/lhiwhat.htm

Valanis, B., Vollmer, W. M., & Steele, P. (1999). Occupational exposure to antineoplastic agents: Self-reported miscarriages and stillbirths among nurses and pharmacists. *Journal of Occupational and Environmental Medicine, 41*(8), 632–638.

Wilburn, S. (1999). Is the air in your hospital making you sick? *American Journal of Nursing. 99*(7), 71.

Wilson, H. (2000). Check out the wellness resolution. *ASNA Reporter, 27*(1), 9.

World Health Organization. (1998). *Health education and promotion.* Retrieved January 19, 2002, from http://www.who.int/m/topics/health_education_promotion/en/indes.html.

Worthington, K. (1999). Toward a latex-safe workplace. *American Journal of Nursing, 99*(11), 71.

SUGGESTED READINGS

Battaglia, C. (1996). *Murmurs.* Long Branch, NJ: Vista.

Battaglia, C. (1997). *Jagged rhythms.* Long Branch, NJ: Vista.

Battaglia, C. (1999). *Drifting among the whales.* Long Branch, NJ: Vista.

Benson, H. (2000). *The relaxation response.* New York: Avon Books.

Boston Women's Health Book Collective. (1998). *Our bodies, ourselves for the new century.* New York: Simon & Schuster.

Breathmach, S. B. (1995). *Simple abundance.* New York: Time Warner.

Chopra, D. (2000). *How to know God.* New York: Harvey Books.

Cox, S. H. (1998). Nixing fix-it syndrome. *Nursing Management, 29*(7), 56.

Greene, B., & Winfrey, O. (1996). *Making the connection.* New York: Hyperion.

Grensing-Pophal, L. (1999). Multitasking made easy. *Nursing99, 29*(2), 55–56.

Haluska, J. (1996). Speak up! Are you getting your ZZZZ's? *RN, 59*(10), 72.

Harris, M. (1991). *Dance of the spirit: The seven steps of women's spirituality.* New York: Bantam Books.

Holzer, B. (2000). *Set for life: Financial peace for people over 50.* New York: Wiley.

Kingma, D. R., & Markova, D. M. (1993). *Random acts of kindness.* Berkeley, CA: Conari Press.

Kobat-Zinn, J. (1994). *Wherever you go, there you are.* New York: Hyperion.

Louden, J. (2000). *The comfort queen's guide to life.* New York: Harmony Books.

Lunden, J. (1997). *Healthy living.* New York: Crown.

Phillips, B., & D'Orso, M. (1999). *Body-for-life.* New York: HarperCollins.

Presley, D. & Robinson, G. (2002). Violence in the Emergency Department. *Nursing Clinic of North America, 37*(1), 161–169.

Redfield, S. M. (1999). *Creating a life of joy: A meditative guide.* New York: Time Warner Trade Publishing.

Richardson, C. (1999). *Take time for your life.* New York: Broadway Books.

Ruiz, D. M. (1999). *The four agreements.* San Rafael, CA: Amber-Allen.

Rupp, J. (1998). *The cup of our life; a guide to spiritual growth.* Notre Dame, IN: Ave Maria Press.

Shriver, M. (2000). *Ten things I wish I'd known.* New York: Time Warner.

Stein, M. K. (1998). *The prosperous retirement.* Boulder, CO, Emstco Press.

Survival of the fittest. (2001). *Consumer Reports, 66*(3), 32–36.

Weil, A. (1997). *Eight weeks to optimum health.* New York: Knopf.

Wright, J., & Basco, M. (2001). *Getting your life back: The complete guide to recovery from depression.* New York: Free Press.

Zukav, G. (1999). *The seat of the soul.* New York: Simon & Schuster.

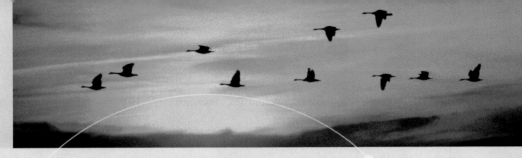

APPENDIX A

Preparation for NCLEX

A new graduate from an educational program that prepares registered nurses will take the NCLEX, the national nursing licensure examination prepared under the supervision of the National Council of State Boards of Nursing. NCLEX is taken after graduation and prior to practice as a registered nurse. The examination is given across the United States. Graduates submit their credentials to the state board of nursing in the state in which licensure is desired. Once the state board accepts the graduate's credentials, the graduate can schedule the examination. This examination ensures a basic level of safe registered nursing practice to the public. The examination follows a test plan formulated on four categories of client needs that registered nurses commonly encounter. The concepts of the nursing process, caring, communication, cultural awareness, documentation, self-care, and teaching/learning are integrated throughout the four major categories of client needs (Table A-1).

TOTAL NUMBER OF QUESTIONS ON NCLEX

Graduates may receive anywhere from 75 to 265 questions on the NCLEX examination during their testing session. Fifteen of the questions are questions that are being piloted to determine their validity for use in future NCLEX examinations. Students cannot determine whether they passed or failed the NCLEX examination from the number of questions they receive during their session. There is no time limit for each question, and the maximum time for the examination is 5 hours. A 10-minute break is mandatory after 2 hours of testing. An optional 10-minute break may be taken after another 90 minutes of testing.

Each test question has a test item and four possible answers. If the student answers the question correctly, a slightly more difficult item will follow, and the

TABLE A-1 NCLEX Test Plan: Client Needs

Client Needs Tested	Percent of Test Questions
Safe, effective care environment:	
Management of care	7–13%
Safety and infection control	5–11%
Physiologic integrity:	
Basic care and comfort	7–13%
Pharmacological and parenteral therapies	5–11%
Reduction of risk potential	12–18%
Physiological adaptation	12–18%
Psychosocial integrity:	
Coping and adaptation	5–11%
Psychosocial adaptation	5–11%
Health promotion and maintenance:	
Growth and development through the life span	7–13%
Prevention and early detection of disease	5–11%

level of difficulty will increase with each item until the candidate misses an item. If the student misses an item, a slightly less difficult item will follow, and the level of difficulty will decrease with each item until the student has answered an item correctly. This process continues until the student has achieved a definite passing or definite failing score. The least number of questions a student can take to complete the exam is 75. Fifteen of these questions will be pilot questions, and they will not count toward the student's score. The other 60 questions will determine the student's score on the NCLEX.

RISK FACTORS FOR NCLEX PERFORMANCE

Several factors have been identified as being associated with performance on the NCLEX examination. Some of these factors are identified in Table A-2.

REVIEW BOOKS AND COURSES

In preparing to take the NCLEX, the new graduate may find it useful to review several of the many NCLEX review books on the market. These review books often include a review of nursing content, or sample test questions, or both. They frequently include computer software disks with test questions for review. The test questions may be arranged in the review book by clinical content area, or they may be presented in one or more comprehensive examinations covering all areas of the NCLEX. Listings of these review books are available at *www.amazon.com*. It is helpful to use several of these books and computer software when reviewing for the NCLEX.

NCLEX review courses are also available. Brochures advertising these programs are often sent to schools and are available in many sites nationwide. The quality of these programs can vary, and students may want to ask former nursing graduates and faculty for recommendations.

TABLE A-2	*Factors Associated with NCLEX Performance*
• HESI Exit Exam	• High school rank and GPA
• Mosby Assesstest	• Undergraduate nursing program GPA
• NLN Comprehensive Achievement test	• GPA in science and nursing theory courses
• NLN achievement tests taken at end of each nursing course	• Competency in American English language
• Verbal SAT score	• Reasonable family responsibilities or demands
• ACT score	• Absence of emotional distress
	• Critical thinking competency

THE NLN EXAMINATION AND THE HESI EXIT EXAM

Many nursing programs administer an examination to students at the completion of their nursing program. Two of these exams are the NLN Achievement test and the HESI Exit Exam. New graduates will want to review their performance on any of these exams because these results will help identify their weaknesses and help focus their review sessions.

Students who examine their feedback from the NLN examination or the HESI Exit Exam have important information that can help them focus their review for the NCLEX. A strategy for examining this feedback and organizing this review is outlined in the following section.

ORGANIZING YOUR REVIEW

In preparing for NCLEX, identify your strengths and weaknesses. If you have taken the NLN examination or the HESI Exit Exam, note any content strength and weakness areas. Additionally, note any nursing program course or clinical content areas in which you scored below a grade of B. Purchase one or more of the NCLEX review books. It is useful to review questions developed by different authors. Review content in the review books in any of your weak content areas. Take a comprehensive exam in the review book or on the computer software disk and analyze your performance. Try to answer as many questions correctly as you can. Be sure to actually practice taking the examinations. Do not just jump ahead to look at the section on correct answers and rationales before answering the questions if you want to improve your examination performance.

Next, once you have completed the comprehensive examination, review the answers and rationales for any weak content areas and take another comprehensive exam. Repeat this process until you are doing well in all clinical content areas and in all areas of the NCLEX examination plan.

Finally, do a general review of the top 10 patient diseases, medications, diagnostic tests, and nursing procedures in each major nursing content area, as well as defense mechanisms, communication tips, and growth and development. Practice visualization and relaxation techniques as needed. These strategies will assist you in conquering the three areas necessary for successful test taking—anxiety control, content review, and test question practice. Table A-3 will help organize your study.

WHEN TO STUDY

Identify your personal best time. Are you a day person? Are you a night person? Study when you are fresh. Arrange to study 1 or more hours daily. Use Table A-4 to organize your study if you have 1 month to go.

Students who use this technique should increase their confidence in their ability to do well on the NCLEX.

TABLE A-3	Preparation for the NCLEX Test

Name: _____

Strengths: _____

Weak content areas identified on NLN examination or HESI Exit Exam:

_____

_____

_____

Weak content areas identified by yourself or others during formal nursing education program (include content areas in which you scored below a grade of B in class or any factors from Table A-2):

_____

_____

_____

Weak content areas identified in any area of the NCLEX test plan, including the following:
Safe, effective care environment
Physiological integrity
Psychosocial integrity
Health promotion and maintenance

Weak content areas identified in any of the top 10 patient diagnoses in each of the following:
Adult health
Women's health
Mental health nursing
Children's health
  (Consider the 10 top medications, diagnostic tools and tests, treatments and procedures used
  for each of the ten diagnoses.)

Weak content areas identified in the following:
Therapeutic communication tools
Defense mechanisms
Growth and development
Other

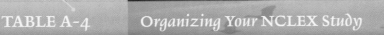

TABLE A-4	Organizing Your NCLEX Study

Note your weaknesses identified in Table A-3.

Take a comprehensive exam from one of the review books and analyze your performance. Then, depending on this test performance and the weaknesses identified in Table A-3, your schedule could look like the following:

Day 1: Practice adult health test questions. Score the test, analyze your performance, and review test question rationales and content weaknesses.

Day 2: Practice women's health test questions. Repeat above process.

Day 3: Practice children's health test questions. Repeat above process.

Day 4: Practice mental health test questions. Repeat above process.

Day 5: Continue with other weak content areas. Continue this process until you are doing well in all areas of the test.

SUGGESTED READING AND RESOURCES

Alexander, J., E., & Brophy, G. H. (1997). A five-year study of graduates' performance on NCLEX-RN. *Journal of Nursing Education, 36,* 443–445.

Arathuzik, D., & Aber, C. (1998). Factors associated with NCLEX-RN success. *Journal of Professional Nursing, 14*(2), 119–126.

Barkley, T. W., Rhodes, R. S., & Dufour, C. A (1998). Predictors of success on the NCLEX-RN. *Nursing and Health Care Perspectives, 19*(3), 132–136.

Beare, P. G. (1995). NCLEX-RN update: Helping your students prepare. *Nurse Educator, 20*(3), 33–36.

Billings, D., Hodson-Carlton, K., Kirkpatrick, J., Aaltonen, P., Dillard, N., Richardson, V., Siktberg, L., & Vinten, S. (1996). Computerized NCLEX-RN preparation programs: A comparative review. *Computers in Nursing, 14*(5), 272–286.

Carpenter, D. R., & Bailey, P. (1999). Predicting success on the registered nurse licensure examination—1999 update. In K. R. Stevens & V. R. Cassidy, Eds. *Evidence-based teaching: Current research in nursing education* (pp. 135–170). Sudbury, MA: Jones and Bartlett.

Drake, C. C., & Michael, W. B. (1995). Criterion-related validity of selected achievement measures in the prediction of a passing or failing criterion on the NCLEX for nursing students in a two-year associate degree program. *Educational and Psychological Measurement, 55*(4), 675–679.

Foti, I., & and DeYoung, S. (1991). Predicting success on the NCLEX-RN: Another piece of the puzzle. *Journal of Professional Nursing, 7*(2), 99–104.

Fowles, E. R. (1992). Predictors of success on NCLEX-RN and within the nursing curriculum: Implications for early intervention. *Journal of Nursing Education, 31*(2), 53–57.

Jenks, J., Selekman, J., Bross, T., & Paquet, M. (1989). Success in NCLEX-RN: Identifying predictors and optimal timing for intervention. *Journal of Nursing Education, 28*(3), 112–118.

Lauchner, K. A., Newman, M., & Britt, R. B. (1999). Predicting licensure success with a computerized comprehensive nursing exam: The HESI Exit Exam. *Computers in Nursing, 17*(3), 120–125.

McClelland, E., Yang, J. C., & Glick, O. J. (1992). A statewide study of academic variables affecting performance of baccalaureate nursing graduates on licensure examination. *Journal of Professional Nursing, 8*(6), 342–350.

McKinney, J. Small, S., O'Dell, N., & Coonrod, B. A. (1988). Identification of predictors of success for the NCLEX and students at risk for NCLEX failure in a baccalaureate nursing program. *Journal of Professional Nursing, 4*(1), 55–59.

National Council of State Boards of Nursing, Inc.; 676 North St. Clair Street, Suite 550; Chicago, Illinois 60611-2921; http://www.ncsbn.org; (312) 787-6555 or (800) 325-9601

Riner, M. E., Mueller, C., Ihrke, B., Smolen, R. A., Wilson, M., Richardson, V., Stone, C., & Zwirn,

E. E. (1997). Computerized NCLEX-RN and NCLEX-PN preparation programs: Comparative review. *Computers in Nursing, 15*(5), 255–267.

Wall, B. M., Miller, D. E., & Widerquist, J. G. (1993). Predictors of success on the newest NCLEX-RN. *Western Journal of Nursing Research, 15*(5), 628–643.

ABBREVIATIONS

AACN — American Association of Critical-Care Nurses

AACN — American Association of Colleges of Nursing

AAHP — American Association of Health Plans

AAN — American Academy of Nursing

AANA — American Association of Nurse Anesthetists

AARP — American Association of Retired Persons

ACLS — advanced cardiac life support

ACNP — acute care nurse practitioner

ACS — American Cancer Society

ADA — American Dietetic Association

ADL — activity of daily living

ADN — associate degree in nursing

AHA — American Hospital Association

AHRQ — Agency for Healthcare Research and Quality

AIDS — Acquired Immune Deficiency Syndrome

AMA — American Medical Association

ANA — American Nurses Association

ANCC — American Nurses Credentialing Center

AONE — American Organization of Nurse Executives

APC — Ambulatory Payment Classification

APHA — American Public Health Association

AWHONN — Association of Women's Health, Obstetric, and Neonatal Nurses

BLS — basic life support

BMI — body mass index

BSN — bachelor of science in nursing

BTIPA — Brooks' Theory of Intrapersonal Awareness

CAMH — Comprehensive Accreditation Manual for Hospitals

CARING — Capital Area Roundtable on Informatics in Nursing

CCQHC — Consumer Coalition for Quality Health Care

CCRN — critical care registered nurse

CCU — coronary care unit

CDC — Centers for Disease Control and Prevention

CEO — chief executive officer

CEU — continuing education unit

CFO — chief financial officer

CHF — congestive heart failure

CINAHL — Cumulative Index to Nursing and Allied Health Literature

CIS — clinical information system

CMP — comprehensive metabolic panel

CMS — Centers for Medicare and Medicaid Services

CN3 — clinical nurse 3

CNA — Canadian Nurses Association

CNM — certified nurse-midwife

CNS — clinical nurse specialist

CNS/NP — clinical nurse specialist/nurse practitioner

CON — certificate of need

COPC — community-oriented primary care

CPR	cardiopulmonary resuscitation
CPR	computerized patient record
CPRI	Computer-based Patient Record Institute
CQI	continuous quality improvement
CRNA	certified registered nurse anesthetist
CU	Consumers Union
CVA	cerebrovascular accident
DM	disease management
DRG	diagnosis-related group
EBC	evidence-based care
EBM	evidence-based medicine
EBNP	evidence-based nursing practice
EBP	evidence-based practice
EMTALA	Emergency Medical Treatment and Active Labor Act
ENIAC	Electronic Numerical Integrator and Computer
ERCP	endoscopic retrograde cholangiopancreatography
ERG	Existence-relatedness-growth theory (Alderfer, 1969)
ET nurse	enterostomal therapy nurse
FTE	full-time equivalent
GI lab	gastrointestinal laboratory
HCFA	Health Care Financing Administration
HIMSS	Health Information and Management Systems Society
HIPAA	Health Insurance Portability and Accountability Act
HIV	human immunodeficiency virus
HMO	health maintenance organization
IADL	instrumental activity of daily living
ICN	International Council of Nurses
ICU	intensive care unit
IOM	Institute of Medicine
IRA	individual retirement account
JBIEBNM	Joanna Briggs Institute for Evidence Based Nursing & Midwifery
JCAHO	Joint Commission on Accreditation of Healthcare Organizations
LOS	length of stay
LPN/LVN	licensed practical nurse/licensed vocational nurse
MBNQA	Malcolm Baldridge National Quality Award
MBTI	Myers-Briggs Type Indicator
MDI	metered-dose inhaler
MEDLARS	Medical Literature Analysis and Retrieval System
MeSH	Medical Subject Headings
MIS	medical information system
MRI	Medical Records Institute
MS-HUG	Microsoft Healthcare Users Group
MSN	master's degree in nursing
NANDA	North American Nursing Diagnosis Association
NANN	National Association of Neonatal Nurses
NAPNAP	National Association of Pediatric Nurses and Practitioners
NAPQ	Nosek-Androwich Profit: Quality Matrix
NCLEX	National Council Licensure Examination
NCQA	National Committee on Quality Assurance
NCSBN	National Council of State Boards of Nursing
NGC	National Guideline Clearinghouse

NHPPD	nursing hours per patient day
NIH	National Institutes of Health
NLM	National Library of Medicine
NLN	National League for Nursing
NNP	neonatal nurse practitioner
NP	nurse practitioner
NRP	neonatal resuscitation program
NWIG-AMIA	Nursing Working Informatics Group of the American Medical Informatics Association
OR	operating room
OSHA	Occupational Safety and Health Administration
PALS	pediatric advanced life support
PC	personal computer
PCA	patient care associate
PCS	patient classification system
PDCA	Plan Do Check Act
PDSA	Plan-Do-Study-Act
PERT	Program Evaluation and Review Technique
P-F-A	purpose-focus-approach
PHN	public health nurse
PI	performance improvement
POD	postoperative day
POS	point of service
POSDCORB	planning, organizing, supervising, directing, coordinating, reporting, and budgeting
PPO	preferred provider organization
QI	quality improvement
RN	registered nurse
RVU	relative value unit
SCHIP	State Children's Health Insurance Program
SPAN	Staff Planning and Action Network
SWOT	strengths, weaknesses, opportunities, threats
TB	tuberculosis
TEFRA	Tax Equity and Fiscal Responsibility Act
TEPP	Tobacco Education and Prevention Program
TQI	total quality improvement
UAP	unlicensed assistive personnel
UC	ubiquitous computing
URL	universal resource locator
USDHHS	United States Department of Health and Human Services
UTI	urinary tract infection
VA	Veterans Affairs
VAK	visual, auditory, kinesthetic
VR	virtual reality
WHO	World Health Organization
WOC nurse	wound, ostomy, continence nurse
WWW	World Wide Web

GLOSSARY

360-degree feedback   System in which an individual is assessed by a variety of people in order to provide a broader perspective.

401K   Account that both employee and for-profit employer contribute to.

403b   Account that both employee and not-for-profit employer contribute to.

accommodating   Satisfying the needs of others, sometimes at the expense of self.

accountability   Liability for actions.

accounting   Activity that nurse managers engage in to record and report financial transactions and data.

acculturation   Process by which individuals adjust and adapt either to their host culture or a subculture by altering their own cultural behaviors.

achievement   Accomplishment of goals through effort.

activities of daily living   Activities related to toileting, bathing, grooming, dressing, feeding, mobility, and verbal and written personal communication.

activity log   Time management technique to assist in determining how time is used by periodically recording activities.

administrative law   Body of law created by administrative agencies in the form of rules, regulations, orders, and decisions to protect the rights of citizens.

administrative principles   General principles of management that are relevant to any organization.

affective domain   Learning domain centered on attitudes, or what the learner feels and believes.

affiliation   Associations and relationships with others.

agnostic   Person who is not committed to belief in the existence or nonexistence of a god or a supreme being, or perhaps believes that no one has effectively proven that a god exists.

altruism   The unselfish concern for the welfare of others.

American Nurses Association   Full-service professional organization representing the nation's entire registered nurse population.

assault   Offer to or threat of touching another in an offensive manner without that person's permission.

atheist   Does not believe in the existence of a god or a supreme being.

attending   Active listening to gain an understanding of the patient's message.

auditory   Pertaining to hearing.

authority   Power and/or right to make decisions.

autocratic leadership   Centralized decision-making style with the leader making decisions and using power to command and control others.

autonomy   An individual's right to self-determination; individual liberty.

avoiding   Retreating.

battery   Touching of another person without that person's consent.

behavioral objective   Statement of specific and measurable behavior that should result from the teaching session.

benchmark   A quantitative or qualitative standard or point of reference used in measuring or judging quality or value.

benchmarking   Management tool for seeking out the best practices in one's industry so as to improve performance.

beneficence   The duty to do good to others and to maintain a balance between benefits and harms.

bioethics   Ethics specific to health care; serves as a framework to guide behavior in ethical dilemmas.

break-even point   That point at which income and expenses are equal.

budget   A plan that provides formal quantitative expression for acquiring and distributing funds over the ensuing time period.

bureaucratic organization   Hierarchy with clear superior-subordinate communication and relations, based on positional authority, in which orders from the top are transmitted down through the organization via a clear chain of command.

capital budget   Accounts for the purchase of major new or replacement equipment.

capitation   Payment of a fixed dollar amount, per person, for the provision of health services to a patient population for a specified period of time (e.g., one month).

care delivery model   Method to organize the work of caring for patients.

case management   Strategy to improve patient care and reduce hospital costs through coordination of care.

certification   Process by which a nongovernmental agency or association asserts that an individual licensed to practice a profession has met certain predetermined standards specified by that profession for practice.

certified registered nurse anesthetist   Advanced clinical nursing specialist who manages the patient's anesthesia needs before, during, and after surgery or other procedures in conjunction with other health care professionals.

change   Making something different from what it was.

change agent   One who is responsible for implementation of a change project.

civil law   That body of law that governs how individuals relate to each other in everyday matters.

clarifying   Restating, rephrasing, or questioning a message as part of a process to help make meaning clear.

clinical information system (CIS)   Collection of software programs and associated hardware that supports the entry, retrieval, update, and analysis of patient care information and associated clinical information related to patient care.

clinical ladder   A promotional model that acknowledges that staff members have varying skill sets based on their education and experience. As such, depending on skills and experience, staff members may be rewarded differently and carry differing responsibilities for patient care and the governance and professional practice of the work unit.

clinical nurse specialist   Advanced practice registered nurse, with either a master's or doctoral degree in a clinical specialty, who functions as health care provider, educator, consultant, researcher, and leader.

clinical pathway   Care management tool that outlines the expected clinical course and outcomes for a specific patient type.

cognitive domain   Learning domain centered on knowledge, or what the learner knows.

collaborating   Resolving conflict so that both parties are satisfied.

collective action   Method to deal with problems by acting as a group with a single voice.

collective bargaining   Practice of employees, in a collective group, bargaining with management in reference to wages, work practice, and other benefits.

collective bargaining agent   Individual who works with employees to formalize collective bargaining though unionization.

committee   Work group with a specific task or goal to accomplish.

common law   Body of law that develops from precedents set by judicial decisions that, over time, have the force of law, as distinguished from legislative enactments.

competing   Engaging in rivalry to meet a goal.

compromising   Finding a middle ground solution where neither party gets all they want.

computer literacy   The knowledge and understanding of computers combined with the ability to use them effectively.

computerized patient record (CPR)   Electronic record that includes all information about an individual's lifetime health status and health care; replacement for the paper medical record as the primary source of information for health care, meeting all clinical, legal, and administrative requirements.

conflict   Disagreement about something of importance to each person involved.

confronting   To work jointly with others to resolve a problem or conflict

connection power   Extent to which nurses are connected with others having power.

consensus   Situation in which all group members agree to live with and support a decision, regardless of whether they totally agree.

consideration   Activities that focus on the employee and emphasize relating and getting along with people.

constitution   A set of basic laws that specifies the powers of the various segments of the government and how these segments relate to each other.

construction budget   Developed when renovation or new structures are planned.

contingency theory   Style that acknowledges that other factors in the environment influence outcomes as much as leadership style and that leader effectiveness is contingent upon or depends upon something other than the leader's behavior.

contract law   Rules that regulate certain transactions between individuals and/or legal entities such as businesses. Also governs transactions between businesses.

cost center   Departmental subsection or unit for tracking of financial data.

culture   Behaviors, norms, belief sets, values, race, traditions, and folkways of a specific group.

dashboard   Documentation tool providing a snapshot image of pertinent information and activity reflecting a point in time.

data capture   Collection and entry of data into a computer system.

decision making   Behavior exhibited in making a selection and implementing a course of action from alternatives.

defamation   Intentionally false communication, either published or publicly spoken.

delegation   Transferring to a competent individual the authority to perform a selected nursing task in a selected situation (NSCBN, 1995).

Delphi technique   Process groups employ to arrive at a decision, though group members never meet face to face; questionnaires are distributed for opinions, then summarized and disseminated with the summaries given to group members until consensus is achieved.

democratic leadership   Style in which participation is encouraged and authority is delegated to others.

deontology   Theory stating that, in determining the ethics of a situation, a person must consider the motives of the actor, not the consequences of the act.

department clinical information system   System that meets the operational needs of a particular department, such as the laboratory, radiology, pharmacy, medical records, or billing.

diagnostic-related groups   Patient groupings established by the federal government for reimbursement purposes; these groupings are sorted by patient disease or condition.

differentiated nursing practice   Care delivery model that sorts the roles, functions, and work of registered nurses according to some identified criteria, commonly education, clinical experience, and competence.

direct care   Time spent providing hands-on care to patients.

direct cost   Cost directly related to patient care within a manager's unit.

direct expenses   Expenses that are directly associated with patient care (e.g., medical and surgical supplies and drugs).

disease management Systematic, population-based approach to identify persons at risk, intervene with specific program of care, and measure clinical and other outcomes (Epstein and Sherwood, 1996)

economics Study of how scarce resources are allocated among possible uses.

egoism The tendency to be self-centered or to consider only oneself and one's own interests.

emotional health How we are feeling in relation to some type of event.

employee-centered leadership Style with a focus on the human needs of subordinates.

empowerment Process by which we facilitate the participation of others in decision making and take action within an environment where there is an equitable distribution of power.

enabling objective Objective that identifies secondary behaviors that contribute to, or enable, achievement of terminal objectives.

enterprise An organization of any size established as a business venture.

episodic care unit Unit that sees patients for defined episodes of care; examples include dialysis or ambulatory care units.

ethical dilemma A conflict between two or more ethical principles for which there is no correct decision.

ethics The doctrine that the general welfare of society is the proper goal of an individual's actions rather than egoism; the branch of philosophy that concerns the distinction between right from wrong on the basis of a body of knowledge, not just on the basis of opinions.

ethnicity Component of cultural identity that includes several factors such as race, geographic identity, physical features, and language.

ethnocentrism Belief that one's own culture or ethnic group is better than all other groups.

evaluation Process of determining the success of teaching; it can measure the patient's learning and the teaching's effectiveness.

evidence-based care Recognized by nursing, medicine, health care institutions, and health policy makers as care based on state-of-the-art science reports. It is a process approach to collecting, reviewing, interpreting, critiquing, and evaluating research and other relevant literature for direct application to patient care.

evidence-based medicine Means to integrate individual clinical medical experience with external clinical evidence using a systematic research approach (Sackett, Rosenberg, Gray, Haynes, & Richardson, 1996).

evidence-based nursing practice Conscientious, explicit, and judicious use of theory-derived, research-based information in making decisions about care delivery to individuals or groups of individuals and in consideration of individual needs and preferences (Ingersoll, 2000, p. 152).

evidence-based practice Conscientious, explicit, and judicious use of current best evidence in making decisions about the care of individual patients (Sackett, et al., 1996, p. 71).

expert power Power derived from the knowledge and skills nurses possess.

false imprisonment Occurs when people are incorrectly led to believe they cannot leave a place.

fee for service reimbursement Reimbursement based on services provided.

feedback A new message generated by the receiver in response to the original message from the sender.

fidelity The principle of promise keeping; the duty to keep one's promise or word.

fixed costs Expenses that are constant and are not related to productivity or volume.

focus groups Small groups of individuals selected because of a common characteristic (e.g., a specific patient population, patients in day surgery, new diabetics, and so on) who are invited to meet in a group and respond to questions about a topic in which they are expected to have interest or expertise.

formal leadership When a person is in a position of authority or in a sanctioned role within an organization that connotes influence.

full-time equivalent Measure of the work commitment of a full-time employee.

functional health status   Ability to care for oneself and meet one's human needs.

functional nursing   Care delivery model that divides the nursing work into functional units that are then assigned to one of the team members.

goal   Specific aim or target that the unit wishes to attain within the time span of 1 year.

Good Samaritan laws   Laws that have been enacted to protect the health care professional from legal liability for actions rendered in an emergency when the professional is giving service without pay.

grapevine   An informal communication channel where information moves quickly and is often inaccurate.

grievance   Situation in which a union member believes that management has failed to meet the terms of the contract or labor agreement and communicates this to management.

group process   Stages that a group progresses through as it matures, consisting of the following: forming, storming, norming, performing, and adjourning.

Hawthorne effect   Phenomenon of being observed or studied, which results in changes in behavior.

health   State of complete physical, social, and mental well-being, and not merely the absence of disease or infirmity (World Health Organization, 1998).

health determinants   Biological, psychosocial, environmental (physical and social), and health system factors or etiologies that may cause changes in the health status of individuals, families, groups, populations, and communities.

health-related quality of life   Those aspects of life that are influenced either positively or negatively by one's health status and health risk factors.

health risk factors   Modifiable and non-modifiable variables that increase or decrease the probability of illness or death; synonym is health determinants.

health status   Level of health of an individual, family, group, population, or community; the sum of existing health risk factors, level of wellness, existing diseases, functional health status, and quality of life.

horizontal integration   Occurs when a health care system contains several organizations of one type, such as hospitals.

indirect care   Time spent on activities that are patient related but are not done directly to the patient.

indirect cost   Cost not explicitly related to patient care within a manager's unit.

indirect expenses   Expenses that are referred to such items as utilities, such as gas, electric, and phones, that are not directly related to patient care.

informal leader   Individual who demonstrates leadership outside the scope of a formal leadership role or as a member of a group, rather than the head or leader of the group.

information communication   Interoperability of systems and linkages for exchange of data across disparate systems.

information power   Nurses who influence others with the information they provide to the group are using information power.

initiating structure   Style that involves an emphasis on the work to be done, a focus on the task and production.

inpatient unit   Hospital unit that is able to provide care to patients 24 hours a day, 7 days a week.

instrumental activities of daily living   Activities related to food preparation and shopping; cleaning; laundry; home maintenance; verbal, written, and electronic community communications; financial management; and transportation, as well as activities to meet social and support needs, manage health care needs, access community services and resources, and meet spiritual needs.

integrated delivery system   Network of health care organizations that provides a coordinated continuum of service to a defined population and is willing to be held clinically and fiscally accountable for the outcomes and the health status of the population served. Networks include hospitals, nursing homes, schools, public health departments, and social and community health organizations.

intellectual health Activities that maintain intellectual curiosity; consists of the knowledge we accumulate and the ability to think.

interdisciplinary team Group composed of members with a variety of clinical expertise.

interpersonal communication Concerned with communication between individuals.

intrapersonal communication Self-talk.

job-centered leaders Style that focuses on schedules, cost, and efficiency with less attention to developing work groups and high-performance goals.

justice The principle of fairness that is served when an individual is given that which he or she is due, owed, deserves, or can legitimately claim.

kinesthetic Pertaining to touching.

knowledge workers Those involved in serving others through their specialized knowledge.

laissez-faire leadership Passive and permissive style in which the leader defers decision making.

leader-member relations Feelings and attitudes of followers regarding acceptance, trust, and credibility of the leader.

leadership Process of influence whereby the leader influences others toward goal achievement.

learner analysis Process of identifying the learner's unique characteristics and needs.

learning domains Taxonomies, or classifications, of learning.

learning style Particular manner in which an individual responds to and processes learning.

legitimate power Power derived from the position a nurse holds in a group; it indicates the nurse's degree of authority.

lesson plan Document that provides the blueprint for the teaching session; it lists the objectives, topics, format, strategies, materials, and evaluation used in the teaching session.

living will Document voluntarily signed by patients that specifies the type of care they desire if and when they are in a terminal state and cannot sign a consent form or convey this information verbally.

maintenance or hygiene factors (Herzberg) Elements such as salary, job security, working conditions, status, quality of supervision, and relationships with others that prevent job dissatisfaction.

malpractice Professional's wrongful conduct in discharge of professional duties or failure to meet standards of care for the profession, which results in harm to another individual entrusted to the professional's care.

management Process of coordinating actions and allocating resources to achieve organizational goals.

management process Function of planning, organizing, coordinating, and controlling.

margin Profit.

MEDLARS (Medical Literature Analysis and Retrieval System) Computerized system of databases and databanks offered by the National Library of Medicine.

message Originating with the sender, consists of verbal and nonverbal stimuli that are taken in by the receiver.

methodology Structured, standardized approach for developing teaching.

mission Call to live out something that matters or is meaningful; an organization's mission reflects the purpose and direction of the health care agency or a department within it.

mission statement A formal expression of the purpose or reason for existence of the organization.

modular nursing Care delivery model that is a kind of team nursing that divides a geographical space into modules of patients with each module having a team of staff led by an RN to care for them.

money market account Similar to a bank checking account though it often requires a larger minimum amount of money to open the account and often has a higher interest rate for your money.

morality Behavior in accordance with custom or tradition; usually reflects personal or religious beliefs.

motivation Whatever influences our choices and creates direction, intensity, and persistence in our behavior.

motivation factors (Herzberg)   Elements such as achievement, recognition, responsibility, advancement, and the opportunity for development that all contribute to job satisfaction.

negligence   Failure to provide the care a reasonable person would ordinarily provide in a similar situation.

networking   Continuous process of initiating and maintaining professional relationships through communication and information sharing.

Nonmaleficence   The principle of doing no harm.

nonproductive hours   Paid time not devoted to patient care; includes benefit time such as vacation, sick time, and education time.

nonverbal communication   Aspects of communication that are outside what is spoken.

nurse practitioner   Advanced practice nurse who has education beyond the bachelor's degree in a clinical specialty area strongly focused on primary care, though two subspecialties are hospital based (NNP and ACNP).

nursing hours per patient day   Standard measure that quantifies the nursing time available to each patient by the available nursing staff.

objective   Measurable step that must be taken to reach a goal.

operational budget   Account for the income and expenses associated with day-to-day activity within a department or organization.

optimal outcomes   Best possible objectives to be achieved given the resources at hand.

organizational change   Planned alteration in an organization to generally improve efficiency.

outcome elements of quality   Outcome elements of quality are the end products of quality care; outcomes review the status of patients that may result from health care. Outcome elements ask the question, "Is the patient better as a result of health care?"

Pareto principle   Principle, developed by Pareto, a 19th century economist, which states that 20% of effort results in 80% of results, or conversely that 80% of unfocused effort results in 20% of results.

patient acuity   Measure of nursing workload that is generated for each patient.

patient care redesign   Initiative in the 1990s to redesign how care was delivered.

patient-centered care   Care delivery model in which care and services are brought to the patient.

patient classification system (PCS)   System for distinguishing among different patients based on their acuity, functional ability, or resource needs.

patient-focused care   A model of differentiated nursing practice that emphasizes quality, cost, and value.

patient-focused clinical information system   System in which automation supports patient care processes; typical applications include order entry, results reporting, clinical documentation, care planning, and clinical pathways.

payer   Third-party reimburser (insurance company or government).

performance improvement   Structured system for creating organization-wide participation and partnership in planning and implementing continuous improvement methods to understand and meet or exceed customer needs and expectations.

personal change   Alteration made voluntarily for one's own reasons, usually for self-improvement.

philosophy   Statement of beliefs based on core values; rational investigations of the truths and principles of knowledge, reality, and human conduct.

philosophy of an organization   A value statement of the principles and beliefs that direct the organization's behavior

physical health   Encompasses nutrition and exercise coupled with a balanced amount of rest; health preventive behaviors such as avoiding smoking; and health screening behaviors that detect health problems early such as an annual Pap smear.

political voice   An increase in the number of voices supporting or opposing an issue.

politics   Process by which people use a variety of methods to achieve their goals.

population-based health care practice Development, provision, and evaluation of multidisciplinary health care services to population groups experiencing increased health risks or disparities, in partnership with health care consumers and the community in order to improve the health of the community and its diverse population groups.

population-based nursing practice Practice of nursing in which the focus of care is to improve the health status of vulnerable or at-risk population groups within the community by employing health promotion and disease prevention interventions across the health continuum.

position power Degree of formal authority and influence associated with the leader.

power Ability to create, get, and use resources to achieve one's goals.

power of attorney Legal document executed by an individual (principal) granting another person (agent) the right to perform certain activities in the principal's name.

practice guideline Descriptive tool or standardized specifications for care of the typical patient in the typical situation; these guidelines are developed by a formal process that incorporates the best scientific evidence of effectiveness and expert opinion. Synonyms or near synonyms include practice parameter, preferred practice pattern, algorithm, protocol, and clinical standard (JCAHO, 1999, p. 113).

preferred provider organization (PPO) Contracts with health care providers (physicians and hospitals) and payers (self-insured employers, insurance companies, government, or managed care organizations) to provide health care services to a defined population for predetermined, fixed fees.

primary health care Services that emphasize the promotion of health and the prevention of illness or disability.

primary nursing Care delivery model that clearly delineates the responsibility and accountability of the RN and places the RN as the primary provider of nursing care to patients.

problem solving Active process that starts with a problem and ends with a solution.

process Set of causes and conditions that repeatedly come together in a series of steps to transfer inputs into outcomes.

process elements of quality Identify what nursing and health care interventions must be in place to deliver quality. Process elements are such things as managing the health care process, utilizing clinical practice guidelines and standards for nursing and medical interventions, passing medications, and so on.

productive hours Hours worked and available for patient care.

professional change Alteration made in position or job such as obtaining education or credentials.

professional health Satisfaction with career choice and belief in continuous opportunity for growth.

profit Determined by the relationship of income to expenses.

progressive discipline System in which the manager and employee's mutual goal is to take steps to correct performance in order to bring it back to an acceptable level; it offers a stepwise process with opportunities for continued feedback and clarification of expectations.

protective factors Patient strengths and resources that the patients can use to combat health threats that compromise core human functions.

psychomotor domain Learning domain centered on skills, or what the learner does.

public law General classification of law, consisting generally of constitutional, administrative, and criminal law. Public law defines a citizen's relationship with government.

quality assurance Inspection approach to ensure that minimum standards of care exist in health care institutions, primarily hospitals.

quality improvement Systematic process to improve outcomes based on customers' needs.

quality of life Level of satisfaction one has with the actual conditions of one's life, including satisfaction with socioeconomic status, education, occupation, home, family life, recreation, and the ability to enjoy life, freedom, and independence.

reasonable outcomes Objectives that can and should be achieved given less-than-optimal circumstances and limited resources.

receiver One who takes in a message and analyzes it.

reengineering Turning an organization upside down and inside out through fundamental rethinking and radical redesign of processes to achieve dramatic improvements in critical performance.

referent power Power derived from how much others respect and like any individual, group, or organization.

reflective thinking Watching or observing ourselves as we perform a task or make a decision about a certain situation.

relative value unit (RVU) Index number assigned to various health care services based on the relative amount of resources (labor and capital) used to produce the service.

religion Organized and public belief system of worship and practices that generally has a focus of a god or supernatural power.

resilience The social and psychosocial capacity of individuals and groups to adapt, succeed, and persereve over time in the face of recurring threats to psychosocial and physiologic integrity.

resources People, money, facilities, technology, and rights to properties, services, and technologies.

respect for others Acknowledgement of the right of people to make their own decisions.

responding Verbally and nonverbally acknowledging a sender's message.

responsibility Reliability, dependability, and the obligation to accomplish work.

resume Brief summary of your background, training, and experience as well as your qualifications for a position.

revenue Income generated through a variety of means (e.g., billable patient services, investments, and donations to the organization).

reward/coercive power Power to reward or punish others, as well as power to instill fear in others to influence them to change their behavior; withholding rewards or achieving a goal by causing others to fear often results in resentment.

risk adjustment Process of statistically adjusting patient data to reflect significant patient variables.

Roth IRA Individual retirement account that is much less restrictive than an IRA; first introduced in 1998.

secondary health care Services that emphasize detection and early intervention in illness to prevent further illness and disability.

self-scheduling Process in which staff on a unit collectively decide and implement the monthly work schedule.

sentinel event Unexpected occurrence involving death or serious physical or psychological injury to a patient.

shared governance Situation where nurses and managers work together to define their roles and expected outcomes, holding everyone accountable for their role and expected outcomes.

shift action plan Written plan based on a shift assessment that includes a global perspective and sets the priorities for the accomplishment of outcomes that are both optimal and reasonable.

situational leadership A framework that maintains that there is no one best leadership style, but rather that effective leadership lies in matching the appropriate leadership style to the individual's or group's level of motivation and task-relevant readiness.

skill mix Percentage of RN staff to other direct care staff, LPNs, and UAP.

social health Ability to relate to and interact with others.

sources of power Combination of conscious and unconscious factors that allow an individual to influence others to do as the individual wants.

spiritual Refers to a belief in a higher power, an awareness of life and its meaning, the centering of a person with purpose in life.

spiritual distress Questioning of the purpose of life and its meaning, refusing to participate in one's usual religious practices, and seeking unusual assistance rather than the usual spiritual or religious support.

spiritual health Human capacity to find strength from within; results from a connection with a higher being or power (Chilton, 1998).

staffing pattern Plan that articulates how many and what kind of staff are needed, by shift and day, to staff a unit or department.

stakeholder Provider, employer, customer, patient, or payer who may have an interest in, and seek to influence, the decisions and actions of an organization.

stakeholders Vested interest groups.

stakeholder assessment A systematic consideration of all potential stakeholders to ensure that the needs of each of these stakeholders are incorporated in the planning phase.

storage Physical location of data in a CPR.

strategic plan The sum total or outcome of the processes by which an organization engages in environmental analysis, goal formulation and strategy development with the purpose of organizational growth and renewal.

strategic planning A process that is designed to achieve goals in dynamic, competitive environments through the allocation of resources.

structure elements of quality Identify what structures must be in place in a health care system/unit to deliver quality health care. Structure elements consist of such things as a well constructed hospital, quality patient care standards, quality staffing policies, environmental standards, and the like.

substitutes for leadership Variables that may influence or have an effect on followers to the same extent as the leader's behavior.

SWOT analysis A tool that is frequently used to conduct environmental assessments. SWOT stands for Strengths, Weaknesses, Opportunities, and Threats.

system Interdependent group of items, people, or processes with a common purpose.

task structure Involves the degree that work is defined, with specific procedures, explicit directions and goals.

team Small number of people with complementary skills who are committed to a common purpose, performance goals and approach for which they hold themselves accountable (Katzenbach & Smith, 1993).

team nursing Care delivery model that assigns staff to teams that then are responsible for a group of patients.

teleology Theory stating that the value of a situation is determined by its consequences; the outcome of an action, not the action itself, is the criterion for measuring the goodness of that action.

terminal objective Objective that identifies major behaviors that contribute to achievement of the overall session goal.

tertiary health care Services that provide restorative or rehabilitation services for patients with chronic or irreversible conditions.

Theory X View that in bureaucratic organizations, employees prefer security, direction, and minimal responsibility; coercion, threats, or punishment are necessary because people do not like the work to be done.

Theory Y View that in the context of the right conditions, people enjoy their work, they can show self-control and discipline, are able to contribute creatively and are motivated by ties to the group, the organization, and the work itself; belief that people are intrinsically motivated by their work.

Theory Z View of collective decision making and a focus on long-term employment that involves slower promotions and less direct supervision.

time management Set of related common-sense skills that helps you use your time in the most effective and productive way possible. (Mind Tools, n.d.-b)

tort A private or civil wrong or injury, including action for bad faith breach of contract, for which the court will provide a remedy in the form of an action for damages.

total patient care Care delivery model in which nurses are responsible for the total care for their patient assignment for the shift they are working.

traditional IRA Individual retirement account.

transcultural nursing   Comparative study and analysis of different cultures and subcultures in the world with respect to their caring behavior, nursing care and health-illness values, beliefs, and patterns of behavior with the goal of developing a scientific and humanistic body of knowledge to provide culture-specific and culture-universal nursing care practices (Leininger, 1997).

transformational leader   Leader who is committed to a vision that empowers others.

ubiquitous computing   Term coined by Mark Weiser of Xerox PARC, it describes the phase of computing in which there are many computers to one person.

union   Formal and legal group that works through a collective bargaining agent and within the context of the National Labor Relations Board to bring forth workers' requests to management.

values   Personal beliefs about the truth of ideals, standards, principles, objects, and behaviors that give meaning and direction to life.

variable costs   Costs that vary with volume and will increase or decrease depending on the number of patients.

variance   Difference between what was budgeted and the actual cost.

veracity   The obligation to tell the truth.

verbal communication   Aspect of communication that relies on spoken words to convey a message.

vertical integration   Occurs when different stages of health care are linked and delivered by one agency.

visual   Pertaining to seeing.

voting block   Group that represents the same political position or perspective.

vulnerable population groups   Sub-groups of a community that are powerless, marginalized, or disenfranchised and are experiencing health disparities.

whistle-blowing   Act in which an individual discloses information regarding a violation of a law, rule or regulation or a substantial and specific danger to public health or safety.

workplace advocacy   Activities nurses undertake to address problems in their everyday workplace setting.

Note:
Page numbers in *italics* reference figures;
page numbers followed by "t" reference tables;
page numbers followed by "b" reference boxed text

Flash! For Nursing Leadership & Management

System Requirements
- 100 MHz Pentium w/24 MB of RAM
- Windows™ 95 or newer
- SVGA 24-bit color display
- 8 megabytes of free disk space

Microsoft® is a registered trademark and Windows™ 95 and NT™ are trademarks of Microsoft Corporation. Netware™ is a trademark of Novell, Inc.

Set Up Instructions
1. Double click My Computer
2. Double click the Control Panel icon
3. Double click Add/Remove Programs
4. Click the Install button and follow the on screen prompts from there.

License Agreement for Delmar Learning, a division of Thomson Learning, Inc.